BM

NEUROLOGICAL DISEASES
AND PREGNANCY

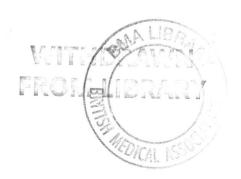

NEUROLOGICAL DISEASES AND PREGNANCY

A Coordinated Care Model for Best Management

EDITED BY

EMMA CIAFALONI, MD, FAAN
Robert C. and Rosalyne H. Griggs
Professor in Experimental Therapeutics of Neurologic Disease
Professor of Neurology and Pediatrics
Director Pediatric Neuromuscular Medicine
University of Rochester Medical Center
Rochester, NY

LORALEI L. THORNBURG, MD
Associate Professor of Obstetrics & Gynecology
James R. Woods, Jr. Professor of Obstetrics & Gynecology
Director Maternal-Fetal Medicine
University of Rochester Medical Center
Rochester, NY

CHERYL D. BUSHNELL, MD, MHS
Professor of Neurology
Director, Wake Forest Baptist Comprehensive Medical Center
Wake Forest School of Medicine
Winston Salem, NC

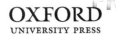

OXFORD
UNIVERSITY PRESS

OXFORD
UNIVERSITY PRESS

Oxford University Press is a department of the University of Oxford. It furthers
the University's objective of excellence in research, scholarship, and education
by publishing worldwide. Oxford is a registered trade mark of Oxford University
Press in the UK and certain other countries.

Published in the United States of America by Oxford University Press
198 Madison Avenue, New York, NY 10016, United States of America.

© Oxford University Press 2018

Library of Congress Cataloging-in-Publication Data
Names: Ciafaloni, Emma, editor. | Bushnell, Cheryl, editor. | Thornburg, Loralei L., editor.
Title: Neurological diseases and pregnancy : a coordinated care model for
best management / edited by Emma Ciafaloni, Cheryl Bushnell, Loralei L. Thornburg.
Description: New York, NY : Oxford University Press, [2018] |
Includes bibliographical references and index.
Identifiers: LCCN 2017056202 | ISBN 9780190667351 (alk. paper)
Subjects: | MESH: Pregnancy Complications—drug therapy | Nervous System
Diseases—drug therapy | Prenatal Care | Perinatal Care | Preconception Care
Classification: LCC RG572 | NLM WQ 240 | DDC 618.3—dc23
LC record available at https://lccn.loc.gov/2017056202

1 3 5 7 9 8 6 4 2

Printed by Sheridan Books, Inc., United States of America

CONTENTS

FOREWORD

Many neurological diseases, such as migraine, multiple sclerosis, and stroke, are more prevalent in women. Despite this increased prevalence of disease, however, women have often been excluded from fundamental research based on concerns that a protocol could contribute to a negative outcome for a current or future pregnancy. As a result, for many years, the fields of neurology and obstetrics were not optimally informed about the impact of neurological disease on pregnancy and vice-versa, or about the impact of pioneering medications to treat these diseases on short- and long-term maternal and fetal health.

In the absence of this critical research, many women with neurological disease or disorders were advised not to become pregnant as their physicians were unsure how to manage their disorders or the medications they would continue to require during the pregnancy. Women who became pregnant with disorders such as epilepsy would often stop taking their anticonvulsant medications for fear that they would cause birth defects, leading to the potential for both maternal and fetal harm. As this book so aptly demonstrates, we have come a long way from these days.

In their own ways, both the fields of neurology and obstetrics have changed significantly over the past 20 to 30 years. Women's health has become increasingly recognized by neurologists as an area of critical importance both clinically and in the research arena. Women now make up almost half of neurology residents and 35% of the neurologists at academic institutions, and while I do not know for sure, I imagine their increased participation in the field is helping to drive more commitment to women's health. Several major academic centers now have "Women's Neurology Centers" to address the unique neurological needs of women throughout their lifespan, particularly during and after pregnancy.

Since the mid-1970s, the subspecialty of obstetrics and gynecology known as maternal-fetal medicine has focused on the care of pregnant women with anticipated and – more often unanticipated – medical complications. Much of the early focus of this subspecialty was on once unanticipated fetal conditions, for which incredible advances have been made. Indeed, prenatal diagnosis of the vast majority of congenital anomalies and major chromosomal disorders is now possible. The development of better ultrasound technology and the spread of Neonatal Intensive Care Units (NICUs) across the country significantly improved fetal and neonatal health, but parallel advances in maternal health and disease management were not made.

While much of my career as a maternal-fetal medicine specialist has focused on fetal conditions, my attention over the last eight years has been on bridging the significant gaps in maternal health, particularly those that lead to preventable maternal mortality and morbidity. A key part of this work with many other colleagues has been to strengthen the role of maternal-fetal medicine in the management of maternal disease—a not insignificant proportion of which is neurological disease.

To optimize outcomes, women need to have their underlying or emergent conditions optimized before, during, and after pregnancy, and that requires considerable collaboration and follow up. There is evidence that younger women with a diagnosis of epilepsy have particularly low rates of contraception, which makes preconception counseling and optimization more challenging for this population. As discussed in Chapters 20 and 21, unplanned pregnancy in a woman with epilepsy can have negative effects on both mom and baby, so prenatal counseling should be viewed as essential to ensure appropriate medication type, dosing, and seizure control. We must do this better.

Not only do we have an increasing number of women with complex neurological disorders achieving pregnancy, but medical conditions that are unique to pregnancy, such as preeclampsia, are known to increase risk for long-term neurological consequences, such as stroke. Once a woman gives birth, her medical conditions during pregnancy are frequently forgotten about as attention turns toward the baby, and the women who have had preeclampsia fail to realize that their risk for stroke and heart disease has doubled. This is a missed opportunity that must be leveraged.

As always, there is still much work to do and the opportunities for collaboration are many. There is now a broad array of treatments for autoimmune diseases, epilepsy, stroke, migraine, and neuromuscular disease, and obstetricians and neurologists must enhance their partnership to achieve optimal outcomes for their shared patients. As more women become pregnant with complex medical histories – and we learn more about what pregnancy can reveal about a woman's future health—the onus is on us to ensure that our fields move forward together to develop and provide new models of care.

Without a doubt, the future of complex neurological disease management in pregnancy is in multidisciplinary collaboration. This timely, comprehensive, and well-referenced text synthesizes expertise from specialists across a broad spectrum of maternal-fetal medicine, obstetric critical care, and neurological subspecialties, offering the most up-to-date evidence to help guide clinicians caring for pregnant women with neurological illness. In fact, it is the first book to address such a wide range of neurological conditions in pregnant women, and I would like to extend my congratulations and thanks to the authors. This book is a tremendous step forward in a long over-due conversation about optimizing maternal health through multidisciplinary collaboration and should be viewed as an essential educational resource in our respective specialties.

Mary E. D'Alton, MD
Willard C. Rappleye Professor
of Obstetrics and Gynecology
Chair, Department of Obstetrics
and Gynecology
Columbia University College
of Physicians & Surgeons

CONTRIBUTORS

Jamie L. Adams, MD
Assistant Professor
Department of Neurology
University of Rochester
Rochester, NY

Ahmed I. Ahmed, MD, MSc, RDMS
Assistant Professor
Department of Obstetrics and Gynecology
Department of Medical Genetics and Genomic
Wayne State University School of Medicine
Detroit, MI

Sarah Aldhaheri, MD, MSc, RDMS
Department of Obstetrics and Gynecology
McGill University
Montréal, QC

Allison Bannick, MS, BSN, RN, CPNP
Division of Genetic
Genomic and Metabolic Disorders, Children's
   Hospital of Michigan
Detroit, MI

Marte Helene Bjørk, MD
Assistant Professor
Department of Clinical Medicine
University of Bergen, and Consultant Neurologist
Department of Neurology
Haukeland University Hospital
Bergen, Norway

Robert D. Brown Jr., MD, MPH
Department of Neurology
John T. and Lillian Mathews Professor of Neuroscience
Mayo Clinic
Rochester, MN

Cheryl D. Bushnell, MD, MHS
Professor of Neurology, Director
Wake Forest Baptist Comprehensive Medical Center
Wake Forest School of Medicine
Winston Salem, NC

Mitchell Chess, MD
Associate Professor of Diagnostic Imaging
Director of Fetal MRI
University of Rochester Medical Center
Rochester, NY

Emma Ciafaloni, MD
Professor of Neurology and Pediatrics
Robert C. and Rosalyne H. Griggs Professor in
   Experimental Therapeutics of Neurologic Disease
Director of Pediatric Neuromuscular Medicine
Department of Neurology
University of Rochester Medical Center
Rochester, NY

Patricia K. Coyle, MD, FAAN, FANA
Professor and Vice Chair (Clinical Affairs)
Director, MS Comprehensive Care Center
Department of Neurology
Stony Brook University Medical Center
Stony Brook, NY

Peter D. Creigh, MD
Senior Instructor of Neurology
Department of Neurology
University of Rochester Medical Center
Rochester, NY

Mary E. D'Alton, MD
Willard C. Rappleye Professor of Obstetrics and
   Gynecology
Chair, Department of Obstetrics and Gynecology
Columbia University College of Physicians &
   Surgeons
New York, NY

Jodi Dodds, MD
Assistant Professor
Department of Neurology
Duke University Medical Center
Durham, NC

Kathryn J. Drennan, MD
Assistant Professor
Department of Obstetrics and
 Gynecology
Division of Maternal-Fetal Medicine
University of Rochester School of Medicine and
 Dentistry
Rochester, NY

Stephanie Dukhovny, MD
Assistant Professor
Oregon Health and Science University
Department of Obstetrics and Gynecology
Division of Maternal Fetal Medicine
Portland, OR

Malin Eberhard-Gran MD, PhD
Professor of Clinical Epidemiology
Institute of Clinical Medicine
University of Oslo and Health Services
 Research Unit
Akershus University Hospital, Lørenskog, and
 Senior Reseacher
Department of Child Health
Norwegian Institute of Public Health
Oslo, Norway

Adam Evans, MD
Resident Physician
Department of Obstetrics and Gynecology
University of Rochester Medical Center
Rochester, NY

Kyle M. Fargen, MD, MPH
Assistant Professor
Department of Neurosurgery
Wake Forest School of Medicine
Winston Salem, NC

William Filer, MD
Assistant Professor
Department of Physical Medicine and
 Rehabilitation
School of Medicine
University of North Carolina
Chapel Hill, NC

Elizabeth Fountaine, MD
Instructor
Department of Obstetrics and Gynecology
University of Rochester Medical Center
Rochester, NY

Deborah I. Friedman, MD, MPH
Professor
Department of Neurology and Neurotherapeutics
 and the Department of Ophthalmology
University of Texas Southwestern Medical Center
Dallas, TX

Dzhamala Gilmandyar, MD
Assistant Professor
Department of Obstetrics and Gynecology
Division of Maternal-Fetal Medicine
Hackensack Meridian Health
Hackensack, New Jersey, NJ

J. Christopher Glantz, MD, MPH
Professor of Obstetrics & Gynecology and Public
 Health Sciences
Divison of Maternal-Fetal Medicine
University of Rochester Medical Center
Rochester, NY

Marjorie Gloff, MD
Assistant Professor of Anesthesiology
Director of the Center for Perioperative
 Medicine
University of Rochester Medical Center
Rochester, NY

David N. Hackney, MD, MS
Division Chief
Maternal Fetal Medicine
UH Cleveland Medical Center
Assistant Professor, Obstetrics and Gynecology,
 CWRU School of Medicine
Cleveland, OH

Johanna Hamel, MD
Senior Instructor of Neurology
Department of Neurology
University of Rochester
Rochester, NY

Amy Robinson Harrington, MD
Associate Professor
Department of Obstetrics and Gynecology
University of Rochester Medical Center
Rochester, NY

Matthew Harris, PhD, ABPP (NC)
Assistant Professor
Department of Physical Medicine and Rehabilitation
School of Medicine
University of North Carolina
Chapel Hill, NC

David N. Herrmann, MBBCh
Professor of Neurology and Pathology
Chief Neuromuscular Division
Department of Neurology
University of Rochester
Rochester, NY

Susan Hutchinson, MD
Director
Orange County Migraine and
 Headache Center
Irvine, California

Chinazom Ibegbu, MD
Senior Instructor of Neurology
Department of Neurology
University of Rochester
Rochester, NY

Melissa Kreso, MD
Assistant Professor of Anesthesiology
Associate Chief of Obstetric Anesthesiology
University of Rochester
Rochester, NY

Ruth A. Lawrence, MD, FAAP, FAACT
Distinguished Alumna Professor of Pediatrics
   and Obstetrics and Gynecology
Medical Director of the Ruth A. Lawrence
   Poison and Drug Information Center and of
   the Breastfeeding and Human Lactation Study
   Center
Northumberland Trust Chair in Pediatrics
University of Rochester Medical Center
Rochester, NY

Michael Y. Lee, MD, MHA, CPE
Professor
Department of Physical Medicine and
   Rehabilitation
School of Medicine
University of North Carolina
Chapel Hill, NC

Heather M. Link, MD, MPH
Instructor
Maternal Fetal Medicine Fellow
University of Rochester Medical Center
Department of Obstetrics and Gynecology
Rochester, NY

Lynn Liu, MD, FAASM
Associate Professor of Neurology
Pediatrics and Anesthesiology & Perioperative
   Medicine
University of Rochester Epilepsy Center
Rochester, NY

Eric Logigian, MD
Professor of Neurology and Physical Medicine
   and Rehabilitation
Department of Neurology
University of Rochester Medical Center
Rochester, NY

Aaron I. Loochtan, DO
Vascular Neurology Fellow
Department of Neurology
Duke University Medical Center
Durham, NC

Tara A. Lynch, MD
Instructor
Maternal Fetal Medicine Fellow
University of Rochester Medical Center
Rochester, NY

Shamin Masrour, MD
Instructor
Department of Neurology and Neurotherapeutics
University of Texas Southwestern Medical Center
Dallas, TX

Lauren A. Miller, MD, MPH
Instructor
Maternal-Fetal Medicine Fellow
Division of Maternal-Fetal Medicine
Department of Obstetrics and Gynecology
University of Rochester Medical Center
Rochester, NY

Nimish A. Mohile, MD
Associate Professor of Neurology and
   Neuro-Oncology
Department of Neurology
Rochester, NY

Courtney Olson-Chen, MD
Assistant Professor Obstetrics Gynecology
Division of Maternal-Fetal Medicine
Department of Obstetrics and Gynecology
University of Rochester Medical Center
Rochester, NY

Michael R. Pichler, MD
Assistant Professor
Department of Neurology
Mayo Clinic
Rochester, MN

Eva K. Pressman, MD
Professor and Chair University of Rochester
   Medical Center
Department of Obstetrics & Gynecology
Henry Theide Professor of Obstetrics Gynecology
University of Rochester Medical Center
Rochester, NY

Tessa L. Reisinger, MD
Clinical Faculty
Department of Obstetrics and Gynecology
FFT Thompson Health
Canandaigua, NY

Jaclyn J. Renfrow, MD
Resident Physician
Department of Neurosurgery
Wake Forest School of Medicine
Winston Salem, NC

Patricia Rogers, RN, C-ANP
Nurse Practitioner
University of Rochester Epilepsy Center
University of Rochester Medical Center
Rochester, NY

Casey Rosen-Carole, MD, MPH, MSEd
Assistant Professor of Pediatrics and Obstetrics
    and Gynecology
Medical Director of Lactation Services and
    Programs
University of Rochester School of Medicine and
    Dentistry
Rochester, NY

Neil S. Seligman, MD, MS
Assistant Professor
Department of Obstetrics and
    Gynecology
Division of Maternal-Fetal Medicine
University of Rochester Medical
    Center
Rochester, NY

Jasmeet Singh, MD
Assistant Professor of Radiology
Wake Forest School of Medicine
Winston Salem, NC

Asha N. Talati, MD
Department of Obstetrics and
    Gynecology
University Hospitals MacDonald Women's
    Hospital
Department of Reproductive Biology
Case Western Reserve University
Cleveland, OH

Christopher G. Tarolli, MD
Senior Instructor
Department of Neurology
University of Rochester
Rochester, NY

Pariwat Thaisetthawatkul, MD
Associate Professor of Neurology
Department of Neurological Sciences
University of Nebraska Medical Center
Omaha, NE

Karla L. Thompson, PhD
Assistant Professor, Director of Psychological
    Services
Department of Physical Medicine and
    Rehabilitation
School of Medicine
University of North Carolina
Chapel Hill, NY

Loralei L. Thornburg, MD
Associate Professor of Obstetrics & Gynecology
James R. Woods, Jr. Professor of Obstetrics &
    Gynecology
Director Maternal-Fetal Medicine
University of Rochester Medical Center
Rochester, NY

Trenton Tollefson, MD
Senior Instructor of Neurology
University of Rochester Medical Center
Rochester, NY

Mary N. Towner, MD
Resident Physician
Department of Obstetrics and Gynecology
University of Rochester Medical Center
Rochester, NY

Maria Vanushkina, MD
Chief Resident
Department of Physical Medicine and Rehabilitation
University of Rochester School of Medicine and
    Dentistry
Rochester, NY

Miriam T. Weber, PhD
Associate Professor
Departments of Neurology and Obstetrics and
    Gynecology
University of Rochester
Rochester, NY

Natalie S. Whaley, MD, MPH
Assistant Professor
Departments of Obstetrics and Gynecology
University of Rochester Medical Center
Rochester, NY

John A. Wilson, MD
Professor and Vice Chair of Neurosurgery
Wake Forest School of Medicine
Winston Salem, NC

Richard Wissler, MD
Professor of Anesthesiology
Director of Perioperative Services
Chief of Obstetric Anesthesiology
University of Rochester
Rochester, NY

Stacey Q. Wolfe, MD
Associate Professor of Neurosurgery
Wake Forest School of Medicine
Winston Salem, NC

Aqib H. Zehri, MD
Resident Physician
Department of Neurosurgery
Wake Forest School of Medicine
Winston Salem, NC

SECTION 1

Reproductive Issues in Women with Neurologic Disease

1

General Approach to Pregnancy Care in the Neurologic Patient

TARA A. LYNCH AND LORALEI L. THORNBURG

ABSTRACT

Caring for the obstetric patient with significant medical problems can be complex. Neurologic diseases in pregnancy can range in severity and therefore vary in the amount of care planning that is required. Certain diseases will require more coordination of care with multidisciplinary teams than others. In these cases, the use of care maps or guidelines can assist practitioners with providing comprehensive care. This chapter will serve as an overview of pregnancy-specific considerations that will be reviewed in subsequent chapters throughout this book. Overall, by focusing attention to the specific needs of the complex obstetric neurologic patient, practitioners can help to optimize outcomes for these women and their pregnancies.

INTRODUCTION

Obstetric care for the patient with a neurologic disease can be complicated. Treatment plans require consideration and balance of the risks to the fetus and the maternal patient. Therefore, multidisciplinary team care planning is often required with high-risk disease processes. Special considerations and preparations may be needed to assist with the differentiation of pathologic and physiologic antepartum symptoms, medication adjustments, anesthesia during labor, and postpartum monitoring. With this in mind, this book will review both common and uncommon neurologic diseases that can impact the management of the obstetric patient. Throughout each chapter, care maps will be provided. Each will outline the recommended and essential components of preconception, antepartum, intrapartum, and postpartum care. This chapter is an overview of the general considerations for the management of a pregnancy with concurrent neurologic disease (see Box 1.1–1.4).

Care maps, also referred to as "clinical pathways" or "checklists" are currently used throughout medicine and outline the important components of care for medically complex patients. The American College of Obstetricians and Gynecologists (ACOG) actively endorses the use of clinical protocols and guidelines. Multidisciplinary care plans have been proven to decrease the length of hospital stay, rate of in-hospital complications, hospitalization costs; they have also improved documentation and enhanced patient care.[1,2] There are published reports on clinical pathways and checklists specific to obstetrics. For example, there are checklists for vaginal delivery,[3] cesarean section,[4] placenta accrete,[5] and oxytocin administration.[6] Based on current evidence, checklists are effective in obstetric scenarios, therefore expansion of this clinical concept to the complex neurologic patient is logical.

PRECONCEPTION

If a patient presents for preconception counseling, or even during annual well-woman or neurologic care, this opportunity should be used to discuss the possibility of pregnancy and to discuss optimizing disease control in anticipation of pregnancy. For those who do not desire pregnancy, medications may influence the effectiveness of their contraception method, and this may be an ideal time to address contraceptive options and prevention of unplanned pregnancy. For those considering pregnancy, preconception (or non-pregnant) visits may include adjusting medications when necessary, initiating folic acid supplementation, and coordinating consultative services. All women considering conception should supplement with 400 mcg of folic acid daily.[7] There is evidence to suggest that preconception counseling may improve adherence to interventions such as folic acid supplementation.[8]

BOX 1.1
CARE MAP FOR PREGNANCY—GENERAL APPROACH

PRECONCEPTION
- Maternal confirmation of the diagnosis
- Preconception control neurologic disease
- Assessment of medication use in pregnancy
- Initiation of prenatal vitamin
- Preconception MFM preconception consultation
- Baseline Assessment
  - Lung function
  - Mobility
  - Concurrent diseases
  - Neurologic symptoms
- Cessation of smoking, recreational drug use, environmental exposures
- Calculation of BMI
- Genetic risk assessment
- Discussion of inheritability
- Discussion of the potential fetal effects of disease
- Preconception imaging if necessary

BOX 1.2
CARE MAP FOR PREGNANCY—GENERAL APPROACH

DURING PREGNANCY (ANTEPARTUM)
- Early initiation of prenatal care with ultrasound
- Medication regimen monitoring and pregnancy safety
- Serum monitoring of drug levels when indicated every trimester (increased frequency as clinically indicated)
- Lactation consultation
- Delivery Planning
  - Anesthesia consultation (based on disease process)
  - Identification of contraindicated medications
  - Timing
  - Assessment of mode of delivery
  - Assessment of ability to Valsalva
- Assessment of the patient's needs (individualized)
  - Urinalysis
  - Mobility
  - Early glucose screening
  - Serial fetal growth assessment
- Preterm labor precautions
- Contraception counseling
- Serial fetal assessment if indicated

BOX 1.3
CARE MAP FOR PREGNANCY—GENERAL APPROACH

DURING DELIVERY (INTRAPARTUM)

- Continue antiepileptic medications
- Potential need for intensive monitoring
- Accommodations for mobility limitations
- Assessment of ability to Valsalva and assisted delivery if needed
- Precautions when indicated (seizure precautions)
- Avoidance of contraindicated medications (such as Magnesium)
- Early anesthesia consult
- Assess candidacy for neuraxial anesthesia
- Coordination of delivery (such as around anticoagulation)

Many neurologic diseases, especially those that are immune mediated (such as multiple sclerosis) may improve during the pregnancy, but others such as myasthenia gravis or epilepsy have a higher risk of exacerbation.[9] Those with limited mobility or physical limitations may need additional counseling on the effects of pregnancy on maternal health and well-being. Careful review of medications being used to control maternal symptoms may allow for the discontinuation of medications contraindicated in pregnancy, such as methotrexate. Although there is no data on the effectiveness of preconception counseling for the reduction of adverse pregnancy outcome in neurologic disease,[10] other studies in pregnancy have demonstrated improvement in knowledge and modification of risky behaviors.[11] Overall, preconception counseling improves pregnancy outcome by allowing for the assessment and optimization of disease control.[9]

Preconception consultation should also focus on the identification of concurrent medical problems, and if applicable, assessment of maternal baseline function, mobility, and neurologic symptoms. Counseling should focus on patient education about potentially modifiable behaviors, such as smoking, illicit drug use, and environmental exposures. Calculation of body mass index (BMI) should be performed and can also allow for discussion of weight-loss options or medical interventions to supplement weight gain. An assessment of genetic risk factors and family history can allow for preconception genetic counseling or testing for diseases.[12] This should also include information regarding the transmission or inheritability of the specific disorder. For example, infants born to mothers with myasthenia gravis have a 10%–20% risk of neonatal myasthenia gravis secondary to the transmission of maternal antibodies across the placenta.[13]

BOX 1.4
CARE MAP FOR PREGNANCY—GENERAL APPROACH

AFTER DELIVERY (POSTPARTUM)

- Medication adjustments
- Contraception counseling
- Neurologic follow
- Lactation consultation
- Monitoring for relapses or exacerbations
- Contraception initiation

DURING PREGNANCY (ANTENATAL)

Specific recommendations for each disease class and for some specific more common or serious diseases are addressed individually throughout each chapter. But as a general approach, the patient with neurologic disease should receive all usual obstetric care; however, they may require additional monitoring, testing, or evaluation.

Once a pregnancy has been confirmed, patients with any medical disorders should be encouraged to establish care early. The physiology of pregnancy can alter the maternal tolerance of neurology disease as well as care for her disease. Medication monitoring is recommended for some conditions because pregnancy alters the pharmacokinetics of many medications. With epilepsy, therapeutic drug level monitoring is recommended in each trimester, with increasing frequency if there is evidence of suboptimal seizure control.[14] If possible, medication adjustments should be made to minimize fetal effects and maximize maternal symptom control, using the lowest dose of the least teratogenic medication (see Chapter 23). With the physiologic changes that occur in the respiratory system, baseline impairment can be exacerbated and require careful monitoring of the patient's oxygen saturation and symptoms. For patients requiring continuation of chronic corticosteroids early glucose tolerance testing should be offered given the association with glucose intolerance.[15] Patients with complex spinal cord injuries may have an increased risk for urinary tract infections, constipation, and orthostatic hypotension.[16] In these cases, urinalysis screening and symptom management should be performed throughout the pregnancy. Certain neurologic disorders will also have significant motor impairment, increasing risks for venous thromboembolism. The hematologic changes that occur during pregnancy further increase these risks, and therefore anticoagulation may be considered. Patients with decreased mobility require careful screening for pressure ulcers and may benefit from physical and occupational therapy throughout the pregnancy. The physical alterations that occur may exacerbate underlying deficits.[17]

Some diseases such as multiple sclerosis are associated with an increased risk of preterm birth and fetal growth restriction and will be discussed in separate chapters.[17] Gestational age dating is most accurate early in the pregnancy, and completion of this will allow for an accurate assessment of fetal growth throughout gestation. Additionally, screening with fundal height, serial ultrasounds

for fetal growth, and patient education of the signs of preterm labor should be performed for those patients at risk.

Neuroimaging is often required for the diagnosis of certain neurologic diseases.[18] During pregnancy there is concern regarding the timing of exposure and fetal risks. In general, computed tomography (CT) scan of the head and neck is considered low to moderate risk with an exposure of (0.1–10 mGy). As a reference point, exposure of 200 mGy during organogenesis has been associated with fetal congenital anomalies.[19] Therefore, CT scan of the head/neck is considered safe at any point in pregnancy (see also Chapter 7). MRI is considered safe in pregnancy but is typically performed without the use of contrast. There is evidence that gadolinium contrast is associated with neonatal demise as well as rheumatologic and inflammatory skin conditions.[20] In general, any neuroimaging needed should be performed if the suspected diagnosis would alter management of the patient or her pregnancy, or allow safety to the maternal-fetal dyad during the delivery process.[19] Therefore contrast may be needed in some cases, especially those with suspected vascular malformations to allow adequate imaging after discussion of risks/benefits with the patient.

With complex neurologic patients, consultation with a maternal fetal medicine specialist will further help with coordination of and determination of additional care needs. It is not unreasonable for a very complex patient to seek a preconception consult and another consult with an established pregnancy. Delivery planning should ideally occur in the antenatal period and will be discussed in the next section and also in Section 4, Chapter 31.

DURING DELIVERY (INTRAPARTUM)

Neurologic diseases are a heterogeneous group of disorders that often require coordination of care and delivery planning. Anesthesia consults during pregnancy may help delivery planning and patient expectations. For example, patients with neuromuscular disorders may have respiratory compromise and limitations to general anesthesia, whereas patients with intracranial tumors may not be candidates for neuraxial anesthesia.[21] During labor, most neurologic diseases are not a contraindication to vaginal delivery. However, there may be cases where a patient's motor limitations or intracranial disease prohibits the ability to valsalva. In these scenarios a multidisciplinary team should determine if cesarean section or operative delivery (assisted second stage) is the better option. Patients with spinal cord injuries and autonomic dysreflexia may benefit from early analgesia[22] (see also chapters on spinal cord injury and anesthesia).

In most instances, medications for chronic disease should be continued during labor.[21] Diseases such as myasthenia gravis preclude the use of medications such as magnesium and this should be identified and clearly delineated for the care team.[13] Additionally, a history of chronic corticosteroid use may necessitate stress dose steroids. Although there is a paucity of data on the indications and dose of stress dose in labor and for cesarean most experts recommend additional supplementation (50–100 mg intravenous) for patients on greater than 20–30 mg prednisone per day.[23]

Some neurologic diseases such as a cerebral venous thrombosis are treated with anticoagulation.[13] Therefore, patients may require coordination of delivery around anticoagulation timing to decrease blood loss and allow for neuraxial anesthesia. Ideally, mode of delivery would be determined prior to the delivery itself; however, based on clinical status, this mode may need to be adjusted. The extent of maternal and fetal monitoring should be based on the clinical situation and disease severity.

AFTER DELIVERY (POSTPARTUM)

Postpartum some patients' may be at risk for disease recurrence or exacerbations and should be counseled accordingly. The usual six-week postpartum visit may need to be supplemented with additional visits based on the patient's needs. For example, about 30% of women with multiple sclerosis will have a relapse postpartum.[17] All women should be screened for postpartum depression.[24] Although there is not specific data that women with neurologic disease have a higher incidence of postpartum depression, there is evidence that women with increased life stressors and chronic disease do have increased risk.[25] Breastfeeding, which has many maternal/infant benefits, should be encouraged and supported when not contraindicated based on medications or comorbidities. Lactation consultation prior to delivery may establish medication safety and postpartum may assist with the initiation and continuation of breastfeeding. Discussion of contraception and potential interactions with medication regimens should be performed to provide pregnancy spacing of at least one year until conception. Medications such as antiepileptics should be titrated to pre-pregnancy doses, and levels may

need to be followed closely during the rapid weight changes of the postpartum period.

CONCLUSIONS

The care of a patient with neurologic disease can vary widely based on the disease type, manifestations, and duration, depending on the treatment regimen being utilized. During pregnancy normal physiologic changes can exacerbate underlying disease processes, which further complicates management. Highly trained specialized care teams such as Centers of Excellence for Neurologic Disease[26] exist and have been shown to improve patient outcomes.[27] Other resources include complex care teams and checklists. All of these coordinated interventions minimize errors and enhance patient care.

Throughout this book, the care of the obstetric patient with a neurologic disease will be outlined. Although many times the severity of the neurologic disease will not require significant coordination of care, there are cases in which the care planning is extremely complex. It is for this latter group of patients that complex care teams and detailed care maps can be of assistance to providers. These care maps should be continually reevaluated based on new evidence and the needs of the individual. Overall, each working toward the common goal of providing comprehensive obstetric care for these patients and their pregnancies.

REFERENCES

1. Rotter T, Kinsman L, James E, et al. Clinical pathways: Effects on professional practice, patient outcomes, length of stay and hospital costs. *Cochrane Database of Systematic Reviews.* 2010(3):Cd006632.
2. Fausett MB, Propst A, Van Doren K, Clark BT. How to develop an effective obstetric checklist. *AJOG.* 2011; 205(3): 165–170.
3. Ransom SB, McNeeley SG, Yono A, Ettlie J, Dombrowski MP. The development and implementation of normal vaginal delivery clinical pathways in a large multihospital health system. *American Journal of Managed Care.* 1998; 4(5): 723–727.
4. Duff P. A simple checklist for preventing major complications associated with cesarean delivery. *Obstetrics and Gynecology.* 2010; 116(6): 1393–1396.
5. El-Messidi A, Mallozzi A, Oppenheimer L. A multidisciplinary checklist for management of suspected placenta accreta. *Journal of Obstetrics and Gynaecology Canada: JOGC.* 2012; 34(4): 320–324.
6. Clark S, Belfort M, Saade G, Hankins G, Miller D, Frye D, Meyers J. Implementation of a conservative checklist-based protocol for oxytocin administration: maternal and newborn outcomes.

American Journal of Obstetrics and Gynecology. 2007; 197(5): 480.e481–485.

7. Harden CL, Pennell PB, Koppel BS, Hovinga CA, Gidal B, Meador KJ, Hopp J, et al. Practice parameter update: Management issues for women with epilepsy—focus on pregnancy (an evidence-based review): vitamin K, folic acid, blood levels, and breastfeeding: report of the Quality Standards Subcommittee and Therapeutics and Technology Assessment Subcommittee of the American Academy of Neurology and American Epilepsy Society. *Neurology.* 2009; 73(2): 142–149.

8. de Weerd S, Thomas CM, Cikot RJ, Steegers-Theunissen RP, de Boo TM, Steegers EA. Preconception counseling improves folate status of women planning pregnancy. *Obstetrics and Gynecology.* 2002; 99(1): 45–50.

9. Kevat D, Mackillop L. Neurological diseases in pregnancy. *The Journal of the Royal College of Physicians of Edinburgh.* 2013; 43(1): 49–58.

10. Winterbottom JB, Smyth RM, Jacoby A, Baker GA. Preconception counselling for women with epilepsy to reduce adverse pregnancy outcome. *The Cochrane Database of Systematic Reviews.* 2008(3): Cd006645.

11. Hussein N, Kai J, Qureshi N. The effects of preconception interventions on improving reproductive health and pregnancy outcomes in primary care: A systematic review. *European Journal of General Practice.* 2016; 22(1): 42–52.

12. ACOG Committee Opinion number 313, September 2005. The importance of preconception care in the continuum of women's health care. *Obstetrics and Gynecology.* 2005; 106(3): 665–666.

13. Karnad DR, Guntupalli KK. Neurologic disorders in pregnancy. *Critical Care Medicine.* 2005; 33(10 Suppl): S362–371.

14. Pennell PB. Antiepileptic drug pharmacokinetics during pregnancy and lactation. *Neurology.* 2003; 61(6 Suppl 2): S35–42.

15. Yildirim Y, Tinar S, Oner RS, Kaya B, Toz E. Gestational diabetes mellitus in patients receiving long-term corticosteroid therapy during pregnancy. *Journal of Perinatal Medicine.* 2006; 34(4): 280–284.

16. Sterling L, Keunen J, Wigdor E, Sermer M, Maxwell C. Pregnancy outcomes in women with spinal cord lesions. *Journal of Obstetrics and Gynaecology Canada: JOGC.* 2013; 35(1): 39–43.

17. Pearce CF, Hansen WF. Headache and neurological disease in pregnancy. *Clinical Obstetrics and Gynecology.* 2012; 55(3): 810–828.

18. Alvis JS, Hicks RJ. Pregnancy-induced acute neurologic emergencies and neurologic conditions encountered in pregnancy. *Seminars in Ultrasound, CT, and MR.* 2012; 33(1): 46–54.

19. Committee Opinion No. 656 Summary: Guidelines for Diagnostic Imaging During Pregnancy and Lactation. *Obstetrics and Gynecology.* 2016; 127(2): 418.

20. Ray JG, Vermeulen MJ, Bharatha A, Montanera WJ, Park AL. Association between MRI exposure during pregnancy and fetal and childhood outcomes. *JAMA.* 2016; 316(9): 952–961.

21. Hopkins AN, Alshaeri T, Akst SA, Berger JS. Neurologic disease with pregnancy and considerations for the obstetric anesthesiologist. *Seminars in Perinatology.* 2014; 38(6): 359–369.

22. ACOG Committee Opinion: Number 275, September 2002. Obstetric management of patients with spinal cord injuries. *Obstetrics and Gynecology.* 2002; 100(3): 625–627.

23. Lindsay JR, Nieman LK. The hypothalamic-pituitary-adrenal axis in pregnancy: challenges in disease detection and treatment. *Endocrine Reviews.* 2005; 26(6): 775–799.

24. ACOG Committee Opinion No. 343: psychosocial risk factors: perinatal screening and intervention. *Obstetrics and Gynecology.* 2006; 108(2): 469–477.

25. Lancaster CA, Gold KJ, Flynn HA, Yoo H, Marcus SM, Davis MM. Risk factors for depressive symptoms during pregnancy: A systematic review. *AJOG.* 2010; 202(1): 5–14.

26. Tinsley N, McCartney LA, Hdeib A, Selman WR. Development of the Neurological Institute: A strategic, improvement, and systems approach. *Journal of Neurointerventional Surgery.* 2011; 3(2): 194–201.

27. Silver RM, Fox KA, Barton JR, et al. Center of excellence for placenta accreta. *AJOG.* 2015; 212(5): 561–568.

2

Pregnancy Safety and Termination

NATALIE S. WHALEY AND ADAM EVANS

ABSTRACT

Access to compassionate, nonjudgmental, and safe abortion care for medically complex women is an important component of obstetric care for high-risk women. The care of women with neurologic disease who seek pregnancy termination or management of pregnancy failure includes consideration of their particular medical, anesthesia, and surgical needs. Counseling regarding pregnancy options is an important first step in helping women achieve their family planning goals. Understanding the safety of abortion, as well as options for medical, surgical, or labor induction termination can help providers discuss pregnancy options with women. Resources are available to help non-obstetric providers ensure their patients have access to medically sound, evidence-based information about pregnancy termination.

INTRODUCTION: EPIDEMIOLOGY AND SAFETY OF LEGAL ABORTION

Improved access to effective contraceptive methods has contributed to declines in abortion rates throughout the United States.[1] Yet, unplanned pregnancy is a continued public health problem in that country. While abortion rates have declined steadily since the late 1970s, half of all pregnancies among American women are unintended and 4 in 10 of these result in termination of pregnancy.[2] In 2011, this amounted to a total of 1.06 million abortions, with 1.7% of reproductive-aged women undergoing abortion annually.[2] Of these, abortions that occur in the first trimester (first 12 weeks of pregnancy) comprise 89% of all abortions in the United States.[2,3] The impact of unplanned and closely spaced pregnancy on maternal and child health is well documented and includes delayed prenatal care, increased maternal mortality, preterm birth, and physical and mental health effects for children.[4,5] Discussions about abortion services are often mired in political

controversy, but it remains that access to safe and evidence-based family planning care is critical to the health and well-being of all women, especially those with chronic medical conditions.

Legal evidence-based abortion procedures pose a low risk to women, with major complication rates less than 0.05% in the first trimester and 0.5% overall.[6] While mortality related to legal abortion is exceedingly rare, gestational age is an important risk factor for abortion-related death. For instance, the risk of death for abortion performed at less than eight weeks estimated gestational age (EGA) is one death per 1 million abortions performed while the risk of death for abortion performed at 21 weeks EGA or later is one death per 11,000.[6,7] Pregnancy is a time of high physiologic stress involving significant changes in maternal physiology to accommodate the growing fetus. Throughout the course of pregnancy, these adaptations can lead to complications, which may pose a significant risk to the health of the mother. In the United States, childbirth is associated with a fourteen-fold increase in risk of death when compared to legal abortion.[8] In women with significant health comorbidities the normal changes of pregnancy have the potential to exacerbate underlying disease processes, thereby increasing the risk of poor outcomes.

Despite their increased risk for adverse pregnancy outcomes and the importance of preconception counseling, women with chronic medical conditions have unmet contraceptive needs.[9–11] Previous research has demonstrated that women who classify themselves as in "poor health" are less likely to be counseled by their medical providers on birth control options. Therefore, unsurprisingly, women over the age of 20 with chronic disease are more likely to have an unplanned pregnancy.[12] This is particularly important, as women with unintended pregnancies are more likely to face poor maternal and fetal outcomes. The explanation for these disparities has been attributed in part to discomfort, on the part of providers, with prescribing birth control to patients with complex medical histories or those taking multiple medications.[13] The U.S. Centers for Disease Control and Prevention publishes the *United States Medical Eligibility Criteria for Contraceptive Use*, which should be used as a resource for physicians and patients to make informed decisions related to birth control[14] (see also Section 1, Chapter 3). Appropriate patient education and access to contraception is critical for family planning in order to allow for medical optimization of a woman's existing medical conditions prior to conception.

Counseling About Pregnancy Options

When faced with an unintended pregnancy, it is critical that women are connected with unbiased and evidenced-based options counseling. While news of a pregnancy can be exciting for some women, for others it may provoke feelings of fear, hopelessness, and uncertainty. Therefore, as a medical provider it is critical to approach news of a new pregnancy with tact and not with the assumption that the pregnancy was planned or desired. At its core, options counseling should be a nonjudgmental and objective discussion between a woman and her provider where she is informed of the three pregnancy options available to women—continuation of the pregnancy with parenthood or adoption, or termination of pregnancy. In discussing these options, healthcare providers have a duty to provide evidence-based resources to help support and guide patients in making this decision. To ensure these needs are met, it is important for primary care providers and subspecialists to be aware of community OB/GYN resources for pregnancy and abortion care. Referrals to established (evidence-based) practices that can effectively counsel patients on all options are critical given the plethora of misinformation and deceptive counseling practices present in some regions. Furthermore, given the medical complexity of some women they may not be candidates for abortion care in the outpatient settings and therefore may require coordinated planning among their providers for safe termination of pregnancy.

When women with significant medical comorbidities have an unintended pregnancy, their options counseling should involve a dialogue between the major providers involved in their care. From a medical standpoint, an assessment should be made regarding how pregnancy, delivery, and medications may impact both the developing fetus and the health of the woman (Box 2.1).[1,16] Given the teratogenicity of certain drugs, alterations or dose adjustments may be needed

should she elect to continue the pregnancy—and ideally should be done prior to conception. If a patient's condition has been well controlled on a teratogenic medication, however, she should be counseled on how stopping or changing a medication may affect her health and the health of the pregnancy. No medication, regardless of fetal effects, should be suddenly halted without a discussion of the risks of this and ideally a bridge to another, safer option. Options counseling should additionally include the economic, psychological, and social needs of the woman and her family. Providers should speak with patients about their current life situation and through nonjudgmental, motivational interviewing assist women in assessing their readiness for a child. This conversation may reveal intimate details such as the circumstances surrounding the conception (including abuse, coercion, or rape), and therefore the provider should be prepared with appropriate resources or referrals if needed. Further resources to assist in decision making and counseling are listed in Box 2.2.

If a patient with an inheritable disorder has an unplanned pregnancy, she may benefit from a referral to a genetic counselor or a specialist in reproductive genetics (see also Chapter 6 and disease-specific chapters for further heritability discussions). These specialists can help women evaluate the likelihood of passing the condition on to their child and its possible severity. For women with chronic medical conditions—those with inheritable disorders or taking teratogenic medications—these discussions should occur prior to conception. Prior to pregnancy, thoughtful planning about management of medications and discussion of risks optimizes a woman's health and understanding about the impact of pregnancy on their health and vice versa. The World Health Organization has identified several conditions that expose a woman to increased health risks as a result of unintended pregnancy—including epilepsy, stroke, and thrombogenic mutations. Women with these conditions should be counseled about the importance of pregnancy planning and use of effective contraceptive methods.

REVIEW OF PREGNANCY TERMINATION OPTIONS

With a complication rate of less than 0.5%, safe abortion care can be provided for most women, even those with most neurologic disorders, in an outpatient setting.[8,17,18] Pregnancy can safely be terminated using medications either surgically or

BOX 2.1
KEYS TO NON-JUDGMENTAL COUNSELING TO PATIENTS REGARDING ABORTION

- Be nonjudgmental. Use of open-ended questions can help the patient's thought process and decision about the pregnancy emerge.

   Tell me how you are feeling about the pregnancy. What things are impacting how you feel about the pregnancy? How would a pregnancy now impact your goals (professional, educational, family)?

- Emphasis of safety of abortion is key. Abortion is a safe option for women with unwanted pregnancy, even women with medical co-morbidities. In fact, pregnancy termination is safer than childbirth.
- Assess how women have come to their decision and discuss their social support in considering pregnancy options.

   Who knows about the pregnancy? Do they know about the abortion decision? How are you feeling about the decision to seek abortion? Do you feel supported by your loved ones in this decision?

- Provide emotional support for women facing unwanted pregnancy or pregnancy loss is an important aspect to their clinical care.

   It sounds like you have thought a lot about this difficult decision. It sounds like you are making the best decision for you and your family at this time.

Adapted from: Upadhyay et al.[16]

BOX 2.2
RESOURCES TO ASSIST WITH DECISION MAKING AROUND ABORTION OR FOR POST-ABORTION CARE

Backline
   Providers confidential and judgment-free support to callers before, during, or after pregnancy, parenting, abortion or adoption.
   https://www.all-options.org
   1-888-493-0092

NAF Hotline
   Provides unbiased information about abortion and other resources for patients.
   1-800-772-9100

Connect & Breathe
   Creates a safe space to talk about abortion experiences by offering a talking staffed by people trained to listen and provide unbiased support and encouragement of self-care.
   1-866-674-1764
   http://www.connectandbreathe.org

via labor induction. Among the most important components of safe abortion care is confirming the location and gestational age and viability of the pregnancy. In the United States, this is typically done with ultrasound. Ensuring the pregnancy is intrauterine and ruling out ectopic pregnancy is important for 2 reasons. First, ruptured ectopic pregnancies can become medical emergencies, and missing the diagnosis increases risk for rupture. And second, medical and surgical approaches to pregnancy termination will be ineffective in treating ectopic pregnancies. Determining the gestational age and viability of the pregnancy are key because this information determines available options for termination and can impact insurance reimbursement and psychosocial reaction to undesired pregnancy. Determining viability of the pregnancy is important because health policy limitations restrict insurance coverage for abortion care for many women but are likely to cover treatment for miscarriage or early pregnancy failure. From a medical standpoint, the management of incomplete abortion (miscarriage) or early pregnancy failure may be identical to pregnancy termination, but the experience for women may be different.

Once an intrauterine pregnancy is confirmed via ultrasound, women with undesired pregnancy should have nonjudgmental, evidence-based options counseling. The options for pregnancy termination differ based on gestational age, availability of trained providers, health policy regulations, and patient preference. Early referral for pregnancy and abortion care decreases complications and morbidity and is particularly important for women with complex medical conditions.[19]

The medications and techniques utilized for early pregnancy failure (miscarriage) and for medical or surgical pregnancy termination in first trimester are the same. Additionally, for the patient experiencing a mid-trimester loss, the options (including labor induction and surgical management) are the same. Therefore the discussion of these medical considerations and approach to safe pregnancy termination in the patient with neurologic disease also applies to the discussion of safe management of the complicated patient with early or mid-trimester pregnancy failure.[13-15]

First Trimester Medical Abortion

Effective up to 10 weeks (70 days) gestation, medication abortion is a safe, evidence-based approach to pregnancy termination.[20-24] With medication abortion, women take a combination of medications to cause the pregnancy to separate from uterine wall, the cervix to soften, and the uterus to expel the pregnancy tissue. For most women, the process of medication abortion is in many ways similar to having a spontaneous miscarriage. The medications most commonly used in the United States for medication abortion are mifepristone and misoprostol. On average women should expect to bleed for approximately 9–16 days after medical abortion. Adverse effects commonly associated with medication abortion with mifepristone and misoprostol include nausea, vomiting, diarrhea, headache, dizziness, and low-grade fever.

Contraindications to medication abortion include: anemia, known or suspected ectopic pregnancy, intrauterine device in place, current long-term systemic corticosteroid use, chronic adrenal failure, inherited porphyria, known coagulopathy or anticoagulant therapy, and intolerance or allergy to mifepristone.

Mifepristone is a synthetic anti-progesterone compound. Because progesterone is an important hormone that supports the growth of early pregnancy, by competitively binding but not activating progesterone receptors, mifepristone leads to withdrawal of hormonal support to the early pregnancy and necrosis of the decidual tissue, cervical softening, and increased contractility 24 to 36 hours after administration. Mifepristone is given orally to women in the clinic at the time of their consultation for abortion. As a steroid blocker, theoretical concerns about co-administration of mifepristone with glucocorticoids exist, and decisions about use of medical abortion in women who chronically take oral steroids should be carefully considered.[24] There are minimal side effects to mifepristone.

The second medication used in medication abortion is misoprostol. Misoprostol is a prostaglandin and is commonly used for cervical preparation and for its uterotonic effects in postpartum hemorrhage. Misoprostol induces strong uterine contractions and softening of the cervix that cause the uterus to expel the pregnancy tissue. Women can take misoprostol buccally, sublingually, or vaginally, typically 6 to 48 hours after the mifepristone (depending on patient preference and route of administration). The misoprostol typically leads to heavy bleeding and cramping within 4 to 6 hours of administration.

Management of pain with non-steroidal anti-inflammatory medications and narcotics and preventing nausea with antiemetic treatment during medication abortion are common. An important component of medication abortion is counseling about risks. The risks of medication abortion include: bleeding requiring transfusion, need for urgent evaluation at a hospital and procedure, infection and incomplete abortion—including risk for ongoing pregnancy. The importance of counseling women regarding these risks and need for follow-up to confirm completion cannot be overstated.

Because of the importance of gestational age as a risk factor for abortion-related morbidity and mortality, the impact of medication abortion in helping shift abortion to earlier gestational ages in the United States supports its promotion as an important public health intervention in safe abortion care.[25] Women have increasingly chosen medication abortion over surgical abortion. The reasons for this include: favoring the option to avoid surgery, increased privacy, and a perception that medication abortion is a safer option than surgical abortion. While the rate of abortion overall has decreased between 2008 and 2011, the proportion of nonhospital abortions that were performed via medication abortion increased from 17% to 23% in the United States.[3] This is important for several reasons, including the lower cost of early abortions, the greater access to providers of first trimester abortion, and the greater public acceptance of abortions performed earlier in pregnancy.

First or Second Trimester Surgical Abortion

First trimester surgical abortion, or a dilation and suction (D&S)—or dilation and curettage (D&C) procedure—is performed using manual or electric vacuum aspiration. Second trimester abortion, or dilation and evacuation (D&E), is performed using instruments to remove fetal parts and placental tissue. There are no contraindications to surgical abortion, although high-risk women may require consultation by specialists trained in advanced abortion care. Surgical abortion, even in the second trimester, is safe with a low complication rate. Risks include bleeding, infection, cervical laceration, and incomplete procedure. Uterine perforation with associated intra-abdominal injury is rare but may require urgent laparotomy. In the United States, most abortion care occurs in the outpatient setting, in freestanding clinics or outpatient surgical centers. Some women have anesthesia needs, medical complexities, or are at risk for complications and require hospital-based procedures.[19] Family planning specialists are best able to determine whether women are candidates for inpatient or hospital-based procedures (see Box 2.3).

BOX 2.3
RESOURCES FOR PROVIDERS OR PATIENTS REGARDING SAFE ABORTION RESOURCES AND REFERRAL OPTIONS TO TRAINED SPECIALISTS

NATIONAL ABORTION FEDERATION

Mission is to ensure safe, legal and accessible abortion care, which promotes health and justice for women. Website and telephone hotlines available that provide referral information and support for patients and evidence-based clinical guidelines for providers.

NAF Hotline for patients seeking resources, including financial assistance with abortion care: 1-800-772-9100

NAF Hotline for patients and providers seeking referral information to quality abortion providers and services: 1-877-257-0012

www.prochoice.org

PLANNED PARENTHOOD

Planned Parenthood is a trusted provider of reproductive health care. Health centers nationwide provide a range of safe, reliable health care—including preventative care, contraceptive services, and abortion care. Website includes information on services, pregnancy, abortion, and contraception as well as resources to find a local clinic.

www.plannedparenthood.org

1-800-230-PLAN

Labor Induction Termination

The final option for pregnancy termination is labor induction. This is an uncommon choice, but some women undergoing termination for fetal indications prefer labor induction because it avoids a procedure and allows for viewing the fetus intact. For fetal anomalies it can also allow for autopsy and fetal evaluation to improve recurrence counseling. Typically this procedure is reserved for later diagnosis of pregnancy in a medical complicated patient, or a fetal anomaly diagnosed later in pregnancy. The access to this service is limited, and gestational age limits vary by state. In the midtrimester labor induction can take 12 to 24 hours or more. Risks of labor induction termination include: bleeding, infection, and need for surgical completion, which is necessary for removal of the placenta in up to 30% of cases.[26]

Post-Abortion Care

Women have a range of experiences with pregnancy termination, and so post-abortion care and services are important. Given the low complication rate, most women will have an uncomplicated recovery after pregnancy termination. However, it is important women know to seek care if they have signs of infection or ongoing significant bleeding. Some women will lactate after undergoing abortion in the second trimester. Counseling these women about this potential and providing anticipatory guidance for help with the physical and psychological discomforts related to this are important. Finally, discussion of contraception is an important component of post-abortion care. Shared decision making that incorporates women's preferences, desires for future pregnancies and her medical problems are all important considerations (see Chapter 3 on contraception). Some women, especially those undergoing pregnancy terminations related to maternal illness and inability to safely complete pregnancy, as well as those with pregnancies complicated by fetal anomalies/syndromes, may benefit from ongoing discussions and care with a mental health professional specializing in women's behavioral health. Connect and Breathe is a national resource that provides a safe space for after abortion support and self-care (Box 2.2), but many pregnancy loss and local mental health services are also available.

Women on Anti-Coagulation

Women receive anti-coagulation or anti-platelet therapies for a variety of neurologic, hematologic, and cardiovascular indications. Bleeding is universal at the time of miscarriage, delivery, or pregnancy termination necessitating discussion of best care practices during these events for all patients on anticoagulation. Often these patients have a significant risk of thrombus formation and are placed on prophylactic therapy to decrease risk of an occlusive vascular event. If these women become pregnant questions may be raised about whether anti-coagulation/anti-platelet therapies need to be held or changed for pregnancy. If there is a pregnancy failure, or the patient is considering abortion then discussion of holding or changing these medications is needed to limit risk of blood loss at the time of the procedure. Women should first consult with their OB/GYN and primary neurologist to evaluate whether medical or surgical termination would be more appropriate based on their gestational age and medical history. This should also include a reevaluation of the reason for initiating anti-coagulation/anti-platelet therapy and whether use is still indicated based on the patient's risk factors as well as institutional guidelines. This decision should also weigh the preferences of the woman, the gestational age of the pregnancy, tolerance of an inpatient surgical procedure, the risk of anesthesia, and the relative risk of hemorrhage while on anti-thrombotic therapy.

Bleeding is expected in all women who choose medical abortion with mifepristone and misoprostol—and unlike surgical techniques will occur in a variable time frame and in the outpatient setting at home. Overall, medical termination is extremely safe and preferred by many women because it allows for privacy and control over the process and avoidance of a procedure. A large multicenter study by Ulmann et al. (1992) examining abortion with mifepristone and a prostaglandin analogue found that only 0.1% of women experienced hemorrhage, which required a blood transfusion.[27,28] However, for the patient on anti-coagulation therapy, understanding the volumes of bleeding and symptoms that should prompt medical evaluation is an important part of the counseling.

It is to be expected that women on therapeutic anti-coagulation will be at a higher risk of prolonged or severe bleeding requiring intervention. Furthermore, Danco Laboratories—the manufacturer of Mifepristone in the United States—identifies active anti-coagulation as a contraindication to medication abortion. As a result, there is limited data in the literature examining medical abortion in such patients, and it is offered in few settings. For this reason, patients on anti-coagulation may benefit from a referral to a hospital-based abortion provider. If the decision is made to pursue medical abortion despite manufacturer warning, providers must assure this aligns with their institutional protocol and that they have the staff support necessary to provide the requisite care to the woman.

Given the elevated risk of hemorrhage and the need for further medical management and observation, surgical termination is generally preferred over medical abortion in patients on therapeutic or prophylactic anti-coagulation. However, in otherwise healthy women, D&S is not associated with an increased risk of bleeding when compared to medical abortion.[6] A second consideration for providers relates to whether or not anti-coagulation needs to be stopped or reversed prior to first trimester surgical abortion. A study by Kaneshiro et al. (2017) found that while women on anti-coagulation undergoing first trimester surgical termination were noted to have increased blood loss relative to healthy peers, they did not have a clinically significant decrease in hemoglobin compared to their pre-procedural value. While underpowered, the findings of this study support that women presenting for pregnancy termination in the first trimester can safely undergo surgical termination while anticoagulated. However, the dearth of evidence in the literature at this time underscores the importance of provider comfort and adherence to institutional protocol in making decisions related to anti-coagulation therapy in the perioperative period.[29,30]

A final consideration for abortion care among women who are anti-coagulated relates to whether the procedure should be performed in a hospital setting or an outpatient setting. The benefits of surgical termination in the hospital setting include access to blood transfusion if needed to correct hematologic status, additional operative equipment, supplies and medication that can be used to manage post-abortion hemorrhage, and careful post-procedural monitoring by trained nursing staff.[31]

Women with Movement Disorders

Parkinson's disease is a movement disorder with low incidence among women of childbearing age. Considerations of management of abortion care among the rare woman experiencing unwanted pregnancy in this population focuses primarily on issues related to the management of anesthesia and risks associated with interruption of medical therapy.

Women with Epilepsy

Epilepsy is a common condition impacting many reproductive-aged women. Considerations of abortion care in women with epilepsy include decisions about where they may safely undergo abortion and drug on drug interactions between medications used in abortion care and anti-epileptic medications. In general, women with well-controlled epilepsy that are stable on anti-epileptic medications may receive outpatient abortion care. Women with recent onset or uncontrolled seizure disorders are likely to benefit from hospital-based care.

When considering medical abortion in this population, medication interactions are important to consider. For women taking anti-epileptic medications that augment the hepatic p450 system, (i.e., phenytoin, phenobarbital, carbamazepine, and oxcabazepine), consideration of a dose increase of the mifepristone may be considered to improve efficacy of medication abortion. This group of patients will also require conceptive adjustments (see Chapter 3, 22, 23).

Women with Neuromuscular Disorders—Myasthenia Gravis

Myasthenia gravis is an autoimmune disease of weakness and fatigue-ability of voluntary muscles. With a mean onset age of 28 years old, this disease is seen most commonly among reproductive-aged women. Smooth muscle remains relatively unaffected by this disease, yet there remains variability in the impact of pregnancy on disease course. Patients with myasthenia have been noted to have symptomatic exacerbation post-abortion. In-hospital termination care may be appropriate for these women given their risk for respiratory compromise in the setting of myasthenia crisis and to allow for careful coordination with anesthesiology[34,35] (see also Section 4, Chapter 24, "Neuromuscular Disorders").

Neurocutaneous Disorders

Neurocutaneous disorders are a group of heterogeneous diseases that differ greatly in their phenotypic presentation and neurologic implications. In many cases, these disorders are heritable and work up is often prompted by the onset of characteristic skin findings. While there are many examples of neurocutaneous disorders, this chapter will focus on Tuberous Sclerosis Complex (TSC). Given the overall low prevalence of these disorders there is limited research examining the management of unintended pregnancy in this patient population.

Therefore, much of the discussion in this section will focus on possible obstetrical and surgical complications and how this can be applied to abortion care.

Tuberous Sclerosis Complex (TSC) is an autosomal dominant disease, which is characterized by the formation of hamartomas in a broad range of organs including the brain, heart, kidney, and skin. The presentation and severity of TSC various dramatically and major complications of this disorder are linked to disruptions in organ function secondary to the presence of these hamartomas. Of particular concern in pregnant patients or those undergoing surgical procedures is the high prevalence of epilepsy in this population (estimated to be as high as 96% in some studies).[36]

Patients with a diagnosed seizure disorder should be managed as discussed in the "epilepsy" section of this chapter. While most cases of TSC related epilepsy present in childhood, up to 10% of patients may experience their first seizure as an adult.[37] As a result, careful surgical planning should take place between anesthesiology and the managing gynecologist. Finally, given that TSC is also associated with cardiac rhabdomyoma, renal angiomyolipoma, and pulmonary lymphangiomyomatosis patients with these findings may benefit from clearance or risk assessment by cardiology, nephrology, or pulmonology respectively prior to medical or surgical abortion[38] (see also Section 5, Chapter 32).

Spinal Cord Injuries

In the United States, an estimated 17,000 Spinal Cord Injuries (SCIs) occur each year, approximately 20% of which affect women.[39] Misconceptions often exist regarding the effect of SCI on fecundity. Immediately following the insult, approximately one in four women experience amenorrhea secondary to stress-induced hyperprolactinemia.[40] However, it remains that there is limited evidence to suggest that the injury affects a woman's ability to conceive once menses return.[41] As a result, contraceptive counseling and discussions about family planning are critical as pregnant women with SCIs face a series of unique risks that both patients and their providers need to be prepared to address (see also Chapter 29).

While there are limited studies that explicitly explore abortion care in women with SCIs, much can be learned from evidence surrounding the care of desired pregnancies in this patient population. A phenomenon known as "autonomic dysreflexia" (AD), can occur in pregnant women with SCI, typically above the level of T5–T6. In this condition,

the afferent inputs derived from simple uterine manipulation during a physical exam, the placement of a urinary catheter, uterine contractions, or even a full rectum or bladder are misinterpreted by the central nervous system, which triggers a sympathetic overdrive. The effects of this response by the CNS range in severity from flushing and hypertension to cerebral hemorrhage and stroke; therefore, careful coordination of care is critical to ensure that abortion care remains safe.[42] Given the risk for serious complications should AD occur, women with SCIs at risk for AD will likely benefit from hospital-based abortion care regardless of gestational age. Because misoprostol and mifepristone cause uterine contractions—a possible trigger of AD—it is likely not safe for women to undergo termination of pregnancy in the outpatient setting. To decrease risk of autonomic dysreflexia during normal labor and delivery, it is recommended that these patients receive a T10 spinal block or epidural regardless of absent sensation of pain (ACOG practice bulletin, exact address above). These guiding principles regarding spinal anesthetic should translate well to the care of abortion patients. For these reasons, women opting for surgical termination, or labor induction an anesthesiologist should be consulted in the preoperative period (see also Chapter 32).

Women with Neurologic Disability/ Brain Injury

Another issue that may arise in women with severe neurological disease relates to the issue of comprehension and consent. For women with history of brain injury or cognitive, linguistic or intellectual disability, ensuring their appropriate participation in medical decision making, particularly around pregnancy decisions, is a cornerstone of ethical medical care. It is important in these challenging situations to consider the context of the pregnancy and the potential for abuse or coercion, as well as be mindful about how to best communicate with the women and those involved in her life. When there is not clarity as to a woman's comprehension, capacity, or ability to consent to decisions about pregnancy and abortion, obtaining an ethics consultation can be helpful to ensure autonomy of the patient and compliance with ethical standards are met.[32,33]

CONCLUSION

Access to compassionate, nonjudgmental, and safe abortion care for medically complex women is an important component of obstetric care for high-risk women. The care of women with neurologic disease who seek pregnancy termination or management of pregnancy failure includes consideration of their particular medical, anesthesia, and surgical needs. Counseling regarding pregnancy options is an important first step in helping women achieve their family planning goals. Resources are available to help non-obstetric providers ensure their patients have access to medically sound, evidence-based information about pregnancy termination.

REFERENCES

1. Jones RK, Kavanaugh ML. Changes in abortion rates between 2000 and 2008 and lifetime incidence of abortion. *Obstetrics and Gynecology.* 2011; 117(6): 1358–1366.
2. Jones RK, Jerman J. Abortion incidence and service availability in the United States, 2011. *Perspectives on Sexual and Reproductive Health.* 2014; 46(1): 3–14.
3. Jones RK, Kooistra K. Abortion incidence and access to services in the United States, 2008. *Perspectives on Sexual and Reproductive Health.* 2011; 43(1): 41–50.
4. Conde-Agudelo A, Rosas-Bermudez A, Kafury-Goeta AC. Effects of birth spacing on maternal health: A systematic review. *American Journal of Obstetrics and Gynecology.* 2007; 196(4): 297–308.
5. Conde-Agudelo A, Rosas-Bermudez A, Kafury-Goeta AC. Birth spacing and risk of adverse perinatal outcomes: a meta-analysis. *JAMA.* 2006; 295(15): 1809–1823.
6. Bartlett LA, Berg CJ, Shulman HB, et al. Risk factors for legal induced abortion-related mortality in the United States. *Obstetrics and Gynecology.* 2004; 103(4): 729–737.
7. Zane S, Creanga AA, Berg CJ, et al. Abortion-related mortality in the United States: 1998-2010. *Obstetrics and Gynecology.* 2015; 126(2): 258–265.
8. Raymond EG, Grimes DA. The comparative safety of legal induced abortion and childbirth in the United States. *Obstetrics and Gynecology.* 2012; 119(2 Pt. 1): 215–219.
9. Perritt JB, Burke A, Jamshidli R, Wang J, Fox M. Contraception counseling, pregnancy intention and contraception use in women with medical problems: an analysis of data from the Maryland Pregnancy Risk Assessment Monitoring System (PRAMS). *Contraception.* 2013; 88(2): 263–268.
10. DeNoble AE, Hall KS, Xu X, Zochowski MK, Piehl K, Dalton VK. Receipt of prescription contraception by commercially insured women with chronic medical conditions. *Obstetrics and Gynecology.* 2014; 123(6): 1213–1220.
11. Phillips-Bell GS, Sappenfield W, Robbins CL, Hernandez L. Chronic diseases and use of contraception among women at risk of unintended pregnancy. *J Womens Health (Larchmt).* 2016; 25(12): 1262–1269.
12. Lee JK, Parisi SM, Schwarz EB. Contraceptive counseling and use among women with poorer health. *Journal of Womens Health Issues Care.* 2013; 2(1): 103.
13. Chor J, Rankin K, Harwood B, Handler A. Unintended pregnancy and postpartum contraceptive use in women with and without chronic medical disease who experienced a live birth. *Contraception.* 2011; 84(1): 57–63.
14. Curtis KM, Tepper NK, Jatlaoui TC, et al. U.S. medical eligibility criteria for contraceptive use, 2016. *MMWR Recomm Rep.* 2016; 65(3): 1–103.
15. Gaffield ML, Kiarie J. WHO medical eligibility criteria update. *Contraception.* 2016; 94(3): 193–194.
16. Upadhyay UD, Cockrill K, Freedman LR. Informing abortion counseling: an examination of evidence-based practices used in emotional care for other stigmatized and sensitive health issues. *Patient Education and Counseling.* 2010; 81(3): 415–421.
17. Renner RM, Brahmi D, Kapp N. Who can provide effective and safe termination of pregnancy care? A systematic review. *BJOG.* 2013; 120(1): 23–31.
18. Cook RJ, Dickens BM, Horga M. Safe abortion: WHO technical and policy guidance. *Internatlinal Journal of Gynaecology and Obstetrics.* 2004; 86(1): 79–84.
19. Guiahi M, Davis A, Society of Family P. First-trimester abortion in women with medical conditions: Release date October 2012 SFP guideline #20122. *Contraception.* 2012; 86(6): 622–630.
20. Sanhueza Smith P, Pena M, Dzuba IG, et al. Safety, efficacy and acceptability of outpatient mifepristone-misoprostol medical abortion through 70 days since last menstrual period in public sector facilities in Mexico City. *Reproductive Health Matters.* 2015; 22(44 Suppl 1): 75–82.
21. Boersma AA, Meyboom-de Jong B, Kleiverda G. Mifepristone followed by home administration of buccal misoprostol for medical abortion up to 70 days of amenorrhoea in a general practice in Curacao. *European Journal of Contraception and Reproductive Health Care.* 2011; 16(2): 61–66.
22. Winikoff B, Dzuba IG, Chong E, et al. Extending outpatient medical abortion services through 70 days of gestational age. *Obstetrics and Gynecology.* 2012; 120(5): 1070–1076.
23. Medical management of first-trimester abortion. *Contraception.* 2014; 89(3): 148–161.
24. ACOG Practice Bulletin No. 143: Medical management of first-trimester abortion. *Obstetrics and Gynecology.* 2014; 123(3): 676–692.

25. ACOG Committee Opinion No 613: Increasing access to abortion. *Obstetrics and Gynecology.* 2014; 124(5): 1060–1065.

26. Borgatta L, Kapp N, Society of Family P. Clinical guidelines. Labor induction abortion in the second trimester. *Contraception.* 2011; 84(1): 4–18.

27. Dubois C, Ulmann A, Aubeny E, et al. Abortion induced by RU 486: importance of its combination with a prostaglandin derivative. *C R Acad Sci III.* 1988; 306(2): 57–61.

28. Barnard J, Ulmann A. Medical abortion. *BMJ.* 1992; 304(6831): 914.

29. Kaneshiro B, Bednarek P, Isley M, Jensen J, Nichols M, Edelman A. Blood loss at the time of first-trimester surgical abortion in anticoagulated women. *Contraception.* 2011; 83(5): 431–435.

30. Kaneshiro B, Tschann M, Jensen J, Bednarek P, Texeira R, Edelman A. Blood loss at the time of surgical abortion up to 14 weeks in anticoagulated patients: a case series. *Contraception.* 2017; 96(1): 14–18.

31. Davey A. Mifepristone and prostaglandin for termination of pregnancy: Contraindications for use, reasons and rationale. *Contraception.* 2006; 74(1): 16–20.

32. ACOG committee opinion No 289:Surgery and patient choice: the ethics of decision making. *International Journal of Gynaecology and Obstetrics.* 2004; 84(2): 188–193.

33. ACOG Committee Opinion No321: Maternal decision making, ethics, and the law. *Obstetrics and Gynecology.* 2005; 106(5 Pt. 1): 1127–1137.

34. Batocchi AP, Majolini L, Evoli A, Lino MM, Minisci C, Tonali P. Course and treatment of myasthenia gravis during pregnancy. *Neurology.* 1999; 52(3): 447–452.

35. Ciafaloni E, Massey JM. Myasthenia gravis and pregnancy. *Neurological Clinics.* 2004; 22(4): 771–782.

36. Yates JR, Maclean C, Higgins JN, et al. The Tuberous Sclerosis 2000 Study: Presentation, initial assessments and implications for diagnosis and management. *Archives of Disease in Childhood.* 2011; 96(11): 1020–1025.

37. Seibert D, Hong CH, Takeuchi F, et al. Recognition of tuberous sclerosis in adult women: Delayed presentation with life-threatening consequences. *Annals of Internal Medicine.* 2011; 154(12): 806–813, W-294.

38. Rabito MJ, Kaye AD. Tuberous sclerosis complex: Perioperative considerations. *The Ochsner Journal.* 2014; 14(2): 229–239.

39. National Spinal Cord Injury Statistical Center. Birmingham, Alabama: Facts and Figures at a Glance 2016. 2016. https://www.nscisc.uab.edu. Accessed September 12, 2017.

40. Trofimenko V, Hotaling JM. Fertility treatment in spinal cord injury and other neurologic disease. *Transl Androl Urol.* 2016; 5(1): 102–116.

41. Jackson AB, Wadley V. A multicenter study of women's self-reported reproductive health after spinal cord injury. *Archives of Physical Medicine and Rehabilitation.* 1999; 80(11): 1420–1428.

42. ACOG Committee Opinion: No 275, September 2002. Obstetric management of patients with spinal cord injuries. *Obstetrics and Gynecology.* 2002; 100(3): 625–627.

3

Contraception Options in Neurologic Disease

TESSA L. REISINGER AND AMY ROBINSON HARRINGTON

Unplanned pregnancy is a prevalent issue in the United States, as 50% of all pregnancies are unplanned.[1] An unplanned pregnancy has potential implications for a woman's social, financial, psychologic (and fetal) well-being, and the health risks of a continuing pregnancy or abortion.[2] For women with chronic medical conditions, pregnancies carry particular risk due to increased likelihood of adverse health events.[3] Additionally, pregnancy itself may impact the course of disease, or may interrupt treatment due to concern for teratogenic effects of medications.[4]

Despite the importance of avoiding unplanned pregnancy in this population, studies suggest suboptimal contraceptive use by women with chronic medical conditions.[3,5] Women with medical problems are more likely to report unintended pregnancy and are less likely to use prescribed methods of contraception than healthy women in spite of more frequent contact with health-care providers.[2] Additionally, these women are more likely to use short acting methods or sterilization rather than highly effective long-acting reversible contraception methods.[3] Provider reluctance to prescribe contraceptive methods in certain conditions, as well as lack of knowledge regarding safe contraceptive options, may play a role in the pattern of contraceptive use in women with chronic medical problems.[3,5]

To help address these concerns, the WHO and the CDC have developed easy reference guidelines: Medical Eligibility Criteria for Contraceptive Use (MEC). These are evidence-based guidelines, published in a chart, that outline the safety of different contraceptive methods as they relate to common medical conditions graded 1 (no restriction) to 4 (unacceptable health risk)[6] (see Figure 3.1). Based on best available evidence, this is meant to be an easy-to-use tool for all health-care practitioners. In addition to general recommendations for each method, recommendations are divided, where appropriate,

into initiation and continuation of existing methods, as a way of guiding providers who diagnose a medical issue while a contraceptive method is in use.

While a useful guide, not all neurological conditions are included in this chart and analysis. This chapter seeks to provide a guide to the full range of contraceptive options for women with a wide variety of neurological disorders. Where available we will discuss data specific to the underlying neurological condition. Unfortunately, there is limited published data for many of these conditions, and therefore our recommendations necessitate looking at not just the disease state but also the associated symptoms, conditions, and medications. Providers of both obstetrics and neurology may therefore need to utilize this and other resources in the medical complex neurologic patient seeking contraceptive counseling. Suggestions for initiating conversations about contraceptive options are included in Table 3.1.

Reversible contraceptives that are currently available in the United States can be broken down into three categories: highly effective, effective, and less effective. Typical compared to perfect use failure rates are the main difference in category of efficacy[7] (see Table 3.2). Highly effective methods include the copper intrauterine device (IUD), progesterone hormonal IUDs, and the progesterone implant. Effective methods include combination estrogen/progesterone-containing pills (COCs), patches and ring, progesterone-only pills (POPs) and depo medroxyprogesterone (DMPA). Less effective methods include diaphragms, condoms, withdrawal, and natural family planning. Patches and rings contain estrogen and are considered to have similar side effects and risk/benefit profiles as COCs.

Selection of contraceptive methods for the immediate post-partum patient with neurological disease who is lactating can be further complicated, as some hormonal methods can interfere with the

Condition	Sub-Condition	Cu-IUD I	Cu-IUD C	LNG-IUD I	LNG-IUD C	Implant I	Implant C	DMPA I	DMPA C	POA I	POA C	CHC I	CHC C
Hypertension	a) Adequately controlled hypertension	1*		1*		1*		2*		1*			3*
	b) Elevated blood pressure levels *(properly taken measurements)*												
	1) Systolic 140 159 or diastolic 90 99	1*		1*		1*		2*		1*			3*
	ii) Systolic ≥160 or diastolic ≥100*	1*		2*		2*		3*		2*			4*
	c) Vascular disease	1*		2*		2*		3*		2*			4*
Inflammatory bowel disease	*(Ulcerative colitis, Crohn's disease)*	1		1		1		2		2			2/3*
Ischemic heart disease	Current and history of	1		2	3	2	3	3		2	3		4
Known thrombogenic mutations*		1*		2		2		2		2			4*
Liver tumors	a) Benign												
	i) Focal nodular hyperplasia	1		2		2		2		2			2
	ii) Hepatocellular adenoma*	1		3		3		3		3			4
	b) Malignant* (hepatoma)	1		3		3		3		3			4
Malaria		1		1		1		1		1			1
Multiple risk factors for atherosclerotic cardiovascular disease	(e.g., older age, smoking diabetes, hypertension, low HOC, high LDL, or high triglyceride levels)	1		2		2*		3*		2*			3/4*
Multiple sclerosis	a) With prolonged immobility	1		1		1		2		1			3
	b) Without prolonged immobility	1		1		1		2		1			1
Obesity	a) Body mass index (BMI) ≥30 kg/m²	1		1		1		1		1			2
	b) Menarche to <18 years and BMI ≥30 kg/m²	1		1		1		2		1			2

Key:

1 No restriction (method can be used)	3 Theoretical or proven risks usually outweigh the advantages
2 Advantages generally outweigh theoretical or proven risks	4 Unacceptable health risk (method not to be used)

* Further details and clarification to this classification score available at: www.cdc.gov/reproductivehealth/contraception/pdf/summary-chart-us-medical-eligibility-criteria_508tagged.pdf

FIGURE 3.1 Summary chart of US Medical Eligibility Criteria for Contraceptive Use.

https://www.cdc.gov/reproductivehealth/contraception/pdf/summary-chart-us-medical-eligibility-criteria_508tagged.pdf

TABLE 3.1 CONTRACEPTIVE COUNSELING: STARTING THE CONVERSATION

Are you planning on trying to get pregnant in the next year?	Yes	Consider referral to an obstetric provider for preconception counselling
	No	Assess current contraception plan and QOL around menstrual symptoms (see below)
Are you using anything to prevent pregnancy?	Vasectomy/Bilateral tubal ligation	Discussion of QOL around menstrual symptoms (see below)
		Discussion of medical eligibility for these services
	IUDs/Implant	Inquire about satisfaction with their method
	Pills/Patch/Ring/Shot	Inquire about satisfaction with their method
		Ask about difficulties with their method (forgetting to take pill daily, unable to get prescription refills on time, difficulty inserting ring due to mobility issues from neurologic condition, etc.)
	Condoms/Diaphragm	Inquire about satisfaction with their method
		Ask about difficulties with their method (forgetting to use every time, difficulty obtaining condoms/spermicide, difficulty inserting the diaphragm due to mobility issues from neurologic condition, etc.)
Are you satisfied with your current method?	No	Consider referral to gynecology provider for contraceptive counseling
	Considering bilateral tubal ligation?	Discussion of risks and benefits of a surgical procedure in the setting of their neurologic condition
Are your menstrual cycles interfering with your quality of life?	If yes, consider referral to a gynecology provider for discussion of menstrual control and/or menstrual suppression	
Does your neurologic condition make it difficult to deal with your menstrual cycles?	If yes, consider referral to a gynecology provider for discussion of menstrual control and/or menstrual suppression	

TABLE 3.2 CONTRACEPTIVE FAILURE RATES

	Method	Percentage of Women Who Become Pregnant in First Year of Use	
		Perfect Use	Typical Use
No method	No method	85	85
Barrier methods	Withdrawal	4	22
	Condoms	2	18
Short-acting hormonal methods	Birth control pills Contraceptive patch Contraceptive vaginal ring	0.3	9
	Injection—depot medroxyprogesterone acetate (Depo Provera)	0.2	6
Long-acting reversible contraception	IUDs — Copper T380A (Paragard)	0.6	0.8
	IUDs — Levonorgestrel	0.2	0.2
	Implants — Etonogestrel implant	0.05	0.05
Surgical sterilization	Tubal ligation	0.5	0.5
	Vasectomy	0.1	0.15

Adapted from Trussell, 2011.

effective establishment of lactation. In general, IUDs, barrier methods, and progesterone-only methods (POPs, DMPA, and the progesterone implant) are considered to have minimal/no effect on lactation. Those methods containing estrogen are not recommended in the first 3 to 6 weeks postpartum due to their thrombogenic risk and the first 4 weeks due to their potential to interfere with lactation. However, all these risks must be balanced against the risk of unintended pregnancy and/or closely spaced pregnancy with its associated risks for poor pregnancy outcomes.

In general, the major medical concern with hormonal contraception is with regard to estrogen-containing methods. Women with cerebrovascular disease, heart disease, diabetes with underlying vessel disease, liver disease, peripheral vascular disease, and smokers above the age of 35 are already at risk for the development or worsening of cardiovascular disease (CVD). The addition of estrogen with these underlying conditions results in an unacceptable increased risk of CVD and is therefore contraindicated.[6,8] Systematic reviews of progestin-only contraception, however, do not suggest increased risk for CVD events and can be used safely with the previously mentioned estrogen contraindications.[9,10] One notable caveat is that US MEC lists DMPA as a category 3 for both initiation and continuation in women who have had a cerebrovascular accident, as the hypoestrogenic effects and reduced HDL levels may increase risk in these patients.[6]

MULTIPLE SCLEROSIS
Multiple sclerosis (MS) is a chronic inflammatory disease that affects the central nervous system that is characterized by damage to myelin sheaths. MS is of particular interest in women's health as the disease is 2.4 times more likely to occur in women than in men and often strikes young patients, with the peak age of onset during childbearing years.[11] The disease does not appear to impact fertility,[12] making contraceptive counseling an important component of the care of women with MS.

Of note, blood levels of sex steroids appear to have an impact on the frequency of relapse in patients with multiple sclerosis, with high-estrogen states being associated with a more benign disease course.[13,14] For instance, patients tend to experience lower frequency of relapse during pregnancy, particularly in the third trimester when estrogen and progesterone are at their highest, followed by more frequent relapses in the relatively low estrogen state during the postpartum period.[15]

Given the potentially beneficial impact of estrogen on multiple sclerosis, studies have examined the relationship between oral contraceptive use and disease progression. Gava et al. performed a retrospective study that noted women using combined oral contraceptives (COCs) tended to have better Expanded Disability Status Scale (EDSS) scores than never users, a difference that remained when the results were adjusted for age and use of disease modifying therapies. The study also noted decreased likelihood of disease progression among COC users, although long-term findings in other studies have been mixed.[12,16] Additionally, Kempe et al collected symptom diaries and found that women experienced worsening symptoms during the hormone-free week of a COC pack. In contrast, there does not appear to be variation in symptoms with the menstrual cycle in patients not on hormonal contraception.[17] While available data indicate a potentially beneficial role for COCs, the body of literature remains limited. In particular, the data may suffer from selection bias, as patients on OCPs identified for the studies generally had less severe disease.[11,14] Further work is needed to more definitively determine whether COC use offers disease-specific benefits for MS patients.

In counseling women with MS regarding contraceptive options, few methods are contraindicated. COCs may have some beneficial effect on symptom control, especially if given in continuous fashion, but further study is needed to more clearly establish this relationship.[14] For patients with more advanced disease and limited mobility, avoidance of estrogen-containing methods is recommended due to the increased risk of venous thromboembolism.[11]

Progesterone-only methods, including POPs and DMPA, are generally safe for women with MS. There is some concern for decreased bone density with DMPA potentially leading to increased fracture risk in MS patients; however, no studies have been performed in this population.[11] Implants and IUDs are highly acceptable options for women with MS, particularly given their excellent contraceptive efficacy and favorable side-effect profiles. Improvement in menstrual bleeding control with the progesterone IUD may be especially beneficial for patients with advanced disease and limited mobility.

While there are no explicit guidelines available for other neurological conditions such as transverse myelitis or neuromyelitis optica, it is reasonable to extrapolate MS recommendations to include these other demyelinating conditions.

EPILEPSY

Family planning is especially important among women with epilepsy (WWE) due to increased maternal and fetal risks in pregnancy. Approximately 15%–30% of WWE will experience increased seizure frequency during pregnancy; women with poor seizure control prior to conception are at highest risk.[18] Pharmacokinetic changes during pregnancy also affect metabolism of certain antiepileptic drugs (AEDs), which can result in therapeutic failure.[21] Additionally, infants born to WWE are at increased risk of congenital malformations (4%–14%), largely secondary to AED exposure, with valproic acid and multidrug therapy posing the greatest risk.[19,21]

Despite these considerations, contraceptive counseling and use among WWE is often suboptimal. Based on data from the Epilepsy Birth Control Registry, approximately 30% of WWE do not use methods of contraception that are considered highly effective. Additionally, a large proportion (47%) of this population use systemic hormones for contraception, which have potential bi-directional interactions with AEDs that may negatively affect the therapeutic efficacy of both medications.[22] While the American Academy of Neurology recognizes the importance of counseling regarding pregnancy and contraception for WWE, only 25% of the women surveyed reported discussing contraception with their neurologist.[22]

AEDs can improve quality of life in WWE by decreasing seizure frequency and are frequently prescribed for reproductive age women. However, the choice of contraceptive in WWE is complicated by potential interactions with these medications. Systemic hormones in the form of oral contraceptive pills (OCPs) are a common contraceptive choice, but WWE using OCPs are more likely to experience contraceptive failure, at rates of 3%–6% with perfect use compared to 1% in healthy women.[23] One study reported OCP failure as the cause in approximately one quarter of unintended pregnancies in WWE.[21] No studies have been performed on the use of emergency contraception (morning-after pill) in women on AED therapy.[23]

The decreased efficacy of systemic hormones in this population is secondary to induction of hepatic enzymes by AEDs, leading to accelerated metabolism of ethinyl estradiol (EE) and progestins.[23] In modern contraceptives, progestin is the component that directly inhibits the LH surge and thus ovulation. If an AED causes more than a 10% decrease of progestins in measured pharmacokinetic studies, it is considered to decrease the efficacy of the contraceptive.[25] Additionally, AEDs have been demonstrated to increase sex hormone binding globulin concentrations, further decreasing biologically active sex steroids.[26] Carbamazepine, phenobarbital, and phenytoin are particularly potent enzyme inducers that may result in OCP failure, while topiramate appears to have a dose-dependent effect hormone metabolism.[23] First line choices for contraception with these medications would include any of the IUDs or DMPA. As DMPA provides a large dose of progesterone, its efficacy is not affected by the increased metabolism caused by AEDs. While second line, the implant, ring, patch and OCPs with the highest progesterone dose can be used as contraception, but duel protection with barrier methods is recommended. AEDs that do not cause hepatic induction, including valproate, gabapentin, levetiracetam, and zonisamide, pose no restrictions on contraceptive choice[23] (see Table 3.3).

Lamotrigine presents several unique issues for women using OCPs for contraception. Lamotrigine appears to decrease levels of the progestin levonorgestrel, with no impact on other progestins.[23] However, the use of estrogen-containing contraceptives accelerates the metabolism of lamotrigine, which can lead to therapeutic failure and increased seizure frequency.[23] Strategies to counteract this effect include increasing the

TABLE 3.3 EFFECT OF COMMON ANTI-EPILEPTIC DRUGS ON METABOLISM OF HORMONAL CONTRACEPTION

AED	Effect on Hormonal Contraception	
	Estrogen Levels	Progesterone Levels
Carbamazepine	Reduced	Reduced
Gabapentin	No effect	No effect
Lamotrigine	No effect	Reduced
Levetiracetam	No effect	No effect
Oxcarbazepine	Reduced	Reduced
Phenobarbital	Reduced	Reduced
Phenytoin	Reduced	Reduced
Topiramate	Reduced*	No effect
Valproate	No effect	No effect
Zonisamide	No effect	No effect

Adapted from Reimers, 2015.
*Dose-dependent.

lamotrigine dose; however, during placebo weeks of the contraceptive, lamotrigine toxicity can occur. This may be counteracted by providing continuous contraception and the avoidance of a hormonal free week. Strict coordination with the contraceptive provider, the AED provider and the patient are critical in preventing either increased seizure activity or AED toxicity. Of note, progestin-only methods of contraception do not impact lamotrigine metabolism,[23] and may therefore be more optimal choices for WWE on this medication.

In general, IUDs are highly acceptable options for women with epilepsy, given their excellent contraceptive efficacy and favorable side-effect profiles. The method is more common among WWE (18.6% report IUD use) than in the general population.[22] No concern exists for AED/IUD interactions, and they can be used in any woman without a known contraindication to an IUD. Improvement in menstrual bleeding control with the progesterone IUD may be especially beneficial for patients with severe cognitive impairment from their epilepsy who struggle with behavioral disturbances or difficulty with hygiene during their menses.

Catamenial epilepsy is an epileptic condition specific to women, with exacerbation of seizures during different phases of the menstrual cycle in women with preexisting epilepsy. The occurrence of changes in estrogen and progesterone levels is thought to be a key factor in catamenial epilepsy, with progesterone being considered an anticonvulsant hormone and estrogen a pro-convulsant.[19] Catamenial seizure activity has been seen both around the time of ovulation and in the week preceding menses, with the sudden surge of estrogen preceding ovulation and the sudden withdrawal of progesterone prior to menstruation as the proposed causative agents. The use of medroxyprogesterone acetate (DMPA) for contraception has the added benefit of potentially decreasing seizure frequency, as the method maintains a high level of progesterone over a 3-month period. The use of combined oral contraceptive pills, while containing estrogen, have not been shown to increase seizure frequency in these patients.[20]

HEADACHE (COMMON, MIGRAINES, PSEUDOTUMOR)

Common Headaches

Headaches are commonly reported with COC use and frequently cited as a reason for discontinuation.[24] Systematic reviews of COCs and headaches are limited by wide variation in COC formulations, endpoints examined, and duration of therapy, as well as differences in studied populations.[28] Based on this limited evidence, it does not appear that there is a strong relationship between COC use and headache symptoms for most women.[29] Additionally, the dose and type of progestin does not appear to impact headache incidence; however, the effect of estrogen is unclear. Headaches that begin or worsen with COC initiation also tend to improve over time.[29] In general, the presence of common headaches should therefore not be the deciding factor in contraceptive choice.

Migraine Headaches

Migraine headaches are common in women, with a lifetime incidence more than two-fold higher than men.[32] Migraine frequency and severity may vary with the menstrual cycle, with many patients experiencing more frequent migraines around the onset of menstruation.[32] Patients with menstrual migraines often experience decreased migraine burden with COCs prescribed in continuous fashion or with a shortened pill-free interval,[32] making the method a useful option for both headache control and contraception. However, some women with migraines experience worsening headache frequency or may have the onset of aura symptoms after initiation of COCs.[32] The development of these worsening symptoms necessitates reevaluation and potential cessation of COC use.

The most notable concern with COC use in patients with migraines, however, is the potential increased risk of cerebrovascular accident. Migraine with aura has been associated with increased risk of ischemic stroke, which may relate to vascular changes in these patients.[30,31] The use of hormonal contraception, specifically estrogen-containing methods, has also been linked to increased stroke risk, prompting concern for further risk elevation in women with migraines that use COCs.[30] Accordingly, combined hormonal contraceptives are a category 4 (unacceptable health risk) in women with migraine with aura in the CDC medical eligibility criteria. In contrast, migraines without aura have not been associated with significantly increased stroke risk[30] and are a category 2 (benefits likely outweigh risks).

Several studies have examined the theoretical concern for increased stroke risk secondary to COC use in women with migraines. A systematic review by Tepper et al found a two- to fourfold increased risk of stroke among women with migraines who used COCs. However, the majority of the studies were of poor-to-fair quality, and many did not distinguish between migraine subtypes. A more recent study that utilized a national health-care claims database found a six-fold increase in ischemic stroke risk among women with migraines with aura that used combined hormonal contraceptives, compared to women with neither risk factor.[31] The use of COCs did not substantially increase stroke risk in women with migraines without aura.

Given these risks, COCs should be avoided in women with history of migraines with aura. However, careful history and distinction between migraine types is essential, as COCs are a safe option in women with migraines without aura, and may be of particular benefit for women who suffer from menstrual migraines. There does not appear to be an association between progesterone-only contraceptive methods and stroke risk.[30] Therefore, methods without estrogen, including POPs, DMPA, implants, and all IUDs, are viable options for women with migraines, either with or without aura.

PSEUDOTUMOR CEREBRI

Pseudotumor cerebri, also known as idiopathic intracranial hypertension (IIH), is a disorder caused by elevated intracranial pressure with normal cerebrospinal fluid composition and no other identified cause of intracranial hypertension.[33,34] The incidence of IIH is approximately 21/100,000.[35] The disorder occurs four times more commonly in women than in men, and is often diagnosed during childbearing years. Obesity is also a significant risk factor, with 90% of affected patients having an elevated BMI.[35]

Minimal data exist to guide contraceptive choice in women with IIH. Thrombogenic abnormalities, such as the presence of antiphospholipid antibiotics, have been noted in 32% of patients with IIH; these findings suggest a possible an increased risk of thrombotic events.[36] However, there are no data indicating that estrogen-containing contraception increases the risk of thrombosis in women with IIH. Of note, there have also been recent case reports of COCs causing the onset of IIH, but no randomized trials have been performed to examine this link.[37]

Progesterone-only methods, including POPs and DMPA, are generally safe for women with headaches of any type. Implants and IUDs are highly acceptable options for women with headaches and migraines, particularly given their excellent contraceptive efficacy and favorable side-effect profiles.

MOVEMENT DISORDERS

Movement disorders include a wide variety of clinical diagnoses and manifestations caused by both hereditary and acquired factors. These can include both hyper- and hypo-activity disorders. There is limited to no literature on the safety of contraception in women with movement disorders. Determining the underlying cause and the associated contraceptive risks of these causes may provide the clearest path to determining contraceptive choice. Particular attention to physical conditions that arise due to these disorders and therapies that may interfere with hormonal contraception also helps guide our recommendations.[6]

One type of movement disorder deserves special discussion due to its association with COCs. Hyperkinetic movement disorders (chorea) are characterized by involuntary brief, random, and irregular contractions. Chorea may be caused by hereditary neurodegenerative diseases; as a result of structural damage to the brain after vascular events like ischemic stroke or hemorrhage; or they may be associated with autoimmune disorders such as lupus, metabolic derangements, or certain medications.[38] Hyperkinetic disorders arising from acquired conditions may be reversed and cured, but there are no current cures for hereditary neurodegenerative disorders.[39]

Use of COCs is an uncommon but well-known cause of chorea. The mechanism is thought to be a reactivation of previous Sydenham's chorea, which is a manifestation of acute rheumatic fever and the most common type of acquired chorea in childhood.[40] Recurrence of chorea may also occur during pregnancy, suggesting a role of estrogen in the disorder. Most patients will have remission in symptoms two to three months after discontinuation of COCs.[40]

Of note, patients with choreiform movements may be treated with anti-epileptic medications, which have implications for contraceptive choice. Carbamazepine and valproic acid may both be used for symptom management.[41,42] These medications have potential teratogenic effects and also have potential pharmacokinetic interactions with hormone therapies (see Epilepsy for further details). Therefore, these patients should receive counseling on alternative contraceptive options when discontinuing COCs.

TABLE 3.4 CLINICAL PEARLS

Clinical Situation	Contraceptive Pearl
Risk of VTE due to immobility	Avoid estrogen. Progesterone is safe
Vascular changes that increase CVA risk	Avoid estrogen. Progesterone is safe
Cognitive deficits that interfere with medication adherence	LARC methods may be a better choice
Antiphospholipid antibodies	Avoid estrogen. Progesterone is safe
Anticoagulation	Avoid estrogen. Progesterone is safe. Consider progesterone IUD for menstrual cycle control.
Need for CT/MRI imaging	IUDs and implants do not measurably affect imaging
Multiple risk factors for osteoporosis (chronic steroids, renal failure, immobility)	Consider avoiding depo medroxyprogesterone
Cancer	Avoid estrogen. Progesterone safe

NEUROMUSCULAR AND METABOLIC DISORDERS

Muscular dystrophies are genetic, progressive, degenerative disorders with the primary symptom of muscle weakness. These can lead to both immobility and respiratory failure.[43] Rarer types can have associated cardiac defects that increase the risk for pre-eclampsia and congestive heart failure during pregnancy.[44]

Patients with metabolic myopathies have underlying deficiencies of energy production in muscle due to a wide variety of defects. These include defects in lipid, glycogen, glucose, adenine nucleotide, and mitochondrial metabolism. Most patients with metabolic myopathies have dynamic rather than static findings, and therefore usually complain of exercise intolerance, muscle pain, and cramps with exercise rather than fixed weakness. Nevertheless, some patients may develop progressive muscular weakness, which is usually proximal, mimicking an inflammatory myopathy or limb girdle muscular dystrophy.[45,46]

The safety of contraception in women with these disorders should be based on the woman's physical condition and underlying risk factors related to the disease. For example, in patients with progression to immobility, avoidance of estrogen containing methods would be necessary.

PERMANENT STERILIZATION

Surgical sterilization is a highly effective method of contraception. It is, however permanent, and the woman must be completely confident that she is done with childbearing. While this may be an optimal contraceptive option for some women with neurologic disease who do not desire future

fertility, it does involve a surgical procedure. The risks and benefits based on their medications and physical state must be taken into consideration. The currently available IUDs (failure rates for copper IUD 0.8% and progesterone IUD 0.2% over one year) are just as effective as vasectomy (0.15%) and are more effective than tubal ligation (0.5%). Implants, with just a 0.05% failure rate over one year, are even more effective than vasectomy.[7] In women whose neurologic condition increases their risk of anesthesia or recovery from surgery, the benefits of LARC methods may outweigh a permanent procedure.

In summary, while literature does exist regarding the interaction of some neurological disorders and contraception, there is limited data for most conditions. Careful attention to the possible underlying causes, medications, and associated conditions in conjunction with US MEC and our summarized clinical pearls will help guide conversations and possible referrals for more contraceptive and family planning counseling (Table 3.4).

REFERENCES

1. Finer LB, Zolna M. Declines in unintended pregnancy in the United States, 2008-2011. *N Engl J Med.* 2016; 374: 843–852.
2. Goossens J, Van Den Branden Y, Van der Sluys L, et al. The prevalence of unplanned pregnancy ending in birth, associated factors, and health outcomes. *Hum Reprod.* 2016 Dec; 31(12): 2821–2833.
3. Champaloux SW, Tepper NK, Curtis KM, et al. Contraceptive use among women with medical conditions in a nationwide privately insured population. *Obstet Gynecol.* 2015; 126: 1151–1159.
4. Houtchens MK, Kolb CM. Multiple sclerosis and pregnancy: Therapeutic considerations. *J Neurol.* 2013; 260(5): 1202–2014.

5. DeNoble AE, Hall KS, Xu X, et al. Receipt of prescription contraception by commercially insured women with chronic medical conditions. *Obstet Gynecol.*2014; 123(6): 1213–1220.

6. Curtis KM, Tepper NK, Jatlaoui TC, et al. U.S. Medical Eligibility Criteria for Contraceptive Use, 2016. *MMWR Recomm Rep* 2016; 65(No. RR-3): 1–104.

7. Trussell J. Contraceptive failure in the United States. In Hatcher RA, Trussell J, Nelson AL, Cates W, Kowal D, Policar MS, eds. Contraceptive Technology. 20th ed. Atlanta, GA: Ardent Media; 2011, 89–96.

8. Lidegaard O, Lokkegaard E, Jensen A, Skovlund CW, Keiding N. Thrombotic stroke and myocardial infarction with hormonal contraception. *N Engl J Med.* 2012; 366: 2257–2266.

9. Westhoff C. Depot-medroxyprogesterone acetate injection (Depo Provera®): a highly effective contraceptive option with proven long-term safety. *Contraception.* 2003; 68: 75–87.

10. Tepper NK, Whiteman MK, Marchbanks PA, James AH, Curtis KM. Progestin-only contraception and thromboembolism: A systematic review. *Contraception.* (2016); 94: 678–700.

11. Zapata LB, Oduyebo T, Whiteman MK, Houtchens MK, Marchbanks PA, Curtis KM. Contraceptive use among women with multiple sclerosis: A systematic review. *Contraception.* 2016; 94(6): 612–620.

12. Hellwig, K. Pregnancy in multiple sclerosis. *Eur Neurol.* 2014; 72(Suppl 1): 39–42.

13. Gava G, Bartolomei I, Constantino A, Berra M, Salvi F, Meriggiola MC.Long-term influence of combined oral contraceptive use on the clinical course of relapsing-remitting multiple sclerosis. *Fertil Steril.* 2014; 102(1): 116–122.

14. Kempe P, Hammar M, Brynhildsen J. Symptoms of multiple sclerosis during use of combined hormonal contraception. *Eur J Obstet Gynecol Reprod Biol.* 2015; 193: 1–4.

15. Vukusic S, Hutchinson M, Hours M, et al. Pregnancy and multiple sclerosis (the PRIMS study). *Brain.* 2004; 127(Pt. 6): 1353–1360.

16. D'Hooghe MB, Haentjens P, Nagels G, D'Hooge T, De Keyser J. Menarche, oral contraceptives, pregnancy and progression of disability in relapsing onset and progressive onset multiple sclerosis. *J Neurol.* 2012; 259: 855–861.

17. Holmqvist P, Hammar M, Landtblom AM, Brynhildsen J. Symptoms of multiple sclerosis in women in relation to cyclical hormone changes. *Eur J Contracept Reprod Health Care.* 2009; 14(5): 365–370.

18. Patel, SI, Pennell PB. Management of epilepsy during pregnancy: An update. *Ther Adv Neurol Disord.* 2016; 9(2): 118–129.

19. Bangar S, Shastri A, El-Sayeh H, Cavanna AE. Women with epilepsy: Clinically relevant issues. *Funct Neurol.* 2016; 31(3): 127–134.

20. Verrotti A, D'Egidio C, Agostinelli S, Verrotti C, Pavone P. Diagnosis and management of catamenial seizures: A review. *Int J Womens Health.* 2012; 4: 535–541.

21. Borgelt LM, Hart FM, Bainbridge JL. Epilepsy during pregnancy: Focus on management strategies. *Int J Womens Health.* 2016; 8: 505–517.

22. Hertzog AG, Mandle HB, Cahill KE, Fowler KM, Hauser WA, Davis AR. Contraceptive practices of women with epilepsy. *Epilepsia.* 2016; 57(4): 630–637

23. Reimers A, Brodtkorb E, Sabers A. Interactions between hormonal contraception and antiepileptic drugs. *Seizure* 2015; 28: 66–70.

24. Fairgrieve SD, Jackson M, Jonas P, et al. Population based, prospective study in the care of women with epilepsy in pregnancy. *BMJ.* 2000; 321: 674–675.

25. Davis A, Pack A, Dennis A. Contraception for women with epilepsy. In: Allen RH, Cwiak CA, eds. *Contraception for the Medically Challenging Patient.* New York: Springer Science+Business Media; 2014: 135–146.

26. Barragry JM, Makin HL, Trafford DJ, Scott DF. Effect of anticonvulsants on plasma testosterone and sex hormone binding globulin levels. *J Neurol Neurosurg Psychiatry.* 1978; 41: 913–914.

27. Rosenberg MJ, Waugh MS. Oral contraceptive discontinuation: A prospective evaluation of frequency and reasons. *Am J Obstet Gynecol.* 1998; 179(3 Pt. 1): 577.

28. Loder EW, Buse DC, Golub JR. Headache as a side effect of combination estrogen-progestin oral contraceptives: A systematic review. *Am J Obstet Gynecol.* 2005; 193(3 Pt. 1): 636.

29. Martin K, Douglas P. Risks and side effects associated with estrogen-progestin contraceptives. In: UpToDate, TW Post, ed. UpToDate, Waltham, MA. Accessed on January 2017. https://www.uptodate.com/contents/overview-of-the-use-of-estrogen-progestin-contraceptives

30. Tepper NK, Whiteman MK, Zapata LB, Marchbanks PA, Curtis KM. Safety of hormonal contaceptives among women with migraine: A systematic review. *Contraception.* 2016; 94(6): 630–640.

31. Champaloux SW, Tepper NK, Monsour M, et al. Use of combined hormonal contraceptives among women with migraines and risk of ischemic stroke. *Am J Obstet Gynecol.* 2017 May; 216(5): 489.e1–489.e7.

32. Sacco S, Ricci S, Degan D, Carolei A. Migraines in women: The role of hormones and their

impact on vascular diseases. *J Headache Pain.* 2012; 13: 177–189.

33. Friendman D, Jacobson D. Diagnostic criteria for idiopathic intracranial hypertension. *Neurology.* 2002; 59(10): 1492–1495.

34. Bousse V, Bruce B, Newman N. Update on the pathophysiology of idiopathic intracranial hypertension. *J Neurol Neurosurg Psychiatry.* 2012; 83: 488–94.

35. Duncan J, Corbett J, Wall M. The incidence of pseudotumor cerebri population studies in Iowa and Louisiana. *Arch Neurol.* 1988; 45(8): 875–877.

36. Sussman J, Leach M, Greaves M, Malia R, Davies-Jones GAB. Potentially prothrombotic abnormalities of coagulation in benign intracranial hypertension. *J Neurol Neurosurg Psychiatry.* 1997; 62: 229–233.

37. Bartz D, O'Neal MA, Edlow A. Contraceptive options for women with headache disease. In Allen RH, Cwiak CA, eds. *Contraception for the Medically Challenging Patient.* New York: Springer Science+Business Media; 2014: 119–134.

38. Cardoso F, Seppi K, Mair KJ, et al. Seminar on choreas. *Lancet Neurol.* 2006; 5: 589–602.

39. Cardoso F, Autoimmune choreas. *J Neurol Neurosurg Psychiatry.* 2017 May; 88(5): 412–417.

40. Miranda M, Cardoso F, Giovannoni G, Church A. Oral contraceptive induced chorea: another condition associated with anti-basal ganglia antibodies. *J Neurol Neurosurg Psychiatry.* 2004;75: 327–328.

41. Genel F, Arslanoglu S, Uran N, et al. Sydenham's chorea: Clinical findings and comparison of the efficacies of sodium valproate and carbamazepine regimens. *Brain Dev.* 2002; 24: 73–76.

42. Postuma RB, Berg D, Stern M, et al. MDS clinical diagnostic criteria for Parkinson's disease. *Mov Disord.* 2015; 30: 1591.

43. Wicklund MP. The muscular dystrophies. *Continuum.* 2013; 19: 1535.

44. Sato M, Shirasawa H, Makino K, et al. Perinatal management of pregnancy complicated by autosomal dominant Emery-Dreifuss muscular dystrophy. *AJP Reports.*2016; 6: 145–147.

45. Gilus N. Myasthenia Gravis. *N Engl J Med.* 2016; 375: 2570–2581.

46. Darras BT, Friedman NR. Metabolic myopathies: A clinical approach; part I. *Pediatr Neurol.* 2000; 22(2): 87–97.

4

Pregnancy Physiology

Effects on Immune and Nervous Systems

LAUREN A. MILLER AND MARY N. TOWNER

In this chapter we review the significant effects pregnancy has on the normal functioning of the nervous and immune systems. Pregnancy tissues themselves, including the placenta, the gravid uterus, the ovaries and the fetus, all secrete physiologically active cytokines, proteins, and other active molecules into the maternal circulation. The specific functions of and maternal physiologic responses to many of these substances remain unknown. We will summarize the current state of knowledge regarding the physiologic effects of pregnancy, focusing on the effects of estrogen, progesterone, and prolactin on the female immune system and central and peripheral nervous systems.

IMMUNE SYSTEM

It was long believed that pregnancy is a state of relative immune-compromise. This belief was based on the notion that immune compromise was necessary to prevent rejection of the "non-self" fetus. These theories were essentially applying the physiology of solid organ transplant and allograft rejection to the science of the maternal-fetal interface.

It is now widely accepted that pregnancy is not in fact a state of immune-compromise. Pregnant women do not have an increased risk of contracting most opportunistic infections. If women were truly immune compromised, the survival of the species would be at significant risk. While it is true that pregnant women are more susceptible to certain infectious agents, such as the intracellular pathogen *Listeria monocytogenes*, it is now known that pregnancy is a complex state of modified immunity, with immune cells playing crucial roles in the implantation process, vasculogenesis, parturition, and fetal tolerance.

It is beyond the scope of this chapter to do an in-depth review of the microscopic role immune cells play in the process of implantation and vasculogenesis. However, in brief, the immune environment within the uterus is a unique microsystem within the body where immune cells take on a range of tasks not known to be performed elsewhere. Immune changes within the uterine microenvironment can be broken down into three phases: an early inflammatory phase, a middle anti-inflammatory phase, and a terminal inflammatory phase.[1]

The early first trimester is a pro-inflammatory phase. There is deliberate damage to the endometrial tissue in order for the embryo to implant. Uterine Natural Killer cells (CD-56 positive; unique to uterine myometrium) infiltrate the endometrium and are necessary for vascular smooth muscle recruitment to provide the implanting embryo with a blood supply.[2,3] Macrophages and dendritic cells also infiltrate the implantation site. The specific action of these monocytes is unknown, however, lack of dendritic cells results in failure implantation (decidualization).[4]

The second immunologic phase encompasses the period of fetal growth and development. This period is a relatively quiescent immunologic period and is believed to be dominated by an anti-inflammatory milieu of cytokines.[5]

The third immunologic phase occurs when fetal development is complete and is characterized by a pro-inflammatory state once again. There is an influx of a large range of varying immune cells into the myometrium. The exact role of this inflammatory assault in parturition onset and timing is an area of active investigation.[6–8]

These immunologic phases are within the uterine micro-environment and do not represent a total body inflammatory or anti-inflammatory state. However, at the systemic level the immune system does experience some alteration in absolute cellular numbers, cellular functions, and cytokine production secondary to the systemic hormonal milieu of the pregnant state.

Nearly all major immune cell types have evidence of possessing a nuclear estrogen receptor (either protein or mRNA evidence). B cells, CD8+ T cell, CD4+ T cells, NK cells, plasma dendritic cells, CNS dendritic cells, macrophages, and hematopoietic stem cells have all demonstrated varying degrees of mRNA or protein expression.[9] Similarly, progesterone receptor mRNA has been found in T-cells, macrophages, dendritic cells, and NK cells.[10,11] Only T cells and macrophages have definitively been found to have membrane-specific progesterone receptors present.[11] The specific function of these estrogen and progesterone receptors in the varying cell types also remain areas of active research.

Innate Immunity

Innate immunity, also known as "natural" immunity, is the primitive immune system that has been conserved across vast mammalian species. The basis of innate immunity is pathogen sequestration and destruction. This is carried out largely via macrophages and granulocytes (neutrophils, eosinophils, natural killer cells, and dendritic cells) (Table 4.1). Through the use of conserved pattern recognition receptors, these cells are able to detect non-self-pathogenic proteins and destroy the pathogens carrying them.

Adaptive Immunity

This is a new evolutionary system, which allows for a learned response to pathogenic entities. The adaptive system works in concert with the innate system during an acute infection to amplify the host response. Simply stated, the adaptive system then retains information regarding the specific infection to quickly control a future exposure. The primary cells involved in adaptive immunity are lymphocytes, including B lymphocytes, CD8+ Cytotoxic T lymphocytes (TCc), CD4+ T helper lymphocytes (THc), Regulatory T cells (Tregs), and Natural Killer T Cells (NKTs) (Table 4.1). During an acute infection the innate system cells present foreign pathogenic proteins to B

TABLE 4.1 ALTERATIONS IN IMMUNE SYSTEM COMPONENTS DURING PREGNANCY

	Increased	Decreased	Neutral
Innate Immune System	# Macrophages		
	# Dendritic Cells IL-12 production IL-4 production Plasma TNF-α Endotoxin Receptor Phagocytosis ability		
	# Granulocytes Phagocytosis ability Alkaline Phosphatase	# NK Cells Cytotoxicity Interferon-γ	
	Complement c1q, c3a, c4a, c4d, c5a		
Adaptive Immune System	# T-Helper-2 Cells IL-2 IL-4 IL-10	# T-Helper-1 Cells IL-5 IL-13 Interferon-γ	#Total T-Helper Cells
	# T-Regulatory Cells	# Type 1 Cytotoxic T-cells	#Type 2 Cytotoxic T-cells
		Pre-B Cell precursors	Mature B Cells

cells, which go on to produce specific antibodies against the presented protein. TCc's and THc's are also presented with information from the innate system leading to enhanced activation of cell lysis mechanisms.

The complement system

It is a non-cellular plasma protein system made up of over 20 proteins that can be activated by either the innate or adaptive immune systems. When activated these proteins lead to enhanced lysis of bacterial pathogens.

Beginning in the first trimester and persisting throughout gestation, there is an increase in the absolute numbers of monocytes (granulocytes, macrophages, and dendritic cells), while there is a decrease in systemic NK cells.[12] The monocytes are in a primed state, with an increased ability to phagocytose potential pathogens and thus protect the mother from infection. The signal to enter this primed state during pregnancy is not yet known. There is also an increase in the total number of complement cascade system proteins. This includes the anaphylatoxins C3a, C4a, C5a, which are normally increased during activation of the system.[13,14]

Absolute numbers of lymphocytes (B cells and T cells) largely remain neutral throughout gestation (though there are multiple conflicting studies).[12,15–20] There is, however, a reduction in pre-B cell precursors and a well-established shift in the relative ratios of specific T-cell types. Lymphocytes have both estrogen and progesterone receptors. Lymphocytes are 100x more sensitive to progesterone binding during pregnancy relative to their non-pregnant state.[21]

T-CELLS

CD4+ T-helper cells differentiate into two subsets of cells, T-Helper 1 (Th1) and T-Helper 2 (Th2), based on the types of cytokines produced. Th1 cells secrete interferon-gamma, Interleukin-2 (IL-2), and TNF-alpha, which increase monocyte activation and the cell-mediated immune response. Th2 cells produce IL-4, IL-5, IL-10 and IL-13, and are important enhancers of antibody production, eosinophil activation and dampen the activation of monocytes.[22,23] During pregnancy there is a shift in the relative ratio of Th1 to Th2 T cell subtypes, with an increase in the Th2 subtype, specifically during the second immunologic phase of pregnancy. The signal to shift toward a Th2 predominance is at least partially triggered by progesterone binding to the undifferentiated T-helper cell.[10,11,23]

The high circulating levels of estrogen and progesterone during pregnancy cause an inhibition in T-cell development in the thymus.[24–26] It is believed that this high level of estrogen contributes to the observation of thymus involution during pregnancy.[25] In murine progesterone receptor knock-out models, when a progesterone receptor null thymus is transplanted into a wild-type mouse the wild-type animal experiences sub-fertility.[26] This suggests a critical role for thymic progesterone receptor activity in controlling T-cell development and subsequent T-cell activity within the uterine implantation micro-environment. T Regulatory cells are highly sensitive to circulating progesterone.[27] It is this subset of T cells that are responsible for producing the anti-inflammatory cytokines TGFB1 and IL-10 that are suspected of maintaining the quiescent second immunologic phase of pregnancy.

B-CELLS

It is notable that progesterone receptors have not been demonstrated in B-cells. However, through indirect mechanisms, progesterone causes an increase in antibody responsiveness, decreased antibody class switching, and decreased T-cell antibody responses.[27]

Estradiol and prolactin are both known to alter B-cell development. B-cells have both alpha and beta-estrogen receptors on their surfaces.[28–30] Activation of these estrogen receptors in the non-pregnant state leads to altered B-cell gene expression, specifically altering genes related to B-cell survival, activation and chain switching.[28–31] It is not known how (if at all) this signaling is altered during the high levels of estrogen experienced during pregnancy.

It is theorized that the estrogen-induced increase in B-cells survival through the complex antibody receptor selection process in the bone marrow is a major contributor to the higher incidence of auto-immune disorders seen in young females compared to males.[32,33] How pregnancy may or may not alter this susceptibility is an area of ongoing research.

Prolactin has a positive effect on B-cell development.[32] The dramatic rise in prolactin postpartum (10–20x normal non-pregnant levels), and its enhancing effect on B-cell release from the bone marrow and subsequent increase in antibody production, has been suggested as an underlying cause of postpartum symptom flairs in women with auto-immune disorders such as lupus, rheumatoid arthritis, and multiple sclerosis.

The Nervous System

The placenta and the fetus function as highly active neuroendocrine organs, secreting many of the hormones normally produced by (or under the influence of) the brain for maintenance and development during the pregnancy. The placenta has been demonstrated to secrete an analogue of every hypothalamic and pituitary hormone. In fact, over the course of gestation, the human placenta is known to produce at least 50 different peptides and hormones, many of which are normally produced by the hypothalamus, pituitary, or their downstream endocrine organs: the adrenal glands and ovaries.[34] Because of the organ's intimate interface with maternal circulation, these hormones readily enter the maternal bloodstream with the ability to act on their respective receptors.

Though there is limited data on how the nervous system adapts to the complex hormonal milieu of pregnancy, much research has been dedicated to the impact individual gestational hormones have on the brain, spinal cord, and peripheral nerves. A review of every identified pregnancy hormone, and the current understanding of its specific impact on the nervous system is beyond the scope of this chapter; however, we will discuss the known physiologic changes that take place in the nervous system during pregnancy and how the major hormones produced throughout gestation impact central and peripheral neurologic activity. We will synthesize the current understanding of the complex relationship between these neuroendocrine substrates and the nervous system in pregnancy and highlight potential areas for future research.

Changes in Uterine Innervation

The gravid uterus undergoes significant alterations in its innervation over the course of gestation.[35] Though this section deals predominantly with the role pregnancy hormones play in the female nervous system, we will first briefly review these structural changes.

In the cervix, the density and branching of afferent nerves increase markedly toward the end of pregnancy.[36] In animal models, this correlates with increased pain signaling from the cervix to the spinal cord, even in the absence of a mechanical stimulus.[37] Interestingly, the uterine fundus undergoes a relative denervation over the course of pregnancy.[36] These changes are likely responsible for the pain profile experienced over the course of pregnancy and labor. Though women may experience contractions of equal strength at different

points in pregnancy, the perceived pain associated with these contractions is often very different. Furthermore, fundal contraction pressures measured postpartum are often significantly higher than those measured intrapartum, though the maternal pain experience does not typically correlate with this.[38]

Pregnancy Hormones: Physiologic Activity

Human chorionic gonadotropin

Human chorionic gonadotropin (HCG) truly is the biochemical sine qua non of pregnancy. The continuation of pregnancy relies solely on its production and secretion by the embryo and placenta. The principle and most well-defined role for HCG is maintenance of the corpus luteum and its production of progesterone. HCG may also serve to support the pregnancy later on, both in downregulating gap junctions and altering calcium channel activity within the uterine myometrium to sustain uterine quiescence.[39,40] Whether HCG partakes in any activity other than its all-important role of maintaining gestation, and whether it specifically has any impact on the human nervous system has not been well studied. There is a paucity of information available to illustrate what effect, if any, this ubiquitous gestational hormone may have on the brain, spinal cord, or peripheral nerves.

Progesterone

Progesterone is normally produced in the postovulatory ovary, predominantly during the second half of the menstrual cycle. The hormone is critical to a normal, healthy pregnancy and is produced in dramatic amounts throughout. Around week 10 of gestation, progesterone production is transferred from the corpus luteum to the placenta; daily secretion levels are 10 to 100 times those of a nonpregnant, menstruating female.[41] Progesterone serves to maintain relaxation of the uterine smooth muscle and to inhibit uterine prostaglandin production. Progesterone may block cell-mediated rejection of pregnancy tissue, decreasing inflammation within the uterus and maintaining myometrial dormancy.[42]

Estrogen

Estrogens are also synthesized during pregnancy in amounts that far exceed those seen in nonpregnant women of the same age. In fact, during a single pregnancy, a woman is estimated to secrete more estrogen than a nulligravid woman could generate in 150 years of regular ovulation.[43] The main estrogen product produced during pregnancy is estriol, which is not made by the non-pregnant female.[41] The main substrate used by the placenta to synthesize this gestational estrogen is dehydroepiandrosterone sulfate (DHEAS), which is made in the fetal adrenal cortex and converted to estrogen in the placenta.

Although the role of progesterone in pregnancy is clear, the exact purpose of these enormous amounts of estrogen is more nebulous. What is appreciated is that estrogen is necessary for the onset of labor; the hormone both increases gap junctions within uterine myometrial cells and uterine prostaglandin production.[41] Pregnancies complicated by estrogen deficiency, such as is seen with cholesterol metabolism disorders (eg, Smith-Lemli-Opitz Syndrome) or enzyme deficiencies (e.g., placental sulfatase deficiency), are usually carried to term.[44] In fact, patients with placental sulfatase deficiency may be diagnosed after carrying a pregnancy far past their due date and failing to respond to labor induction medications.[44]

Prolactin

Estrogen released by the placenta provokes prolactin production and secretion by inhibiting hypothalamic release of dopamine and promoting activity in the prolactin cells of the anterior pituitary.[44] The gravid endometrium is also a major source of prolactin, which is produced and secreted there in response to progesterone stimulation. Prolactin's main function is to stimulate lactation, although animal studies would suggest the hormone also facilitates parental behavior, possibly by mediating stress responses within the hypothalamic-pituitary-adrenal axis.[45]

At full-term, the gravid woman's serum prolactin levels are 10 to 20 times those of a non-pregnant, premenopausal woman.[46,47] This tremendous increase in prolactin production is made possible by a physiologic hypertrophy of the pituitary during pregnancy. Compared to their non-pregnant, menstruating female counterparts, the pregnant woman's pituitary increases in size by approximately 136% and in height by 4–5 mm, differences appreciable on imaging, which should not be mistaken for a pituitary macroadenoma.[47,48] These elevations persist postpartum in the lactating patient, with levels at least twice those of a non-pregnant, premenopausal woman.

Pregnancy Hormones: Effects on Central and Peripheral Nervous Systems

Central nervous system

A great deal of research has been dedicated to progesterone and its activity within the brain. Nuclear progesterone receptors can be found within every cell type in the central nervous system (CNS); many cells express genes for transmembrane receptors as well.[49] Progesterone has an overall protective effect within the brain. It has been shown to improve neuroplasticity by mitigating damage from free radicals, as well as ischemic insult.[50,51] In addition, progesterone facilitates remyelination of the CNS.[49] In animal models of traumatic brain injury, progesterone has been demonstrated to attenuate the inflammatory response to such damage.[52] Progesterone also mitigates cerebral edema in the animals, at least partially by preventing breakdown of the blood-brain barrier.[49] Interestingly, these neuroprotective effects of progesterone have not been seen with administration of synthetic progestins, such as those found in oral contraceptive pills.[49] Because of this observed protection offered by progesterone, much research has gone into evaluating the utility of progesterone therapy after neurologic injury in humans—which while well tolerated has failed to produce clinical benefit.[53]

Just as progesterone serves to decrease activity within the uterus, an overall quieting effect is seen in the brain as well. Progesterone serves to decrease cAMP signaling within cells and prolongs conductance of γ-aminobutyric acid (GABA) signals, both of which result in overall inhibition of neurotransmission and a decrease in seizure activity[49] (see also Chapter 20). Just as there was with traumatic brain injury, there is currently a hope that progesterone may have a role in the treatment of epilepsy; a Phase III clinical trial of the progesterone metabolite, allopregnenolone, for the treatment of refractory status epilepticus is currently underway.[54]

Conversely, estrogen enhances neuronal activity via several mechanisms. In animal models, the hormone has been shown to potentiate glutamate signaling and transiently quell GABA pathways.[55–58] In addition, estrogen causes an increase in dendritic spine density.[58] Unfortunately, this increase in neurotransmission is the culprit behind the lowered seizure threshold seen with estrogen exposure[59] (see also Chapter 20).

Prolactin also has potential to alter neurosignaling. The hormone self-regulates by stimulating dopamine signaling pathways from the hypothalamus. Animal models have shown that administration of intravenous prolactin leads to increased hypothalamic GABA activity as well.[60] The distinction between prolactin activating and inhibiting neurotransmission appears to depend on the biochemical milieu and specific neuron in question.[61]

These alterations in neurotransmission have effects on cognition. The culmination of estrogen effects mentioned above (increased glutamate signaling, inhibited GABA pathways, and increased dendritic spine density) has been associated with sharpened memory and enhanced learning ability.[58] Interestingly, studies assessing progesterone's impact on cognition, learning, and memory have demonstrated a detectable negative impact on subjects' abilities to memorize and recognize faces,[62] presumably due to decrease neuronal communication. The net result of these changes in learning and memory during pregnancy, when estrogen and progesterone are in high levels, but also in a complex biochemical environment, is not well understood; and the impact of pregnancy on cognition is an area of ongoing research.

Besides its effect on seizure activity, progesterone's ability to decrease neuronal activity has other sequelae. Some studies have shown progesterone to have anxiolytic properties, thought to be a result of its effect on GABA signaling.[63] Analgesic properties of progesterone have also been demonstrated, not only as a result of presumably decreased transmission of pain signals but also as a result of activation of endogenous opioid mechanisms within the spinal cord.[49,64] In fact, pain thresholds rise late in pregnancy, which some attribute to increasing serum levels of progesterone.[65]

The pronounced increase in systemic estrogens has many notable sequelae in the CNS. Along with alterations in production and response to coagulation factors, the gestational rise in estrogens creates the well-known hypercoagulable state of pregnancy.[66] This propensity toward thrombosis is proposed to be one of the major rationalizations for the gravid woman's increased risk of ischemic stroke and cerebral venous thrombosis.[66,67] The risk of stroke during pregnancy or the postpartum period is two to three times that of a non-pregnant woman of childbearing age, though this number does include hemorrhagic stroke, which is generally a result of processes other than hypercoagulation.[66,68]

A true example of evolutionary elegance, estrogen brings with it both a higher likelihood of cerebrovascular events but also defense against the damaging consequences of such events. Just like progesterone, estrogen has an overall protective effect on the brain. In fact, estrogen has been shown to decrease ischemic injury and even enhance neuronal recovery after a stroke.[69] Estrogen promotes expression of both anti-apoptotic and pro-survival factors within brain tissue and exert antioxidant effects.[69,70] The hormone is thought to offer protection against neurodegenerative disorders such as Alzheimer's disease and Parkinson's disease.[69]

Perhaps not surprisingly, prolactin may also have neuroprotective properties. Prolactin promotes neurogenesis in the maternal brain during gestation.[71] It has also been shown to attenuate neurologic cell death after a variety of insults.[72] Just like progesterone, studies have demonstrated that prolactin has the ability to support remyelination in damaged neurons.[73] Data is not consistent on this last point, however and the relationship between prolactin and multiple sclerosis is still a convoluted one[74] (see also Chapter 10).

Peripheral nervous system

It will come as no surprise that progesterone functions as a generally inhibitory hormone in the peripheral nervous system, including within the myenteric plexus. Progesterone results in diminished contractility of gastrointestinal smooth muscle and is implicated in the many gastrointestinal complaints associated with pregnancy, such as gastric reflux, nausea, and constipation. Progesterone decreases lower esophageal sphincter tone, especially in an environment where estrogen is also present.[75] In various other studies, progesterone impeded smooth muscle activity within the stomach and colon—effects not seen with estrogen.[76]

As mentioned above, both progesterone and prolactin are known to promote remyelination in the CNS and the same is true peripherally. Progesterone acts on Schwann cells to incite remyelination of damaged nerves, which has important implications for patients with multiple sclerosis (see also Chapter 10) or nerve damage of other origins.[77,78] Progesterone may even be useful for patients suffering from neuropathic pain due to diabetes and chemotherapeutic agents.[79,80]

The relationship between progesterone, estrogen, and nociception is complex.[59] As mentioned before, progesterone seems to possess anti-nociceptive qualities, presumed due to its inhibition of neuronal signaling and activation of the endogenous opioid system in the spinal cord.

Studies looking at estrogen's connection with pain detection and perception have yielded mixed and often contradictory results.[80] In animal models, behavior associated with pain are seen more frequently after prolonged exposure to estradiol.[81] When estrogen is combined with progesterone in levels meant to simulate gestation, however, pain thresholds increase.[82] Perplexingly, though, pain from fibromyalgia has been shown to actually worsen during the luteal phase of menstruation, another period marked by high levels of both estrogen and progesterone.[83] The association is clearly not perfectly understood, but it would seem both estrogen and progesterone modulate the sensation and perception of pain in some capacity.

SUMMARY

Pregnancy is a magnificent physiologic feat. The mother, placenta, and fetus create an unimaginably complex but carefully orchestrated hormonal environment that allows the remarkable accomplishment of supporting foreign life until the precisely correct moment. The symphony of hormones facilitating this circulate throughout the mother's body, altering not only her physiology but also the way she thinks and feels. Though much research has been dedicated to eliciting how and in what way these hormones affect the female immune and nervous systems, there is more knowledge to be acquired. Notably, many studies do not include the synthetic progestins found in contraception. Animal studies do suggest that these also have detectable effects, so further investigation is indicated.[84] Finally, while understanding individual hormones and their sequelae offers important insight, appreciating the intricate interaction between pregnancy hormones and clarifying how their cumulative presence alters the immunologic and neurologic function of the gravid patient is an as-yet unexplored universe.

REFERENCES

1. Mor G. Pregnancy reconceived. *Nat History.* 2007; 116: 36–41.
2. Hanna J, Goldman-Wohl D, Hamani Y, et al. Decidual NK cells regulate key developmental processes at the human fetal-maternal interface. *Nature Med.* 2006; 12(9): 1065–1074.
3. Manaster I, Mandelboim O. REVIEW ARTICLE: The unique properties of uterine NK cells. *American Journal of Reproductive Immunology.* 2010; 63(6): 434–444.
4. Mor G, Cardenas I, Abrahams V, Guller S. Inflammation and pregnancy: The role of the immune system at the implantation site. *Annals of the New York Academy of Sciences.* 2011; 1221(1): 80–87.
5. Mor G, Cardenas I. Review article: The immune system in pregnancy: a unique complexity. *American Journal of Reproductive Immunology.* 2010; 63(6): 425–433.
6. Romero R, Espinoza J, Kusanovic JP, et al. The preterm parturition syndrome. *BJOG: An International Journal of Obstetrics and Gynaecology.* 2006; 113 (Suppl 3): 17–42.
7. Romero R, Espinoza J, Goncalves LF, Kusanovic JP, Friel LA, Nien JK. Inflammation in preterm and term labour and delivery. *Seminars in Fetal & Neonatal Medicine.* 2006;11(5):317–326.
8. Gomez-Lopez N, Romero R, Arenas-Hernandez M, et al. In vivo T-cell activation by a monoclonal alpha CD3 epsilon antibody induces preterm labor and birth. *American Journal of Reproductive Immunology.* November 2016; 76(5): 386–390.
9. Kovats, S. Estrogen receptors regulate innate immune cells and signaling pathways. *Cellular Immunology.* 2015; 294(2): 63–69.
10. Szekeres-Bartho J, Barakonyi A, Par G, Polgar B, Palkovics T, Szereday L. Progesterone as an immunomodulatory molecule. *International Immunopharmacology.* June 2001; 1(6):1037–1048
11. Dressing GE, Goldberg JE, Charles NJ, Schwertfeger KL, Lange CA. Membrane progesterone receptor expression in mammalian tissues: A review of regulation and physiological implications. *Steroids.* 2011; 76(1–2): 11–17.
12. Luppi P. How immune mechanisms are affected by pregnancy. *Vaccine.* 2003; 21(24): 3352–3357.
13. Richani K, Soto E, Romero R, et al. Normal pregnancy is characterized by systemic activation of the complement system. *Journal of Maternal-Fetal & Neonatal Medicine.* 2005; 17(4): 239–245.
14. Sacks G, Sargent I, Redman C. An innate view of human pregnancy. *Immunology Today.* 1999; 20(3): 114–118.
15. Watanabe M, Iwatani Y, Kaneda T, et al. Changes in T, B, and NK lymphocyte subsets during and after normal pregnancy. *Am J Reprod Immunol.* 1997; 37: 368–377.
16. Matthiesen L, Berg G, Ernerudh J, Skogh T. Lymphocyte subsets and autoantibodies in pregnancies complicated by placental disorders. *American Journal of Reproductive Immunology.* 1995; 33(1): 31–39.
17. Fiddes TM, O'Reilly DB, Cetrulo CL, et al. Phenotypic and functional evaluation of suppressor cells in normal pregnancy and in chronic aborters. *Cellular Immunology.* 1986; 97(2): 407–418.
18. Kühnert M, Strohmeier R, Stegmüller M, Halberstadt E. Changes in lymphocyte subsets

during normal pregnancy. *European Journal of Obstetrics & Gynecology and Reproductive Biology.* 1998; 76(2): 147–151.

19. Sabahi F, Rola-Plesczcynski M, O'Connell S, Frenkel LD. Qualitative and quantitative analysis of T lymphocytes during normal human pregnancy. *American Journal of Reproductive Immunology.* 1995; 33(5): 381–393.

20. Luppi P, Haluszczak C, Trucco M, Deloia J. Normal pregnancy is associated with peripheral leukocyte activation. *American Journal of Reproductive Immunology.* 2002; 47(2): 72–81.

21. Romagnani S. Th1/Th2 cells. *Inflammatory Bowel Diseases.* November 1999; 5(4): 285–294.

22. Sykes L, MacIntyre DA, Yap XJ, Ponnampalam S, Teoh TG, Bennett PR. Changes in the Th1 & Th2 cytokine bias in pregnancy and the effects of the anti-inflammatory cyclopentenone prostaglandin 15-deoxy--prostaglandin. *Mediators of Inflammation.* 2012; 2012: 12.

23. Piccinni M-P, Giudizi M-G, Biagiotti R, et al. Progesterone favors the development of human T helper cells producing Th2-type cytokines and promotes both IL-4 production and membrane CD30 expression in established Th1 cell clones. *Journal of Immunology.* 1995; 155(1): 128–133.

24. Miyaura, H. and M. Iwata. Direct and indirect inhibition of Th1 development by progesterone and glucocorticoids. *Journal of Immunology.* 2002; 168(3): 1087–1094.

25. Rijhsinghani AG, Thompson K, Bhatia SK, Waldschmidt TJ. Estrogen blocks early T cell development in the thymus. *American Journal of Reproductive Immunology.* 1996; 36(5): 269–277.

26. Tibbetts TA, DeMayo F, Rich S, Conneely OM, O'Malley BW. Progesterone receptors in the thymus are required for thymic involution during pregnancy and for normal fertility. *Proceedings of the National Academy of Sciences.* 1999; 96(21): 12021–12026.

27. Tan IJ, Peeva E, Zandman-Goddard G. Hormonal modulation of the immune system—A spotlight on the role of progestogens. *Autoimmunity Reviews.* 2015; 14(6): 536–542.

28. Grimaldi CM, Cleary J, Dagtas AS, Moussai D, Diamond B. Estrogen alters thresholds for B cell apoptosis and activation. *Journal of Clinical Investigation.* June 15, 2002; 109(12): 1625–1633

29. Bynoe MS, Grimaldi CM, Diamond B. Estrogen up-regulates Bcl-2 and blocks tolerance induction of naïve B cells. *Proceedings of the National Academy of Sciences.* March 14, 2000; 97(6): 2703–2708

30. Hill L, Jeganathan V, Chinnasamy P, Grimaldi C, Diamond B. Differential roles of estrogen receptors α and β in control of B-cell maturation and selection. *Molecular Medicine.* 2011;17(3–4):211–220.

31. Jones BG, Penkert RR, Xu B, et al. Binding of estrogen receptors to switch sites and regulatory elements in the immunoglobulin heavy chain locus of activated B cells suggests a direct influence of estrogen on antibody expression. *Molecular Immunology.* 2016; 77: 97–102.

32. Cohen-Solal JFG, Jeganathan V, Hill L, et al. Hormonal regulation of B-cell function and systemic lupus erythematosus. *Lupus.* June 1, 2008; 17(6): 528–532.

33. Ngo ST, Steyn FJ, McCombe PA. Gender differences in autoimmune disease. *Frontiers in Neuroendocrinology.* 2014; 35(3): 347–369

34. Mesiano S. The endocrinology of human pregnancy and fetoplacental neuroendocrine development. In: Strauss JF, Barbieri RL, eds. *Yen and Jaffe's Reproductive Endocrinology.* 6th ed. Philadelphia: W.B. Saunders; 2009: 249–281

35. Tingaker BK, Irestedt L. Changes in uterine innervation in pregnancy and during labour. *Curr Opin Anaesthesiol.* June 2010; 23(3): 300–303.

36. Stjernholm Y, Sennstrom M, Granstrom L, Ekman G, Liang Y, Johansson O. Neurochemical and cellular markers in human cervix of late pregnant, postpartal and non-pregnant women. *Acta Obstet Gynecol Scand.* July 2000; 79(7): 528–537.

37. Liu B, Tong C, Eisenach JC. Pregnancy increases excitability of mechanosensitive afferents innervating the uterine cervix. *Anesthesiology.* June 2008; 108(6): 1087–1092.

38. Cibils LA, Hendricks CH. Uterine contractility on the first day of the puerperium. *Am J Obstet Gynecol.* January 15, 1969; 103(2): 238–243.

39. Ambrus G, Rao CV. Novel regulation of pregnant human myometrial smooth muscle cell gap junctions by human chorionic gonadotropin. *Endocrinology.* December 1994; 135(6): 2772–2779.

40. Doheny HC, Houlihan DD, Ravikumar N, Smith TJ, Morrison JJ. Human chorionic gonadotrophin relaxation of human pregnant myometrium and activation of the BKCa channel. *J Clin Endocrinol Metab.* September 2003; 88(9): 4310–4315.

41. Liu JH. Endocrinology of pregnancy. In: *Creasy and Resnik's Maternal-Fetal Medicine: Principles and Practice.* 7th ed. Ed: Robert Resnik, Robert Creasy, Jay Iams, Charles Lockwood, Thomas Moore, Michael Greene. Philadelphia: Elsevier/Saunders; 2014: 100–111.

42. Siiteri PK, Febres F, Clemens LE, Chang RJ, Gondos B, Stites D. Progesterone and maintenance of pregnancy: is progesterone nature's immunosuppressant? *Ann N Y Acad Sci.* March 11, 1977; 286: 384–397.

43. Tulchinsky D, Hobel CJ. Plasma human chorionic gonadotropin, estrone, estradiol, estriol, progesterone, and 17 alpha-hydroxyprogesterone

in human pregnancy. 3. Early normal pregnancy. *Am J Obstet Gynecol.* December 1, 1973; 117(7): 884–893.

44. Fritz MA, Speroff L. *Clinical gynecologic endocrinology and infertility.* 8th ed. Philadelphia: Wolters Kluwer Health/Lippincott Williams & Wilkins; 2011.

45. Gangestad SW, Grebe NM. Hormonal systems, human social bonding, and affiliation. *Horm Behav.* 2017 May; 91: 122–135.

46. Berga S, Nitsche J, Braunstein G. Endocrine changes in pregnancy. *Williams Textbook of Endocrinology.* Eds: Melmed, S, Polonsky, KS, Larsen, PR, Kronenberg, HM. 13th ed. Philadelphia: Elsevier Health Sciences; 2015: 832–848.

47. Nader S. Other endocrine disorders of pregnancy. In: *Creasy and Resnik's Maternal-Fetal Medicine: Principles and Practice.* Ed: Robert Resnik, Robert Creasy, Jay Iams, Charles Lockwood, Thomas Moore, Michael Greene. 7th ed. Philadelphia: Elsevier/Saunders; 2009: 1038–1058.

48. Osborn A. *Osborn's brain: Imaging, pathology, and anatomy.* Salt Lake City, UT: Amirsys; 2013.

49. Brinton RD, Thompson RF, Foy MR, et al. Progesterone receptors: Form and function in brain. *Front Neuroendocrinol.* May 2008; 29(2): 313–339.

50. Cervantes M, Gonzalez-Vidal MD, Ruelas R, Escobar A, Morali G. Neuroprotective effects of progesterone on damage elicited by acute global cerebral ischemia in neurons of the caudate nucleus. *Arch Med Res.* January–Feburary 2002; 33(1): 6–14.

51. Roof RL, Hoffman SW, Stein DG. Progesterone protects against lipid peroxidation following traumatic brain injury in rats. *Mol Chem Neuropathol.* May 1997; 31(1): 1–11.

52. Pettus EH, Wright DW, Stein DG, Hoffman SW. Progesterone treatment inhibits the inflammatory agents that accompany traumatic brain injury. *Brain Res.* July 5, 2005; 1049(1): 112–119.

53. Zeng Y, Zhang Y, Ma J, Xu J. Progesterone for acute traumatic brain injury: A systematic review of randomized controlled trials. *PLoS One.* 2015; 10(10): e0140624.

54. A study with SAGE-547 for super-refractory status epilepticus. *ClinicalTrials.gov,* https://clinicaltrials.gov/ct2/show/NCT02477618. Accessed February 15, 2017.

55. Cyr M, Ghribi O, Di Paolo T. Regional and selective effects of oestradiol and progesterone on NMDA and AMPA receptors in the rat brain. *J Neuroendocrinol.* May 2000; 12(5): 445–452.

56. Smith SS, Waterhouse BD, Woodward DJ. Locally applied estrogens potentiate glutamate-evoked excitation of cerebellar Purkinje cells. *Brain Res.* December 20, 1988; 475(2): 272–282.

57. Rudick CN, Woolley CS. Estradiol induces a phasic Fos response in the hippocampal CA1 and CA3 regions of adult female rats. *Hippocampus.* 2000; 10(3): 274–283.

58. Woolley CS, Schwartzkroin PA. Hormonal effects on the brain. *Epilepsia.* 1998; 39(Suppl 8): S2–8.

59. Aloisi AM, Bonifazi M. Sex hormones, central nervous system and pain. *Horm Behav.* June 2006; 50(1): 1–7.

60. Locatelli V, Apud JA, Gudelsky GA, et al. Prolactin in cerebrospinal fluid increases the synthesis and release of hypothalamic gamma-aminobutyric acid. *J Endocrinol.* September 1985; 106(3): 323–328.

61. Patil MJ, Henry MA, Akopian AN. Prolactin receptor in regulation of neuronal excitability and channels. *Channels (Austin).* 2014; 8(3): 193–202.

62. van Wingen G, van Broekhoven F, Verkes RJ, et al. How progesterone impairs memory for biologically salient stimuli in healthy young women. *J Neurosci.* October 17, 2007; 27(42): 11416–11423.

63. Majewska MD, Harrison NL, Schwartz RD, Barker JL, Paul SM. Steroid hormone metabolites are barbiturate-like modulators of the GABA receptor. *Science.* May 23, 1986; 232(4753): 1004–1007.

64. Dawson-Basoa ME, Gintzler AR. Estrogen and progesterone activate spinal kappa-opiate receptor analgesic mechanisms. *Pain.* March 1996; 64(3): 608–615.

65. Gintzler AR, Liu N-H. The maternal spinal cord: Biochemical and physiological correlates of steroid-activated antinociceptive processes. In: Russell JA, Douglas AJ, Windle RJ, Ingram CD, eds. *The Maternal Brain.* 1st ed. London: Elsevier; 2001: 83–97.

66. Grear KE, Bushnell CD. Stroke and pregnancy: Clinical presentation, evaluation, treatment, and epidemiology. *Clin Obstet Gynecol.* June 2013; 56(2): 350–359.

67. James AH, Bushnell CD, Jamison MG, Myers ER. Incidence and risk factors for stroke in pregnancy and the puerperium. *Obstetrics and Gynecology.* September 2005; 106(3): 509–516.

68. Tate J, Bushnell C. Pregnancy and stroke risk in women. *Womens Health (Lond).* May 2011; 7(3): 363–374.

69. Scott E, Zhang QG, Wang R, Vadlamudi R, Brann D. Estrogen neuroprotection and the critical period hypothesis. *Front Neuroendocrinol.* January 2012; 33(1): 85–104.

70. Zhang QG, Wang R, Khan M, Mahesh V, Brann DW. Role of Dickkopf-1, an antagonist of the Wnt/beta-catenin signaling pathway, in

estrogen-induced neuroprotection and attenuation of tau phosphorylation. *J Neurosci.* August 20, 2008; 28(34): 8430–8441.

71. Shingo T, Gregg C, Enwere E, et al. Pregnancy-stimulated neurogenesis in the adult female forebrain mediated by prolactin. *Science.* January 3, 2003; 299(5603): 117–120.

72. Costanza M, Pedotti R. Prolactin: Friend or foe in central nervous system autoimmune inflammation? *Int J Mol Sci.* December 2, 2016; 17(12).

73. Gregg C, Shikar V, Larsen P, et al. White matter plasticity and enhanced remyelination in the maternal CNS. *J Neurosci.* February 21, 2007; 27(8): 1812–1823.

74. Zhornitsky S, Yong VW, Weiss S, Metz LM. Prolactin in multiple sclerosis. *Mult Scler.* January 2013; 19(1): 15–23.

75. Fisher RS, Roberts GS, Grabowski CJ, Cohen S. Inhibition of lower esophageal sphincter circular muscle by female sex hormones. *Am J Physiol.* March 1978; 234(3): E243–247.

76. Kumar D. In vitro inhibitory effect of progesterone on extrauterine human smooth muscle. *American Journal of Obstetrics and Gynecology.* 1962; 84: 1300–1304.

77. Baulieu EE, Schumacher M, Koenig H, Jung-Testas I, Akwa Y. Progesterone as a neurosteroid: actions within the nervous system. *Cell Mol Neurobiol.* April 1996; 16(2): 143–154.

78. Schumacher M, Guennoun R, Ghoumari A, et al. Novel perspectives for progesterone in hormone replacement therapy, with special reference to the nervous system. *Endocr Rev.* June 2007; 28(4): 387–439.

79. Coronel MF, Labombarda F, Gonzalez SL. Neuroactive steroids, nociception and neuropathic pain: A flashback to go forward. *Steroids.* Jun 2016; 110: 77–87.

80. Patte-Mensah C, Meyer L, Taleb O, Mensah-Nyagan AG. Potential role of allopregnanolone for a safe and effective therapy of neuropathic pain. *Prog Neurobiol.* Feb 2014; 113: 70–78.

81. Aloisi AM, Ceccarelli I. Role of gonadal hormones in formalin-induced pain responses of male rats: modulation by estradiol and naloxone administration. *Neuroscience.* 2000; 95(2): 559–566.

82. Dawson-Basoa M, Gintzler AR. Gestational and ovarian sex steroid antinociception: synergy between spinal kappa and delta opioid systems. *Brain Res.* May 25, 1998; 794(1): 61–67.

83. Korszun A, Young EA, Engleberg NC, et al. Follicular phase hypothalamic-pituitary-gonadal axis function in women with fibromyalgia and chronic fatigue syndrome. *J Rheumatol.* June 2000; 27(6): 1526–1530.

84. Pluchino N, Cubeddu A, Giannini A, et al. Progestogens and brain: An update. *Maturitas.* April 20, 2009; 62(4): 349–355.

5

Fetal Imaging for the Neurologist

NEIL S. SELIGMAN AND MITCHELL CHESS

INTRODUCTION

Imaging of the fetus and the mother may present some unique challenges for the woman with neuromuscular disorders. Provides must consider the potential complications of both the disease process and the treatment to the fetus and how to detect them. Some Therapeutic agents have teratogenic effects that may require more careful or more frequent screening. In addition, the patient require imaging to aid in treatment of her underlying neuromuscular disorder, and this imaging needs to take into account the safety of the developing baby. Finally, the birth process may be compromised in certain disease entities presenting some unique issues. In this chapter, we outline current best practice to best serve both mother and child to optimize care. A general protocol for imaging will be discussed. This chapter is not meant as an exhaustive outline of care for each individual entity.

ROLE OF FETAL ULTRASOUND

Modern diagnostic ultrasound, which was introduced in the 1970s, was originally used as a technique for locating submarines in World War II. In only a little more than 4 decades, real-time ultrasound has become a standard part of pregnancy, playing a critical role in nearly every area of obstetrics (Table 5.1).[1]

Nearly every pregnant woman in the United States has at least one ultrasound, including those women who have had little or no prenatal care.[1] Estimates of the annual cost of prenatal ultrasound exceeds $1 billion based on an average of 1.5 ultrasounds per pregnancy; however, insurance claims data indicates that the average woman receives 4 to 5 ultrasounds per pregnancy.[1,2] There is substantial clinical variation in the indications for, and number of, ultrasounds per pregnancy. National guidelines are lacking in this area.[3] According to the American College of Obstetricians and Gynecologists (ACOG), the benefits of ultrasound include: accurate determination of gestational age, fetal number, viability, and placental location, detection of fetal anomalies, growth disturbances, and abnormalities in amniotic fluid volume.[4]

ULTRASOUND SAFETY

There are no documented adverse fetal effects for diagnostic sonography. However, while ultrasound is generally believed to be safe for the fetus, potential and theoretical risks include erroneous diagnosis and thermal or mechanical damage (due to vibration). The harmful effects of heat in pregnancy on the fetus (particularly in the first trimester) are well documented. During ultrasound, an increase in temperature for the fetus may be as high as 2°C (35.6°F) which is within FDA allowable parameters for sonography examination performance and it is unlikely that this degree of temperature elevation will occur at any single fetal anatomic site.[5] The risk of temperature elevation is higher with color Doppler and spectral Doppler applications. Chick embryos exposed to up to 5 minutes of pulsed-wave Doppler showed significant impairment in memory and learning when assessed post-hatch; however, adverse effects in humans have not been demonstrated.[6] When used appropriately for valid obstetric indications, Doppler does not produce changes that would potentially harm the fetus but should be avoided/limited in the first trimester when possible.[7] Mechanical damage is less of a concern; cavitational bubbles that can cause damage require air or gas that is not present in the fetal tissues.[8] In any case, practicing according to the ALARA (As Low As Reasonably Achievable) principle should be considered in all imaging exams.[9] This principle states that unindicated procedures (in this case, unneeded obstetric ultrasound) should be avoided, even when not proven harmful, until safety is clearly established. The energy delivered

TABLE 5.1 COMMON INDICATIONS AND USAGES OF ULTRASOUND IN PREGNANCY

Possible Indication	Example	Typical Gestational Age
Pregnancy location	Ectopic pregnancy	4–10 weeks
Viability	Miscarriage	5–42 weeks
Dating	Due date	5–42 weeks
Aneuploidy Screening	Nuchal translucency	11–13 weeks
	intracardiac echogenic focus	18–22 weeks
Anatomy and Gender	Anencephaly	11–13 weeks (40% of lethal anomalies detectable)
	Clubbed foot	18–20 weeks typical
Echocardiogram	Ventricular septal defect	22 weeks
Cervical length	Preterm labor	16–34 weeks
Growth	Macrosomia	5–42 weeks
Amniotic fluid	Polyhydramnios	16–27 weeks (single deepest pocket), 28–42 weeks (fluid volume)
Fetal number	Monochromic twins	5–12 weeks ideal
Fetal position	Vertex, breech	36+ weeks
Evaluation of the placenta	Previa, placenta accreta	16–42 weeks
Fetal well-being	Biophysical profile	28+ weeks
Doppler	Umbilical artery	18–42 weeks
Guidance for invasive procedures	Karyotype	11–13 weeks (chorionic villus sampling), 15 weeks (amniocentesis)
Maternal structures	Myomas, ovarian masses	Any
	Cervical length	16–24 weeks (screening), 24–34 weeks (preterm labor)

to the fetus cannot be assumed to be completely innocuous since it is "possible" that adverse effects may be identified in the future.[9,10] This applies mainly to "vanity" ultrasounds performed to capture a 3-dimensional picture of the face or to create a keepsake video but also applies to first trimester ultrasound during which time additional precautions should be taken to limit energy exposure by avoiding the use of pulsed-wave and color Doppler.[8] Overall, ultrasound is believed to be safe for the fetus but should only be used when medical information about the pregnancy is needed (ie, when a valid medical indication exists).

ULTRASOUND IN UNCOMPLICATED PREGNANCIES

While prenatal ultrasounds are not *required*, it would be the exception, rather than the rule, for a woman to complete a pregnancy without ever having had an ultrasound. Prenatal ultrasound is so ubiquitous in obstetric practice that a patient presenting to labor and delivery with no record of an ultrasound should prompt careful review for factors that may put the mother or fetus at risk (no prenatal care, substance abuse). A typical ultrasound schedule is shown in Figure 5.1.

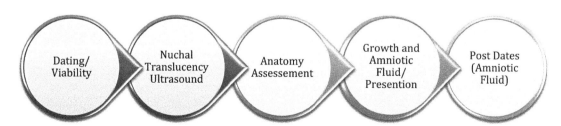

FIGURE 5.1 Typical schedule of prenatal ultrasound by indication. Order (left to right) represents the common chronology of prenatal ultrasounds.

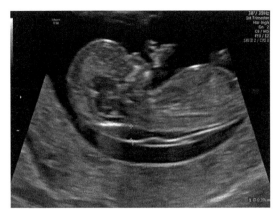

FIGURE 5.2 Sonographic measurement of the nuchal translucency (NT) thickness. Normal is typically <3mm. A thickened NT is associated with an increased risk of aneuploidy, other genetic syndromes, and congenital anomalies (most commonly congenital heart disease) (ISUOG 2013).

Gestational age is most accurately determined by first trimester measurement of the crown-rump length (midsagittal length of the whole fetus).[10,11] Accurate dating may facilitate optimal timing of intervention and reduce the need for postterm induction (medically induced delivery after 42 weeks).[12] Although important, first trimester ultrasound for dating or viability is not recommended unless the last menstrual period is unknown or unreliabe (eg, recently stopped contraception). Likewise, ultrasound for viability is only recommended when there is an indication (bleeding, history of multiple miscarriages).[13] Transvaginal probes are frequently used during early pregnancy. These probes operate at a higher frequency than abdominal probes permitting higher resolution albeit with lower penetrance.

Chromosomal abnormalities, of which sex chromosome aneuploidies (ie, Turner syndrome) and autosomal trisomies (ie, Down's syndrome) are the most common causes of concern, occur in approximately 1 in 150 live births.[14] According to ACOG, "all women should be offered the option of aneuploidy screening or ultrasound-guided diagnostic testing (amniocentesis or chorionic villus sampling) for genetic disorders". Although technologies which isolate fragments of fetal DNA circulating in maternal serum are quickly replacing analyte-based screening tests, the first trimester screen (FTS) remains a popular option (typically due to insurance coverage) especially among average risk women (those without additional risk factors: age

>35 years old, other abnormal screening, abnormal ultrasound, family history of congenital anomalies). The FTS combines maternal serology (beta hCG and pregnancy-associated plasma protein A) with measurement of the nuchal translucency (NT) between 11–14 weeks (Figure 5.2). The FTS detects 82–87% of fetuses with Down's syndrome with a 5% screen positive rate and also detects fetuses at increased risk of trisomy 18. In women who decline aneuploidy screening, an ultrasound solely for the purpose of measurement of the NT, is not recommended.[15]

DATA ABOUT DIAGNOSIS OF CONGENITAL ANOMALIES

In the United States, the rate of congenital anomalies was 3.5% in 2009 or approximately 1 in 28 births.[16] Ultrasound significantly increases the detection of congenital anomalies compared to no screening ultrasound (RR 3.46).[17] Overall sensitivity for the diagnosis of congenital anomalies is approximately 40% (15%–80%) and varies considerably with experience (eg, tertiary care center), organ system (eg, heart), severity of the anomaly (eg, major vs. minor), gestational age, and maternal factors (eg, gestational age; Table 5.2). Detection of major anomalies is proportional to maternal habitus. In a study by Dashe et al, for normal BMI, overweight, and class I, II, and III obesity, standard ultrasound was able to detect 66%, 49%, 48%, 42%, and 25% of major anomalies.[18]

On the other hand, while screening ultrasound increases the detection of congenital anomalies, whether this translates into improved outcomes is less clear; decreases in perinatal mortality are not universally reported and may be attributable to elective termination of pregnancy. Likewise, the cost effectiveness of screening ultrasound is unclear, although it has become standard of care for most pregnancies.[19]

TABLE 5.2 FACTORS THAT CAN INFLUENCE SENSITIVITY OF PRENATAL ULTRASOUND

Maternal	Fetal	System
Obesity	Gestational Age	Sonographer
Pain/	Fetal Position	Experience
Discomfort	Fetal Movement	Interpreting
	Hydramnios (Oligo-	Provider
	or Poly-)	Experience
		Equipment

Despite recent advances in ultrasound technology, ultrasound cannot diagnose all structural anomalies or genetic conditions; however, strict adherence to ACOG and American Institute of Ultrasound in Medicine (AIUM) recommendations will maximize the possibility of detecting abnormalities. While the gestational age at which an anomaly can be visualized varies by the defect, the optimal gestational age at which to evaluate the anatomy is between 18–22 weeks. However about 40% of lethal anomalies can be detected as early as the first trimester.[20] Additionally, some abnormalities, such as microcephaly, may only become evident in the third trimester. Three-dimensional (3D) and 4-dimensional (4D) ultrasound are being used almost routinely during the screening anatomy ultrasound but frequently for keepsake pictures. Three-dimensional ultrasound has 3 main purposes: (1) reconstruction of a difficult to visualize (or unconventional) orthogonal two-dimensional (2D) plane, (2) surface rendering, and/or (3) calculating volume. Four-dimensional ultrasound (3D ultrasound in real-time) allows, among other things, evaluation of fetal activity. Despite the technological advance, it is unclear whether the use of 3D and 4D imaging provides an advantage over traditional 2D imaging in prenatal diagnosis. Three-dimensional ultrasound has the potential to increase the speed of image acquisition by reducing operator dependence since reconstruction can be performed post-hoc after the fact. Demonstrating an anomaly in multiple planes increases the confidence in the diagnosis.[21] In a screening anatomy ultrasound, 3D ultrasound may be superior to 2D ultrasound for obtaining images of some parts of the anatomy (eg, heart, spine, brain) but is most useful for screening as an adjunct when 2D scanning is incomplete.[22] In a study by Lacroix et al, 3D ultrasound was helpful in >85% of cases where information was missed with 2D ultrasound.[22]

If no other ultrasounds are being performed, then the single best time for an ultrasound in between 18–20 weeks.[10] Most ultrasounds performed after this are to complete the screening anatomy ultrasound (if some anatomy was poorly seen on a previous ultrasound), check presentation (vertex, breech), or to assess growth and amniotic fluid. After 40 weeks, standard practice is to assess amniotic fluid volume (measured as the amniotic fluid index) in women who are being expectantly managed.

THE ROLE OF FETAL MRI

Fetal MRI is becoming more common in clinical practice. In most circumstances ultrasound will give the needed information; however, indications are expanding as techniques improve to allow better definition of structures that may not be well visualized sonographically. MRI may be used in evaluation of abnormalities visualized by ultrasound that need further definition, especially if this will result in formulating advice to the family concerning either delivery or therapy. Specific structures in the brain may not have impedance differences to adequately view with ultrasound but may be clearly visualized on MRI.[23,24] Breathing motion and fetal movement may be evaluated with cine MRI, but ultrasound is quicker, cheaper, and more readily available. MRI may also be helpful in postnatal planning. Recent FDA guidelines and multiple articles suggest harmful effects of prolonged sedation in children under 3.[25] Prenatally, the fetus does not require sedation and is in an "incubator." Concerns for warmth and respiration are eliminated.

In cases of maternal obesity, oligohydramnios, or advanced gestational age, MRI may be especially useful as these scenarios lead to limitations in sonography.[26,27] Oligohydramnios and more advanced gestational ages (>25 weeks) are ideal for MRI as the decreased ability for fetal movement helps in the acquisition of clear images. Maternal obesity may present an issue with fetal MRI if the overall weight exceeds table limitations. Claustophobia may be an issue in some cases as well.

During organogenesis in the first trimester MRI is not recommended, although there are no specific FDA guidlelines. Additionally, prior to 16 weeks gestation the small size of the fetus, large amounts of fetal movement, and associated organ developmental changes limit MRI benefits. The American College of Radiology (ACR) suggests imaging after 18 weeks because the effects of higher magnetic field strength and potentially prolonged imaging times are unknown. There is no evidence that MRI without contrast is detrimental to the fetus (see also Chapter 7).[28]

COMPLICATIONS OF NEUROLOGIC DISEASE: MATERNAL IMAGING

In general, ultrasonography and MRI are not associated with maternal or fetal risks and are the imaging techniques of choice for the pregnant patient. Nevertheless, imaging should be used only when needed. Non-obstetrical ultrasound is useful in evaluation of neuromuscular entities such as carpal tunnel and other nerve compression disorders but plays a limited role in evaluation of most other neuromuscular disease entities and is used primarily for fetal evaluation. Rather,

MRI will be the primary imaging modality for the mother with a neuromuscular disorder.

MRI is not operator dependent and does not use ionizing radiation. There are no precautions or contraindications specific to pregnancy and no evidence of harm to the fetus. Tissue heating is proportional to the tissue's proximity to the scanner and, therefore, is negligible near the uterus.[29] In addition there are no documented cases of acoustic injury to the fetus during prenatal MRI.[30] The American College of Radiology concludes that MRI is safe during pregnancy (see also Chapter 7).[31]

MRI evaluation may be performed to evaluate status or progression of neuromuscular and neurology disorders, with careful consideration as to the need for contrast. In most cases MRI may be diagnostic without the use of contrast. However, gadolinium may be useful in imaging of the nervous system.[32] Although gadolinium-based contrast can help define tissue margins and invasion in the setting of placental implantation abnormalities, non-contrast MRI still can provide useful diagnostic information regarding placental implantation and is sufficient in most cases.[29] Even though it can increase the specificity of MRI, the use of contrast during pregnancy is controversial. Gadolinium is water soluble and can cross the placenta to the fetus and amniotic fluid. Gadolinium is teratogenic at high and repeated doses in animal studies.[30,33] In humans, the principal concern arises because duration of fetal exposure is not known. Contrast in the amniotic fluid is swallowed by the fetus, reenters the fetal circulation, and is then excreted into the amniotic fluid. The longer contrast remains in the amniotic fluid, the greater the potential for dissociation of gadolinium from the chelate resulting in exposure to "free" gadolinium, which is toxic, thereby increasing the risk to the fetus.[31] However, there have been no adverse perinatal or neonatal outcome reported. Nonetheless, gadolinium administration should be limited and only utilized if it significantly improves diagnostic capability and will affect clinical decision.[33]

Postpartum, it should also be noted that minimal contrast is excreted in breast milk and then absorbed by the fetus. Breastfeeding should continue without interruption after both gadolinium or CT contrast administration.[34]

While ultrasound and MRI are the safest ways to image the mother, in some cases, other imaging technologies may be necessary. However, these potentially expose the fetus to ionizing radiation. Radiation exposure with X-ray, computed tomography (CT), or nuclear imaging is at a dose much lower than associated with fetal harm. Computed tomography use during pregnancy has increased by 25% per year from 1997 to 2006.[30] Radiation exposure from CT procedures varies and using a low-dose technique that is adequate for diagnosis is optimal. Oral contrast agents are not absorbed by the patient and cause no harm. Intravenous contrast is iodinated and carries a low risk of adverse effects. No teratogenic or mutagenic effects have been from its use.[31] CT contrast should only be used during pregnancy if the additional information will impact the clinical course. However, if CT scan is warranted to evaluate or care for the acute neurologically ill pregnant woman, and awaiting other imaging modalities will result in significant delay in care, then it should be utilized.

EVALUATION OF FETAL WELL-BEING IN MATERNAL NEUROLOGY AND NEUROMUSCULAR DISEASE

For non-inherited and treated neurologic diseases (eg, stroke) fetal imaging and evaluation outside of the standard care is unlikely to be needed. For those diseases that have ongoing medical needs and/or heritability, further evaluation of the fetus during pregnancy may be needed.

With any condition, it always important to consider 2 questions: 1) What are the effects of pregnancy on the disease? and 2) What are the effects of the disease on the pregnancy? Specific disorders come with their own risks of fetal involvement—and this is covered within each disease chapter for those inheritable disorders. Additionally each therapeutic agent used to manage maternal symptoms and disease comes with its own risks. While many have low risks, a few are quite teratogenic and will have imaging implications. A careful understanding of each entity by the neurologist will be important in determining if special screening or genetic testing will be necessary.

In the second and third trimesters, fetal weight is estimated based on measurement of head (circumference and biparietal diameter), abdomen (circumference), and femur (length). The margin of error of an estimated weight is generally regarded as +/− 10% but varies somewhat with gestational age, fetal weight, and many of the other factors listed in Table 5.2. Given this error rate, fetal weight is not as helpful as a single measure but instead for following fetal growth trajectory and potential effects on the fetus from both intrinsic disorders resulting in growth failure (aneuploidy, genetic disorders), extrinsic factors effecting fetal growth (maternal nutrition, medications, viral infections), and factors effecting the placental development and resulting in growth failure.

Amniotic fluid index (AFI) is measured by adding the deepest pocket in each of four quadrants using the umbilicus as a horizontal and vertical reference. As such, an AFI is typically reserved for pregnancies that are 28 weeks gestational or later, but fluid volume can be assessed at any time in the second or third trimester using the single deepest pocket (normal 2–8cm). Any neurologic disease that is heritable and potentially manifest in the fetus may result in impaired fetal swallowing and therefore polyhydramnios.

Fetal tests of wellbeing include nonstress testing (NST) and biophysical profile (BPP). In the United States, the risk of stillbirth is approximately 6 per 1,000.[35] When the risk of fetal demise is greater than the risk in the general population then additional surveillance is recommended. This can be accomplished with weekly or twice weekly NST, which is an assessment of the pattern of the fetal heart rate. Two "accelerations," 10–15 beat increases in the fetal heart above baseline lasting at least 10–15 seconds reliably predicts the absence of fetal academia. Alternatively, a BPP, which includes assessment of fetal movement, tone, breathing and amniotic fluid volume serves a similar purpose though relying on ultrasound.

MEDICATION EFFECTS ON FETAL GROWTH AND DEVELOPMENT

Fetal complications may result not only from the maternal disease entity itself but also from the treatment, specifically medications. Minimizing medication risks during pregnancy starts with appropriate selection of medications, preferably during the preconception period. Ideally, medications with the least reproductive risk should be used. The most common resource for drug safety information is the FDA letter category (Table 5.3). Unfortunately, the letter category can be misleading since a category C medication used extensively during pregnancy may be a better choice than a category B medication that is new to the market. This system was replaced in June of 2015 with more informative labeling and will apply to drugs approved after this time; drugs approved between 2001 and 2015 will be gradually phased in, while drugs produced before 2001 are exempt. Further discussion of medications utilized and risks and benefits can be found in individual disease chapters, as well as in Chapter 21 (antiepileptic therapies).

Additional resources that are commonly used by perinatologists to assess medication risk are shown in Table 5.4. MotherToBaby not only provides downloadable medication fact sheets but also has e-mail, phone, and online chat access to teratology experts. All women should be encouraged to participate in medication registries when one is available for medications with limited pregnancy experience.

When there are no "safe" but equally effective options, potentially teratogenic medications can be used, but caution should be taken to ensure that an effective contraceptive plan is in place and that the woman is properly counseled about the risks (see also Chapter 3). Preconception consultation can help with discussion of medication risks and help with selecting medications with the best safety profile. Unfortunately, many pregnancies are unplanned, and counseling after

---

TABLE 5.3 CURRENTLY USED FDA CATEGORIES

Category A	Adequate and well-controlled studies have failed to demonstrate a risk to the fetus in the first trimester of pregnancy (and there is no evidence of risk in later trimesters).
Category B	Animal reproduction studies have failed to demonstrate a risk to the fetus and there are no adequate and well-controlled studies in pregnant women.
Category C	Animal reproduction studies have shown an adverse effect on the fetus and there are no adequate and well-controlled studies in humans, but potential benefits may warrant use of the drug in pregnant women despite potential risks.
Category D	There is positive evidence of human fetal risk based on adverse reaction data from investigational or marketing experience or studies in humans, but potential benefits may warrant use of the drug in pregnant women despite potential risks.
Category X	Studies in animals or humans have demonstrated fetal abnormalities and/or there is positive evidence of human fetal risk based on adverse reaction data from investigational or marketing experience, and the risks involved in use of the drug in pregnant women clearly outweigh potential benefits.

TABLE 5.4 RESOURCES FOR ASSESSMENT OF MEDICATION RISKS IN PREGNANCY

Tool	Examples
Research databases	PubMed (www.ncbi.nlm.nih.gov/pubmed/) Google Scholar (scholar.google.com)
Teratology databases	Reprotox (www.reprotox.org) Teris (depts.washington.edu/terisdb/)
Online resources	MotherToBaby (www.mothertobaby.org)
Breastfeeding	Lactmed (toxnet.nlm.nih.gov/newtoxnet/lactmed.htm)

medication exposure is somewhat different since the exposure has already occurred. The first step in this scenario is determining the timing of exposure since susceptibility to congenital anomalies varies significantly with gestational age (Figure 5.3).

A few general rules apply:

- Exposure in the first four weeks is unlikely to cause congenital anomalies. Significant effects during this time would result in miscarriage.
- Stopping in a medication in the first trimester (after the first month) rarely reduces fetal risk since the exposure has already occurred.

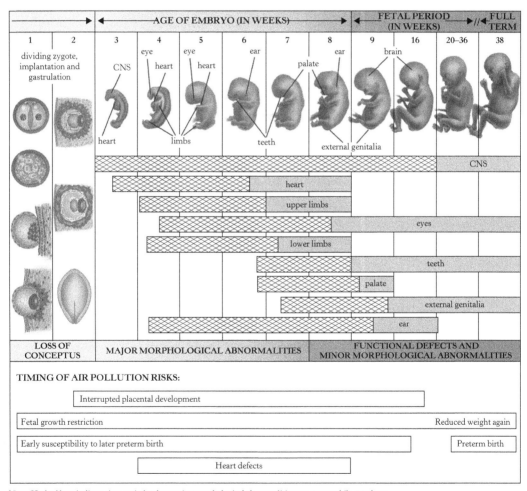

Note: Hashed bars indicate time periods when major morphological abnormalities can occur, while grey bars correspond to periods at risk for minor abnormalities and functional defects.

FIGURE 5.3 Gestational age and risk of congenital anomalies. Most major congenital anomalies occur by the 10th week of gestation (8th week of embryologic development).

Adapted from: https://www.epa.gov/sites/production/files/2014-04/childrens_health_1.gif

Adapter from Ritz B. and Wilhelm, M. 2008, " 'Air pollution impacts on infants and children'. Southern California Environmental Report Card. University of California-Los Angeles, Institute of the Environment and Sustainability. Retrieved April 28, 2015 (http://www.environ-ment.ucla.edu/reportcard/article1700.html)"

TABLE 5.5 COMMON NEUROLOGIC MEDICATIONS AND ASSOCIATED CONGENITAL ANOMALIES (SEE ALSO CHAPTER 23 SECTION ON ANTI-EPILEPTICS)

Medication	FDA Category	Attributed Congenital Anomalies
Acetazolamide	C	Not expected to increase the risk of congenital malformations[c]
Agalsidase alpha	*	No data in humans
Agalsidase beta	B	A limited number of successful pregnancies reported[c]
Alemtuzumab	C	Not expected to increase the risk of congenital malformations
Amitriptyline	C	Not expected to increase the risk of congenital malformations[c]; third trimester use associated with neonatal withdrawal
Antiepileptic Drugs	B-D	Risk varies with the drug from no increased risk of congenital malformations (levetiracetam) to well-characterized patterns of malformations (valproic acid); open neural defects are the most commonly associated congenital anomaly[c]
Aspirin (low-dose, 81mg)	*	Not expected to increase the risk of congenital malformations
Azathioprine	D	Possible association with septal defects
		Other possible associations include preterm birth, intrauterine growth restriction, and neonatal hematologic and immune impairment
Cyclosporine	C	Not expected to increase the risk of congenital malformations[c]
Everolimus	C	A limited number of successful pregnancies reported[c]
Daclizumab	*	Not increased the risk of congenital malformations in studies in which exposures was defined as pregnancy within 6 months of the last dose[c]
Flecainide	C	A limited number of successful pregnancies reported
		More commonly used for fetal arrhythmias but typically later than would be expected to cause congenital anomalies
Furosemide	C	Not expected to increase the risk of congenital malformations
Gabapentin	C	Not expected to increase the risk of congenital malformations[c]
Glatiramer	B	Not expected to increase the risk of congenital malformations
Glycopyrrolate	B	Not expected to increase the risk of congenital malformations[a]
Hyoscyamine	C	Data based on experience with atropine (isomer)
		Not expected to increase the risk of congenital malformations
Imatinib	*	Both normal and abnormal pregnancies have been reported with anomalies in 9.6–21.4% including bony defects, hypospadias, exomphalos, and gastrointestinal and heart anomalies
Immune globulin	C	Not expected to increase the risk of congenital malformations[b]
Methazolamide	C	Causes skeletal abnormalities in rats; no human data
Mexilitine	C	Not expected to increase the risk of congenital malformations[b]
		May cause fetal bradycardia
Modafinil	C	Not expected to increase the risk of congenital malformations[b]
Mycophenolate mofetil	D	Myocophenolate embryopathy (ear, eye, and lip/palate abnormalities); additional anomalies: distal limb, heart, esophagus, kidney, and nervous system
Ocrelizumab	*	Causes harm in animals; no human data
Natalizumab	C	Not expected to increase the risk of congenital malformations (limited transfer across the placenta in the first trimester)
		Possible hematologic effects in the neonate
NSAIDs (Ibuprofen, Naproxen)	*	third trimester use may cause ductal constriction, persistent pulmonary hypertension, oligohydramnios, necrotizing enterocolitis, renal dysfunction/failure, intracranial hemorrhage
Nusinersen	*	Not expected to increase the risk of congenital malformations[a]
Pazopanib	*	Not expected to increase the risk of congenital malformations[a]

TABLE 5.5 CONTINUED

Medication	FDA Category	Attributed Congenital Anomalies
Prednisone	C/D	Possible small increase in oral clefts[c]
		Also associated with preterm premature rupture of membranes, preterm birth, and low birth weight though possible due to the mother's illness rather than the medication
Pregabalin	*	Causes bony and craniofacial anomalies in rats as well as abnormal behavior in surviving offspring[c]
Propafenone	C	Not expected to increase the risk of congenital malformations[a]
Propantheline	C	Not expected to increase the risk of congenital malformations[b]
Pyridostigmine	B/C	Not expected to increase the risk of congenital malformations
Selumtinib	*	Reproductive risk unknown
Sirolimus	C	Not expected to increase the risk of congenital malformations[b,c]
SSRI/SNRI	*	Not expected to increase the risk of congenital malformations with the exception of paroxetine which has been associated with an increase in congenital heart defects
		Second and third trimester use associated with pulmonary hypertension (risk <1%) and neonatal withdrawal
		The risks of untreated depression generally outweigh the risks of these medications
Sunitinib	D	Reproductive risk unknown
Vigabatrin	C	Cardiac defects, limb defects, male genital malformations, fetal anticonvulsant syndrome, renal and ear abnormalities

[a]Data limited to animal studies; [b]Data limited to a small number of cases in humans; [c]A registry to monitor pregnancy outcomes is currently enrolling patients; *Data not available or category not assigned.

- Starting medications in the second trimester, in general, is unlikely to result in major malformations since the organs are largely formed by this time. Rather, medications effects in the second and third trimester include effects on fetal growth, renal function, and brain development.

A list of commonly used medications in the treatment of neuromuscular disorders and associated congenital anomalies are shown in Table 5.5.

ULTRASOUND FINDINGS IN FETUSES WITH NEUROLOGIC AND NEUROMUSCULAR DISORDERS

In familial syndromes, prenatal diagnosis is largely dependent on family history and detection of disease causing gene mutations through preimplantation genetic diagnosis or prenatal diagnosis (chorionic villus sampling or amniocentesis). Compared to cytogenetics, ultrasound findings are generally less valuable, and only a few cases have been diagnosed by prenatal ultrasound (Table 5.6). In some cases,

the maternal and fetal manifestations of disease may show significant variation. Two concepts that can be used to explain this are variable expressivity and anticipation. Variable expressivity refers to phenotypic variation from person to person with the same condition, while anticipation refers to progressive worsening (early onset, more severe manifestations) with each successive generation.

A few neurologic diseases that can strongly affect fetal development deserve special mention and discussion are outlined here.

Myathesenia gravis (MG) antibodies (IgG anti-acetylcholine receptor antibodies) can cross the placenta and result in fetal and neonatal manifestations of the disease. Antenatal findings may include polyhydramnios (due to impaired swallowing), decreased fetal movement, and decreased swallowing.[36] Myasthenia gravis is a rare cause of arthrogryposis multiplex congenita in which lack of movement results in multiple joint contractures and occasionally can also lead to neonatal demise due to pulmonary hypoplasia.

Transient neonatal MG happens in 10–20% of pregnancies (risk is higher with a previously affected sibling).[37] Symptoms (eg, muscle weakness,

TABLE 5.6 COMMON ULTRASOUND FINDINGS IN HERITABLE AND NON-HERITABLE FETAL NEUROLOGIC DISEASES AND CONDITIONS

Condition	Ultrasound Findings	Comments	Reference
Prenatal Findings Likely			
Tuberous Sclerosis Complex	Cardiac rhabdomyoma (CR) Ventriculomegaly (possible obstructive tumors) Astrocytoma Renal tumors	CR may grow (hydrops possible)/ regress or cause dysrhythmia Possible additional fetal MRI findings (subependymal nodules, cortical tumors) Renal tumors may hemorrhage	40,41
Congenital Myotonic Dystrophy Type 1	Talipes equinovarus Polyhydramnios Ventriculomegaly (posterior horns) Myopathic facies ("tent mouth")	Polyhydramnios secondary to impaired swallowing	42
Inborn errors of metabolism	Skeletal abnormalities (stippled epiphyses, hypomineralization, synostosis, lytic lesions, calcifications, limb shortening, limb reduction, brachytelephalangy, syndactyly, polydactyly, micro/macrocephaly) Nasal bone hypoplasia Facial dysmorphism (midface hypoplasia, micrognathia) Hydrops Arthrogryposis Ambiguous genitalia Neural tube defects Renal cysts Hepatomegaly Congenital heart disease (cardiomegaly, left ventricular non-compaction) Central Nervous System (CNS) anomalies (abnormal gyration, holoprosencephaly, hydrocephaly, absence of the corpus callosum, posterior fossa abnormalities)	Skeletal abnormalities may be isolated or not, symmetrical or not Pattern of anomalies may be unique to a specific diagnosis	
Intracranial hemorrhage, hemorrhagic stroke	Irregularly shaped, hyperechoic lesions in ventricles and/or parenchyma	Variable appearance Later findings include porencephalic cysts and intracranial calcifications	
Hemangiomas	Hypoechoic mass with low velocity flow Polyhydramnios	Cutaneous, intracranial, hepatic	
Aneurysm, vascular malformations	Hypoechoic cystic space with high velocity, turbulent flow Cardiomegaly Hydrops	Feeder vessels seen with careful evaluation Cardiac dysfunction and hydrops secondary to high output cardiac failure Can rupture and cause hemorrhage Vein of Galen malformation most common	

TABLE 5.6 CONTINUED

Condition	Ultrasound Findings	Comments	Reference
Prenatal Findings Rare			
Neurofibromatosis 1 (NF 1)	Cardiac and craniofacial anomalies CNS tumors (e.g., neurofibromas, astrocytomas) Other tumors (e.g., congenital epulis)	Generally not useful Anomalies not typical of NF1, diagnosis not considered prenatally in all but 1 case.	43,44
Autoimmune-Myasthenia Gravis	Arthrogryposis Polyhydramnios Fetal Akinesia Deformation Sequence (FADS)	Due to transplacental passage of anti-acetylcholine receptor antibodies FADS includes: akinesia, Intrauterine growth restriction (IUGR), cystic hygroma, pulmonary hypoplasia, cleft palate, cryptorchidism, cardiac defects and intestinal malrotation, limb pterygia	45-47
Sturge-Weber Syndrome	Polymicrogyria and gyriform calcifications	Case report only	48
Congenital Myasthenia Gravis	Reduced movement, akinesia		
Spinal Muscular Atrophy Type 1	Reduced movement	Typically third trimester	49
Hereditary Hemorrhagic Telangiectasia	Cardiomegaly Hepatic arteriovenous malformation		50
Fetal seizures	Rapid, repetitive fine movement of the whole body Rapid myoclonic jerking of fetal extremities Episodic	Maternal perception of abnormal movement Most commonly secondary to fetal CNS anomalies Duration consistent with seizure	51

Not Diagnosed Prenatally

Neurofibromatosis type 2/3, schwannomatosis
Nondystrophic myotonia
Spinal muscular atrophy type 2/3
Von-Hippel Lindau
Ataxia telangiectasia
Fabry disease
Epidermal nevus, linear sebaceous nevus
Fetal ischemic stroke

impaired swallowing) may begin hours after birth, are always present by 3 days and resolve within a few weeks with supportive care and occasionally with neostigmine.[38] A complete discussion of neonatal MG is outside the scope of this chapter, but see also Section 4 of Chapter 24 on neuromuscular disorders.[36–38]

Maternal myotonic dystrophy—DM1—brings a high risk of fetal disease, even when the mother is subclinical.[27] Complications of pregnancy include high perinatal mortality, placental anomalies, polyhydramnios, and preterm delivery.[23] Maternal complications include respiratory and cardiac issues, including infection. Brain involvement may lead to apathy and can hinder involvement with medical care. Both DM1, DM2 are inherited in an autosomal dominant fashion, and there is a tendency to worsen with each generation. However, should a woman with DM2 pass the gene to their child, there can be significant maternal anticipation of the effects leading to congenital myotonic dystrophy (Steinert's disease). This disorder can also occur when inherited from the father but much more rarely. Unlike the typical onset of myotonic dystrophy is in later childhood, or even in adulthood, with this disorder infants will manifest weakness, muscular wasting, and respiratory insufficiency from birth. Typical findings include need for ventilatory support at delivery, "floppy" muscle tone, facial weakness, and poor head control. In utero ultrasound may show polyhydramnios due to poor swallowing, decreased or absent fetal movements, and stiffened, contractures of the limbs with poor movement. Premature labor is common in affected pregnancies as well. With DM2 congenitally affected children have not been reported.[25]

The benign tumors that form in a number of organs in patients with tuberous sclerosis (TSC) are the result of inactivation of the TSC gene, which normally functions as a tumor suppressor. Based on mode of inheritance (autosomal dominant), 50% of fetuses of an affected parent can be expected to have the disease; however, in many there is no family history (two-thirds); these cases represent new mutations. In a review that included 43 fetuses, the most common findings were central nervous system lesions (47.5%), cardiac rhabdomyomas (32.8%), and renal lesions (13.2%).[39] Cardiac rhabdomyomas, depending on their size and location, can cause obstruction or dysrhythmia, which can lead to hydrops and possibly fetal demise.[39]

FETAL COMPLICATIONS OF MATERNAL NEUROMUSCULAR DISORDERS

The effects of neuromuscular disorders on the fetus during pregnancy, though varied, can be divided into 3 categories: (1) growth and development, (2) congenital anomalies secondary to medications, and (3) manifestations of fetal neuromuscular disorders. An in-depth review of the effects of each specific disorder is outside the scope of this review (additionally specific maternal and fetal effects and complications are covered in individual neuromuscular disease—Chapters 24–25), but there is a somewhat limited range of potential complications, which are shown in Table 5.7.

TABLE 5.7 POTENTIAL EFFECTS ON THE FETUS FROM NEUROMUSCULAR DISORDERS

Findings
Abnormal growth
Intrauterine growth restriction (fetal weight <10th percentile)
Macrosomia (fetal weight >90th percentile)
Hydramnios
Oligohydramnios (amniotic fluid volume <5cm or maximum vertical pocket <2cm)
Polyhydramnios (amniotic fluid volume >25cm or maximum vertical pocket >8cm)
Preterm labor
Preterm premature rupture of membranes
Non-reassuring fetal status
Stillbirth
Abnormal brain or renal development
Presentation
Vertex
Transverse
Breech

SUMMARY

In pregnant women with neuromuscular disorders, imaging, either maternal or fetal, requires special consideration. Ultrasound is commonly utilized in the evaluation of pregnancy. It has been shown to be safe, without documented adverse effects on the fetus. First trimester ultrasound is frequently utilized to establish pregnancy location, viability, and dating. Screening for aneuploidy should be offered to all women by ACOG guidelines and frequently involves ultrasound. If a single ultrasound is to be performed, a study between 18 and 20 weeks gestation is suggested since most congenital anomalies can be detected by this time.

MRI may be utilized in the fetal evaluation, typically in the second and third trimesters, in cases where ultrasound is ambiguous or if further definition of an abnormality is warranted. This may be the case when sonographic limitations, including low amniotic fluid volume and maternal obesity are present. There are no detrimental effects to the fetus documented with MRI.

For maternal evaluation MRI is ideal for imaging. The adverse effects from radiation that accompany CT evaluation are not present with MRI. Use of contrast with MRI remains controversial; although teratogenic at high and repeated doses, gadolinium has no reported effect on the fetus when used diagnostically. However, gadolinium should only be used if it would significantly improve the diagnostic capability and such information will affect management. Postpartum gadolinium can be excreted in breast milk but only minimally, and this should not affect breast feeding. Furthermore, if other imaging modalities, including CT or X-ray are better for assessment of the mother's or fetus's condition, these should not be excluded from consideration.

REFERENCES

1. Hobbins JC. Overview of imaging in pregnancy: History to the present, including economic impact. *Seminars in Perinatology.* 2013; 37(5): 290–291.
2. O'Keeffe DF, Abuhamad A. Obstetric ultrasound utilization in the United States: Data from various health plans. *Seminars in Perinatology.* 2013; 37(5): 292–294.
3. Reddy UM., Abuhamad, A, Saade GR. Fetal imaging. *Seminars in Perinatology.* 2013; 37(5).
4. American College of Obstetricians and Gynecologists. ACOG Practice Bulletin No. 101: Ultrasonography in pregnancy. *Obstetrics and Gynecology.* 2009; 113(2): 451.
5. American Institute of Ultrasound in Medicine. Statement on Mammalian Biological Effects of Heat. Laurel, MD: AIUM; 2015.
6. Schneider-Kolsky M E, Lombardo P, et al. Ultrasound exposure of the foetal chick brain: effects on learning and memory. *International Journal of Developmental Neuroscience.* 2009; 27(7): 677–683.
7. Abramowicz JS. Benefits and risks of ultrasound in pregnancy. *Seminars in Perinatology.* 2013; 37(5).
8. American Institute of Ultrasound in Medicine. Statement on the safe use of Doppler ultrasound during 11-14 week scans (or earlier in pregnancy). Laurel (MD): AIUM; 2011
9. AIUM Practice Parameter for the Performance of Obstetrical Ultrasound Examinations. *J Ultrasound Med.* 2013; 32(6):1083–1101
10. American College of Obstetricians and Gynecologists. ACOG Practice Bulletin No. 175: Ultrasonography in pregnancy. *Obstetrics and Gynecology.* 2016; 128(6): e241–256.
11. Salomon LJ, et al. ISUOG practice guidelines: Performance of first-trimester fetal ultrasound scan. *Ultrasound in Obstetrics & Gynecology: The Official Journal of the International Society of Ultrasound in Obstetrics and Gynecology.* 2013; 41(1): 102.
12. American College of Obstetricians and Gynecologists. ACOG Committee Opinion No. 700: Methods for estimating the due date. *Obstetrics and Gynecology.* 2017; 129(5): 967–968.
13. Demianczuk NN, Van den Hof MC. The use of first trimester ultra- sound. SOGC Clinical Practice Guidelines. No. 135. October 2003. *Obstet Gynaecol Can.* 2003; 25(10): 864–869.
14. American College of Obstetricians and Gynecologists. Screening for fetal aneuploidy. ACOG Practice bulletin no. 163. *Obstetrics and Gynecology.* 2016; 27(5): e123–e137.
15. Norton ME, Biggio JR, Kuller JA, et al. The role of ultrasound in women who undergo cell-free DNA screening. *American Journal of Obstetrics and Gynecology.* 2017; 216(3): B2–B7.
16. Hill LM. Timing of ultrasound in pregnancy—How often? At what intervals?. *Seminars in Perinatology.* 2013; 37(5).
17. Whitworth M, Bricker L, Mullan C. Ultrasound for fetal assessment in early pregnancy. *Cochrane Library* (2015).
18. Dashe, JS, McIntire, DD, Twickler, DM. Effect of maternal obesity on the ultrasound detection of anomalous fetuses. *Obstetrics & Gynecology.* 2009; 113(5): 1001–1007.
19. Roberts T, Henderson J, Mugford M, et al. Antenatal ultrasound screening for fetal abnormalities: A systematic review of studies of cost and cost effectiveness. *BJOG.* 2002; 109: 44.
20. Obican S, Brock C, Berkowitz R, Wapner RJ. Multifetal pregnancy reduction. *Clinical Obstetrics and Gynecology.* September 1, 2015; 58(3): 574–584.
21. Merz E, Abramowicz JS. 3D/4D ultrasound in prenatal diagnosis: Is it time for routine use? *Clinical Obstetrics and Gynecology.* 2012; 55(1): 336–351.
22. Roy-Lacroix ME, Moretti F, Ferraro ZM, et al. A comparison of standard two-dimensional ultrasound to three-dimensional volume sonography for routine second-trimester fetal imaging. *Journal of Perinatology.* 2017; 37(4): 380–386.
23. Rudnik-Schöneborn S, Zerres K. Outcome in pregnancies complicated by myotonic dystrophy: A study of 31 patients and review of the literature. *Eur J Obstet Gyn.* 2004; 114: 44–53.

24. Prayer D, Kasprian G, Krampl E, et al. MRI of normal fetal brain development. *Eur J Radiol.* 2006; 57(2): 199–216.

25. Norwood F, Rudnil-Schoneborn S. 179th ENMC international workshop: Pregnancy in women with neuromuscular disorders. *Neuromuscular Disorders.* 2012; 22: 183–190.

26. Prayer D, Brugger PC, Krampl E, et al. Indications for fetal magnetic resonance imaging (MRI). *Radiologe.* 2006; 46(2): 98–104.

27. Redman JB, Fenwick RG, Fu YH, Pizzuti A, Caskey CT. Relationship between parental trinucleotide GCT repeat length and severity of myotonic dystrophy in offspring. *JAMA.* 1993; 269: 1960–1965.

28. Strizek B, Jani JC, Mucyo E, et. al. Safety of MR imaging at 1.5 T in fetuses: A retrospective case-control study of birth weights and the effects of acoustic noise. *Radiology.* 2015; 275(2): 530–537.

29. Leyendecker JR, Gorengaut V, Brown JJ. MR imaging of maternal diseases of the abdomen and pelvis during pregnancy and the immediate postpartum period. *Radiographics.* 2004; 24: 1301–16.

30. Chen MM, Coakley FV, Kaimal A, Laros RK Jr. Guidelines for computed tomography and magnetic resonance imaging use during pregnancy and lactation. *Obstet Gynecol.* 2008; 112: 333–40.

31. Kanal E, Barkovich AJ, Bell C, et al. ACR guidance document on MR safe practices: 2013. Expert panel on MR safety. *J Magn Reson Imaging.* 2013; 37: 501–530.

32. Adam A, Dixon AK, Gillard JH, Schaefer-Prokop CM, eds. *Grainger & Allison's Diagnostic Radiology: A Textbook of Medical Imaging.* 6th ed. New York, NY: Churchill Livingstone/Elsevier; 2015.

33. Guidelines for diagnostic imaging during pregnancy and lactation. Committee Opinion No. 656. American College of Obstetricians and Gynecologists. *Obstet Gynecol.* 2016; 127: e75–80.

34. Sachs HC. The transfer of drugs and therapeutics into human breast milk: An update on selected topics. Committee on Drugs. *Pediatrics.* 2013; 132: e796–809.

35. MacDorman MF, Gregory EC. Fetal and Perinatal Mortality: United States, 2013. *Natl Vital Stat Rep.* July 2015; 64(8): 1–24

36. Ferrero S,Esposito F, Biamonti M, et al. Myasthenia gravis during pregnancy. Expert review of neurotherapeutics. 2008; 8(6): 979–988.

37. Berlit S, et al. Myasthenia gravis in pregnancy: A case report. *Case Reports in Obstetrics and Gynecology.* 2012.

38. Papazian O. Topical review article: Transient neonatal myasthenia gravis. *Journal of Child Neurology.* 1992; 7(2): 135–141.

39. Isaacs H. Perinatal (fetal and neonatal) tuberous sclerosis: A review. *American Journal of Perinatology.* 2009; 26(10): 755–760.

40. Bader RS, Chitayat D, Kelly E, et al. Fetal rhabdomyoma: prenatal diagnosis, clinical outcome, and incidence of associated tuberous sclerosis complex. *Journal of Pediatrics.* 2003; 143(5): 620–624.

41. King JA, Stamilio DM. Maternal and fetal tuberous sclerosis complicating pregnancy: A case report and overview of the literature. *American Journal of Perinatology.* 2005; 22(2): 103–108.

42. Zaki M, Boyd PA, Impey L, et al. Congenital myotonic dystrophy: Prenatal ultrasound findings and pregnancy outcome. *Ultrasound in Obstetrics & Gynecology.* 2007; 29(3): 284–288.

43. Radtke HB, Sebold CD, Allison C, et al. Neurofibromatosis type 1 in genetic counseling practice: recommendations of the National Society of Genetic Counselors. *Journal of Genetic Counseling.* 2007; 16(4): 387–407.

44. McEwing, R, Joelle R, Mohlo M, et al. Prenatal diagnosis of neurofibromatosis type 1: Sonographic and MRI findings. *Prenatal Diagnosis.* 2006; 26(12): 1110–1114.

45. Polizzi A, Huson, SM, Vincent A. Teratogen update: Maternal myasthenia gravis as a cause of congenital arthrogryposis. *Teratology.* 2000; 62(5): 332–341.

46. Chen C-P. Prenatal diagnosis and genetic analysis of fetal akinesia deformation sequence and multiple pterygium syndrome associated with neuromuscular junction disorders: A review. *Taiwanese Journal of Obstetrics and Gynecology.* 2012; 51(1): 12–17.

47. Verspyck E, Mandelbrot L, Dommergues M, et al. Myasthenia gravis with polyhydramnios in the fetus of an asymptomatic mother. *Prenatal Diagnosis,* 1993; 13(6): 539–542.

48. Cagneaux M, Paoli V, Blanchard G, et al. Pre- and postnatal imaging of early cerebral damage in Sturge-Weber syndrome. *Pediatric Radiology.* 2013; 43(11): 1536–1539.

49. Parra J, Martinez-Hernandez R, Also-Rallo E, et al. Ultrasound evaluation of fetal movements in pregnancies at risk for severe spinal muscular atrophy. *Neuromuscular Disorders.* 2011; 21(2): 97–101.

50. Saleh M, Miron I, Al-Rukban H, et al. Prenatal presentation of hereditary hemorrhagic telangiectasia—a report of two sibs. *Prenatal Diagnosis.* 2016; 36(9): 891–893.

51. Jung E, Lee BY, Huh, CY. Prenatal diagnosis of fetal seizure: A case report. *Journal of Korean Medical Science.* 2008; 23(5): 906–908.

6

Prenatal Genetics for Women with Neurology Disease

Pregnancy, Preimplantation, and Newborn Screening

STEPHANIE DUKHOVNY

INTRODUCTION

Screening and detection for neurologic diseases of the fetus and newborns have received a great deal of attention in the 21st century. Screening options have expanded from detection of neural tube defects to the identification of couples at risk for rare autosomal recessive neurologic conditions. Timing of diagnosis has moved from identifying affected neonates at the time of birth to now being able to recognize families at risk during pregnancies, and even to prevention of the birth of an affected child with preimplantation genetic diagnosis. Newborn screening has allowed for the identification of affected children early in the neonatal period, with the hopes of early intervention to improve the long-term outcome of the neonatal and child. All of these advances have allowed for improved care for families at risk for neurologic diseases in the fetus and newborn infants.

Genetic Screening
General approach to screening
The initial concept of prenatal screening for fetal disease began in the 1970s using maternal serum alpha fetoprotein (AFP) for detection of neural tube defects.[1] Prenatal screening in the modern era has evolved to the use of maternal serum cell free fetal DNA for detection of aneuploidy and expanded carrier screening panels for detection of rare autosomal recessive disorders. Additionally, advances in ultrasound have allowed for more sensitive and earlier detection of fetal anatomic malformations and is often called the "genetic sonogram."

The detection of neurologic diseases prenatally has received special attention since the 1980s. Anatomic abnormalities of the central nervous system and spinal cord can be detected by maternal serum alpha-fetoprotein and by prenatal ultrasound. Also many autosomal recessive disorders that can be detected on expanded carrier screening panels have neurologic consequences for the newborn and child.

Prenatal ultrasound screening
Advances in prenatal ultrasound have allowed for a more detailed screening assessment of the fetal central nervous system. The American College of Radiology, American College of Obstetrics and Gynecology, American Institute of Ultrasound in Medicine, and the Society of Radiologists in Ultrasound have suggested practice parameters for fetal ultrasound of the CNS and fetal spine in order to screen for anomalies in these structures (Table 6.1).

Once a neurologic concern is detected on screening prenatal ultrasound, a patient may be referred for a more detailed workup, including invasive diagnostic testing via amniocentesis, and consideration of a fetal MRI for further delineation of the area of concern.[2] Patients can then be appropriately counseled regarding the diagnosis, prognosis, and reproductive choice options including pregnancy termination. Referral can also be made to subspecialists in pediatric neurology and pediatric neurosurgery for detailed counseling (see also Chapter 5).

Carrier screening
The goal of carrier screening is to identify women who are not experiencing symptoms of a genetic disorder but are carriers of a pathogenic mutation that could lead to affected offspring if they mate

TABLE 6.1 RECOMMENDED ULTRASOUND SCREENING FOR CENTRAL NERVOUS SYSTEM

Anatomic Structure	Disease Detection (Example)
Biparietal diameter	Microcephaly, Macrocephaly
Head circumference	Microcephaly, Macrocephaly
Lateral cerebral ventricles	Ventriculomegaly, Hydrocephalus
Choriod plexus	Choriod plexus cysts
Midline falx	Holoprosencephaly
Cavum septi pellucidi	Corpus callosal and midline defects
Cistern magna	Neural tube defects
Spine	Neural tube defects

with an individual with a pathogenic mutation in the same gene.

Ethnicity-based carrier screening

Carrier screening was initially proposed in the 1970s as ethnic carrier screening specifically in the Ashkenazi Jewish population and in the Mediterranean population.[3,4] Initial proposals for choosing diseases was based on the Wilson and Junger principles of screening, which require that, among other things, the condition is severe, the test is acceptable to the population, and that it is cost effective. Professional organizations, including the American College of Medical Genetics and Genomics (ACMGG) and the American College of Obstetrics and Gynecology (ACOG) have made recommendations for conditions to include when performing carrier screening in a patient with Ashkenazi Jewish heritage, although the choice of what diseases to screen for has been controversial.[5] Screening panels in the Ashkenazi Jewish population include a number of disorders with severe neurologic consequence, including Tay-Sachs disease, and while the disease lists are not identical, both include other neurologic diseases such as familial dysautonomia, Canavan disease, Niemann-Pick (type A), Mucolipidosis IV, and Gaucher disease.[5]

Pan-ethnic carrier screening

Pan-ethnic screening is screening all women regardless of ethnic background and is recommended for diseases with high population prevalence where ethnic background is less predictive of carrier status.

Genetic screening is suggested for all women of reproductive age contemplating pregnancy for cystic fibrosis as well as spinal muscular atrophy (SMA). ACOG recommends that screening for SMA be offered to all women who are pregnant or planning to become pregnant. They also emphasize that for patients with a family history of SMA that a clinician review the molecular testing of the affected patient and the carrier testing for the partner, and if those records are not available for review, that deletion testing for the SMN1 gene be performed.[6] Additionally, Fragile X premutation carrier screening is recommended by ACOG for women with disorders related to Fragile X, including premature ovarian failure or a family history of intellectual disability.[6]

Expanded carrier screening

As technology has advanced and cost has decreased, it is now possible to screen for hundreds of conditions simultaneously. This screening method is called Expanded Carrier Screening and is now considered to be an acceptable screening strategy by ACOG.[7] A number of commercial and academic labs are now offering panels of both autosomal recessive and X-linked disorders—with changes to these panels frequently as new mutations and diseases become available. The ordering clinician can also customize panels. Methods include mutation testing and sequencing, and often the partner is tested simultaneously in order to assess fetal risk. Ideally this testing occurs preconception. Of the hundreds of disorders, dozens of them have neurologic symptoms, which vary from mild to severe and from congenital to later onset.

Preimplantation Genetic Diagnosis

Preimplantation genetic diagnosis (PGD) is a procedure that can be performed on an embryo for families with a known genetic disorder. This can be performed for genetic conditions of all inheritance patterns (autosomal dominant, autosomal recessive, or X-linked) as well as for families with a known balanced chromosome rearrangement in one of the parents.[8] PGD allows a couple to avoid the risk of having a child affected with a specific genetic disorder, rather than becoming pregnant and undergoing traditional prenatal diagnosis (chorionic villus sampling or amniocentesis). The advantage of PGD is that it allows the couple to avoid the risk of diagnosing an affected fetus in-utero and thus consider issues regarding continuation versus termination of pregnancy.[9] In order to perform PGD, DNA is obtained from the polar body, blastomere, or blastocyst from the embryo prior to implantation at a point at which it does not impact embryonic development.[10–12] The DNA is then evaluated for the gene of interest, and while this occurs the embryo is frozen until results can be obtained. Once unaffected embryos are identified, the patient will then need in-vitro fertilization (IVF) to transverse the unaffected embryo(s). PGD has not been identified as associated with increased risks for fetal anomalies or adverse outcomes, although long-term data are limited.[13] IVF itself is associated with increased risks for multiple births (twins, triplets), however, and the associated adverse perinatal outcomes with multiples. PGD is costly, although the cost varies from institution to institution, the combination of PGD and the necessary IVF can be prohibitive for many patients. Generally, these procedures (PGD or IVF) are not covered by health insurance even for women with genetic conditions/indications.

Identification of a neurologic disorder within a family can present in a number of different scenarios. One parent may be affected with a neurologic condition that may be inherited by the offspring, such as myotonic dystrophy. The couple may have a history of an affected child and desire future unaffected children, such as parents who have a child with Duchenne Muscular Dystrophy or SMA. Alternatively, the parents may have been identified preconception as both carriers of an autosomal recessive neurologic condition, such as Tay Sachs, on a carrier screening panel and would like to ensure they do not have an affected fetus prior to conception.

Importantly, not all neurologic genetic disorders will present in the neonatal or childhood period. The ethics of offering PGD for adult onset neurodegenerative diseases can be complex. These diseases are often autosomal dominant, such as Huntington's disease. Counseling is particularly complicated in couples when one partner is at risk of the disorder but does not know their own status. In this case all available embryos can be tested for the relevant familial mutation and can be discarded if they are affected. However, PGD and IVF are expensive, and in this scenario the couple may have undergone this extensive testing for no reason (ie, the parent at risk may not carry the mutated gene).[14] Further, if all embryos are noted to be carriers, the infertility team will need to communicate that there are no embryos available,

although they cannot disclose the reason why. The American Society for Reproductive Medicine has stated that PGD for serious adult onset conditions can be ethically justified and that it can also be allowed for conditions with "lesser severity or penetrance."[15] This recommendation would apply to both life limited and non-lethal neurologic genetic disorders. Because of both the scientific and ethical complexity, the patient must to meet with a genetic counselor with expertise in this area. Further, in order to be a candidate for PGD for any disorder, a family must have had molecular genetic testing to identify the specific mutation in the gene of interest, and should receive extensive genetic counseling for options counseling in this setting prior to proceeding with any screening or PGD testing.

Newborn Screening

The goal of newborn screening programs across the world is to identify infants in the newborn period who are at risk of having disorders that may have early interventions that could impact the long-term health of the child. Most children born in the United States today receive a combination of "blood spot" screening as well as screening for congenital heart disease using oxygen saturation and a newborn hearing screen.

Serum newborn screening was first introduced in the 1960s for phenylketonuria and now with advances in technology has been expanded in many states to include dozens of disorders. The current recommendations by the United States Department of Health and Human Services includes 31 core conditions ("Recommended Uniform Screening Panel"), as well as additional diseases that may be detected at the time of screening (Table 6.2). The decision to include a disease on the newborn screen depends on a number of criteria, including the following: the disorder should be serious, there is effective treatment in the pre-symptomatic or early stages that would impact outcome, the test must have a low false negative rate, the test must be simple and inexpensive, the results must be able to be obtained in a timely fashion, and conformatory testing must be available.[16] Of the 31 disorders included are a number of metabolic disorders, including fatty acid oxidation disorders, organic acid disorders, and amino acid disorders. Many of these metabolic disorders can have serious neurologic complications if not detected early, such as organic acid and amino acid disorders.[17–19]

TABLE 6.2 RECOMMENDED UNIFORM SCREENING PANEL CORE CONDITIONS

Propionic Acidemia	Very Long-chain Acyl-CoA Dehydrogenase Deficiency	S, S Disease (Sickle Cell Anemia)
Methylmalonic Acidemia (methylmaloic academia mutase)	Long-chain L-3 Hydroxyacyl-CoA Dehydrogenase Deficiency	S, Beta-Thalassemia
Methylmalonic Acidemia (co-balamin disorders)	Trifunctional Protein Deficiency	S, C Disease
Isovaleric Acidemia	Arginosuccinic Aciduria	Biotinidase Deficiency
3-Methylcrotonyl-CoA Carboxylase Deficiency	Citrullinemia, Type I	Critical Congenital Heart Disease
3-Hydroxy-3-Methyglutaric Aciduria	Maple Syrup Urine Disease	Cystic Fibrosis
Holocarboxylase Synthase Deficiency	Homocystinuria	Classic Galactosemia
B-Ketothiolase Deficiency	Classic Phenylketonuria	Glycogen Storage Disease Type II (Pompe)
Glutaric Acidemia Type I	Tyrosinemia, Type I	Hearing Loss
Carnitine Uptake Defect/ Carnitine Transport Defect	Primary Congenital Hypothyroid	Severe Combined Immunodeficiencies
Medium chain Acyl-CoA Dehydrogenase Deficiency	Congenital Adrenal Hyperplasia	Mucopolysaccaradiosis Type I
X-Linked Adrenoleukodystrophy		

CONCLUSION

Developments in maternal serum screening, ultrasound, expanded carrier screening, pre-implantation genetic diagnosis, and newborn screening have given families at risk for neurologic diseases the opportunity for early identification, intervention, and in some cases, even prevention for future affected children. Once a family has been identified to be at risk, the approach to their care should be individualized for pregnancy or preconception, for the disease at hand, and if prenatal or PGD molecular testing is available or desired (Table 6.3).

TABLE 6.3 APPROACH TO THE PREGNANT PATIENT AT RISK FOR NEUROLOGIC DISEASES IN THE NEWBORN

Questions to Ask	Follow Up to Consider
Is the patient pregnant, or pre-conception? Is she considering pregnancy?	Referral to prenatal consultation with a genetic counselor and Maternal-Fetal Medicine
What is the disease of concern?	How was the disease diagnosed? Who is the affected family member?
Has molecular genetic testing been performed for the disease of interest?	Obtain laboratory reports of molecular testing
If not pregnant, but considering pregnancy, would she be interested in PGD?	Referral to an infertility clinic
If pregnant, would she be interested in diagnostic testing during pregnancy (Chorionic Villus Sampling (CVS) or amniocentesis)?	Referral to center that performs diagnostic procedures

REFERENCES

1. Wald NJ, Cuckle H, Brock JH, Peto R, Polani PE, Woodford FP. Maternal serum-alpha-fetoprotein measurement in antenatal screening for anencephaly and spina bifida in early pregnancy. Report of U.K. collaborative study on alpha-fetoprotein in relation to neural-tube defects. *Lancet.* 1977; 1: 1323–1332.

2. Prayer D, Malinger G, Brugger PC, et al. ISUOG Practice Guidelines: Performance of fetal magnetic resonance imaging. *Ultrasound Obstet Gynecol.* 2017 May; 49(5): 671–680.

3. Cao A, Furbetta M, Galanello R, et al. Prevention of homozygous beta-thalassemia by carrier screening and prenatal diagnosis in Sardinia. *Am J Hum Genet.* 1981; 33: 592–605.

4. Kaback MM. Population-based genetic screening for reproductive counseling: The Tay-Sachs disease model. *Eur J Pediatr.* 2000; 159 (Suppl 3): S192–195.

5. Edwards JG, Feldman G, Goldberg J, et al. Expanded carrier screening in reproductive medicine-points to consider: A joint statement of the American College of Medical Genetics and Genomics, American College of Obstetricians and Gynecologists, National Society of Genetic Counselors, Perinatal Quality Foundation, and Society for Maternal-Fetal Medicine. *Obstet Gynecol.* 2015; 125: 653–662.

6. Committee on G. Committee Opinion No. 691: Carrier screening for genetic conditions. *Obstet Gynecol.* 2017; 129: e41–e55.

7. Committee on G. Committee Opinion No. 690: Carrier screening in the age of genomic medicine. *Obstet Gynecol.* 2017; 129: e35–e40.

8. Practice Committee of Society for Assisted Reproductive T, Practice Committee of American Society for Reproductive M. Preimplantation genetic testing: A Practice Committee opinion. *Fertil Steril.* 2008; 90: S136–143.

9. Traeger-Synodinos J. Pre-implantation genetic diagnosis. *Best Pract Res Clin Obstet Gynaecol.* 2017; 39: 74–88.

10. Cieslak-Janzen J, Tur-Kaspa I, Ilkevitch Y, Bernal A, Morris R, Verlinsky Y. Multiple micromanipulations for preimplantation genetic diagnosis do not affect embryo development to the blastocyst stage. *Fertil Steril.* 2006; 85: 1826–1829.

11. Handyside AH, Pattinson JK, Penketh RJ, Delhanty JD, Winston RM, Tuddenham EG. Biopsy of human preimplantation embryos and sexing by DNA amplification. *Lancet.* 1989; 1: 347–349.

12. Verlinsky Y, Rechitsky S, Verlinsky O, et al. Prepregnancy testing for single-gene disorders by polar body analysis. *Genet Test.* 1999; 3: 185–190.

13. Desmyttere S, Bonduelle M, Nekkebroeck J, Roelants M, Liebaers I, De Schepper J. Growth and health outcome of 102 2-year-old children conceived after preimplantation genetic diagnosis or screening. *Early Hum Dev.* 2009; 85: 755–759.

14. Stark Z, Wallace J, Gillam L, Burgess M, Delatycki MB. Predictive genetic testing for neurodegenerative conditions: How should conflicting interests within families be managed? *J Med Ethics.* 2016; 42: 640–642.

15. Ethics Committee of American Society for Reproductive M. Use of preimplantation genetic diagnosis for serious adult onset conditions: A committee opinion. *Fertil Steril.* 2013; 100: 54–57.

16. Zinn A. Inborn errors of metabolism. In R. J. Martin, A. Fanaroff, & M. C. Walsh (Eds), Fanaroff and Martin's neonatal-perinatal medicine: Disease of the fetus and infant (9th ed. pp. 1621–1679). Philadelphia: Mosby.

17. Guthrie R, Susi A. A simple phenylalanine method for detecting phenylketonuria in large populations of newborn infants. *Pediatrics.* 1963; 32: 338–343.

18. Kaye CI, Committee on G, Accurso F, et al. Introduction to the newborn screening fact sheets. *Pediatrics.* 2006; 118: 1304–1312.

19. American Academy of Pediatrics Newborn Screening Authoring C. Newborn screening expands: Recommendations for pediatricians and medical homes—implications for the system. *Pediatrics.* 2008; 121: 192–217.

7

Radiation Exposure and Neuroimaging During Pregnancy

DZHAMALA GILMANDYAR

INTRODUCTION

Ideally, non-emergent radiologic studies should be performed prior to conception. However, situations can arise during pregnancy that require immediate evaluation.

Sometimes maternal neurologic and other medical conditions can complicate pregnancy. With the increasing obesity prevalence as well as delayed childbearing, the rate of concurrent medical diseases seen during pregnancy is increasing. As an example, the incidence of breast cancer diagnosed during pregnancy and in the immediate postpartum period has increased, and approximately 11% of newly diagnosed breast cancers are among women of reproductive age of 45 or younger.[1-3] Women with neurologic diseases, such as multiple sclerosis (MS) can also first present in the antepartum period, and it has been reported that up to 10% of women with MS will first develop concerning symptoms during pregnancy.[4] This, in turn, leads to a dilemma not only about safety of treatment options, but about safe diagnostic tests as well.

Concern for fetal well-being and exposure related risk is a topic of frequent discussion among providers from various medical specialties and can be a cause of maternal hesitation in consenting to the recommended imaging study. Although the risk to the fetus should always be considered, it is frequently perceived by medical providers and mothers as being higher than it actually is.[5-6] While it is expected that both mother and physicians should be concerned about unnecessary radiation exposure, unfortunately many physicians and patients approach the topic in a similar, non-evidence-based manner.[5,6] This can lead to inadequate patient care and inappropriate advice, which further enhances a patient's fear. Delaying or missing maternal diagnosis of life-threatening pathology out of fear of exposing the fetus to an X-ray or CT scan poses a much higher risk to the mother and the entire pregnancy than the small risk from typical doses of radiation utilized in these tests.

Data from the Chernobyl disaster and Hiroshima bombing illustrate some of the teratogenic effects from high-dose radiation exposure in utero.[7-9] These reports illustrate some of the more common embryopathies (such as CNS changes, disturbances of fetal development and growth as well as increased risk of neoplasms) seen with higher levels of radiation exposure. While some discussion of data obtained from above catastrophes will be presented, this chapter will mainly focus on amount of radiation and possible fetal effects seen with diagnostic imaging tests commonly utilized during pregnancy.

BIOLOGIC EFFECTS OF IONIZING RADIATION

Radiation is a physical process where energy travels through space in a form of particles or waves. Radiation containing particles that have adequate energy to remove electrons from an atom of a body it is traveling through is called "ionizing" radiation. Alpha particles, beta particles, neutrons, gamma rays, and X-rays are all examples of ionizing radiation. Diagnostic imaging is one of the sources of ionizing radiation. Nonionizing radiation is not robust enough to excite atoms but has its own effect on an organism through transfer of heat. Examples of this include microwave, visible light, radio/TV waves, and ultraviolet light.

Ionizing radiation can cause tissue damage through several mechanisms. When radiation comes into contact with cells and atoms, it produces excitation and ionization of those elements. This, in turn, can produce free radicals, break chemical bonds, produce new bonds, and cause DNA/RNA damage. Since cells possess the inherent ability to repair themselves, low levels of radiation (such as everyday background radiation) are likely of no significant consequence. With higher doses, the DNA damage can begin to accumulate and result in cell death.[9] Sensitivity to radiation damage is not only based on dose but also on tissue type. In general, proliferating cells are more sensitive to radiation exposure. Hence, erythropoietic organs and reproductive organs are some of the more vulnerable ones, while muscle, bone, and CNS are more resistant. Because the developing fetus is highly proliferative, it is a sensitive organism, especially in the first trimester.

Several terms are used to define radiation dose and exposure. Absorbed dose is the amount of energy taken up by a kilogram of tissue and is measured in rads (1 rad = 0.01 gray [Gy] = 0.01sievert [Sv] and hence 0.001rad = 0.01mGy). Effective dose is the most commonly used term in medical literature and clinical use. It is the combination of radiation dose and the assessment of effectiveness of the type and energy of radiation on the particular tissue or organ that absorbs it. In short, it provides a way to quantify potential harm from ionized radiation exposure to a patient. As a reference, it is estimated that annual effective radiation dose from natural sources is 3mSv.[10] According to International Commission on Radiologic Protection (IRCP) a whole body radiation dose of 1 Sv (1Sv = 1000mSv) is needed to significantly increase a person's cancer risk.[11] As per the recommendations of US Nuclear Regulatory Commission, pregnant women should limit their total occupational radiation exposure over the course of the entire pregnancy to < 5mGy, which is equivalent to 5 mSv or 5 rads.[12]

PREGNANCY AND RADIATION

The first 2–4 weeks after fertilization is when the embryo is most sensitive to lethal effects of ionizing radiation. This is sometimes known as a period of "all or nothing."[13] If exposed, the embryo will either go on unharmed or not survive the insult. Embryopathies are not seen during this period of exposure. After this time, however, organogenesis begins to take place, and the fetus is much more susceptible to teratogenic effects of radiation through various mechanisms described earlier (DNA damage, cell death, etc.). From the reports on survivors of Hiroshima and Chernobyl we know that the fetus is most susceptible prior to 16 weeks of gestation.[7-9] These effects include growth restriction and CNS

TABLE 7.1 ESTIMATED DOSES OF RADIATION TO THE UTERUS/ FETUS FROM COMMON RADIOLOGY PROCEDURES DURING PREGNANCY

Type of Imaging	mGy	mRad
CT Scan		
Chest	0.16	16
Abdomen	30	3,000
Head	0	0
Radiograph		
Chest (PA & lateral)	0.002	0.2
Abdominal/KUB (Kidney, Uterer, Bladder)	2.5	250
Extremities	<0.001	<0.1
Cervical Spine	<0.001	<0.1
Thoracic Spine	<0.001	<0.1

Adapted and condensed from: Wagner et al, Parry et al, McCollough et al.

anomalies, particularly microcephaly. According to CDC, prior to 16 weeks, a dose of 0.10– 0.20 Gy (10–20 rads) is needed to induce fetal malformations. After 16 weeks, the dose that will result in harm is estimated to be much higher at 0.5–0.7 Gy (50–70 rads).[14] The risks and severity of mental disability and growth restriction seem to follow the same trend as malformations: the threshold for notable effect between 8–15 weeks appears to be lower than at > 16 weeks.[6-8] For mental disability, the threshold between 8–15 weeks appears to be 12 rads, and 21 rads after 16 weeks.[14,15] Estimated doses to the uterus from common radiologic procedures are shown in Table 7.1.[16-18]

COMMON NEUROIMAGING PROCEDURES USING IONIZING RADIATION

Many of the frequently used diagnostic procedures employ ionizing radiation. The utility of plain film X-rays in neuroimaging is low. However, X-rays of other parts of the body may be necessary for comprehensive evaluation and are frequently used to rule out gross pathology. Studies of maternal limbs, chest, head, or neck cause almost no dissemination to the fetus. Nonetheless, when possible, maternal abdominal shielding is recommended. On average, a plain chest X-ray (combination of lateral and postero-anterior views) is estimated to produce < 1 mrad of fetal exposure. Similarly, low radiation doses are seen with head or dental X-rays. It is estimated that the fetus receives about 0.01mrad from standard head or dental X-ray views.[19] This radiation dose is low enough that it is unlikely to have any effect on the fetus and therefore should be considered safe in pregnancy, especially when shielding is used.[20,21]

Computed tomography (CT) is another frequently utilized study when ruling in/out life-threatening maternal pathology. CT is a widely available and quick initial imaging tool. Fetal exposure depends on the location of the CT scan. CT of the head with abdominal shielding produces fetal exposure dose of 10 mrads. Non-contrast CT (NCCT) is an ideal first test for diagnosing many neuropathologies such as confirmation of intracranial hemorrhage, bony abnormalities and large masses. In addition, NCCT can demonstrate some early signs of stroke including hypoattenuation and swelling.[22] In 2004, a study found that immediate CT scanning for patients with symptoms concerning for possible acute stroke is cost effective and increases independent survival.[23]

The assessment of pregnant women should be no different than that of non-pregnant adults and should not be delayed due to fear of radiation exposure. This has been confirmed by both American College of Obstetrics and Gynecology and American College of Radiology.[11,20,21] Certain procedural modifications can be made to reduce the dose of radiation (such as moving the mother through the scanner quicker and shielding the abdomen) as long as the timing and quality of imaging is not compromised. Specific pregnancy protocols exist in many tertiary care institutions. Contrast material is frequently utilized during CT scans to improve visualization of vasculature and soft tissue. The contrast used is an iodinated media, which has been shown to cross the placenta. To date, however, no clinical fetal sequelae have been reported. Breastfeeding does not need to be interrupted for CT imaging regardless of contrast use in the post-partum patient.

ULTRASOUND

Ultrasound utilizes sound waves instead of ionizing radiation to obtain images. This is the most common modality of imaging a pregnant woman, and hence its safety profile is important. Data from mice that were exposed to extreme levels of ultrasound showed suboptimal neuronal migration.[24] Several studies in humans, however, showed no adverse effects on the fetus from multiple ultrasound exposures.[25,26] Recently conducted meta-analyses with a total of 41 studies (16 controlled studies, 13 cohort reports, and 12 case control studies) found no association between ultrasound exposure in pregnancy and adverse maternal or neonatal outcomes.[25] Specifically, there was no evidence of impaired physical/neurological development, increased risk of childhood malignancy, increased rate of mental disease, or lower intellectual performance among the offspring of women who received ultrasounds during their gestation. Regardless, all ultrasound imaging should follow the "ALARA" principle (as low as reasonably achievable) in order to minimize high-energy ultrasound forms (Doppler assessment, color flow), especially in the first trimester, unless necessary for diagnosis or evaluation.[27]

MRI (MAGNETIC IMAGING RESONANCE)

MRI is a frequently utilized neuroimaging modality that does not utilize ionizing radiation but instead utilizes a combination of electromagnetism and radio waves to create an image. Theoretical fetal risk exists due to generation of electric currents and heat in biological tissues from radiofrequency waves and magnets. However, human data do not suggest fetal risk from MRI studies.[28,29] While ultrasound is excellent in showing bony structures and vasculature, it is suboptimal when it comes to soft organs and differentiating certain pathologies. MRI is far superior to ultrasound in visualizing soft tissue. American College of Obstetrics and Gynecology suggests that "no special consideration is recommended for the first (versus any other) trimester in pregnancy" when utilizing MRI. Therefore, if necessary for complete evaluation, MRI imaging should be recommended in pregnancy just like outside of pregnancy with a single exception in the discussion of contrast material.

Just like in a CT scan, contrast material is sometimes necessary to enhance MR imagining. Gadolinium is the most commonly used enhancing agent and is necessary for certain neuropathologies such as tumors or demyelinating diseases. It has been shown to cross the placenta and is expelled by the fetus into the amniotic fluid. Since the fetus is normally in constant homeostasis with intrauterine environment, including amniotic fluid, and continuously swallows the fluid, some of the contrast material will end up in the fetal circulation. Most recent study found no adverse effects on the fetus from MRI alone, but it reported significant and concerning association of gadolinium exposure in pregnancy and postnatal outcomes. Multiple conditions were noted in children exposed to gadolinium in utero including rheumatological, inflammatory, and infiltrative skin conditions. In addition, the rate of stillbirth and neonatal death was increased in the gadolinium cohort.[30] For this reason, if possible, it is recommended that gadolinium be avoided in pregnancy if an alternative exists. However, just like with all procedures during pregnancy, if maternal (and therefore fetal) benefit from the information obtained clearly outweighs the theoretical fetal risk, then use of the contrast material may become necessary. In diseases that can only be effectively diagnosed and treated with contrast MRI, where the treatment has the potential to benefit the dyad, contrast should be utilized if necessary after discussion of risks and benefits with the patient. Just like with iodinated contrast, gadolinium can be given without interrputing breast feeding.[31,32]

CONCLUSION

Not infrequently, maternal medical conditions, including neuropathologies, can complicate pregnancy. Similar to the non-pregnant patients, each situation should be individualized. Counseling frequently depends on the seriousness of the medical condition suspected, gestational age, and confounding medical problems. If radiologic testing is needed, then risks, benefits, and alternatives should be discussed with the mother. If maternal risk from an undiagnosed condition is deemed greater than the benefit the fetus would receive from avoiding minute amount of radiation then a recommendation for an appropriate diagnostic test should be made by the health-care professional. While studies on some of the diagnostic imaging procedures during pregnancy are limited, the data that is available is overwhelmingly reassuring. Most tests deliver far less radiation than is considered harmful during pregnancy and some even less than background radiation we are all exposed to on daily basis. Maternal anxiety over fetal safety is understandable, but it is important to note that deterioration in her health from untreated disease will directly affect fetal well-being as well. Therefore, appropriate counseling by the healthcare professionals and provision of evidence based data is important when a radiologic test to evaluate for neurologic involvement during pregnancy is deemed necessary.

REFERENCES

1. Lambertini M, Anserini P, Fontana V, et al. The PREgnancy and FERtility (PREFER) study: An Italian multicenter prospective cohort study on fertility preservation and pregnancy issues in young breast cancer patients. *BMC Cancer.* May 19, 2017; 17(1): 346

2. Stensheim H, Moller B, van Dijk T, et al: Cause-specific survival for women diagnosed with cancer during pregnancy or lactation: A registry-based cohort study. *J Clin Oncol.* 2009; (27): 45–51.
3. Ranstam J, Janzon L, Olsson H: Rising incidence of breast cancer among young women in Sweden. *Br J Cancer.* 1990; 61(1): 120–122.
4. Bennet KA. Pregnancy and multiple sclerosis. *Clinical Obstetrics and Gynecology.* 2005; 48: 38–47.
5. Ratnapalan S, Bona N, Chandra K, Koren G. Physicians' perceptions of teratogenic risk associated with radiography and CT during early pregnancy. *AJR Am J Roentgenol.* 2004; 182: 1107.
6. Bentur Y, Horlatsch N, Koren G. Exposure to ionizing radiation during pregnancy: perception of teratogenic risk and outcome. *Teratology.* 1991; 43: 109.
7. Blot WJ, Miller RW. Mental retardation following in utero exposure to the atomic bombs of Hiroshima and Nagasaki. *Radiology.* 1973; 106: 617–619.
8. Yamazaki JN, Schull WJ. Perinatal loss and neurological abnormalities among children of the atomic bomb: Nagasaki and Hiroshima revisited, 1949 to 1989. *JAMA.* 1990; 264: 605–609.
9. Fucic A, Brunborg G, Lasan R, et al. Genomic damage in children accidentally exposed to ionizing radiation: A review of the literature *Mutat Res.* January-Feburary 2008; 658(1-2): 111–123.
10. United Nations Scientific Committee on the Effects of Atomic Radiation, Sources and Effects of Ionizing Radiation, UN Publication E.94. IX.2. New York, NY: UN Publications, United Nations; 1993.
11. The 2007 Recommendations of the International Commission on Radiological Protection. ICRP publication 103. *AUSOAnn ICRP.* 2007; 37(2-4): 1.
12. http://www.nrc.gov/reading-rm/doc-collections/cfr/part020/full-text.html. Accessed October, 31, 2012.
13. De Santis M, Cesari E, Nobili E, et al. Radiation effects on development. *Birth Defects Res C Embryo Today.* 2007; 81: 177.
14. http://www.bt.cdc.gov/radiation/prenatalphysician. asp. Accessed October 31, 2012.
15. Hall EJ. Scientific view of low-level radiation risks. *Radiographics.* 1991; 11: 509.
16. Wagner LK, Lester RG, Saldana LR. Exposure of the Pregnant Patient to Diagnostic Radiations: A Guide to Medical Management. 2nd ed. Madison, WI: Medical Physics Publishing; 1997.
17. Parry RA, Glaze SA, Archer, BR. *The AAPM/RSNA Physics Tutorial for Residents RadioGraphics.* 1999; 19: 5, 1289–1302.
18. McCollough CH, Schueler BA, Atwell TD, et al. Radiation exposure and pregnancy: When should

we be concerned? *RadioGraphics*. 2007; 27: 4, 909–917

19. Guidelines on diagnosis and management of acute pulmonary embolism. Task Force on Pulmonary Embolism, European Society of Cardiology. *Eur Heart J*. 2000; 21: 1301.

20. American College of Obstetrics and Gynecology Committee Opinion No. 656: Guidelines for diagnostic imaging during pregnancy and lactation. *Obstet Gynecol*. 2016; 127: e75–80.

21. Brent RL. Saving lives and changing family histories: Appropriate counseling of pregnant women and men and women of reproductive age, concerning the risk of diagnostic radiation exposures during and before pregnancy. *Am J Obstet Gynecol*. 2009; 200: 4.

22. Wardlaw JM, Mielke O. Early signs of brain infarction at CT: observer reliability and outcome after thrombolytic treatment--systematic review. *Radiology*. May 2005; 235(2): 444–453.

23. Wardlaw JM, Seymour J, Cairns J, et al. Immediate computed tomography scanning of acute stroke is cost-effective and improves quality of life. *Stroke*. 2004; 35(11): 2477.

24. Ang ES Jr, Gluncic V, Duque A, et al. Prenatal exposure to ultrasound waves impacts neuronal migration in mice. *Proc Natl Acad Sci USA*. 2006; 103: 12903.

25. Torloni MR, Vedmedovska N, Merialdi M, et al. Safety of ultrasonography in pregnancy: WHO systematic review of the literature and meta-analysis. *Ultrasound Obstet Gynecol*. 2009; 33: 599.

26. Whitworth M, Bricker L, Neilson JP, Dowswell T. Ultrasound for fetal assessment in early pregnancy. *Cochrane Database Syst Rev*. 2010; CD007058.

27. American Institute of Ultrasound Medicine http://www.aium.org/resources/guidelines/obstetric.pdf

28. Duncan KR. The development of magnetic resonance imaging in obstetrics. *Br J Hosp Med*. 1996; 55: 178.

29. Kirkinen P, Partanen K, Vainio P, Ryynänen M. MRI in obstetrics: A supplementary method for ultrasonography. *Ann Med*. 1996; 28: 131.

30. Ray JG1, Vermeulen MJ2, Bharatha A, et al. Association between MRI exposure during pregnancy and fetal and childhood outcomes. *JAMA*. September 2016; 316(9): 952–961.

31. Webb JA, Thomsen HS, Morcos SK, (ESUR) MoCMSCoESoUR. The use of iodinated and gadolinium contrast media during pregnancy and lactation. *Eur Radiol*. 2005; 15(6): 1234–1240.

32. Ito S. Drug therapy for breast-feeding women. *N Engl J Med*. 2000; 343(2): 118–126.

8

Cognitive Changes in Pregnancy

MIRIAM T. WEBER

INTRODUCTION

The hormones of the hypothalamic-pituitary-gonadal (HPG) axis have effects on the central nervous system beyond those of reproduction, and there has been tremendous growth in research into their role in regulating brain structure and function. Of particular interest to the neurologist is how reproductive states impact psychological and cognitive health in women. Some enduring changes in pregnancy are related to maternal behaviors that enable survival of offspring. For instance, compared to non-mothers, mothers demonstrate increased activity in limbic regions in response to infant cries[1] and increased neural responsivity in visual-processing areas in response to infant facial expressions.[2] Other changes relate to cognitive and psychological function. In animals, pregnancy is associated with increased dendritic spine density in the hippocampus,[3,4] a brain region critical for memory, and altered spine density in the amygdala,[5] a brain region critical for emotion processing. In humans, pregnancy has been shown to decrease physiological and psychological responses to stress,[6,7] but rates of depression increase in pregnancy and the postpartum period.[8,9]

It was in the context of early studies of postpartum psychiatric disturbance (depression and psychosis) that the first studies of cognitive changes in pregnancy appeared nearly 50 years ago.[10,11] In a survey of obstetrical patients on the third postpartum day, 64% of patients showed subjective evidence of anxiety and/or depression and cognitive dysfunction. Several patients were described as distractible and having deficits in sustained attention and recent memory on mental status exam. A follow-up study found that compared to non-pregnant controls, pregnant women (and to a lesser degree, postpartum women) had decreased performance on measures of executive function (concentration and planning), and that women with postpartum anxiety were less likely to show

improvement on these measures from pregnancy to postpartum.[11] Since that time, over 40 original studies and two meta-analyses have been published; however, there is considerable equipoise in the field, including whether or not there are objective cognitive declines during pregnancy and the postpartum, what cognitive domains are affected, when these declines begin, how long they last, and what factors contribute to them. The vast majority of published studies are small, with group sizes of 10–50 women. Many are cross-sectional, and the longitudinal studies do not include evaluations of women prior to pregnancy. Several studies do not include a non-pregnant control group, making it difficult to determine if changes are due to a change in pregnancy status or a result of repeated exposures to the tests (commonly referred to as "practice effects"). Finally, many studies combine women at different stages in pregnancy and with different pregnancy histories. The aim of this chapter is to (1) review the literature on the effects of pregnancy and the postpartum on domains of cognitive function (2) explore contributions to cognitive changes in pregnancy and postpartum, and (3) outline a care pathway for practitioners encountering pregnant women with cognitive concerns.

SELF-REPORTED COGNITIVE COMPLAINTS IN PREGNANCY

Numerous studies have demonstrated that pregnancy is accompanied by a subjectively experienced decline in memory. Reports vary, but typically between 50–80% of women report memory difficulties in pregnancy and the postpartum period.[12,13] In the scientific literature, this has been referred to as "benign encephalopathy of pregnancy"[14,15] or "gestational memory impairment"[13]; colloquially, it is described as "baby brain" or "pregnancy brain." Cognitive symptoms most frequently reported are forgetfulness and poor memory, but distractibility, poor concentration, poor concentration, confusion, word finding difficulties, difficulty reading, and cognitive slowing have all been noted.[13] These subjective memory complaints (SMC) are reported in both the second and third trimesters,[16,17] the postpartum,[18] and in both primigravid and multigravid women.[12] Some studies have linked SMC to higher levels of education[12] or having a profession.[14] SMC are unrelated to self-reported physical health, emotional health, or anxiety[14,19] but are related to self-reported sleep difficulties.[10,20] While the literature on SMC is fairly consistent and suggests that pregnancy is associated with a subjectively experienced decline in cognition, the data on objective cognitive changes are more equivocal.

OBJECTIVE COGNITIVE CHANGES IN PREGNANCY

In reviewing the literature on objective cognitive function in pregnancy and the postpartum period, we focused on studies that included standardized neuropsychological measures of verbal memory, visual memory, attention, working memory, processing speed, executive function, and language. As education and/or intellectual function are often highly correlated with these measures, they are important covariates to consider. When a non-pregnant control group was utilized, the vast majority of studies matched subjects on education level, or found no significant differences between groups on either education level, or measures of estimated intellectual function. When there were significant differences between groups, the statistical models included education as a covariate.

Verbal Memory

Most studies of cognitive function in pregnancy have focused on explicit verbal memory. In a typical testing paradigm, subjects are presented with a list of words or a short story to recall immediately, and then after some period of delay (typically 20–30 minutes). A forced-choice recognition task may be given as well, in which as subject is asked to differentiate target words from foils, or to answer yes/no questions about the story. In this way, one can separate out the encoding, retention, and retrieval components of memory.

Cross-sectional studies of the effects of pregnancy on immediate verbal memory have produced mixed results, with some demonstrating a deleterious effect[21,22] and others showing no differences between pregnant women and non-pregnant controls.[23,24,25] Longitudinal studies are similarly mixed, with several showing a negative impact of pregnancy when performance between pregnancy and postpartum is compared[26–30] while others showed no such change.[17,31,32,33] The pattern is the same with studies of delayed verbal memory, with many cross-sectional and longitudinal studies showing a deleterious effect of pregnancy[21,22,27,30,33,34] and a similar number showing no effect.[16,19,23,24,26,31,32,35] Three studies report a differential effect of pregnancy on immediate versus delayed verbal memory. One found that women's delayed verbal memory performance improved when 3–12 months postpartum compared to when they were pregnant (suggesting a negative effect of pregnancy), but immediate verbal memory did not improve,[33] whereas a second found that immediate verbal memory improved from pregnancy to postpartum, and delayed verbal memory did not.[26] The third included a non-pregnant control group, and found that both immediate and delayed verbal memory improved in the early postpartum, but that the latter did not meet statistical significance.[29] Notably, in one study, women performed well below normative values on both measures at both times.[26] Together, these findings suggest that there is a deleterious effect of pregnancy on both immediate and delayed verbal memory but that they recover at different rates in the postpartum. Studies of recognition memory are similarly equivocal with some showing a negative effect of pregnancy,[22,33,36] some no effect,[23,35] and some a positive effect, at least for pregnancy-related material.[16]

These differences may be due to methodological issues such as type and sensitivity of memory tests used, heterogeneity of the study sample (varied stages of pregnancy, varied pregnancy history), cross-sectional or limited longitudinal design (only assessing at one point in pregnancy and comparing to postpartum), small sample sizes, and/or the lack of a healthy, non-pregnant control group. In an attempt to counter these limitations, Henry and Rendell (2007) conducted a meta-analysis of 14 cross-sectional and longitudinal studies published between 1991 and 2007 that included an appropriate control group and found significant deficits in both immediate and delayed free recall for pregnant women. No significant differences were seen in recognition memory tasks; however, only 2 studies included measures of recognition memory.[37] An updated meta-analysis in 2012 of 21 studies reported similar findings, with pregnant women performing significantly worse than non-pregnant controls on tests of immediate and delayed free recall.[38] The effect sizes reported in both meta-analyses were in the small to medium range. However, in

2 studies that compared women's performance to published normative data, pregnant women's scores were well below normative values, in the mild to moderately impaired range.[26,39] Currently, the bulk of the literature suggests that there is a significant but subtle negative effect of pregnancy on encoding and recall of verbal information. At this time, there are too few studies comparing free recall and recognition, but the evidence suggests that it is a retrieval, rather than a retention-based deficit.

Visual Memory

Similar to verbal memory, explicit visual memory is assessed by paradigms that involve presenting visual information and asking a subject to recall it immediately and then after some period of delay (typically 20–30 minutes). In these paradigms, subject may be exposed to pictures of faces or designs and then asked to recognize them from a group of targets and foils, or asked to reproduce the designs. Compared to verbal memory, far fewer studies have examined the effect of pregnancy on episodic visual memory. One small cross-sectional study found no differences between women in the first and third trimesters of pregnancy and non-pregnant controls on measures of visual memory,[22] whereas another found pregnant women outperformed non-pregnant controls on a visual memory task.[40] Results from two small longitudinal studies are also mixed, with one demonstrating declines in visual memory beginning in the second trimester,[41] and another showing no differences between pregnant women and never pregnant controls when tested in the third trimester.[18] In all of these studies, sample sizes were very small, with 20–25 women per group. A much larger longitudinal study involving over 300 women revealed no differences between pregnant women and non-pregnant controls on measures of visual memory.[28] Thus, the most compelling data suggests no effect of pregnancy on visual memory, but the existing data is very limited.

Attention and Working Memory

After episodic memory, the cognitive domains most frequently studied in pregnancy are attention and working memory. The former refers to the ability to focus awareness on a stimulus or task, or to shift awareness. Attentional capacity may be assessed by asking a subject to repeat increasing longer strings of digits, whereas selective attention may be assessed in paradigms in which a subject is asked to search for a target in an array of foils.

Working memory refers to the ability to store and manipulate information over brief periods of time. In a typical testing paradigm, a subject may be asked to sequence strings of letters and numbers according to a specified pattern. An early study that examined attentional capacity found no change in performance from the last month of pregnancy to 2–6 weeks postpartum, but a non-pregnant control group was not included.[26] In the meta-analyses described above, there were no differences between pregnant women, postpartum women, or healthy controls on tests of basic attentional capacity, which the authors refer to as the "storage component of working memory,"[37] a finding confirmed in more recent studies.[18] However, pregnant women performed worse than controls on measures of working memory, which the authors refer to as the "executive components of working memory."[37] The 2012 meta-analysis, which included several additional studies, reported similar findings in working memory, with pregnant women performing worse than non-pregnant women.[38] The magnitude of the reported effects sizes in both meta-analyses was small, suggesting that alterations in working memory are subtle. A more recent study showed no effect of pregnancy on working memory in non-depressed women, but this study had fewer than 30 women in each group.[42] The largest longitudinal study to date, which was not included in either meta-analysis, showed no effect of pregnancy on working memory.[28] Thus, the bulk of the literature suggests no effect of pregnancy on attention, and a modest effect of pregnancy on working memory.

Processing Speed and Executive Function

Other cognitive domains that have been studied in pregnancy are processing speed and executive function. Processing speed refers to the speed at which cognitive operations can be completed or executed. It is often assessed by timed tests requiring a motor output, such as drawing a line connecting numbers in circles across a page or substituting numbers for symbols according to a code. Executive function refers to a number of cognitive processes necessary for the control of behavior. Components of executive function include cognitive flexibility, inhibitory control, goal setting and selection and monitoring of behavior to attain the goal, planning, reasoning, and problem solving. Tests of executive function are varied, depending on the process being assessed. Cognitive flexibility tasks are often timed and may include visual scanning, sequencing, and motor output, whereas non-verbal reasoning and problem-solving tasks may involve using feedback to identify a card sorting strategy.

Compared to episodic memory, fewer studies have examined the effect of pregnancy on processing speed, but the findings in this domain are much more consistent. Two early cross-sectional studies found a negative effect of pregnancy on processing speed,[11,26] a finding confirmed in a later longitudinal study.[18] A meta-analysis of 6 studies found a significant moderate negative effect of pregnancy on processing speed, and the effect size for processing speed was the largest of any cognitive domain examined.[38] Several studies have assessed the impact of pregnancy on executive function, and nearly universally, no significant effect has been found.[11,17,18,21,24–27,29,32,41,43] Thus, the literature supports a moderate negative effect of pregnancy on processing speed and no effect on executive function.

Language
There is no suggestion that pregnancy is associated with aphasia, a disruption of expressive or receptive speech; however, there are many anecdotal reports of more subtle changes in language, such as word-finding difficulties. This may be measured objectively through tests of confrontation naming, in which a subject is shown pictures of objects and asked to name them, or through tests of fluency, in which a subject is asked to come up with words that begin with a certain letter or that fit a certain category over a specified period of time. Few studies have specifically assessed the impact of pregnancy on language function. Two cross-sectional studies found a negative effect of pregnancy on verbal fluency,[21,25] whereas one longitudinal study found no effect.[18] Only one study has examined confrontation naming, and it found no effect.[26] The sample sizes in all of these studies are small, and thus no definitive conclusions can be made regarding the effect of pregnancy on language function.

TIMING OF COGNITIVE DECLINES
Although the bulk of the evidence suggests that there are moderate declines in processing speed and more subtle declines in working memory and verbal episodic memory during pregnancy, it is less clear when in pregnancy these changes occur. Many cross-sectional studies have included women at various stages of pregnancy, and many longitudinal studies have only compared one stage in pregnancy to postpartum, thus the ability to detail when cognitive difficulties begin

in pregnancy is limited. Numerous studies have found deficits in processing speed in the third trimester of pregnancy,[11,18,26,29] but these studies only included women in late pregnancy and did not compare earlier stages. One small study that included a mixture of women in the second and third trimesters demonstrated a negative effect on processing speed,[25] and another found that women in the second and third trimesters were slower than non-pregnant controls but did not differ from one another.[27] However, another found processing speed to be worse in the final 4 months of pregnancy compared to earlier stages.[31] The finding of a negative effect of pregnancy on working memory comes primarily from the meta-analyses that combined effects of multiple studies. These included mixed groups of women in all trimesters[19,20,23] and ones that focused only on women in the last trimester of pregnancy.[29,44] Thus the existing data suggests that deficits in processing speed and working memory are apparent in the latter half of pregnancy, but given limitations in available data, declines earlier in pregnancy cannot be ruled out.

There is more data examining a timing effect in episodic memory. One longitudinal study reported no differences in verbal memory between pregnant women in the second trimester and non-pregnant women, but found differences emerged in the third trimester.[28] Similarly, other studies have found verbal memory to be worse in the third trimester compared to postpartum.[29,30,42] Other studies, however, have found declines in verbal memory at 14 weeks of pregnancy,[21] and at 17, 29 and 36 weeks of pregnancy.[27] Together, this data suggests that the memory declines begin early, and persist throughout all trimesters.

DURATION OF COGNITIVE DECLINES
Data is mixed on what happens to these cognitive declines in the postpartum period. A small longitudinal study found that processing speed improved at 1-month postpartum, compared to the month prior to delivery, but this study did not include a non-pregnant control group.[26] Longitudinal studies that included such a control group report decreased processing speed at ranges of 3–8 months postpartum.[27,29] The 2012 meta-analysis found a small negative effect of the postpartum period on processing speed and working memory, though these did not reach statistical significance.[38] The one study examining long-term changes in cognition postpartum found

improvements in attention and working memory at 2 years postpartum (compared to early postpartum), but this improvement was not independent of improvements in mood.[46]

Findings on episodic memory suggest the negative effect continues into the postpartum period. One small study found that the difference between pregnant women and controls ameliorates at 3 months postpartum,[30] whereas others find the negative effect persists at 3 months postpartum.[28,29] Both meta-analyses described above found significant deficits in both immediate and delayed free recall for postpartum women compared to non-pregnant controls,[37,38] though in the latter this did not reach statistical significance.[38] There were no studies of recognition memory in the postpartum period.

Fewer studies have examined verbal memory performance in the later postpartum period. One longitudinal study reported improved verbal memory when women were tested 6–12 months postpartum compared to their performance in late pregnancy (36 weeks).[46] However, other studies suggest that pregnancy-related verbal memory declines may be of longer duration, with decreased verbal encoding and retrieval persisting at 8 months postpartum.[27] The one long-term study showed improved verbal memory at 2 years postpartum compared to performance in the early postpartum; however, this improvement was not independent of improvements in mood.[45]

CONTRIBUTIONS TO COGNITIVE CHANGES IN PREGNANCY

Pregnancy is associated with several other symptoms known to affect cognitive function. For instance, irritability, mood lability, anxiety, and depression are common during pregnancy and the postpartum period.[11,47,48] Subjectively reported memory difficulties are associated with psychiatric illness, particularly depression,[49,50] negative affect,[51] and stress,[52] all of which have been independently associated with cognitive performance.[53,54] Thus an important clinical question is whether a woman's perceived or actual deficits are due to changes in mood. Several studies have found that symptoms of depression are related to subjectively reported memory difficulties,[23,55,56] but the vast majority have found no effect on objectively measured cognitive function.[18,22,26,31,41,57,58] Two small studies found that depression was related to working memory performance,[42,59] and one found that depression was related to processing speed and executive function.[32]

Results are similar when anxiety has been specifically measured separately from depression. Anxiety has been shown to be associated with subjective cognitive function,[60] but the majority of studies find no relationship between anxiety and objectively measured cognition.[19,26,41] One small study found that anxiety is related to processing speed and executive function,[11] and another found it related to verbal fluency—but only in those with low levels of anxiety.[18] Thus, changes in mood do not seem to account for the observed pregnancy associated deficit in verbal episodic memory but may be related to pregnancy-related changes in working memory and processing speed.

Another possible contributor to cognitive changes in pregnancy is sleep disturbance. Sleep difficulties are common in pregnancy and the postpartum, beginning in the second trimester and extending into the first several postpartum months.[30,61] Typical changes include prolonged sleep latency,[62] fewer hours of sleep per night,[63] and reduced sleep efficiency.[64,65] The role of sleep in memory consolidation has long been appreciated,[66] but impaired sleep is also associated with declines in attention, working memory, and executive functions.[67] In studies of pregnant women, self-reported sleep difficulties have been found to be a significant predictor of subjective memory complaints[19,55] and in early studies have been associated with worse memory,[19,56] processing speed, and executive function.[11,56] However, many other studies find no relationship between subjectively reported sleep difficulties and objectively measured cognitive function.[25,31,42,58] Thus, the literature suggests that sleep is related to SMC and may account for some but not all objective changes in cognitive function in pregnancy.

CLINICAL CARE

The existing literature demonstrates that pregnancy is associated with SMC and objective declines in working memory, processing speed, and episodic memory that are notable in the second and third trimesters and that may persist through the first postpartum year. Although changes in mood and sleep may account for SMC and some objective changes in working memory and processing speed, they do not account for the observed changes in memory. A key question, then, is how should a neurologist proceed when a patient presents with concerns about changes in cognitive function during pregnancy.

A pregnant woman presenting with SMC should be carefully assessed to rule out any treatable conditions that may be causing cognitive dysfunction. This includes a thorough screening for mood and/or sleep disturbance. Clinically significant, as well as subsyndromal, anxiety and depression can be treated effectively with psychotherapy. Cognitive-behavioral therapy (CBT) and intrapersonal therapy (IPT) are well-validated treatments with demonstrated efficacy[68,69] and pose no risk for the fetus. Milder dysthymia, worry, and adjustment issues may be managed with these approaches or mindfulness-based stress reduction. If there is concern about insomnia or sleep apnea, referral to a sleep disorders clinic for a formal sleep evaluation is most appropriate. Milder sleep difficulties may be treated with cognitive-behavioral approaches, such as CBT for Insomnia (CBTI) or improving sleep hygiene.

If careful screening suggests no anxiety, depression, or sleep disturbance, it may be helpful to normalize the patient's experience. Providing education about the typical nature and duration of cognitive changes may do much to alleviate a patient's concern that there is a more significant underlying problem. Patients should be counseled to try lifestyle modifications, such as engaging in physical exercise, which has a significant positive impact on brain structure and function.[70] Patients may find it helpful to use strategies to compensate for cognitive lapses, such as using lists and notes, reducing distractions when working on complex tasks, and mono- rather than multi-tasking. If the patient's concerns are significant, and she performs poorly on a screening measure such as the Mini-Mental State Exam (MMSE)[71] or Montreal Cognitive Assessment (MoCA),[72] a referral to a clinical neuropsychologist may be warranted for an in-depth examination of her cognitive function. If deficits are interfering with daily function, referral for cognitive rehabilitation, usually by a speech language pathologist, occupational therapist, or neuropsychologist, may also be helpful (Box 8.1).

BOX 8.1
CARE MAP FOR PREGNANCY PATIENT WITH COGNITIVE CONCERNS

DURING PREGNANCY
Assess for depression
  refer for Cognitive Behavioral Therapy or other evidence-based psychotherapy
Assess for sleep disturbance
  educate on sleep hygiene
  refer for sleep evaluation
  refer for Cognitive Behavioral Therapy for Insomnia
Normalize experience
Encourage exercise
Refer for neuropsychological evaluation
Refer for cognitive rehabilitation for compensatory strategies

POSTPARTUM
Assess for depression
  refer to psychiatry or psychology
Assess for sleep disturbance
  educate on sleep hygiene
  refer for sleep evaluation
  refer for Cognitive Behavioral Therapy for Insomnia
Normalize experience
Encourage exercise
Refer for neuropsychological evaluation
Refer for cognitive rehabilitation for compensatory strategies

REFERENCES

1. Seifritz E, Esposito F, Neuhoff JG, et al. Differential sex-independent amygdala response to infant crying and laughing in parents versus nonparents. *Biol Psychiatry.* 2003; 54:1367–1374.

2. Proverbio AM, Brignone V, Matarazzo S, Del Zotto M, Zani A. Gender and parental status affect the visual cortical response to infant facial expression. *Neuropsychologia.* 2006; 44: 2987–2999.

3. Kinsley CH, Lambert KG. The maternal brain. *Sci Am.* 2006; 294: 72–79.

4. Pawluski JL, Galea LA. Hippocampal morphology is differentially affected by reproductive experience in the mother. *J Neurobiol.* 2006; 66: 71–81.

5. Rasia-Filho AA, Fabian C, Rigoti, KM, Archaval M. Influence of sex, estrous cycle and motherhood on dendritic spine density in the rat medial amygdala revealed by the Golgi method. *Neuroscience.* 2004; 126: 839–847.

6. Glynn LM, Schetter CD, Wadhwa PD, Sandman CA. Pregnancy affects appraisal of negative life events. *J Psychosom Res.* 2004; 56: 47–52.

7. de Weerth C, Buitelaar JK. Physiological stress reactivity in human pregnancy—a review. *Neurosci Biobehav Rev.* 2005; 29: 295–312.

8. O'Hara MW, Swain AM. Rates and risk of postpartum depression: A meta-analysis. *Int Rev Psychiatr.* 1996; 8: 37–54.

9. Bennett HA, Einarson A, Taddio A, Koren G, Einarson TR. Prevalence of depression during pregnancy. *Obstet Gynecol.* 2004; 103: 698–709.

10. Kane FJ Jr., Harmon WJ Jr., Keeler MH, Ewing JA. Emotional and cognitive disturbance in the early puerperium. *Brit J Psychiatry.* 1968; 114: 99–102.

11. Jarrahi-Zadeh A, Kane FJ Jr, Van De Castlf RL, Lachenbruch PA, Ewing JA. Emotional and cognitive changes in pregnancy and early puerperium. *Brit J Psychiatry.* 1969; 115: 797–805.

12. Parsons C, Redman S. Self-reported cognitive change during pregnancy. *Aust J Adv Nurs.* 1991; 9: 20–29.

13. Brett M, Baxendale S. Motherhood and memory: A review. *Psychoneuroendocrinology.* 2001; 26: 339–362.

14. Poser CM, Kassirer MR, Peyser JM. Benign encephalopathy of pregnancy. Preliminary clinical observations. *Acta Neurol Scand.* 1986; 73: 39–43.

15. Purvin VA, Dunn DW. Caffeine and the benign encephalopathy of pregnancy. *Acta Neurol Scand.* 1987; 75: 76–77.

16. Christiansen H, Poyser C, Pollitt P, Cubis J. Pregnancy may confer a selective cognitive advantage. *J Reprod Infant Psychol.* 1999; 17: 7–25

17. Crawley RA, Dennison K, Carter C. Cognition in pregnancy and the first year post-partum. *Psychol Psychother.* 2003; 76: 69–84.

18. Logan DM, Hill KR, Jones R, Holt-Lunstad, Larson MJ. How do memory and attention change with pregnancy and childbirth? A controlled longitudinal examination of neuropsychological functioning in pregnant and postpartum women. *J Clin Exp Neuropsychol.* 2014; 36: 528–539.

19. Janes C, Casey P, Huntsdale C, Angus G. Memory in pregnancy. I: Subjective experiences and objective assessment of implicit, explicit and working memory in primigravid and primiparous women. *J Psychosom Obstet Gynecol.* 1999; 20: 80–87.

20. Casey, P, Huntsdale C, Angus G, and Janes C. Memory in pregnancy II: Implicit, incidental, explicit, semantic, short term, working, and prospective memory in primigravid, multigravida and postpartum women. *J Psychosom Obstet Gynecol.* 1999; 20: 158–164.

21. de Groot RH, Hornstra G, Roozendaal N, Jolles J. Memory performance but not information processing speed, may be reduced during pregnancy. *J Clin Exp Neuropsychol.* 2003; 25; 482–488.

22. Wilson DL, Barnes M, Ellett L, Permezel M, Jackson M, Crowe SF. Compromised verbal episodic memory with intact visual and procedural memory during pregnancy. *J Clin Exp Neuropsychol.* 2011; 33: 680–691.

23. Cuttler C, Graf P, Pawluski JL, Galea LAM. Everyday life memory deficits in pregnant women. *Can J Exp Psychol.* 2011; 65: 27–37.

24. Crawley R, Grant S, Hinshaw K. Cognitive changes in pregnancy: Mild decline of societal stereotype? *Appl Cognitive Psych.* 2008; 22: 1142–1162.

25. Onyper SV, Searleman A, Thacher PV, Maine EE, Johnson AG. Executive functioning and general cognitive ability in pregnancy women and matched controls. *J Clin Exp Neuropsychol.* 2010; 32: 986–995.

26. Buckwalter JG, Stanczyk FZ, McCleary CA, et al. Pregnancy, the postpartum, and steroid hormones: Effects on cognition and mood. *Psychoneuroendocrinology.* 1999; 24: 69–84.

27. de Groot RH, Vuurman EF, Hornstra G, Jolles J. Differences in cognitive performance during pregnancy and early motherhood. *Psychol Med.* 2006; 36: 1023–1032.

28. Glynn, LM. Giving birth to a new brain: Hormone exposures of pregnancy influence human memory. *Psychoneuroendocrinology.* 2010; 35: 1148–1155.

29. Henry JF, Sherwin BB. Hormones and cognitive functioning during late pregnancy and postpartum: A longitudinal study. *Behav Neurosci.* 2012; 126: 73–85.

30. Keenan PA, Yaldoo DT, Stress ME, Fuerst DR, Ginsburg KA Explicit memory in pregnancy women. *Am J of Obstet Gynecol.* 1998; 179: 731–737.

31. Christiansen H, Leach LS, Mackinnon A. Cognition in pregnancy and motherhood: prospective cohort study. *Brit J Psychiatry*. 2010; 196: 126–132.

32. Harris ND, Deary IJ, Harris MB, Lees MM, Wilson JA. Peripartal cognitive impairment: secondary to depression? *Brit J Health Psych*. 1996; 1: 127–136.

33. Mickes L, Wixted JT, Shapiro A, Scarff JM. The effects of pregnancy on memory: recall is worse but recognition is not. *J Clin Exp Neuropsychol*. 2009; 31: 754–761.

34. Lurie S, Gidron Y, Piper I, et al. Memory performance in late pregnancy and erythrocyte indices. *J Soc Gynecol Investig*. 2005; 12: 293–296.

35. Brindle PM, Brown MW, Brown J, Griffith HB, Turner GM. Objective and subjective memory impairment in pregnancy. *Psychol Med*. 1991; 21: 647–653.

36. Sharp K, Brindle PM, Brown MW, Turner GM. Memory loss during pregnancy. *Br J Obstet Gynaecol*. 1993; 100: 209–215.

37. Henry JF, Rendell PG. A review of the impact of pregnancy on memory function. *J Clin Exp Neuropsychol*. 2007; 29: 793–803.

38. Anderson MV, Rutherford MD. Cognitive reorganization during pregnancy and the postpartum period: An evolutionary perspective. *Evol Psychol*. 2012; 10: 659–687.

39. Rana S, Lindheimer M, Hibbard J, Pliskin N. Neuropsychological performance in normal pregnancy and preeclampsia. *Am J Obstet Gynecol*. 2006; 195: 186–191.

40. Anderson MV, Rutherford MD. Recognition of novel faces after single exposure is enhanced during pregnancy. *Evol Psychol*. 2011; 9: 47–60.

41. Farrar D, Tuffnell D, Neil J, Scally A, Marshall K. Assessment of cognitive function across pregnancy using CANTAB: A longitudinal study. *Brain Cogn*. 2014; 84: 76–84.

42. Hampson E, Phillips SD, Duff-Canning SJ, et al. Working memory in pregnant women: Relation to estrogen and antepartum depression. *Horm Behav*. 2015; 74: 218–227.

43. De Groot RH, Adam JJ, Hornstra G. Selective attention deficits during human pregnancy. *Neurosci Lett*. 2003; 340: 21–24.

44. Rendell PG, Henry JD. Prospective-memory functioning is affected during pregnancy and postpartum. *J Clin Exp Neuropsychol*. 2008; 30: 913–919.

45. Buckwalter JG, Buckwalter DK, Bluestein BW, Stanczyk FZ. Pregnancy and post partum: Changes in cognition and mood. *Prog Brain Res*. 2001; 133: 303–319.

46. Silber M, Almkvist O, Larsson B, Unvas-Moburg K. Temporary peripartal impairment in memory and attention and its possible relation to oxytocin concentration. *Life Sci*. 1990; 47(1): 57–65.

47. Andersson L, Sundstrom-Poromaa I, Wulff M, Astrom M, Bixo M. Depression and anxiety during pregnancy and 6 months postpartum: A follow-up study. *Acta Obstet Gynecol Scand*. 2006; 85: 937–944.

48. Heron J, O'Connor TG, Evans J, et al. The course of anxiety and depression through pregnancy and the postpartum in a community sample. *J Affect Disord*. 2004; 80: 65–73.

49. Feehan M, Knight RG, Partridge FM. Cognitive complaint and test performance in elderly patients suffering depression or dementia. *Int J Ger Psych*. 1991; 6: 287–293.

50. Kahn RL, Zarit SH, Hilbert NM, Niederehe G. Memory complaint and impairment in the aged. The effect of depression and altered brain function. *Arch Gen Psychiatry*. 1975; 32: 1569–1573.

51. Derouesne C, Lacomblez L, Thibault S, LePoncin M. Memory complaints in young and elderly subjects. *Int J Geriatr Psychiatry*. 1999; 14: 291–301.

52. Elfgren C, Gustafson L, Vestberg S, Passant U. Subjective memory complaints, neuropsychological performance and psychiatric variables in memory clinic attendees: A 3-year follow-up study. *Arch Gerontol Geriatr*. 2010; 51: e110–e114.

53. Gagnon SA, Wagner AD. Acute stress and episodic memory retrieval: neurobiological mechanisms and behavioral consequences. *Ann NY Acad Sci*. 2016; 1369: 55–75.

54. Thomas AJ, Gallagher P, Robinson LJ et al. A comparison of neurocognitive impairment in younger and older adults with major depression. *Psychol Med*. 2009; 39: 725–733.

55. Stark MA. Directed attention in normal and high-risk pregnancy. *J Obstet Gynecol Neonatal Nurs*. 2006; 35: 241–249.

56. Swain AM, O'Hara MW, Starr KR, Gorman, LL. A prospective study of sleep, mood, and cognitive function in pregnancy and the postpartum. *Obstet Gynecol*. 1997; 90: 381–386.

57. Parsons TD, Thompson E, Buckwalter DK, Bluestein BW, Stanczyck FZ, Buckwalter JG. Pregnancy history and cognition during and after pregnancy. *Int J Neusrosci*. 2004; 9: 1099–1110.

58. Vanston CM, Watson NV. Selective and persistent effect of foetal sex on cognition in pregnant women. *Neuroreport*. 2005; 16: 779–782.

59. Kataja EL, Karlsson L, Huizink AC, et al. Pregnancy-related anxiety and depressive symptoms are associated with visuospatial working memory errors during pregnancy. *J Affect Disord*. 2017; 218: 66–74.

60. Casey P. A longitudinal study of cognitive performance during pregnancy and new motherhood. *Arch Women Ment Hlth*. 2000; 3: 65–76.

61. Hunter LP, Rychnovsky JD, Yount, SM. A selective review of maternal sleep characteristics in the postpartum period. *J Obstet Gynecol Neonatal Nurs*. 2009; 38: 60–68.

62. Mindell JA, Jacobson BJ. Sleep disturbances during pregnancy. *J Obstet Gynecol Neonatal Nurs*. 2000; 29: 590–597.

63. Mindell JA, Cook RA, Nikolovski J. Sleep patterns and sleep disturbances across pregnancy. *Sleep Med*. 2015; 16: 483–488.

64. Shinkoda H, Matsumoto K, Park YM. Changes in sleep-wake cycle during the period from late pregnancy to puerperium identified through the wrist actigraph and sleep logs. *Psychiatry Clin Neurosci*. 1999; 53: 133–135.

65. Karacan I, Heine W, Agnew HW, Williams RL, Webb WB, Ross JJ. Characteristics of sleep patterns during late pregnancy and the postpartum periods. *Am J Obstet Gynecol*. 1968; 101: 579–586.

66. Rasch B, Born J. About sleep's role in memory. *Physiol Rev*. 2013; 93: 681–766.

67. Alhola P, Polo-Kantola P. Sleep deprivation: Impact on cognitive performance. *Neuropsychiatr Dis Treat*. 2007; 3: 553–567.

68. Hollon SD, Jarrett RB, Nierenberg AA, Thase ME, Trivedi M, Rush AJ. Psychotherapy and medication in the treatment of adult and geriatric depression: which monotherapy or combined treatment? *J Clin Psychiatry*. 2005; 66: 455–468.

69. Hoffman SG, Smits JA. Cognitive-behavioral therapy for adult anxiety disorders: A meta-analysis of randomized placebo-controlled trials. *J Clin Psychiatry*. 2007; 69: 621–632.

70. Hillman CH, Erickson KI, Kramer AF. Be smart, exercise your heart: Exercise effects on brain and cognition. *Nat Rev Neurosci*. 2008; 9: 58–65.

71. Folstein MF, Folstein SE, McHugh PR. Mini-mental state. A practical method for grading the cognitive state of patients for the clinician. *J Psychiatr Res*. 1975; 12: 189–198.

72. Nasreddine ZS, Phillips NA, Bedirian V, et al. The Montreal Cognitive Assessment, MoCA: A brief screening tool for mild cognitive impairment. *J Am Geriatr Soc*. 2005; 53: 695–699.

9

Principles of Reproductive Healthcare in Chronic Neurologic Disease

KATHRYN J. DRENNAN AND MARIA VANUSHKINA

Disability is defined as the consequence of physical, sensory, intellectual, and cognitive impairments that affect a person's ability to perform normal activities.[1] An estimated 15% of the global population live with at least one disability.[1] Many patients with neurologic illnesses or injury have some form of chronic disability, whether limitations of sensation (as sometimes seen with multiple sclerosis), cognitive disability, intellectual disability, and/or physical impairments (such as seen in spinal cord injury, muscular dystrophy, or cerebral palsy). People with physical, sensory, intellectual, or cognitive disabilities are sexually active and have similar sexual and reproductive health (SRH) needs as individuals without disabilities but often experience multiple structural and social barriers to adequate health information and services.[1-5] Examples of structural barriers to adequate health services include examining tables that do not accommodate the patient's disability or the lack of appropriate assistive devices that allow mobility on to or off of the exam table. Social barriers include the failure of health-care providers to assess the sexual and/or reproductive health needs and address the questions of patients with various disabilities.

All of these barriers to care have significant impact on the reproductive health of women living with neurologic illness or injury.[6] To adapt a phrase from Fiona Williams, women with disabilities are women, too.[7] Women with disability experience barriers to reproductive care including: sexual health and wellness, preconception care, prenatal care, and care during labor and delivery and in the postpartum period.[8] Providers often report barriers to providing care to patients with disabilities. Barriers to care occur at the level of the practitioner, the clinic, the health-care system, scientific evidence, and society (Figure 9.1).[9] The barriers to patients and the barriers to

providers act synergistically to decrease access to care and subsequently increase the risk of adverse outcomes and dissatisfaction with care in this patient population.

Women with physical disabilities due to neurologic disorders, including spinal cord injury or disorders (SCI/D), are a particularly at-risk group for marginalization, with literature suggesting that their sexual and reproductive health (SRH) needs are not being adequately addressed in the United States and on a global scale.[10-12] This issue has been identified as a definite area for improvement by almost every publication on the topic. Over the past several decades, dramatic advances in medical management have led to improvement in overall health outcomes for these patients, allowing many women to live successfully with congenital or acquired neurologic injuries or illnesses that would have been fatal just a few years earlier.[13] As risk factors related to morbidity and mortality in spinal cord disorders are better controlled, motherhood is slowly but increasingly becoming a sought-after option for this patient population.[14]

PRECONCEPTUAL BARRIERS

Women with chronic medical conditions are at higher risk of unintended pregnancy.[15] This may be because women with neurological injury or illness, cognitive, or mobility-related disability are often viewed by society as asexual or sexually innocent,[16] which often leads to exclusion from sexual counseling and can result in lower levels of sexual knowledge, especially for individuals with congenital conditions or injuries during childhood due to overprotective parents.[5] While we know that unintended pregnancies are associated with adverse maternal and perinatal outcomes,[17,18] these assumptions form a barrier to appropriate reproductive care. Sexual and reproductive health

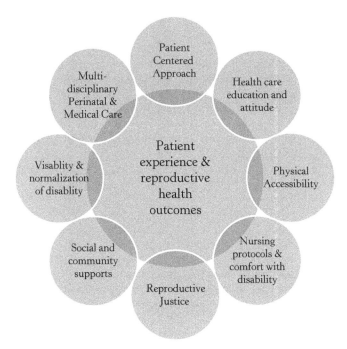

FIGURE 9.1 Principles in the reproductive care of women with neurologic illnesses or injury.

(SRH) topics may be unaddressed by health-care providers due to underlying negative attitudes towards sexuality in the context of disability.[5,19] WWDs are at a significant and unique disadvantage because of intersectional discrimination of gender and disability resulting in a higher likelihood of experiencing exclusion when compared with women without disability or men with disability.[1,20] This social and medical marginalization compromises critical outcomes in WWD including education, employment, and attainment of health including SRH.[21] With regard to SRH, many women may not know how their medical condition will impact their ability to have children or may encounter providers who advise them to practice abstinence or terminate their pregnancy because of their disability. And they often struggle to find providers who are able to manage both their SRH care while also addressing medical issues associated with their disabilities.[5,22] WWDs are also less likely to receive SRH maintenance and preventative services such as cervical and breast cancer screening, contraceptive counseling, preconception counseling, and testing for sexually transmitted infections.[2,4,23,24] It is not clear if this is because providers that typically see WWD for maintenance care are less comfortable discussing these aspects of care, do not view this areas of care as urgent/needed in WWD, or

a lack of knowledge by these providers of the potential for sexual activity in WWD. WWD may not have additional visits with general obstetrics/gynecology (ob/gyn) providers, even in adulthood, and addressing these issues or referral for visits with ob/gyn providers with experience caring for WWD are key to assuring that reproductive needs are met and discussed. This is especially true for the woman with disability that began in childhood as she transitions into adulthood. Both her and her family/partner will likely have questions and needs regarding puberty, sexuality, and reproductive health that need to be addressed as part of whole patient-centered care. Additionally, the fact that women with all sorts of disability seek sexual intimacy for pleasure and fulfillment is counternormative in today's society as is the concept that women with disability seek pregnancy intentionally.[25] These assumptions create further barriers to both sexual reproductive health and perinatal care for women with disabilities, including neurologic illness or injury.[14,25,26]

Interestingly, approximately half of all women with disability report some degree of sexual dysfunction,[27] yet high-quality research remains lacking. Opening the conversation and addressing these issues may improve the ability of WWD to have happy and healthy sexual relationships and interactions. Assumptions of heteronormity of the sexual experience should be avoided, as women (and men) with disability may choose to (or be primarily able to) experience sexuality without traditional penetration modalities. WWD even without partners may still be interested in sexuality and discussion of options and ways to achieve sexual satisfaction without partnered sex.

Women with neurologic illness and injury often desire pregnancy and should be allowed to consider it a possibility. Many women feel that their providers do not consider pregnancy an option for them or review the positive aspects of this choice with them as well as the risks. As stated in her study of disabled women's experiences of pregnancy, birth and motherhood by Walsh-Gallagher et al, "The women in this study welcomed pregnancy as affirming their identity and worth as women and as mothers. They encountered mixed reactions from partners and families, while professionals tended to view them as liabilities, regarding most as 'high risk.'"[28]

The predominant expert opinion is that fertility in women, unlike men, is only minimally impacted by their neurologic injury or illness, if at all. Studies of women with spinal cord injury suggest that only a minority are counseled about the possibility of pregnancy.[26] This lack of counseling and anticipatory guidance may, in part, be one of the reasons pregnancy is uncommon in the spinal cord injury population. The motivational speaker Muniba Mazari, who was is in a wheelchair after a traumatic spine injury in a car accident, often speaks about being told that she would be unable to have children immediately after her injury and the devastating effect this had on her recovery despite the fact that the fertility is not generally affected by spinal injury.[29] Additionally, while optimization of medical status prior to pregnancy is one of the primary principles of management of pregnancy in this population,[30,31] without proactive counseling the opportunity for such medical optimization is missed.

BARRIERS TO PERINATAL CARE

Studies of barriers to prenatal care have cited lack of provider experience, negative provider and medical professional attitude, and lack of accessibility as the most common barriers to perinatal care.[32] These barriers act synergistically with barriers to providers, including lack of accessibility, lack of education, and lack of experience providing care to this group of women.[9] WWD have lower rates of employment, which may lead to insurance barriers, as well as to lower rates of social engagement and limited social supports for assistance and advocacy.[33] WWD may experience extreme societal isolation in some cases. Overall, the dearth of research in issues around women with various disabilities and medical care creates a sense of erasure,[32] which does not foster excellent perinatal care.

Survey data has suggested that poor experiences with the medical system are common in women with physical disability. The prenatal care providers' office is usually the first location of perinatal care. Inaccessible offices are a common barrier to perinatal care cited by both patients and practitioners.[9,32] The physical office would ideally be designed with doorways wide enough to allow a wheelchair to easily pass through, with motorized beds allowing the bed to be placed at a low height to allow transfer from a wheelchair to a bed—and slightly higher to allow for ease of transfer from bed to wheelchair. Additionally, scales that allow weight to be taken with a wheelchair are important for monitoring of weight.[26] Women with relapsing/remitting or progressive neurologic diseases, such as MS, may have fluctuations in their abilities and needs for these assistive devices and adaptations, and their prior needs should not be assumed to be the same at every visit.[34] Pregnancy weight gain and body changes may also change adaptive needs through pregnancy, and occupational/physical therapy should likely be involved on an ongoing basis.[35] Providers are typically unaware that WWD are at increased risk for domestic violence and other forms of abuse. WWD have higher rates of intimate partner violence than other groups, and screening for this is key to assuring safety and improving perinatal outcomes.[15] Additionally, physical and sexual abuse are common in WWD, and assessment and sensitivity to this possibility are needed for health care providers when caring for these women.

A more difficult barrier to address includes the attitudes of staff and providers caring for patients with disabilities intersecting with pregnancy. In studies of patient experience, many patients report negatively biased healthcare worker attitudes.[6] This forms a barrier to even the initiation of care. In one study, 44% of gynecology offices refused to accept a patient with limited mobility who could not self-transfer onto examination tables and lacked any assistive devices.[26] Additionally, in surveys of patients with mobility-limiting disabilities, negative reactions from health-care workers (such as "I asked for help twice and got a lecture by the head nurse about how the heck are you going to take care of a baby?")[32] were cited as a difficulty encountered in perinatal care. Some of this bias can be attributed to a lack of knowledge and expertise. When objective data is reviewed, most women with physical disability perform a wide variety of childcare for their child, often with assistance from their partner or mother, but are generally satisfied with both their ability to maintain care and the amount of assistance received.[36]

Most survey participants reported that it was difficult to access information about pregnancy and disability either from providers or community resources.[32] In a recent survey, almost all practitioners, including experienced clinicians, describe a lack of education and training related to maternity care and perinatal needs of women with disabilities.[9] Providers report a desire for this education, training, and for clinical guidelines and tools to aid in the care of these patients,[9] and it does not escape the people providing perinatal and sexual/reproductive health care for women with disabilities that accessibility, knowledge, and training is important while caring for this population. The lack of evidence around best practices in this population provides additional barriers,[9] and one of the goals of this volume is to provide evidence around best practices in women with chronic neurologic illness or injury.

System level barriers for the perinatal care of women with various disability include time and scheduling constraints as well as insurance reimbursement policies.[9] Providers report that the pressure to confine care to the 10–15 minute time slot allotted per patient per prenatal visit potentially compromises care particularly in women with disabilities, whose visit may take up to 3–4 times the allotted appointment time, and when this is combined with low payment rates for maternity care with complex needs, this does make it difficult to provide high-quality perinatal care for patients with disabilities.[9] Additionally, the medical care system is not set up to encourage multidisciplinary management, which is important in the management of many neurologic injuries or illnesses during pregnancy. Utilization of complex care services, medical homes, and maternal-fetal medicine services prior to and during pregnancy may assist in removing some of these barriers.

OPTIMIZING CARE

While there are many barriers to the care of patients with the various forms of disability frequently encountered in patients with neurologic illness or injury, these barriers are not insurmountable. Exposure and education can improve

both knowledge- and attitude-based barriers for people with disabilities in various settings.[37] Educational strategies that show promise to improve the care of individuals with disabilities include the following: (1) framing disability as part of the spectrum of human diversity, (2) skills training for assessment of disability, (3) learning about the roles of the spectrum of health-care practitioners to form integrated teams focused around individual patient needs, (4) understanding how to accommodate disability in health-care settings as well as the requirement to do so, and (5) emphasis on and competency in approaches consistent with patient-centered care.[38] Additionally, there is evidence that exposure to a curriculum about patient-centered care in a disability context improves attitudes of medical students as well as other health-care students.[39,40]

While the erasure of women with disability from society[41]—including restricted media portrayals, reduced employment, lower rates of social engagement,[33,42] and reduced access to health care, has created health disparities[28] and barriers to accessing care, those barriers are surmountable. Education aimed at caring for women with specific illnesses and injuries and a patient-centered approach toward both, the medical care will improve access to care and experiences interacting with the health-care system (Figure 9.1). Providing an appropriately accessible physical environment is essential to delivering high-quality perinatal care in this population.[26] Ultimately, the care of women with neurologic illness or injury, including perinatal care, contraception, sexuality care, and health care in general will benefit from research that addresses the specific health needs of these women and results in evidence-based approaches to help optimize outcomes in this population.

REFERENCES

1. World Health Organization, Research DoRHa, Fund UNP. *Promoting sexual and reproductive health for persons with disabilities: WHO/UNFPA guidance note.* 2009. http://www.who.int/reproductivehealth/publications/general/9789241598682/en/
2. McRee AL, Haydon AA, Halpern CT. Reproductive health of young adults with physical disabilities in the U.S. *Prev Med.* 2010; 51(6): 502–504.
3. Becker H, Stuifbergen A, Tinkle M. Reproductive health care experiences of women with physical disabilities: a qualitative study. *Arch Phys Med Rehabil.* 1997; 78(12 Suppl 5): S26–33.
4. Cheng MM, Udry JP. Sexual behaviour of physically disabled adolescents in the United States. *Journal of Adolescent Health.* 2002; 31: 48–58.

5. Personal experiences of pregnancy and fertility in individuals with spinal cord injury. *Sex Disabil.* 2014; 32(1): 65–74.

6. Iezzoni LI, Wint AJ, Smeltzer SC, Ecker JL. Effects of disability on pregnancy experiences among women with impaired mobility. *Acta Obstet Gynecol Scand.* 2015; 94(2): 133–140.

7. Williams F. Women with learning disabilities are women too. In M. Langan and L. Day (Eds.), *Women, oppression and social work.* London: Routledge; 2002.

8. Smeltzer SC. Pregnancy in women with physical disabilities. *Journal of Obstetric, Gynecologic, and Neonatal Nursing.* 2007; 36(1): 88–96.

9. Mitra M, Smith LD, Smeltzer SC, Lonb-Bellil LM, Moring MS, Iezzoni LI. Barriers to providing maternity care to women with physical disabilities: Perspectives from health care practitioners. *Disabil Health J.* 2017; 10: 445–450.

10. Bertschy S, Pannek J, Meyer T. Delivering care under uncertainty: Swiss providers' experiences in caring for women with spinal cord injury during pregnancy and childbirth—an expert interview study. *BMC Pregnancy Childbirth.* 2016; 16(1): 181.

11. Iezzoni LI, Yu J, Wint AJ, Smeltzer SC, Ecker JL. Prevalence of current pregnancy among US women with and without chronic physical disabilities. *Med Care.* 2013; 51(6): 555–562.

12. Lipson JG, Rogers JG. Pregnancy, birth, and disability: Women's health care experiences. *Health Care Women Int.* 2000; 21(1): 11–26.

13. Ward J, Walker C. Caring for reproductive-aged women with spinal cord injuries: a case report. *Obstet Med.* 2012; 5(3): 133–134.

14. Iezzoni LI, Chen Y, McLain AB. Current pregnancy among women with spinal cord injury: Findings from the US national spinal cord injury database. *Spinal Cord.* 2015; 53(11): 821–826.

15. Barranti CCR, Yuen FKO. Intimate partner violence and women with disabilities: Toward bringing visibility to an unrecognized population. *Journal of Social Work in Disability & Rehabilitation.* 2008; 7(2): 115–130.

16. Dotson LA, Stinson J, Christian L. People tell me I can't have sex. *Women & Therapy.* 2008; 26(3–4): 195–209.

17. Kost K, Landry D, Darroch J. The effects of pregnancy planning status on birth outcomes and infant care. *Fam Plann Perspect.* 1988; 30: 223–230.

18. Mohllajee A, Curtis K, Morrow B, Marchbanks P. Pregnancy intention and its relationship to birth and maternal outcomes. *Obstet Gynecol.* 2007; 109: 678–686.

19. Wolfe PS. The influence of personal values on issues of sexuality and disability. *Sexuality and Disability.* 1997; 15(2): 69–90.

20. Astbury J, Walji F. The prevalence and psychological costs of household violence by family members against women with disabilities in Cambodia. *J Interpers Violence.* 2014; 29(17): 3127–3149.

21. Lee K, Devine A, Marco MJ, Zayas J, Gill-Atkinson L, Vaughan C. Sexual and reproductive health services for women with disability: A qualitative study with service providers in the Philippines. *BMC Womens Health.* 2015; 15: 87.

22. Nosek MA, Howland CA, Rintala DH, Young ME, Chanpong GF. National study of women with physical disabilities: Final report. *Sexuality and Disability.* 2001; 19(1): 5–39.

23. Armour BS, Thierry JM, Wolf LA. State-level differences in breast and cervical cancer screening by disability status: United States, 2008. *Womens Health Issues.* 2009; 19(6): 406–414.

24. Nosek MA, Howland CA. Breast and cervical cancer screening among women with physical disabilities. *Arch Phys Med Rehabil.* 1997; 78(12 Suppl 5): S39–44.

25. Iezzoni LI, Mitra M. Transcending the counternormative: Sexual and reproductive health in persons with disability. *Disabil Health J.* 2017; 10: 369–370.

26. Iezzoni LI, Wint AJ, Smeltzer SC, Ecker JL. Physical accessibility of routine prenatal care for women with mobility disability. *J Womens Health (Larchmt).* 2015; 24(12): 1006–1012.

27. Coyle CP, Santiago MC, Shank JW, Ma GX, Boyd R. Secondary conditions and women with physical disabilities: A descriptive study. *Archives of Physical Medicine and Rehabilitation.* 2000; 81(10): 1380–1387.

28. Walsh-Gallagher D, Sinclair M, McConkey R. The ambiguity of disabled women's experiences of pregnancy, childbirth, and motherhood: A phenomenological understanding. *Midwifery.* 2012; 28(2): 156–162.

29. Turning Adversity into Opportunity. *TEDx Islamabad*: YouTube; 2015. https://www.youtube.com/watch?v=I68Y81ZpjNM. Accessed 1/8/2017

30. Pereira L. Obstetric management of the patient with spinal cord injury. *Obstet Gynecol Surv.* 2003; 58(10): 678–687.

31. ACOG Committee Opinion: Number 275, September 2002. Obstetric management of patients with spinal cord injuries. *Obstet Gynecol.* 2002; 100(3): 625–627.

32. Tarasoff LA. 'We don't know. We've never had anybody like you before': Barriers to perinatal care for women with physical disabilities. *Disabil Health J.* 2017; 10: 426–433.

33. Hanna WJ, Rogovsky B. Women with disabilities: Two handicaps plus. *Disability, Handicap & Society.* 1991; 6(1): 49–63.

34. Peters SL. Having a disability 'sometimes.' *Canadian Woman Studies.* 1993; 13(4): 26–27.

35. Ghai A. *(Dis)embodied form: Issues of disabled women.* Har-Anand; 2003. Har Anand Publications (June 30, 2007). New Delhi: Shakti Books, ©2003.

36. Jacob J, Kirschbaum M, Preston P. Mothers with physical disabilities caring for young children. *Social Work in Disability & Rehabilitation.* 2017; 16(2): 95–115.

37. Vornholt K, Uitdewilligen S, Nijhuis FJN. Factors affecting the acceptance of people with disabilities at work: A literature review. *Journal of Occupational Rehabilitation.* 2013; 23(4): 463–475.

38. Iezzoni LI, Long-Bellil LM. Training physicians about caring for persons with disabilities: 'Nothing about us without us!' *Disabil Health J.* 2012; 5: 136–139.

39. Robey KL, Minihan PM, Long-Bellil LM, Hahn JE, Reiss JG, Eddey GE. Teaching health care students about disability within a cultural competancy context. *Disabil Health J.* 2013; 6: 271–297.

40. Symons AB, Morley CP, McGuigan D, Akl EA. A curriculum on care for people with disabilities: Effects on medical student self-reported attitudes and comfort level. *Disabil Health J.* 2014; 7: 88–95.

41. Zitzelberger H. (In)visibility: accounts of embodiment of women with physical disabilities and differences. *Disability & Society.* 2010; 20(4): 389–403.

42. Zayid M. I got 99 problems . . . palsy is just one. *TedWomen* 2013; https://www.ted.com/talks/maysoon_zayid_i_got_99_problems_palsy_is_just_one, accssed 1/8/2018.

SECTION 2

Central Nervous System Neurologic Diseases

10

Immune-mediated Disorders of the Central Nervous System

PATRICIA K. COYLE

This chapter will cover pregnancy issues in two diseases, multiple sclerosis (MS) and neuromyelitis optica spectrum disorder (NMOSD), and one syndrome, acute transverse myelitis (ATM). All three disorders are immune-mediated and pathologically confined to the central nervous system (CNS). The CNS encompasses the brain, spinal cord, and optic nerves.

Emerging understanding of the immunology of pregnancy supports dynamic and changing immune interactions between the mother and fetus.[1] These occur over the entire 9 months. During the first trimester there is inflammation that helps to promote blastocyst implantation and development. During the second trimester an anti-inflammatory T helper 2 (Th2) milieu is promoted, to support fetal growth. During the third trimester there is an inflammatory switch to a Th1 background, to prepare for labor and delivery. In addition to the systemic immune system, there is increasing evidence that the maternal microbiota of the gut, uterus and placenta also play a role in fetal health.[1,2]

Such data highlights that special concerns may be raised about the impact of pregnancy in the setting of women with preexisting immune-mediated disorders, particularly when they involve the CNS. This is because hormonal and micro-biota changes, via neuroendocrine and gut-brain axis connections, would be expected to have particular consequences for the CNS. The following summarizes current information on pregnancy in the three selected disorders, with a care map based on distinct time periods (Box 10.1).

MULTIPLE SCLEROSIS (MS): BACKGROUND

MS is considered the major CNS disease of young adults, short of trauma. It is estimated to affect at least 947,000 Americans,[3A] and over 2.5 million individuals worldwide.[3] These numbers are likely underestimates. MS has several characteristic features. The disease is not evenly distributed. Globally there are low, medium, and high-risk zones (classically there are low rates of MS at the Equator, but affected individuals become increasingly common as you move away geographically either north or south). There is a current female to male ratio of about 3:1. This is rising because MS has been documented to be increasing among women.[4] Although it largely affects individuals with a Caucasian Northern European background (>90%), MS is being seen in diverse groups including African Americans, Asians, and Hispanics. In fact, in one recent study the risk for MS was found to be highest in African American females.[5] The disease affects young people: 90% present between the ages of 15 to 50 years. MS is extremely variable clinically. No two patients are alike. MS ranges from those who have pathologic but silent disease, to those that present clinically with a disease course that can be mild, severe, or anything in between.

The major clinical phenotype is relapsing MS, where patients experience episodic neurologic abnormalities (also referred to as attacks, flare-ups, exacerbations, or relapses), but are clinically stable in between these attacks.[6] This is how 85% to 90% of MS patients start out. The neuroimaging biomarker for relapse is a contrast positive lesion on magnetic resonance imaging (MRI). Relapses are associated in particular with young age and early disease. There is also a progressive form of MS, which shows gradual clinical worsening (typically in the form of a myelopathy). There are two progressive phenotypes. Slow worsening from onset is primary progressive MS. Patients present a decade later than their relapsing MS counterparts (late 30s, early to mid-40s), and show an equal sex ratio. Relapsing patients can also transition to

---

BOX 10.1
CARE MAP FOR PREGNANCY IN THE IMMUNE-MEDIATED DISORDER PATIENT

BEFORE PREGNANCY/PRE-PREGNANCY/NON-PREGNANT

Confirm the neurologic diagnosis
Assess disease severity (clinical and MRI disease activity profile; prognostic indicators)
Explain genetics (in the case of MS)
Discuss need for planned pregnancy timing
Contraception counseling
Correct low vitamin D levels
Avoid smoking
Discuss DMT washout plans

DURING PREGNANCY

Folic acid
Routine monitoring (ultrasound can be done in high risk situations)
Review criteria to recognize disease relapses
If there is disease activity, evaluate and treat if necessary

DELIVERY

No special precautions necessary (unless a woman is significantly disabled)

POSTPARTUM

Must have discussion about breastfeeding vs. resumption of DMT, and whether DMT can be used while breastfeeding
If breastfeeding is done, it should be exclusive
Contraception counseling
Periodic monitoring of vitamin D levels

---

the secondary progressive phenotype, typically at midlife (around menopause/perimenopause). In such patients relapses become less and less frequent and ultimately (typically) cease. However, the prototypic MS patient remains a young woman of childbearing age with relapsing disease. This is why pregnancy is such a major concern in MS. Pregnancy issues have been complicated by the development of multiple disease modifying therapies (DMTs) that modulate or suppress the immune system. As a general rule, they are not used during pregnancy.

The precise cause of MS remains unknown. There are several hundred disease-associated genes, important environmental risk factors, and ultimately an organ-specific immune-mediated disease process. In MS the host immune system is continually attacking the CNS, to cause ongoing damage.

MS: PREGNANCY

MS shows interesting links to hormonal states. Disease onset starts to rise at puberty and then increases over the next 10 to 15 years. It is at this time that the female predominance becomes evident. In the rare pediatric onset individual before puberty, no sex preference is appreciated. In contrast onset of the progressive phenotype shows an age-related link to perimenopause/menopause, with no sexual preference. With regard to the menstrual cycle, MS symptoms are often reported to worsen around the time of menstruation.

Pregnancy is the best studied hormonal state in MS. There are key counseling issues that arise before, during, and after pregnancy (Table 10.1). First, it is important to reassure individuals with MS that it is not an inherited disease. Most people with MS (80%) have no other family member affected. Although there are many genes that slightly

---

TABLE 10.1 KEY PREGNANCY COUNSELING ISSUES FOR MS

Pre-Pregnancy
- You do not inherit MS
  - 80% of MS individuals have no positive family history
  - Risk of MS rises from 0.13% to 2%-2.5% with affected parent, 2.7% with affected sib[81]
- Pregnancy does not worsen MS (may be beneficial for relapsing MS)
- MS does not cause issues with ability to conceive, pregnancy itself, or fetal health; it does not produce a high risk pregnancy
- Assisted reproductive technology/in vitro fertilization techniques which use gonadotropin releasing hormone agonists, and which fail, are associated with a 3-month period of increased risk of MS (clinical/MRI) disease activity
- Maternal vitamin D levels should be normalized
- Typically effective contraception should be used in female MS patients on DMTs (see Table 10.2 for exceptions)

Pregnancy
- MS disease activity goes down, particularly in the last trimester
- Relapses can occur during pregnancy; it is safe to treat with short term corticosteroids
- MRI scans can be done during pregnancy, but gadolinium-based contrast agents should be avoided
- Any form of delivery and anesthetic can be used in MS

Post-Partum
- The 3 months postpartum are a time of increased clinical and MRI disease activity
- Exclusive breastfeeding decreases MS disease activity (but it is unclear how it compares to effective DMT use)
- There is no need to avoid breastfeeding after contrast MRI; breastfeeding should be delayed ≥one hour after corticosteroid treatment
- For most DMTs (see Table 10.2) the option is to resume the DMT, or to breastfeed

---

increase risk of the disease, and there are likely other linked protective and disease severity genes, there is no single gene that can pass on MS to a child. Environmental factors (such as vitamin D deficiency, smoking, adolescent obesity, Epstein-Barr virus infection) contribute to MS occurrence in unexplained ways and may be more important than genetic factors.

Up until the 1950s women with MS were advised not to get pregnant because it would worsen their MS. This turned out to be untrue. At least 87% to 97% of pregnant MS patients have the relapsing form of the disease and are typically without significant disability.[7,8] There is now convincing data that pregnancy does not worsen the long-term prognosis of relapsing MS,[9,10] and in some studies in fact seems to improve it.[11-14] In a multicenter case control study of a first demyelinating event, higher parity for women was associated with a decreasing risk for development of a first clinical attack.[15] Other studies found that giving birth, or even having a terminated pregnancy, protected against MS, at least for the next 5-year period.[16,17] In contrast there is no robust data for the impact of pregnancy on progressive MS. One study hinted that it may be distinct from relapsing MS.[18] Anecdotal concerns have been raised about

pregnancy in progressive MS, and it would be expected that the rare pregnancy in a disabled individual would at least influence choice of delivery methods.

Pregnancy may have an activating effect on silent MS. Radiologically isolated syndrome (RIS) involves individuals with an abnormal brain MRI compatible with MS but with no prior suggestive neurologic history and a normal examination. In a study of 7 RIS individuals who became pregnant, 57% had a postpartum clinical attack.[19] In the RIS control group (N = 53), only 41.5% showed clinical conversion. T2 lesion development was significantly higher in the pregnancy cohort.

MS itself is not associated with infertility, abnormal fetal development, or ability to carry to term. In a small series of 115 consecutive French women who became pregnant, there was no impact of clinical phenotype or prior DMT use.[20] MS has no increase in spontaneous abortions, still births, cesarean delivery, premature delivery, or birth defects.[21,22] Some studies have reported that MS babies are a bit smaller in weight and length, but other studies do not confirm this. In summary, having MS does not put the fetus at any extra risk and does not constitute a high-risk pregnancy.

There has been controversy about whether MS shows poorer ovarian reserve. One study used transvaginal ultrasound to examine mean ovarian volume, antral follicle number, and ovarian stromal artery blood flow, in 19 MS and 25 control subjects.[23] They concluded that the MS group had lower ovarian reserve, based on lower mean ovarian volume and antral follicle numbers. A later study raised concerns that relapsing MS women may have decreased ovarian reserve, based on low serum anti-Müllerian hormone levels compared to healthy controls.[24] This was not due to detectable anti-ovarian antibodies, or abnormalities in interleukin (IL)-1 α or β levels.[25] A subsequent study of 25 relapsing MS women and 25 matched controls did not confirm low hormone levels.[26] In addition, antral follicle count on ultrasound was normal in the MS group as a whole. However, those with higher versus lower disease activity did show poorer ovarian reserve (lower anti-Müllerian hormone levels, total antral follicle count, and ovarian volume).

Approximately 10% of all women encounter problems getting pregnant, and may seek assisted reproductive technology/in vitro fertilization. Although overall numbers are small, 3 independent groups found that MS women who go through such a procedure and fail to get pregnant are at risk during the three months following the procedure for increased disease activity (both clinical and MRI).[27-29] One group reported this risk was associated with use of gonadotropin releasing hormone agonists rather than antagonists. Based on this preliminary data, it would seem reasonable to recommend preferential use of antagonists in MS women undergoing fertility treatment.

Because vitamin D deficiency is identified as an environmental risk factor for development of MS, it is standard practice to check vitamin D 25 hydroxy levels in MS patients and replace any deficiency to normal range.[30] Several thousand units of over-the- counter vitamin D3 is easy to use for this. Therefore one would think that most pregnant MS women are likely to have normal levels. However, a recent small study found that deficient levels were common.[31] Maternal hypovitaminosis D is associated with adverse neonatal outcomes, providing further rationale for normalizing levels.[32,33] There is conflicting evidence as to whether maternal vitamin D deficiency increases risk of MS in the offspring.[34,35] In a recent Danish study, neonatal vitamin D levels inversely correlated with risk of MS.[36]

Contraception is an important topic to discuss with at-risk MS women of reproductive age. The goal is always a planned versus unexpected pregnancy. A recent systematic review of contraception use in MS found no evidence that oral contraceptives, or combined oral contraceptives, worsened the disease course.[37] Only 4 studies met the criteria for inclusion, however, and the level of evidence was considered limited. Among all the diverse methods that women can use, long acting reversible contraception (also referred to as LARC) is preferred based on efficacy (>99%), safety, and convenience.[38] This involves an intrauterine device, or implanted rod, that lasts several years. In 2016 the Centers for Disease Control and Prevention provided contraception guidance for the first time ever for women with MS.[39] They stated that all of the various methods appeared to be safe. However, combined hormonal contraceptives were not recommended for MS women with prolonged immobility, due to concerns about venous thromboembolism. These combined hormonal methods involved low dose combined oral contraceptives (≤35 mcg ethinyl estradiol), the hormonal patch, and the vaginal ring. They also noted a concern that bone health should be assessed and followed if depo medroxyprogesterone was used.

Pregnancy itself has an impressive impact on MS. The relapse rate is reduced by as much as 60% to 70% during the third trimester. This effect on disease activity is not as strong in the first two-thirds of pregnancy, and it is certainly possible to see clinical attacks. In a recent series relapse during pregnancy occurred in 15% to 22.6% of women.[40] There are two issues that arise when a pregnant woman experiences an acute relapse. The first involves the evaluation, and the second involves treatment. MRI scans, if they are deemed necessary and helpful, can be done during pregnancy.[41,42] MRI scans are considered safe, with no radiation exposure. Use of a gadolinium-based contrast agent is more controversial because it is known to deposit into human brain tissue. Contrast agents involve fairly large water-soluble molecules that cross the placenta somewhat slowly. Contrast will appear in the fetal bladder by 11 minutes after maternal injection. Contrast is generally cleared into the amniotic fluid, where it is swallowed by the fetus and then undergoes gastrointestinal reabsorption.[42] A recent review of this issue included summary guidelines and suggested that contrast be used during pregnancy on a case-by- case basis only if benefits outweighed the poorly defined risks.[42] The standard treatment for an acute relapse, to speed up recovery, is an optional short (3- to 5-day) course of high-dose corticosteroids. This can be either intravenous or oral because of high corticosteroid bioavailability. The most common dose is one gram of methylprednisolone, or its equivalent per day. Use of corticosteroids does not affect the ultimate degree of recovery, so they do not have to be used; however, they can jump-start the improvement phase. It is accepted that corticosteroids can be given at any time during the pregnancy, including the first trimester. Earlier concerns about increased risk for orofacial clefts with first trimester use have not been confirmed.[43] Short-acting agents such as prednisone or methylprednisolone are metabolized by the placental enzyme 11-β-hydroxysteroid, so that fetal exposure is reduced to about 10% of the maternal dose.[44] In contrast, fluorinated agents such as dexamethasone or betamethasone cross the placenta relatively intact and should be avoided.

There is no limitation on choice of delivery anesthetic (including epidural or spinal anesthesia) or delivery procedure for a woman with MS. The one exception is the unusual case of the pregnant MS individual who is disabled, with significant motor limitations and/or respiratory dysfunction. This would likely influence available options.

The postpartum period, particularly the first 3 months, is recognized to carry risk for increased MS disease activity. High relapse rate and greater disability before pregnancy, as well as relapse during pregnancy, are associated with increased risk for postpartum activity.[8,45,46] In contrast, low maternal vitamin D levels were not predictive in a small scale study.[47] In the large MSBase pregnancy registry study, use of DMTs prior to pregnancy decreased risk for postpartum relapses.[8] This led the authors to recommend that it might be better to treat newly diagnosed women for 1 to 2 years, before they attempted pregnancy. This seems particularly important in the face of active, poor prognosis MS. In the historic Pregnancy in MS (PRIMS) study, 30% of MS women had a postpartum relapse within 3 months.[7] In the more recent MSBase registry study, 14% of MS women had such a postpartum relapse.[8] This is consistent with the general observation that the attack rate is diminishing in modern-era MS.

Traditionally, postpartum MS individuals usually decide either to breastfeed or to initiate/resume a DMT. However, recent evidence suggests that some agents can be used safely while breastfeeding (see Section 5, Chapter 35). Pediatrics recommends that women breastfeed exclusively (less than 1 bottle daily) for at least 6 months for the health of both the mother and infant. There have been a number of prospective studies, as well as a meta-analysis of breastfeeding by MS mothers, that have predominantly focused on the impact of breastfeeding on postpartum attacks.[7,46,48,49] No study has reported a negative effect of breastfeeding in MS. Although the evidence is not conclusive, it does appear that exclusive breastfeeding suppresses disease activity while nonexclusive breastfeeding may not. Exclusive breastfeeding produces a lactational amenorrhea, with increased prolactin levels and low nonpulsatile luteinizing hormone levels. One could hypothesize that these changes are somehow beneficial to reduce MS disease activity. Prolactin is considered an immune system stimulant, but it impacts on both innate and acquired immune responses and promotes both oligodendrocyte and neuronal precursor cells.[50] Prior studies reported that breastfeeding for an extended period (over 4 months) lowers the risk of subsequent MS in the child,[51] while breastfeeding for over 15 months lowers risk of subsequent MS in the mother.[52]

With regard to evaluating and treating postpartum relapses in a woman who is breastfeeding, gadolinium-based contrast agent excretion into breast milk in the first 24 hours is <0.04% of the IV dose.[41] Less than 1% of this is absorbed by the infant's GI tract. Therefore, the recommendation is not to interrupt breastfeeding after contrast is given for either MRI or CT evaluations. With regard to breastfeeding during IV methylprednisolone therapy for relapse, a recent study found the relative infant dose was only 0.71% of the weight-adjusted maternal dose.[53] They noted a low infant exposure by simply delaying breastfeeding for 1 hour after infusion; waiting 2 to 4 hours limits exposure even more dramatically.

Prior accepted guidelines have indicated that DMTs should not be used in women who are pregnant, trying to become pregnant, or who are breastfeeding. However, accumulating data is leading to modifications in such guidelines to make them less rigid. Table 10.2 updates the latest information on the currently approved MS DMTs with regard to reasonable washouts prior to attempting pregnancy, as well as the feasibility of their use in pregnant women and breastfeeding women. There have now been sufficient human pregnancy exposures for glatiramer acetate, as well as the interferon betas as a class, to judge them as safe. They require no washout prior to an MS individual trying to become pregnant. Once pregnancy is confirmed, the DMTs are discontinued. However, a pregnant MS woman could choose to continue on treatment if she felt strongly about it. These DMTs are likely compatible with breastfeeding since they are safe and relatively

TABLE 10.2 APPROVED MS DMTS AND THEIR PREGNANCY AND BREASTFEEDING CONCERNS

DMT		Class, Dosing, and Brands	Pregnancy Washout	Pregnancy Use	Breastfeeding	Comments
Needle Injectables	Interferon Betas (IFNβs)	Regulatory cytokine; IFNβ-1b 250 mg SC every other day (Betaseron, Extavia); IFNβ-1a 44 (22) mcg SC 3x weekly (Rebif); IFNβ-1a 30 mcg IM weekly (Avonex); pegylated IFNβ-1a 125 mcg SC Q14 days (Plegridy)	None needed	Acceptable	Probably compatible; breast milk levels of drug 0.06%[82]	Over 1,000 human pregnancy exposures without teratogenic signal[83,84,85]
	Glatiramer acetate	Random polymers of 4 AAs; 40 mg SC 3x weekly (Copaxone); 20 mg SC daily (Copaxone, Glatopa)	None needed	Acceptable	Probably compatible	Over 7,000 human pregnancy exposures without teratogenic signal[86]
Orals	Fingolimod	Sphingosine-1 phosphate receptor modulator; 0.5 mg PO daily (Gilenya)	2 months, T ½ 6–9 days	No	Not recommended No human data; excreted into rat milk	Pregnancy outcomes from clinical development program raised concerns[87]; S1P receptor involvement in vascular formation during embryogenesis
	Teriflunomide	Mitochondrial enzyme inhibitor to block de novo pyrimidine pathway, cytostatic for activated lymphocytes; 14 (7) mg PO daily (Aubagio)	Accelerated elimination procedure up to 11 days using cholestyramine (or activated charcoal) to get blood level <0.02 mcg/ml	No	Not recommended No human data	Human exposures to date do not support teratogenicity or other issues (unlike animal models)[88]
	Dimethyl fumarate	Fumaric acid ester; 240 mg PO twice daily (Tecfidera)	Likely none needed, T ½ 1 hour	No	Not recommended No data	Human exposures to date do not suggest any issues[89]

	Drug	Mechanism	Washout/Half-life	Can be considered for highly active disease	Breastfeeding	Breast milk excretion	Pregnancy
Monoclonals	Natalizumab	Anti-α4 integrin humanized IgG4 monoclonal antibody: blocks adhesion molecule, interferes with cell trafficking; 300 mg IV Q4 weeks (Tysabri)	Ideally minimal to no washout (0–4 weeks), T½ 7–15 days	Can be considered for highly active disease	Use with caution	Excreted into breast milk 5.3% by day 50[90]	Maternal pregnancy exposure may produce temporary hematologic abnormalities in infant; human exposures to date appear safe[91,92]
	Alemtuzumab	Anti-CD52 cytolytic humanized IgG1 monoclonal antibody lyses CD4+ and CD8+ T cells; more transient lysis of B cells and monocytes; induction therapy with two cycles of treatment (Lemtrada)	4 months, T½ 2 weeks	No	Use with caution	No human data; excreted in monkey milk at <0.122%; should be at low level, likely destroyed in infant GI tract	Human pregnancy exposures to date appear safe[94]
	Daclizumab	Daclizumab Anti-CD25 humanized IgG1 monoclonal antibody; binds to high affinity IL2-receptor; 150 mg SC Q4 weeks (Zinbryta)	4 months, T½ 21 days No Use with caution	No		human data; excreted in monkey milk at <0.122%; should be at low level, likely destroyed in infant GI tract	Human pregnancy exposures to date appear safe[94]
	Ocrelizumab	Anti-CD20 cytolytic humanized IgG1 monoclonal antibody; 600 mg IV Q6 months (Ocrevus)	Label recommends 6 months, T½ 26 days	No	Use with caution	No human data; excreted in monkey milk	Based on other anti-CD20s, infants exposed during pregnancy may show transient B cell depletion, lymphopenia
Other	Mitoxantrone	Anthracenedione chemotherapy agent; intercalates into DNA, inhibits repair enzyme; 12 mg/m² IV Q3 months to lifetime maximum 140 mg/m² (Novantrone)	6 months, mean T½ 75 hours	No	Not acceptable	Excreted into breast milk at 2%–12%	This DMT is now rarely, if ever used in MS

large molecules, have negligible blood levels, and are likely to be degraded in the infant's gut.

The 3 oral agents are all small molecules. They do not have sufficient human pregnancy exposures to make definitive statements on safety. With regard to their washout periods, fingolimod requires approximately 2 months. The half-life of dimethyl fumarate is so short (1 hour) that one could choose no washout, since animal studies found no evidence of teratogenicity, and human exposures to date have not been associated with adverse outcomes.[54] Teriflunomide, because of its prolonged half-life, requires an 11-day elimination procedure with oral cholestyramine (8 grams three times daily) or oral activated charcoal (50 grams twice daily for 11 days). This is taken until the plasma level is <0.02 mcg/ml. Cholestyramine appears more efficient than charcoal and can be reduced to 4 grams if it is not well tolerated. Both cholestyramine and charcoal bind teriflunomide in the small intestine to prevent reabsorption and enterohepatic recirculation. Sometimes less than 11 days will be sufficient. In addition, the days do not have to be in a row. In the case of pregnancy, elimination is documented by confirming negligible plasma levels. With regard to breastfeeding on the oral agents, since clear human data is not available it should be avoided. One recent review on breastfeeding labeled fingolimod and teriflunomide as hazardous and dimethyl fumarate as possibly hazardous.[55]

Among the monoclonal antibodies, natalizumab has actually been maintained or restarted during pregnancy in small numbers of highly active patients.[56–58] Some have recommended treating through the second trimester.[59] In addition, extended dosing (every 6 to 8 weeks) could be done during pregnancy. This is one of two DMTs (fingolimod is the other) where a minority of MS subjects who discontinue therapy may experience rebound disease activity. It is interesting that both of these agents with risk of rebound interfere with lymphocyte trafficking. The major issue with use of natalizumab during pregnancy has been temporary hematologic disturbances (anemia, thrombocytopenia, pancytopenia) in the newborn. Since natalizumab is associated with rebound activity and is essentially gone after 3 months, as short a washout as possible is desirable prior to attempting pregnancy. Some practitioners even recommend no washout before trying to become pregnant. For the other monoclonals washouts of 4 (alemtuzumab, daclizumab) and 6 months (ocrelizumab) are recommended, although based on ocrelizumab's half-life one might consider approximately 4 months is reasonable as well. With regard to breastfeeding, transmission of IgG into breast milk can occur. There are receptors in the infant gut that could transport such IgG into the blood.[60] The monoclonals have limited human data on passage into breast milk. Natalizumab does enter breast milk, and infants show detectable levels.[90A] Of course IgG may be degraded in the infant's gastrointestinal tract. Since safety evidence is lacking, they should be used with caution. Mitoxantrone, a chemotherapeutic anthracenedione, is now rarely if ever used to treat MS. A 6-month washout is recommended for pregnancy. Since it is excreted into breast milk, breastfeeding is best avoided.

NMOSD: BACKGROUND

For many years NMOSD was considered a variant of MS. It is now recognized to be a unique neuroimmune CNS channelopathy that typically targets aquaporin 4 (AQP4), a water channel expressed on astrocyte foot processes. This astrocytopathy results in CNS inflammation and demyelination, mediated by antibody and complement, with neutrophil and eosinophil infiltrations. Th17 cells, and IL-17 and IL-23, are elevated in the blood and believed to play a role in disease pathogenesis.[61] The immunopathogenesis of NMOSD is quite different from MS, with an identified autoantigen target and autoantibody biomarker. NMOSD involves a much more destructive neuropathology than is seen in MS, and it carries a worse prognosis; often there is incomplete recovery from disease attacks. Unlike MS, NMOSD is uncommon in Caucasians. It accounts for only 1.5% of their demyelinating diseases. A significant proportion of affected individuals are Asians and blacks. They show an older age at onset (near 39 years), and a higher female- to-male ratio (7:1, to as high as 9:1) than MS. NMOSD can also occur in association with connective tissue diseases.

Formal diagnostic criteria were proposed in 2015.[62] Patients present with optic neuritis, transverse myelitis with a longitudinally extensive spinal cord lesion (>3 vertebral segments), area postrema syndrome (with acute persistent nausea, vomiting, and hiccups), or a variety of brainstem, diencephalon, and cerebral syndromes that can include posterior reversible encephalopathy syndrome. At least 60% to 80% of NMOSD patients are positive for serum IgG antibodies to AQP4. This is both a diagnostic and prognostic biomarker, which predicts risk for future attacks requiring maintenance therapy. There are many different assays to detect these autoantibodies, but cell-based assays are the most sensitive. A number of the MS DMTs (IFNβs, fingolimod, dimethyl fumarate, natalizumab, alemtuzumab) appear to worsen NMOSD, which emphasizes how important it is not to misdiagnose these patients as MS. Acute NMOSD attacks are treated with high dose corticosteroids, with plasma exchange routinely added for severe attacks. Plasma exchange has been used safely in pregnancy and lactation for a variety of conditions. Maintenance therapy involves anti-CD20 monoclonal antibodies, or other immunosuppressives such as azathioprine or mycophenolate mofetil. There are phase III trials in NMOSD currently investigating monoclonal antibodies against CD19, C5 and the IL-6 receptor. NMOSD involves a humoral (Th2-mediated) pathogenetic mechanism, with increasing data that the antibodies are pathologic. T cells also play a role. A subset of AQP4 IgG negative patients are positive for anti-myelin oligodendrocyte glycoprotein (MOG) antibodies. Perhaps 5% of NMOSD patients have a monophasic disorder and do not go on to later attacks; they would be in the AQP4 antibody negative group.

NMOSD: PREGNANCY

Because this is a much less common disease than MS, pregnancy data is more limited. However, NMOSD is even more enriched for women, and a good proportion of patients are within childbearing age. AQP4 is expressed on the syncytiotrophoblast of human and mouse placenta and is highest on the placenta during mid-gestation, peaking at 21 weeks.[63] Mice injected intraperitoneally with anti-AQP4 IgG develop a complement-dependent placentitis, followed by necrosis.[63] This would raise concern that pregnancy, which includes a period of shift from Th1 to Th2, could worsen a humorally-mediated disease such as NMOSD. Virtually no study to date reports any significant decrease in attacks during pregnancy, and in contrast to MS there is no meaningful and consistent decrease in disease activity during the third trimester. Two studies found increased attack rates during pregnancy.[64] One study reported no negative impact of epidural anesthesia or breastfeeding on the disease.[64A] There has been evidence for an increase in negative consequences in pregnant NMOSD women, such as miscarriages, pre-eclampsia, and prematurity.[65,66,66A] A recent review of pregnancy outcome in an international cohort of AQP4 antibody positive patients concluded that NMOSD is an independent risk factor for miscarriage. This is especially notable in the 3 years before and

after disease onset.[65] In particular pregnancies that occur at times of high disease activity are at increased risk for miscarriage. Women with NMOSD and additional autoimmune disorders are at increased risk for preeclampsia.[65] It appears that controlling disease activity before and during pregnancy improves pregnancy outcome. There is a consistent increased risk for attacks postpartum for at least 6 months, including in the first postpartum trimester.[66] This is similar to MS, and these postpartum relapses can be associated with increase in disability.[67,68] This is the basis for generally resuming maintenance therapy quickly after birth.[69] In one study of Japanese AQP4 antibody positive women, a relapse in the year before pregnancy, or discontinuing therapy or using low dose (versus high dose) immunosuppressive therapy during pregnancy, were associated with pregnancy-related relapses.[70] Nearly half of their pregnancy cohort had a pregnancy-related relapse. With regard to therapy during pregnancy, steroids (prednisone 10 mg daily) and plasma exchange have been used during pregnancy, and were reported to be well tolerated, while in one study azathroprine and cyclophosphamide were associated with issues.[67,71]

Therapies for NMOSD used to treat the mother may impact the fetus. In one case a pregnant woman, who had last received rituximab seven months prior to conception, gave birth to an otherwise healthy newborn with detectable anti-AQP4 antibodies and reduced B lymphocytes in cord blood.[72] Counts normalized by 3 months. In this case rituximab was restarted successfully 2 days after delivery. Rituximab and other monoclonals have limited to no human data on passage into breast milk (see earlier MS monoclonal antibody discussion). However, since they are large molecules, they are similarly unlikely to pass in breast milk and likely to be destroyed in the infant's gastrointestinal tract. However, since there is no evidence for their safety, they should be used with caution.

To summarize, women with NMOSD should be counseled that miscarriage rate is elevated; attacks can occur during pregnancy, but can be treated. Their pregnancy should be monitored closely. The postpartum period is associated with increased risk for disease activity and disability, so that maintenance therapy should be resumed after delivery. Ideally, it would be preferable to avoid any prolonged treatment-free period prior to pregnancy. That would favor trying to time pregnancy around an infrequently dosed disease therapy agent such as the anti-CD20 monoclonal antibody rituximab. This is most commonly used at an initiation dose of 1,000 mg IV twice (spaced 15 days apart), followed by 1,000 mg IV every 6 months. This can be restarted postpartum (see above regarding monoclonals and breastfeeding, as well as Section 5, Chapter 35). Among the immunosuppressants, azathioprine has classically been considered the safest to use.[73]

TRANSVERSE MYELITIS: BACKGROUND

ATM is an acute inflammatory syndrome that targets the spinal cord. It is estimated there is at least one severe case per million population per year and up to 8 milder cases per million per year.[74] ATM affects all ages, with peaks from ages 10 to 19 years, and 30 to 39 years.[75] The clinical presentation involves acute or subacute onset of motor, sensory, and autonomic (bladder, bowel) issues referable to the spinal cord.[75] There is often an identifiable sensory level, and abnormalities are typically bilateral but can be asymmetric. It is always critical to rule out spinal cord compression in suspected cases, typically by performing MRI scanning of the cord. The timespan from onset to the worst clinical point ranges from 4 hours to 21 days; more rapid onset to nadir would support a vascular etiology. Prognosis is broadly divided into thirds: one-third recover just about back to normal, one-third are left with some permanent disability, and one-third have severe disability.[75] Poor prognosis indicators include rapid clinical worsening, severe back pain, and complete loss of function with spinal shock.[75]

ATM is a syndrome. It can be idiopathic, or secondary to a neurologic or systemic disease. MS and NMOSD are both in the differential diagnosis. It is estimated that about 70% of ATM cases turn out to have relapsing MS. MS typically produces a partial myelitis and rarely causes a complete transverse myelitis (loss of all function below the lesion site). NMOSD would be highly likely in the setting of a longitudinally extensive spinal cord lesion (>3 vertebral segments in length). Other causes include connective tissue disorders, sarcoidosis, direct infection (herpes viruses, flaviviruses, Lyme disease), a monophasic post infectious process, paraneoplastic process, or vascular disorder. In one series idiopathic ATM, where no etiology could be established, accounted for 15.6% of cases.[76]

Standard workup based on the differential diagnosis includes selected blood studies, MRI of the spinal cord and brain with and without contrast, CSF evaluation, and assessment of optic nerves via visual evoked potentials and optical coherence tomography.[77] Spinal cord inflammation is demonstrated by contrast enhancement on MRI, or by CSF pleocytosis or elevated CSF IgG index.

TRANSVERSE MYELITIS: PREGNANCY DATA

There is very limited data on ATM and pregnancy. Two situations can arise. First, ATM can occur during pregnancy. It should be worked up and treated. Blood work, MRI, and lumbar puncture are all safe procedures for a pregnant woman. Gadolinium-based contrast is not an absolute requirement and would typically be avoided. The attack could be treated with a standard short course of high-dose corticosteroids, and plasma exchange can be done during pregnancy for severe attacks. A recent trial (STRIVE) planned to randomize transverse myelitis patients to IV corticosteroids, or IV corticosteroids plus 5 days of intravenous immunoglobulin (IVIG) (total 2 g/kg) but failed to recruit.[78] IVIG offers an alternative therapy (albeit with limited data) that is safe during pregnancy. The second situation involves a patient with a history of ATM, who asks about future pregnancy and delivery issues. Counseling would be guided by the underlying cause of the ATM, and the extent of any fixed deficits. However, even paraplegic patients have had successful vaginal deliveries (for more on spinal cord injury see Section 4, Chapter 29).[79,80]

SUMMARY

The Care Map outlines major points to raise in women with an immune-mediated disorder who are facing pregnancy [Box 10.1]. The most important issue remains effective and ongoing communication, counseling, and management, as well as a rapid and appropriate response if there is an acute neurologic episode.

REFERENCES

1. Mor G, Aldo P, Alvero AB. The unique immunological and microbial aspects of pregnancy. *Nat Rev Immunol.* 2017; 17(8): 469–482.
2. Macpherson AJ, de Agüero MG, Ganal-Vanarburg SC. How nutrition and the maternal microbiota shape the neonatal immune system. *Nat Rev Immunol.* 2017; 17(8): 508–517.
3. Chen AY, Chonghasawat AM, Leadholm KL. Multiple sclerosis: Frequency, cost, and economic burden in the United States. *J Clin Neurosci.* 2017; 45: 180–186. doi: 10.1016/j.jocn.2017.06.005.
3A. Wallin MT. The Prevalence of Multiple Sclerosis in the United States: A Population-Based Healthcare Database Approach. *ECTRIMS* 2017; Abstract P344.

4. Jobin C, Larochelle C, Parpal H, et al. Gender issues in multiple sclerosis: An update. *Womens Health (Lond).* 2010; 6(6): 797–820.

5. Langer-Gould A, Brara SM, Beaber BE, et al. Incidence of multiple sclerosis in multiple racial and ethnic groups. *Neurology.* 2013; 80(19): 1743–1749.

6. Lublin FD, Reingold SC, Cohen JA, et al. Defining the clinical course of multiple sclerosis: The 2013 revisions. *Neurology.* 2014; 83(3): 278–286.

7. Confavreux C, Hutchinson M, Hours MM, et al. Rate of pregnancy-related relapse in multiple sclerosis. Pregnancy in multiple sclerosis group. *N Engl J Med.* 1998; 339(5): 285–291.

8. Hughes SE, Spelman T, Gray OM, et al. Predictors and dynamics of postpartum relapses in women with multiple sclerosis. *Mult Scler.* 2014; 20(6): 739–746.

9. Karp I, Manganas A, Sylvestre MP, et al. Does pregnancy alter the long-term course of multiple sclerosis? *Ann Epidemiol.* 2014; 24(7): 504–508.

10. Ramagopalan S, Yee I, Byrnes J, et al. Term pregnancies and the clinical characteristics of multiple sclerosis: a population based study. *J Neurol Neurosurg Psychiatry.* 2012; 83(8): 793–795.

11. Keyhanian K, Davoudi V, Etemadifar M, et al. Better prognosis of multiple sclerosis in patients who experienced a full-term pregnancy. *Eur Neurol.* 2012; 68(3): 150–155.

12. Masera S, Cavalla P, Prosperini L, et al. Parity is associated with a longer time to reach irreversible disability milestones in women with multiple sclerosis. *Mult Scler.* 2015; 21(10): 1291–1297.

13. Runmarker B. and Anderson O. Pregnancy is associated with a lower risk of onset and a better prognosis in multiple sclerosis. *Brain.* 1995; 118(Pt. 1): 253–261.

14. Verdu P, Theys P, D'Hooghe MB, et al. Pregnancy and multiple sclerosis: The influence on long term disability. *Clin Neurol Neurosurg.* 1994; 96(1): 38–41.

15. Ponsonby AL, Lucas RM, van der Mei IA, et al. Offspring number, pregnancy, and risk of a first clinical demyelinating event: the AusImmune Study. *Neurology.* 2012; 78(12): 867–874.

16. Hedström AK, Hillert J, Olsson T, et al. Reverse causality behind öe association between reproductive history and MS. *Mult Scler.* 2014; 20(4): 406–411.

17. Magyari M. Role of socio-economic and reproductive factors in the risk of multiple sclerosis. *Acta Neurol Scand.* 2015; 132(199): 20–23.

18. D'hooghe MB, Haentjens P, Nagels G, et al. Menarche, oral contraceptives, pregnancy and progression of disability in relapsing onset and progressive onset multiple sclerosis. *J Neurol.* 2012; 259(5): 855–861.

19. Lebrun C, Le Page E, Kantarci O, et al. Impact of pregnancy on conversion to clinically isolated syndrome in radiologically isolated syndrome cohort. *Mult Scler.* 2012; 18(9): 1297–1302.

20. Roux T, Courtillot C, Debs R, et al. Fecundity in women with multiple sclerosis: an observational mono-centric study. *J Neurol.* 2015; 262: 957–960.

21. Alwan S, Yee IM, Dybalski M, et al. Reproductive decision making after the diagnosis of multiple sclerosis (MS). *Mult Scler.* 2013; 19(3): 351–358.

22. Ramagopalan SV, Guimond C, Criscuoli M, et al. Congenital abnormalities and multiple sclerosis. *BMC Neurol.* 2010; 10: 115.

23. Çil AP, Leventoğlu A, Sönmezer M, et al. Assessment of ovarian reserve and Doppler characteristics in patients with multiple sclerosis using immunomodulating drugs. *J Turk Ger Gynecol Assoc.* 2009; 10(4): 213–219.

24. Thöne J, Kollar S, Nousome D, et al. Serum anti-Müellerian hormone levels in reproductive-age women with relapsing-remitting multiple sclerosis. *Mult Scler.* 2015; 21(1): 41–47.

25. Thöne J, Kleiter I, Stahl A, et al. Relevance of endoglin, IL-1α, IL-1β and anti-ovarian antibodies in females with multiple sclerosis. *J Neurol Sci.* 2016; 362: 240–243.

26. Sepulveda M, Ros C, Martinez-Lapiscina EH, et al. Pituitary-ovary axis and ovarian reserve in fertile women with multiple sclerosis: A pilot study. *Mult Scler.* 2016; 22(4): 564–568.

27. Correale J, Farez MF and Ysrraelit MC. Increase in multiple sclerosis activity after assisted reproduction technology. *Ann Neurol.* 2012; 72(5): 682–694.

28. Hellwig K and Correale J. Artificial reproductive techniques in multiple sclerosis. *Clin Immunol.* 2013; 149(2): 219–224.

29. Michel L, Foucher Y, Vukusic S, et al. Increased risk of multiple sclerosis relapse after in vitro fertilization. *J Neurol Neurosurg Psychiatry.* 2012; 83(8): 796–802.

30. Pierrot-Deseilligny C and Souberbielle JC. Vitamin D and multiple sclerosis: An update. *Mult Scler Relat Disord.* 2017; 14: 35–45.

31. Jalkanen A, Kauko T, Turpeinen U, et al. Clinical Commentary: Multiple sclerosis and vitamin D during pregnancy and lactation. *Acta Neurol Scand.* 2015; 131: 64–67.

32. Hollis BW, Wagner CL. Vitamin D supplementation during pregnancy: Improvements in birth outcomes and complications through direct genomic alteration. *Mol Cell Endocrinol.* 2017; 453: 113–130.

33. Wagner CL, Hollis BW, Kotsa K, et al. Vitamin D administration during pregnancy as prevention for pregnancy, neonatal and postnatal complications. *Rev Endocr Metab* Disord. 2017; 18: 307–322.

34. Munger KL, Aivo J, Hongell K, et al. Vitamin D status during pregnancy and risk of multiple

sclerosis in offspring of women in the Finnish maternity cohort. *JAMA Neurol.* 2016; 73(5): 515–519.

35. Salzer J, Hallmans G, Nyström M, et al. Vitamin D as a protective factor in multiple sclerosis. *Neurology.* 2012; 79: 2140–2145.

36. Nielsen NM, Munger KL, Koch-Henriksen N, et al. Neonatal vitamin D status and risk of multiple sclerosis. *Neurology.* 2017; 88: 44–51.

37. Zapata LB, Oduyebo T, Whiteman MK, et al. Contraceptive use among women with multiple sclerosis: a systematic review. *Contraception.* 2016; 94: 612–620.

38. Committee on Gynecologic Practice Long-Acting Reversible Contraception Working Group. Committee Opinion No. 642: Increasing access to contraceptive implants and intrauterine devices to reduce unintended pregnancy. *Obstet Gynecol.* 2015; 126(4): e44–48.

39. Houtchens MK, Zapata LB, Curtis KM, et al. Contraception for women with multiple sclerosis: Guidance for healthcare providers. *Mult Scler.* 2017; 23(6): 757–764.

40. Benoit A, Durand-Dubief F, Amato MP, et al. History of multiple sclerosis in 2 successive pregnancies: A French and Italian cohort. *Neurology.* 2016; 87(13): 1360–1367.

41. American College of Obstetricians and Gynecologists' Committee on Obstetric Practice. Committee Opinion No. 656 Guidelines for Diagnostic Imaging During Pregnancy and Lactation. *Obstet Gynecol.* 2016; 127(2): e75–80.

42. Fraum TJ, Ludwig DR, Bashir MR, et al. Gadolinium-Based Contrast Agents: A Comprehensive Risk Assessment. *J Magn Reson Imaging.* 2017; 46: 338–353.

43. Hviid A and Mølgaard-Nielsen D. Corticosteroid use during pregnancy and risk of orofacial clefts. *CMAJ.* 2011; 183(7): 796–804.

44. Levy RA, de Jesús GR, de Jesús NR, et al. Critical review of the current recommendations for the treatment of systemic inflammatory rheumatic diseases during pregnancy and lactation. *Autimmun Rev.* 2016; 15: 955–963.

45. Vukusic S, Hutchinson M, Hours M, et al. Pregnancy and multiple sclerosis (the PRIMS study): clinical predictors of post-partum relapse. *Brain.* 2004; 127(Pt. 6): 1353–1360.

46. Portaccio E, Ghezzi A, Hakiki B, et al. Breastfeeding is not related to postpartum relapses in multiple sclerosis. *Neurology.* 2011; 77(2): 145–150.

47. Runia TF, Neuteboom RF, de Groot CJ, et al. The influence of vitamin D on postpartum relapse and quality of life in pregnant multiple sclerosis patients. *Eur J Neurol.* 2015; 22(3): 479–484.

48. Pakpoor J, Disanto G, Lacey MV, et al. Breastfeeding and multiple sclerosis relapses: a meta-analysis. *J Neurol.* 2012; 259: 2246–2248.

49. Langer-Gould A and Beaber B. Effects of pregnancy and breastfeeding on the multiple sclerosis disease course. *Clin Immunol.* 2013; 149: 244–250.

50. Costanza M, Binart N, Steinman L, et al. Prolactin: A versatile regulator of inflammation and autoimmune pathology. *Autoimmun Rev.* 2015; 14: 223–230.

51. Conradi S, Malzah U, Paul F, et al. Breastfeeding is associated with lower risk for multiple sclerosis. *Mult Scler.* 2012; 19(5): 553–558.

52. Langer-Gould A, Smith JB, Hellwig K, et al. Breastfeeding, ovulatory years, and risk of multiple sclerosis. *Neurology.* 2017; 89: 1–7.

53. Boz C, Terzi M, Zengin Karahan S, et al. Safety of IV pulse methylprednisolone therapy during breastfeeding in patients with multiple sclerosis. *Mult Scler.* 2017. doi: 10.1177/1352458517717806.

54. Gold R, Phillips JT, Havrdova E, et al. Delayed-release dimethyl fumarate and pregnancy: Preclinical studies and pregnancy outcomes from clinical trials and postmarketing experience. *Neurol Ther.* 2015; 4: 93–104.

55. Almas S, Vance J, Baker T, et al. Management of multiple sclerosis in the breastfeeding mother. *Mult Scler Int.* 2016; article ID 6527458.

56. Haghikia A, Langer-Gould A, Rellensmann G, et al. Natalizumab use during the third trimester of pregnancy. *JAMA Neurol.* 2014; 71(7): 891–895.

57. De Giglio L, Gasperini C, Tortorella C, et al. Natalizumab discontinuation and disease restart in pregnancy: A case series. *Acta Neurol Scand.* 2015; 131: 336–340.

58. Théaudin M, Elefant E, Senat MV. Natalizumab continuation during pregnancy in a patient with previous severe IRIS syndrome. *J Neurol Sci.* 2015; 359: 211–212.

59. Amato MP, Bertolotto A, Brunelli R, et al. Management of pregnancy-related issues in multiple sclerosis patients: The need for an interdisciplinary approach. *Neurol Sci.* 2017. doi: 10.1007/s10072-017-3081-8.

60. Voskuhl R, Momtazee C. Pregnancy: Effect on multiple sclerosis, treatment considerations, and breastfeeding. *Neurotherapeutics.* 2017; 14: 974–984. doi: 10.1007/s13311-017-0562-7.

61. Davoudi V, Keyhanian K, Bove RM, et al. Immunology of neuromyelitis optica during pregnancy. *Neurol Neuroimmunol Neuroinflamm.* 2016; 3(6): e288.

62. Wingerchuk DM, Branwell B, Bennett JL, et al. International consensus diagnostic criteria for neuromyelitis optica spectrum disorders. *Neurology.* 2015; 85: 177–189.

63. Saadoun S, Waters P, Leite MI, et al. Neuromyelitis optica IgG causes placental inflammation and fetal death. *J Immunol.* 2013; 191(6): 2999–3005.

64. Bourre B, Marignier R, Zéphir H, et al. Neuromyelitis optica and pregnancy. *Neurology.* 2012; 78(12): 875–879.

64A. Klawiter EC, Bove R, Elsone L, et al. High risk of postpartum relapses in neuromyelitis optica spectrum disorder. *Neurology.* 2017; 89(22): 2238–2244.

65. Nour MM, Nakashima I, Coutinho E, et al. Pregnancy outcomes in aquaporin-4-positive neuromyelitis optica spectrum disorder. *Neurology.* 2016; 86: 79–87.

66. Huang Y, Wang Y, Zhou Y, et al. Pregnancy in neuromyelitis optica spectrum disorder: A multicenter study from South China. *J Neurol Sci.* 2017; 372: 152–156.

66A. Shosha E, Pittock SJ, Flanagan E, et al. Neuromyelitis optica spectrum disorders and pregnancy: Interactions and management. *Mult Scler.* 2017; 23(14): 1808–1817.

67. Shi B, Zhao M, Geng T, et al. (2017) Effectiveness and safety of immunosuppressive therapy in neuromyelitis optica spectrum disorder during pregnancy. *J Neurol Sci.* 2017; 377: 72–76.

68. Fragoso YD, Adoni T, Bichuetti DB, et al. Neuromyelitis optica and pregnancy. *J Neurol.* 2013; 260: 2614–2619.

69. Jurewicz A, Selmaj K. Case report: Relapse of neuromyelitis optica during pregnancy-treatment options and literature review. *Clin Neurol Neurosurg.* 2015; 130: 159–161.

70. Shimizu Y, Fujihara K, Ohashi T, et al. Pregnancy-related relapse risk factors in women with anti-AQP4 antibody positivity and neuromyelitis optica spectrum disorder. *MSJ.* 2016; 22(11): 1413–1420.

71. Rubio Tabares J., Amaya Gonzalez P.F. Plasma exchange therapy for a severe relapse of Devic's disease in a pregnant woman: A case report and concise review. *Clin Neurol Neurosurg.* 2016; 148: 88–90.

72. Ringlestein M, Harmel J, Distelmaier F, et al. Neuromyelitis optica and pregnancy during therapeutic B cell depletion: infant exposure to anti-AQP4 antibody and prevention of rebound relapses with low-dose rituximab postpartum. *MSJ.* 2013; 19(11): 1544–1547.

73. Leroy C, Rigot JM, Leroy M, et al. Immunosuppressive drugs and fertility. *Orphanet J Rare Dis.* 2015; 10: 136.

74. Scott TF, Frohman EM, De Seze J, et al. Evidence-based guideline: Clinical evaluation and treatment of transverse myelitis. *Neurology.* 2011; 77: 2128–2134.

75. Transverse Myelitis Consortium Working Group. Proposed diagnostic criteria and nosology of acute transverse myelitis. *Neurology.* 2002; 59: 499–505.

76. De Seze J, Lanctin C, Lebrun C, et al. Idiopathic acute transverse myelitis: Application of the recent diagnostic criteria. *Neurology.* 2005; 65: 1950–1953.

77. Greenberg BM. and Frohman EM. Immune-mediated myelopathies. *Continuum.* 2015; 21(1): 121–131.

78. Absoud M, Brex P, Ciccarelli O, et al. A multicenter randomiSed controlled Trial and IntraVEnous immunoglobulin compared with standard therapy for the treatment of transverse myelitis in adults and children (STRIVE). *Health Technol Assess.* 2017; 21(31): 1–50.

79. Sharpe EE, Arendt KW, Jacob AK, et al. Anesthetic management of parturients with pre-existing paraplegia or tetraplegia: a case series. *Int J Obstet Anesth.* 2015; 24(1): 77–84.

80. Walsh P, Grange C. and Beale N. Anaesthetic management of an obstetric patient with idiopathic acute transverse myelitis. *Int J Obstet Anesth.* 2010; 19(1): 98–101.

81. O'Gorman C, Lin R, Stankovich J, et al. Modelling genetic susceptibility to multiple sclerosis with family data. *Neuroepidemiology.* 2013; 40: 1–12.

82. Hale TW, Siddiqui AA and Baker TE. Transfer of interferon β-1a into human breast milk. *Breastfeed Med.* 2012; 7(2): 123–125.

83. Coyle PK, Sinclair SM, Scheuerle AE, et al. Final results from the Betaseron (interferon β-1b) Pregnancy Registry: A prospective observational study of birth defects and pregnancy-related adverse events. *BMJ Open.* 2014; 4: e004536.

84. Romero RS, Lünzmann C, Bugge JP. Pregnancy outcomes in patients exposed to interferon beta-1b. *J Neurol Neurosurg Psychiatry.* 2015; 86: 587–589.

85. Thiel S, Langer-Gould A, Rockhoff M, et al. Interferon-beta exposure during first trimester is safe in women with multiple sclerosis—A prospective cohort study from the German Multiple Sclerosis and Pregnancy Registry. *Mult Scler.* 2016; 22(6): 801–809.

86. Sandberg-Wollheim M, Neudorfer O, Grinspan A, et al. Pregnancy outcomes from the Branded Glatiramer Acetate Pregnancy Database. *Int J MS Care.* 2017. doi: 10.7224/1537-2073.2016-079.

87. Karlsson G, Francis G, Koren G, et al. Pregnancy outcomes in the clinical development program of fingolimod in multiple sclerosis. *Neurology.* 2014; 82: 674–680.

88. Kieseier BC, Benamore M. Pregnancy outcomes following maternal and paternal exposure to Teriflunomide during treatment for relapsing-remitting multiple sclerosis. *Neurol Ther.* 2014; 3: 133–138.

89. Gold R, Phillips JT, Havrdova E, et al. Delayed-release dimethyl fumarate and

pregnancy: Preclinical studies and pregnancy outcomes from clinical trials and postmarketing experience. *Neurol Ther*. 2015; 4: 93–104.

90. Baker TE, Cooper SD, Kessler L, et al. Transfer of natalizumab into breast milk in a mother with multiple sclerosis. *J Hum Lact*. 2015; 31(2): 233–236.

90A. Proschmann U, Thomas K, Thiel K, et al. Natalizumab during pregnancy and lactation. *Mult Scler*. 2017.

91. Friend S, Richman S, Bloomgren G, et al. Evaluation of pregnancy outcomes from the Tysabri (natalizumab) pregnancy exposure registry: a global, observational, follow-up study. *BMC Neurol*. 2016; 16: 150.

92. Ebrahimi N, Herbstritt S, Gold R, et al. Pregnancy and fetal outcomes following natalizumab exposure in pregnancy. A prospective, controlled observational study. *Mult Scler*. 2015; 21(2): 198–205.

93. Lemtrada® [package insert] Genzyme Corporation. Cambridge, MA; 2016.

94. Gold R, Stefoski D, Selmaj K, et al. Pregnancy experience: Nonclinical studies and pregnancy outcomes in the Daclizumab Clinical Study Program. *Neurol Ther*. 2016; 5(2): 169–182.

11

Neurologic Infections in Pregnancy

COURTNEY OLSON-CHEN

ABSTRACT

Despite advances in prevention, diagnosis, and treatment, infectious diseases continue to be a major cause of maternal, fetal, and neonatal morbidity and mortality. Immunologic changes in pregnancy can increase both susceptibility to certain infections and the severity of infection. Infectious diseases in pregnancy contribute to the development of congenital fetal syndromes in addition to adverse outcomes including preterm birth, stillbirth, and intrauterine growth restriction. While infections of the maternal central nervous system, or CNS, are rare during pregnancy, the potential impact can be critical.[1] This chapter will cover both the types of infections within the CNS and the potential organisms that cause these infections. The chapter will also provide general management recommendations for pregnancy in order to both prevent and maintain awareness about CNS infections.

MENINGITIS

Meningitis involves inflammation of the meninges, or the membranes surrounding the brain and spinal cord. This most often occurs secondary to the presence of an infectious organism in the cerebrospinal fluid, or CSF. Meningitis can be caused by a variety of different organisms including bacteria, viruses and fungi (see Table 11.1)[1]. The clinical presentation and optimal treatment depend on the infectious etiology.[2] Fetal effects differ based on the organism and its potential to be vertically transmitted. In general, meningitis does not present differently in pregnant women as compared to non-pregnant patients, and the evaluation and management of meningitis is similar in all patients.[3]

Viral Meningitis

Viruses are the most common cause of meningitis with an incidence of 7.6 per 100,000 adults each year.[1] In the United States, viral meningitis is most often due to enteroviruses. Other potential etiologies include herpes simplex virus, varicella-zoster virus, mumps, measles and influenza. Symptoms of viral meningitis in adults include fever, headache, neck stiffness, photophobia, drowsiness, nausea, vomiting, anorexia and lethargy. Most cases of viral meningitis resolve within 7–10 days without treatment.[2] Antipyretics may be required for high fever in addition to pain management for severe headaches.[1] Certain infections, like herpes simplex virus and influenza, benefit from antiviral treatment.[2] CSF testing in viral meningitis shows normal opening pressure, low white cell count and normal glucose and protein levels. PCR assays and serology can be used to distinguish the virus of origin.[1] Immunization, hand washing and avoidance of sick contacts are key strategies for prevention of viral meningitis.[2,4]

The overall risk of viral meningitis in pregnancy is low, but viruses have the most potential to cause fetal or neonatal damage. The risk of potential teratogenicity cannot be overlooked. Outcomes can include spontaneous abortion, fetal demise and congenital viral syndromes.[5] To optimize maternal and fetal outcomes, antiviral treatment with acyclovir should be initiated as soon as meningitis is suspected during pregnancy.[6]

Bacterial Meningitis

Acute bacterial meningitis can evolve in a short period of time and requires prompt evaluation and treatment.[1] While most people recover from bacterial meningitis, it has the potential to cause severe outcomes, including permanent neurologic disabilities and death. The incidence of bacterial meningitis is estimated to be 2.6 to 6 per 100,000 adults each year. The most common causes of bacterial meningitis in adults in the United States are *Streptococcus pneumoniae, Neisseria meningitides, Haemophilus influenza type* and *Listeria monocytogenes*. Pregnant women have increased susceptibility to infection with *Listeria*

TABLE 11.1 CLASSES OF NEUROLOGIC INFECTIONS

CNS Infection	Symptoms	Common Causes
Viral Meningitis	Fever, headache, neck stiffness, photophobia, nausea, vomiting, lethargy, lack of appetite	Enteroviruses Herpes simplex virus Varicella zoster virus Mumps
Bacterial Meningitis	Fever, headache, neck stiffness, photophobia, nausea, vomiting, altered mental status	*Streptococcus pneumoniae* *Neisseria meningitides* *Haemophilus influenza type b* *Listeria monocytogenes*
Fungal Meningitis	Fever, headache, neck stiffness, photophobia, nausea, vomiting, altered mental status	*Cryptococcus* *Candida* *Histoplasmosis* *Blastomyces* *Coccidiodes*
Encephalitis	Fever, headache, rapid-onset altered mental status, behavioral changes, seizures, focal neurological deficits	Herpes simplex virus Cytomegalovirus Varicella zoster virus
Brain Abscess	Headache, seizures, confusion, focal neurological deficits	Rare and variable

monocytogenes, which can lead to meningitis and adverse pregnancy outcomes.[7]

Women with bacterial meningitis often present with new onset fever, headache, and neck stiffness. Other symptoms can include nausea, vomiting, photophobia, and altered mental status. The diagnosis involves collection of blood and CSF samples.[2] CSF demonstrates increased opening pressure, predominant neutrophils, elevated protein levels, and decreased glucose concentration. Gram stain is useful with a high sensitivity and specificity for community-acquired forms of bacterial meningitis.[8]

A case review of 42 pregnant women with bacterial meningitis found a 28% overall maternal mortality rate and a 37% risk of fetal or neonatal loss.[3] Due to the risk of severe complications, it is crucial to maintain a high clinical suspicion for bacterial meningitis in pregnancy. Empiric treatment should begin immediately if bacterial meningitis is suspected.[8] In pregnant women, empiric treatment should also include coverage for listeria. The optimal regimen involves a third- or fourth-generation cephalosporin, vancomycin, and ampicillin. The addition of dexamethasone is also recommended in adults with bacterial meningitis.[9]

Risk factors for bacterial meningitis include residing in a community setting where large groups of people frequently gather, like college campuses, and travel to other countries with an increased burden of meningitis.[2] Vaccines are important for prevention of many of the major causes of bacterial meningitis including *Neisseria meningitidis, Streptococcus pneumoniae* and *Hemophilus influenza b*. These are part of the standard Centers for Disease Control and Prevention (CDC)-recommended immunization schedule in children and adolescents. Pregnancy should not preclude meningococcal vaccination if it is indicated. There is limited data regarding the safety of the pneumococcal vaccine during pregnancy, but no adverse consequences have been reported.[4]

Fungal Meningitis

Fungal organisms are rarely found in the CSF, but fungal meningitis can occur in patients with weakened immune systems. Symptoms include fever, headache, neck stiffness, nausea, vomiting, photophobia, and altered mental status. The most common causes in the United States are *Cryptococcus, Candida, Histoplasmosis, Blastomyces,* and *Coccidiodes*.[2] CSF may demonstrate an elevated opening pressure, moderate increase in white blood cell count, low glucose, and elevated protein.[1] Those at risk include patients with cancer, HIV infection, or using immunomodulators for autoimmune conditions or post-transplant. Pregnant women are at increased risk of *Coccidiodes* infection, particularly in the third trimester in the southwestern United States. Treatment of fungal meningitis involves long courses of intravenous antifungal medications such as Amphotericin B. Amphotericin B has not been associated with adverse events in pregnancy, and it is recommended for the treatment of serious systemic fungal infections in pregnant women. Prevention includes avoidance of environmental causes such as soil and bird droppings, especially in geographic areas of increased prevalence.[2]

ENCEPHALITIS

Encephalitis involves inflammation of the brain and clinical neurologic dysfunction. Patients with encephalitis have many of the same symptoms as those with meningitis including fever and headache. Rapid-onset altered mental status is more common in encephalitis, but this presentation does not rule out bacterial meningitis. Additional neurologic manifestations of encephalitis include behavioral changes, focal neurologic signs, and seizures. It is possible to have a combination of meningeal inflammation and encephalitis, known as meningoencephalitis. Clinical findings can include rash, respiratory symptoms, and lymphadenopathy.[10]

Identification of the infectious etiology is important for prognosis, counseling, and treatment. The evaluation of patients with suspected encephalitis should include cultures and infectious analysis of blood and CSF, serologic testing, and magnetic resonance imaging (MRI). Neuroimaging is important because it can reveal findings indicative of specific infectious etiology.[10] (See also Section 1, Chapter 7 for discussion of imaging safety in pregnancy.) Many patients may require imaging studies prior to lumbar puncture because of clinical contraindications to immediate lumbar puncture.[11] Herpes simplex virus (HSV) is the most common cause of encephalitis in both the general population and pregnant women.[1] One case series found that pregnant women with HSV encephalitis may have less significantly impaired consciousness when compared to non-pregnant patients perhaps secondary to earlier presentation.[11] All patients with suspected encephalitis should have HSV PCR of CSF. Acyclovir for coverage of herpes simplex virus is recommended in all patients with suspected encephalitis until this virus is ruled out and is considered safe throughout pregnancy.[2] The mortality of HSV encephalitis can be reduced from more than 70% to less than 20–30% when acyclovir is used so treatment should be started immediately.[11] Other potential causes include cytomegalovirus and varicella zoster virus.[1] If transmitted to the fetus, these viruses can also cause congenital infection and other complications depending on the timing of the infection (under the "Cytomegalovirus" and

"Varicella Zoster Virus" sections).[8] While there is no evidence to support anti-epileptic seizure prophylaxis in pregnant women with encephalitis, anti-epileptic medications should be given as needed for management of encephalitis-associated seizures in order to avoid fetal risks of seizures.[11]

BRAIN ABSCESS

There are less than 15 case reports of cerebral abscess during pregnancy, but this is a potentially life-threatening condition.[1] In some cases during pregnancy, cerebral abscess has been seen in association with infections of the ear and sinuses.[12,13] Patients with underlying infection, foreign bodies, or immunosuppression are at increased risk of cerebral abscesses. Symptoms of an abscess may include headache, seizures, confusion, and focal neurological deficits. MRI can be used for diagnosis and localization. Surgical drainage is sometimes needed for large abscesses.[1] Given the limited data, care and evaluation should be focused on maximizing maternal outcomes and survival for this serious condition.

ORGANISMS CAUSING NEUROLOGIC INFECTIONS IN PREGNANCY

The effect of neurologic infections in pregnant women can vary depending on the specific organism. The impact on the fetus also differs based on the organism, timing of infection, and the selected treatment. Many infectious diseases are more likely to be transmitted to the fetus later in gestation, but the most severe fetal effects can occur when infection occurs in early pregnancy.[1] Preventive steps are key for each organism in order to avoid potentially devastating outcomes.[9] Below, we will discuss each of the common organisms leading to neurologic infection in pregnancy in further detail. It is also possible for some infections to be transmitted to the neonate through breastfeeding, but the risk depends on the specific organism and the timing of infection as discussed below.

Listeria

Listeria monocytogenes is an intracellular bacteria that enters the gastrointestinal tract through ingestion of contaminated foods.[8,14] While this infection is rare in the general population with approximately 0.7 cases in 100,000 people each year, listeria is up to 20 times more common in pregnant women.[1,15] The clinical presentation can range from asymptomatic to flu-like symptoms.[16] Listeria infection of the CNS causes meningitis or meningoencephalitis with fever, headache, changes in mental status, and seizures.[1] However, meningismus is less common in listeria meningitis than other bacterial cases of meningitis.[9] CSF testing can show a predominance of neutrophils or lymphocytes, elevated protein concentration, and normal or decreased glucose levels.[1,15] The gram stain is frequently negative in the setting of listeria, and therefore, clinicians must have a high index of suspicion.[9] Diagnosis is made using listeria culture of blood or CSF. Treatment should begin in pregnant women who are symptomatic and have been exposed to listeria without waiting for culture results, which can take several days. At least three weeks of high-dose ampicillin is used for treatment of listeria meningitis.[9,16] Listeria is associated with an increased risk of pregnancy complications including miscarriage, preterm birth, stillbirth, and neonatal sepsis.[1] The CDC recommends avoidance of certain foods that have been linked to listeriosis including soft cheeses, raw sprouts, cold hot dogs, and lunch meats.[17] The incidence of listeriosis in pregnant women has decreased due to educational efforts around avoidance of these high risk foods.[7] CDC recommendations are updated regularly at www.cdc.gov.[17]

Herpes Simplex Virus

Both HSV-1 and HSV-2 are common in the general population and in pregnant women.[18] Primary infections with HSV acquired during pregnancy, especially in the third trimester, are more likely to progress to a disseminated form of the infection that can involve hepatitis, encephalitis and coagulopathy.[9,19] Up to one-third of all women with primary genital HSV-2 infection have meningeal symptoms.[1] The maternal mortality rate of disseminated HSV is as high as 70% without treatment.[19] MRI can demonstrate T2 hyperintensity in the medial temporal lobes, insula, and cingulate gyri (see Chapter 7 for discussion of safety of neuroimaging in pregnancy). Diagnosis is made using CSF PCR for HSV, which has high sensitivity and specificity.[9,10] Treatment for herpes encephalitis is acyclovir for 2–3 weeks.[9]

Transplacental intrauterine infection of the fetus can occur with HSV infection, especially when it is disseminated in the mother. Congenital HSV can cause microcephaly, intracranial calcifications, seizures, skin scarring, arthrogryposis, and cataracts. In addition, neonatal HSV infection can occur due to exposure to maternal genital herpes infection at the time of delivery.[20] This can lead to disseminated infection

in the newborn with CNS involvement and a high risk of mortality.[8] While cesarean delivery does not completely prevent vertical transmission, it is indicated in women with active genital lesions or prodromal symptoms at the time of labor or ruptured membranes near term as this can decrease the risk of transmission by up to 85%. Cesarean delivery is not recommended for women with non-genital HSV lesions.[21] The management of patients with suspected primary HSV lesions in the third trimester, particularly within 6 weeks of delivery, is a subject of much debate. Prolonged viral shedding can occur, and the risk of vertical transmission remains until the development of maternal antibodies, which may take 6 to 12 weeks.[22] The Royal College of Obstetricians and Gynecologists recommends delivery by cesarean section in all women with their first episode of genital herpes within 6 weeks of delivery unless maternal testing shows the presence of antibodies to the same type of HSV causing the lesion.[23] While HSV cannot be transmitted through breast milk, infants can become infected by making contact with an exposed herpes lesion. The American College of Obstetricians and Gynecologists recommends covering HSV lesions while breastfeeding and washing hands with soap and water before and after breastfeeding. Infants should not be breastfed from breasts with active HSV lesions.[21]

Varicella Zoster Virus

Varicella zoster virus, or VZV, is a herpes virus transmitted through respiratory droplets and contact with skin lesion.[1] Although VZV in pregnancy is rare due to immunity in most adults, there is high maternal and fetal morbidity and mortality associated with this infection. The virus is 5 times more likely to cause death in pregnant women as compared to the general population.[8] Prodromal symptoms can occur after initial infection including fever, headache, and malaise in addition to rash. Pneumonia occurs in up to 20% of cases, and in rare cases, the virus can lead to encephalitis.[1,24] Less common neurologic manifestations of varicella include cerebellar ataxia, transverse myelitis and Guillian-Barre syndrome. Up to 20% of survivors of CNS varicella infection have epilepsy.[9]

Fetal infection can lead to congenital varicella syndrome or intrauterine demise. Congenital varicella syndrome involves skin lesions, limb hypoplasia, and contractures in addition to neurologic abnormalities including microcephaly, hydrocephalus, and seizures. Severe neonatal varicella infections are possible when maternal varicella occurs between 5 days before and 2 days after delivery. Immunization prior to pregnancy is important for prevention but is not recommended during pregnancy, as this is a live vaccination. Pregnant women without immunity to varicella should avoid contact with those with active infection. Varicella zoster immune globulin should be given as soon as possible for post-exposure prophylaxis in non-immune women, and acyclovir is used when patients develop signs and symptoms of varicella.[1,8] Newborns at risk for neonatal infection should receive post-exposure prophylaxis with varicella zoster immune globulin and be isolated from the mother until she is no longer has infectious lesions.[25] Outside of maternal varicella infection in the critical window 5 days before delivery to 2 days postpartum, breastfeeding is encouraged due to the presence of protective antibodies in breast milk.[26]

Cytomegalovirus

The seroprevalence of cytomegalovirus, or CMV, in the United States is approximately 60%, with most infections acquired in childhood.[27] Infections are frequently asymptomatic, and transmission occurs through both respiratory droplets and contact with infected urine where the CMV is concentrated and excreted. Pregnant women who have contact with young children and have not previously had CMV are at risk of seroconversion. Due to the method of transmission, women with children in daycare settings (especially those with children still utilizing diapers) are at the highest risk for exposure.[27]

Maternal primary cytomegalovirus infection, reinfection with a new strain or reactivation of a prior infection, can lead to congenital CMV.[28] Approximately 1% of all live births in the United States are affected by congenital CMV. The highest risk of transmission to the fetus occurs when infection is acquired in the third trimester, but fetal infection in the first half of pregnancy has the highest chance of severe neonatal sequelae. Neurologic manifestations of congenital CMV include chorioretinitis, microcephaly, seizures, and hearing loss. Severe CMV inclusion disease in fetuses can cause cerebral atrophy, ventriculomegaly, and periventricular calcifications.[29] There is a 20% risk of long-term neurologic sequelae, including sensorineural deafness and psychomotor delay. Diagnosis is made using serologic testing with conversion of CMV IgG antibodies from negative to positive.[1]

CMV testing is recommended for pregnant women with mononucleosis-like symptoms including prolonged fever, lymphadenopathy, and mild pharyngitis in addition to those with sonographic fetal abnormalities concerning for congenital CMV. Antiviral agents such as ganciclovir can be used for treatment of cytomegalovirus in pregnancy, and clinical trials are currently underway for the optimal treatment and for the potential use of CMV immunoglobulin and vaccines.[8,30] More information regarding active randomized trials for the prevention of congenital CMV can be found at https://clinicaltrials.gov/ct2/show/NCT01376778. Of note, CMV can be transmitted through breast milk, but healthy infants who acquire CMV after birth typically have few complications. Caution is advised for mothers with active CMV infection against breastfeeding very preterm infants as this can lead to symptomatic neonatal infection.[31]

Human Immunodeficiency Virus

Human Immunodeficiency virus, or HIV, is a retrovirus that targets the immune system leading to increased occurrence of opportunistic infections.[1] HIV can involve neuronal damage leading to neurocognitive disorders and distal sensory polyneuropathy.[32] While these conditions are typically indolent, acute neurologic illness in HIV patients during pregnancy is usually caused by opportunistic infections covered elsewhere in this chapter.[9] However, acute HIV infection immediately after seroconversion can cause meningeal symptoms in up to 17% of patients.[1] Combination antiretroviral therapy should be used to manage HIV infection in pregnancy, and treatment should be started as soon as possible. Delaying the initiation of combination antiretroviral therapy in pregnancy can increase the risk of perinatal transmission.[33] Selection of a particular antiretroviral regimen should consider viral resistance profiles and the likelihood of adherence. Women on antiretroviral therapy before the diagnosis of pregnancy should continue their current treatment regimen with the exception of stavudine, didanosine, or full-dose ritonavir.[34] Intravenous zidovudine is recommended at the time of delivery to decrease perinatal transmission. Breastfeeding should be avoided in women with HIV in order to minimize the risk of transmission to the neonate.[35]

Influenza Virus

Influenza viral infection can lead to neurologic complications with a range of severity. Neurologic manifestations include encephalopathy, necrotizing encephalitis, transverse myelitis, movement disorders, myositis, Guillain-Barre syndrome and acute disseminated encephalomyelitis.[9,36] Neurologic findings may occur due to direct infection, immune-mediated mechanisms, or cytokine dysregulation.[37] Influenza RNA is rarely detected in the CSF so a negative result does not rule out the possibility of infection.[9,36] Transplacental infection is rare due to lack of viremia and is generally not harmful to the fetus outside of the effects of maternal illness. Pregnant women with acute influenza have a higher rate of serious illness and hospitalization than their non-pregnant counterparts. Treatment involves neuraminidase inhibitors and supportive care to improve outcomes for both fetus and mother.[8,9] Of note, these medications have limited penetration of the CSF.[7] Seasonal vaccination is recommended in all pregnant women for prevention of influenza, as pregnancy increases vulnerability to infection.[8] Antiviral medications and influenza vaccination are not contraindications to breastfeeding. Breastfeeding should be encouraged, though during active maternal influenza infection, the CDC recommends that pumped milk be fed to the infant by a healthy adult to limit exposure.[38]

West Nile Virus
The West Nile virus, a flavivirus, is transmitted to humans through an arthropod vector.[39] It is becoming increasingly prevalent in North America.[9] The majority of infections are asymptomatic. Clinical symptoms can include rash, fever, headache, malaise, nausea, vomiting, and lymphadenopathy.[9,39] It can progress to neurologic disease with meningitis, encephalitis, or acute paralysis. Diagnosis occurs through West Nile virus IgM serology in blood and CSF.[39] There are reports of suspected congenital West Nile virus leading to chorioretinitis, lissencephaly, and white matter loss, but this seems to be a rare complication.[8,40] There are no approved treatments for West Nile virus. Prevention is important by reducing exposure to infected mosquitoes.[8] While West Nile virus has been detected in breast milk, there are no reported cases of transmission and breastfeeding is not contraindicated.[41]

Zika Virus
Zika virus is an arbovirus transmitted by mosquito bite from the vector *Aedes* species.[42] There is also evidence that Zika virus persists in semen and can be sexually transmitted.[43] While up to 80% of cases are asymptomatic, symptoms can include maculopapular rash, fever, conjunctivitis and arthralgia. Zika virus can affect the central nervous system cause complications such as Guillain-Barre syndrome.[42] There is no evidence that pregnant women experience more severe disease from Zika virus.[43] Zika virus RNA and serology can be detected in maternal serum, CSF, urine, and amniotic fluid. The proper testing depends on the patient's symptoms and travel history.[43] Up-to-date information regarding testing recommendations can be found on the CDC's website (https://www.cdc.gov/zika/). Zika virus has been linked to fetal microcephaly, defined by a head circumference more than two standard deviations below the mean. More than 90% of cases of microcephaly are associated with intellectual disability. Zika cases in Brazil showed additional neurologic complications including seizures and hearing and vision impairment.[42] The pattern of birth defects known as congenital Zika syndrome has been defined by severe microcephaly, decreased brain tissue, damage to the back of the eye, limited range of joint motion, and increased muscle tone restricting movement after birth.[43] The timing of placental transmission is still uncertain. Thus, it is crucial that pregnant women avoid travel to Zika-endemic areas, use condoms, or avoid sexual intercourse with partners who have traveled to Zika-endemic areas. Pregnant women should take steps to prevent mosquito bites when they reside within such an area.[42,43] There are no reported cases of Zika transmission through breastfeeding.[43]

Cryptococcus
Cryptococcus neoformans is a fungal infection that can cause meningitis. The symptoms of cryptococcal meningitis are similar to other forms of meningitis, though visual symptoms and papilledema are seen more commonly.[8] The severity of this infection may be greater in pregnant women, with mortality rates as high as 25%.[44] Cryptococcus can also cause focal abscesses and stroke. Cryptococcus is more common in immunocompromised patients, yet it is not clear whether pregnant women are at increased risk.[9] Analysis of CSF shows elevated protein, decreased glucose, lymphocytic pleocytosis, and high opening pressure.[8,9] Brain imaging is usually unremarkable but can be used to exclude other diagnoses. Definitive diagnosis can be made through detection of the cryptococcal antigen in CSF.[9] Amphotericin B is used for treatment of Cryptococcus meningitis in pregnancy. Case series of Amphotericin B treatment in all trimesters of pregnancy have not demonstrated an increase in adverse fetal outcomes.[45]

Toxoplasmosis

Toxoplasma gondii is a protozoan parasite that becomes dormant in humans after exposure.[46] Maternal infections are usually asymptomatic, but they can involve fever, malaise, and lymphadenopathy. Transmission occurs through ingestion of infected foods or sporocysts from cat feces. Toxoplasma can become reactivated in the setting of poor cell-mediated immunity, such as concurrent HIV infection, leading to severe encephalitis. Imaging shows rim-enhancing lesions in the basal ganglia with surrounding edema. Diagnosis in pregnancy is made through serology studies.[9]

The risk of congenital toxoplasmosis seems to increase with gestational age at time of maternal infection. Fetal neurologic outcomes are most severe after first trimester infection. The parasite has an affinity for neurologic tissue and can cause chorioretinitis, hydrocephalus, and intracranial calcifications leading to eventual learning and visual deficits.[8] Congenital infection is confirmed with amniotic fluid testing. There is weak evidence that spiramycin can be used for prevention of vertical transmission. Fetal infection is managed with pyrimethamine, sulfadiazine, and folic acid. While there is evidence that prenatal treatment reduces serious childhood neurologic complications and postnatal death, treatment has not been shown to decrease the risk of intracranial lesions or retinochoroiditis in children with congenital toxoplasmosis. Transmission of toxoplasmosis through breast milk is unlikely. Immunosuppressed HIV patients with low CD4 counts are treated with trimethoprim/sulfamethoxazole to prevent reactivation of toxoplasmosis. Prevention of toxoplasmosis occurs through maternal avoidance of raw meat and cat feces.[47]

Lyme Disease

Lyme disease is a tick-borne infection caused by the *Borrelia burgdorferi* spirochete. A tick feeding period of more than 36 hours is considered to be required for transmission of the spirochete.[48] Approximately 10–15% of those acutely infected with *Borrelia* have CNS involvement. Acute manifestations can include meningitis, facial neuritis, and radiculitis.[49] CSF testing shows a lymphocytic pleocytosis and mild elevation in protein levels. Blood serology can be tested for the presence of Lyme antibodies. Lyme disease in pregnancy can be treated with oral amoxicillin, but doxycycline is contraindicated. CNS involvement is managed with parenteral ceftriaxone or penicillin.[9] Transplacental infection has been documented in isolated cases, but there is no consensus on the effects of Lyme disease on pregnancy outcomes. There are no reported cases of Lyme disease transmission through breast milk. Pregnant women should avoid tick-infected environments. Following exposure to ticks, close inspection of the skin surface should be performed with removal of ticks and bathing as soon as possible to reduce the risk of Lyme disease.[48]

Prion Disease

Prions are infectious protein particles that can accumulate in the CNS.[50] Creutzfeldt-Jakob disease, or CJD, is the most common human prion disease. The majority of the cases are sporadic, but there are also autosomal dominant familial, variant, and iatrogenic forms of the disease. Variant CJD is caused by ingestion of contaminated meat. Iatrogenic CJD occurs after exposure to contaminated surgical equipment or organ transplants. The disease presents with rapidly progressive dementia, ataxia, myoclonus, and eventual death within approximately 1 year.[8] It remains unknown if the non-familial varieties of the disease can be vertically transmitted during pregnancy. Among 4 pregnancy cases reported, there was no evidence of transmission to the offspring with children up to 22 years of age.[50] There are no reports of CJD transmission through breast milk. Preconception genetic testing or prenatal diagnosis in the first trimester can be performed for women with a history of the autosomal dominant familial form of CJD.[8]

PREGNANCY MANAGEMENT PLAN

The CDC recommends infectious disease screening and counseling during preconception visits. All women should be offered HIV testing.[51] In addition, vaccinations should be up to date according to the CDC immunization schedule.[4] Once pregnant, all women should undergo screening for HIV, syphilis, hepatitis B, and if risk factors are present, hepatitis C.[52] Immunizations can also be performed during pregnancy, though live or live-attenuated vaccines are contraindicated. All pregnant women should be offered the inactivated influenza vaccine during the appropriate season as complications of influenza in pregnancy can be severe.[1,51]

In addition, counseling should take place early in the pregnancy regarding preventative measures, particularly for infections that could cause neurologic infection. This includes CMV prevention by encouraging universal precautions in women exposed to young children, listeriosis prevention by teaching safe food preparation techniques and avoidance of high-risk foods, and toxoplasmosis prevention through avoidance of cat feces and raw meat. Counseling should take place regarding the importance of avoiding unprotected intercourse for prevention of sexually transmitted infections. Women should be given travel precautions if they plan to travel to Zika virus-endemic areas during the pregnancy. In addition, appropriate management of herpes simplex virus in symptomatic patients should be initiated including both antiviral treatment and prophylaxis.[51] A screening anatomic ultrasound is performed in the majority of pregnancies at 18–20 weeks of gestation. Sonographic findings

that could represent a congenital infectious syndrome should be discussed with patients and serologic and/or amniotic fluid testing offered as indicated. This could provide evidence of an underlying maternal infection. Given the rarity of some of these infections, involvement of infection disease physicians may be needed, and much of the testing may be performed at an outside reference laboratory.

Women presenting with signs or symptoms potentially concerning for an infection of the CNS should be adequately evaluated and examined. Alarming symptoms include headache, neck stiffness, fever, photophobia, nausea, and altered mental status. It is important to inquire about recent exposure to an infection as well as vaccination history. If the clinical suspicion is high for a neurologic infection, prompt neurology

---

BOX 11.1
CARE MAP FOR NEUROLOGIC INFECTIONS IN PREGNANCY

BEFORE PREGNANCY/PRE-PREGNANCY/NON-PREGNANT
Ensure vaccinations up to date
Accurate history and physical examination
Offer HIV screening for all women

DURING PREGNANCY
Update vaccinations as appropriate, but avoid live and live-attenuated vaccines
Provide influenza vaccination during influenza season
Standard infectious disease screening in pregnancy
    HIV, syphilis, hepatitis B, and hepatitis C if high risk
CMV prevention counseling including universal precautions in those exposed to children
Listeriosis prevention by teaching safe food preparation and avoidance of high-risk foods
Travel precautions for Zika virus-endemic areas
Toxoplasmosis prevention through avoidance of cat feces and raw meat
Counseling about risks of unprotected intercourse
Antiviral treatment and prophylaxis of HSV as indicated
Screening anatomic ultrasound at 18–20 weeks
Maintain suspicion for neurologic infection in appropriate clinical scenario
Prompt neurology consult for patients with high clinical suspicion of neurologic infection

DELIVERY
Alert Neonatologist/NICU team and notify pediatrician if anticipated fetal involvement

POSTPARTUM
Consider consultation with specialists as needed for comorbidities prior to discharge
Contraception counseling
Lactation consult

consultation is indicated. Therapy appropriate for the suspected infection without delay is the general rule in order to avoid sequelae for the mother and fetus.

CONCLUSION

Neurologic infections in pregnancy are uncommon, but they can be associated with high maternal, fetal, and neonatal morbidity and mortality. Pregnant women are more susceptible to certain infectious diseases due to immunologic adaptations. Antenatal screening and maintenance of recommended immunizations are key for prevention of infections during pregnancy, see Box 11.1. It is important to have a low threshold for neurology consultation when patients present with neurologic symptoms that cannot be easily explained by another diagnosis.

REFERENCES

1. Azwa I, Marsh MS, Hawkins DA. Infections in pregnancy. In: Marsh MS, Nashef LAM, Brex BA, ed. Neurology and pregnancy: Clinical management. London: Informa Healthcare; 2012: 134–145.
2. CDC. *Meningitis*. 2016. Available from https://www.cdc.gov/meningitis/index.html (last accessed 12 February 2017).
3. Adriani KS, Brouwer MC, van der Ende A, van de Beek D. Bacterial meningitis in pregnancy: Report of six cases and review of the literature. *Clin Microbiol Infect*. 2012; 18(4):345–351.
4. CDC. *Immunization Schedules*. 2017. Available from https://www.cdc.gov/vaccines/schedules/index.html (last accessed 12 February 2017).
5. Ornoy A, Tenenbaum A. Pregnancy outcome following infections by coxsackie, echo, measles, mumps, hepatitis, polio and encephalitis viruses. *Repro Tox*. 2006; 21(4): 446–457.
6. Jayakrishnan A, Vrees R, Anderson B. Varicella zoster meningitis in a pregnant woman with acquired immunodeficiency syndrome. *Am J Perinatol*. 2008; 25(9): 573–575.
7. Thigpen MC, Whitney CG, Messonnier NE, et al. Emerging infections programs network. Bacterial meningitis in the United States, 1998-2007. *N Engl J Med*. 2011; 364: 2016–2025.
8. Baldwin KJ, Roos Kl. Neuroinfectious diseases in pregnancy. *Semin Neurol*. 2011; 31: 404–412.
9. Mukerji SS, Lyons JL. Neurologic infections in pregnancy. In: Klein AK, O'Neal A, Scifres C, Waters JFR, Waters JH, eds. Neurologic Illness in Pregnancy: Principles and Practice.1st ed. Chichester, UK: John Wiley; 2016: 213–233.
10. Tunkel AR, Glaser CA, Bloch KC, et al. The management of encephalitis: Clinical practice guidelines by the Infectious Diseases Society of America. *Clin Infect Dis*. 2008; 47(3): 303–327.
11. Dodd KC, Michael BD, Ziso B, et al. Herpes simplex virus encephalitis in pregnancy—a case report and review of reported patients in the literature. *BMC Res Notes*. 2015; 8: 118. doi: 10.1186/s13104-015-1071-6.
12. Jacob CE, Kurien M, Varghese AM, et al. Treatment of otogenic brain abscess in pregnancy. *Otol Neurotol*. 2009; 30(5):602–603.
13. Wax JR, Mancall A, Cartin A, et al. Sinogenic brain abscess complicating pregnancy. *Am J Obstet Gynecol*. 2004; 191(5):1711–1712.
14. Baud D, Greub G. Intracellular bacteria and adverse pregnancy outcomes. *Clin Microbiol Infect*. 2011; 17(9):1312–1322.
15. Southwick FS, Purich DL. Intracellular pathogenesis of listeriosis. *N Engl J Med*. 1996; 334(12):770–776.
16. Janakiraman V. Listeriosis in pregnancy: Diagnosis, treatment, and prevention. *Rev Obstet Gynecol*. 2008; 1(4): 179–185.
17. CDC. *Listeria: Prevention*. 2016. Available from https://www.cdc.gov/listeria/prevention.html (last accessed 5 May 2017).
18. Anzivino E, Fioriti D, Mischitelli M, et al. Herpes simplex virus infection in pregnancy and in neonate: Status of art of epidemiology, diagnosis, therapy and prevention. *Virol J*. 2009; 6: 40. doi: 10.1186/1743-422X-6-40.
19. Young EJ, Chafizadeh E, Oliveira VL, Genta RM. Disseminated herpesvirus infection during pregnancy. *Clin Infect Dis*. 1996; 22(1): 51–58.
20. Hutto C, Arvin A, Jacobs R, et al. Intrauterine herpes simplex virus infections. *J Pediatr*. 1987; 110(1): 97–101.
21. American College of Obstetricians and Gynecologists. Management of herpes in pregnancy. ACOG Practice Bulletin No. 82. *Obstet Gynecol*. 2007; 109: 1489–1498.
22. Brown ZA, Selke S, Zeh J, et al. The acquisition of herpes simplex virus during pregnancy. *N Engl J Med*. 1997; 337(8): 509–516.
23. Foley E, Clarke E, Beckett VA, et al. Royal College of Obstetricians and Gynaecologists. Management of genital herpes in pregnancy. October 2014. Available from https://www.rcog.org.uk/globalassets/documents/guidelines/management-genital-herpes.pdf (last accessed May 5, 2017).
24. Gardella C, Brown ZA. Managing varicella zoster infection in pregnancy. *Cleve Clin J Med*. 2007; 74(4): 290–296.
25. Tebruegge M, Pantazidou A, Curtis N. Towards evidence based medicine for paediatricians. How effective is varicella-zoster immunoglobulin (VZIG) in preventing chickenpox in neonates following perinatal exposure? *Arch Dis Child*. 2009; 94(7): 559.

26. Grumach AS, Carmano RC, Lazarotti D, et al. Immunological factors in milk from Brazilian mothers delivering small-for-date term neonates. *Acta Paediatr*. 1993; 82(3): 284.

27. Kenneson A, Cannon MJ. Review and meta-analysis of the epidemiology of congenital cytomegalovirus (CMV) infection. *Rev Med Virol*. 2007; 17(4): 253–276.

28. Cannon MJ, Davis KF. Washing out hands of the congenital cytomegalovirus disease epidemic. *BMC Pub Health*. 2005; 5(70). doi: 10.1186/1471-2458-5-70.

29. Syggelou A, Iacovidou N, Kloudas S, Christoni Z, Papaevangelou V. Congenital cytomegalovirus infection. *Ann NY Acad Sci*. 2010; 1205: 144–147.

30. Pass RF, Zhang C, Evans A, et al. Vaccine prevention of maternal cytomegalovirus infection. *N Engl J Med*. 2009; 360(12): 1191–1199.

31. CDC. *Cytomegalovirus and Congenital CMV Infection*. 2017. Available from https://www.cdc.gov/cmv/clinical/features.html (last accessed 21 October 2017).

32. McArthur JC, Steiner J, Sacktor N, Nath A. Human immunodeficiency virus-associated neurocognitive disorders: Mind the gap. *Ann Neurol*. 2010; 67(6): 699–714.

33. Read PJ, Mandalia S, Khan P, et al. When should HAART be initiated in pregnancy to achieve an undetectable HIV viral load by delivery? *AIDS*. 2012; 26(9): 1095–1103.

34. Panel on Antiretroviral Guidelines for Adults and Adolescents. Guidelines for the use of antiretroviral agents in HIV-1-infected adults and adolescents. Department of Health and Human Services. Available from http://www.aidsinfo.nih.gov/contentfiles/adultandadolescentGL.pdf. (last accessed May 5, 2017).

35. Briand N, Warszawski J, Mandelbrot L, et al. Is intrapartum intravenous zidovudine for prevention of mother-to-child HIV-1 transmission still useful in the combination antiretroviral therapy era? *Clin Infect Dis*. 2013; 57: 903–914.

36. Atkins PT, Belko J, Uyeki TM, Axelrod Y, Lee KK, Silverthorn J. H1N1 encephalitis with malignant edema and review of neurologic complications from influenza. *Neurocrit Care*. 2010; 13(3): 396–340.

37. Sejvar JJ, Uyeki TM. Neurologic complications of 2009 influenza A (H1N1): heightened attention on an ongoing question. *Neurology*. 2010; 74(13): 1020–1021.

38. CDC. *CDC Guidance on Influenza and Infant Feeding*. 2017. Available from https://www.cdc.gov/breastfeeding/disease/influenza.htm (last accessed 21 October 2017).

39. Davis LE, Debiasi R, Goade DE, et al. West Nile virus neuroinvasive disease. *Ann Neurol*. 2006; 60(3):286–300.

40. Alpert SG, Fergerson J, Noel LP. Intrauterine West Nile virus: Ocular and systemic findings. *Am J Ophthalmol*. 2003; 136(4):733–735.

41. CDC. West Nile virus: Pregnancy & Breastfeeding. 2017. Available from https://www.cdc.gov/westnile/faq/pregnancy.html (last accessed 21 October 2017).

42. De Carvalho NS, De Carvalho BF, Fugaca CA, Doris B, Biscaia ES. Zika virus infection during pregnancy and microcephaly occurrence: A review of literature and Brazilian data. *Braz J Infect Dis*. 2016; 20(3): 282–289.

43. CDC. *Zika Virus*. 2017. Available from https://www.cdc.gov/zika/ (last accessed 6 May 2017).

44. Ely EW, Peacock JE, Haponik EF, Washburn RG. *Cyptococcal pneumonia complicating pregnancy*. *Medicine*. 1998; 77(3): 153.

45. Perfect JR, Dismukes WE, Dromer F, et al. Clinical practice guidelines for the management of cryptococcal disease: 2010 update by the infectious disease society of America. *Clin Infect Dis*. 200; 50(3): 291–22.

46. Boyer KM, Holfels E, Roizen N, et al. Toxoplasmosis Study Group. Risk factors for *Toxoplasma gondii* infection in mothers of infants with congenital toxoplasmosis: Implications for prenatal management and screening. *Am J Obstet Gyencol*. 2005; 192(2): 564–571.

47. Montoya JG, Remington JS. Management of *Toxoplasma gondii* infection during pregnancy. *Clin Infect Dis*. 2008; 47(4): 554–566.

48. Stanek G, Wormser GP, Gray J, Strle F. Lyme borreliosis. *Lancet*. 2012; 379(9814): 461–473.

49. Pachner AR, Steiner I. Lyme neuroborreliosis: infection, immunity and inflammation. *Lancet Neurol*. 2007; 6(6): 544–552.

50. Xiao X, Miravalle L, Yuan J, et al. Failure to detect the presence of prions in the uterine and gestational tissues from a gravida with Creutzfeldt-Jakob disease. *Am J Pathol*. 1999; 174(5): 1602–1608.

51. CDC. *Preconception Health and Health Care: Infectious Disease*. 2014. Available from https://www.cdc.gov/preconception/careforwomen/disease.html (last accessed 12 February 2017).

52. CDC. *2015 Sexually Transmitted Diseases Treatment Guidelines*. 2015. Available from https://www.cdc.gov/std/tg2015/screening-recommendations.htm (last accessed 12 February 2017).

12

Headache

Migraine, Pseudotumor Cerebri Syndrome, and Postnatal Headache

DEBORAH I. FRIEDMAN, SHAMIN MASROUR, AND SUSAN HUTCHINSON

ABSTRACT

In most cases, women with headache disorders have normal pregnancy and delivery outcomes and should not be discouraged from becoming pregnant. Pre-pregnancy planning includes weaning of contraindicated medications. Most women with migraine without aura improve during pregnancy. Although there are limitations, various acute and preventive treatments may be employed, including non-pharmacologic options. Anti-epileptic medications should be avoided. For pseudotumor cerebri, the mainstay of treatment includes diuretics and therapeutic lumbar punctures, avoiding topiramate. Surgical treatment may be necessary if vision is threatened. Close monitoring and collaboration between an ophthalmologist, neurologist and obstetrician are critical. New-onset pseudotumor cerebri requires an investigation for secondary causes such as cerebral venous thrombosis. In the absence of a pre-existing primary headache disorder, new headaches in the postnatal period warrant evaluation for secondary headache disorders, including post-dural puncture headache, stroke, cerebral venous thrombosis, pre-eclampsia, eclampsia, reversible cerebral vasoconstriction syndrome (RCVS), and pituitary apoplexy.

MIGRAINE

Background

Migraine is common among females. The prevalence rate in the United States is 18% of women (versus 6% of men) but peaks to 25–30% in mid-life during childbearing years.[1] Given that 50% of pregnancies are unplanned, the choice of migraine medications for women in this population is important to protect against maternal and fetal complications of pregnancy.

Fortunately, most women with migraine experience improvement during pregnancy especially if they have migraines without aura. Migraine with aura is less likely to improve with pregnancy. New onset migraine with or without aura during pregnancy needs further investigation with an appropriate work-up to rule out a secondary headache condition such as preeclampsia, stroke, cerebral venous thrombosis, pituitary tumor, and choriocarcinoma.

The stage of pregnancy is an important consideration for the treatment of migraine during pregnancy. For example, ondansetron is no longer advised during the first trimester due to concerns about cardiac defects and other birth defects in the developing fetus but may be used in the second and third trimesters after organ formation has occurred. A narcotic may be necessary for a severe migraine during the second trimester but should be avoided closer to delivery to prevent withdrawal symptoms in the infant.

For the purposes of this section on treatment, it will be assumed that the diagnosis of migraine was established prior to pregnancy and that there is no secondary headache condition. Treatment will be divided into acute and preventive categories and further divided into pharmacologic and non-pharmacologic. Specific comments will address the appropriateness of treatment for the three trimesters of pregnancy when a distinction is important.

For years, clinicians have become accustomed to looking at the pregnancy category ratings of medications by the letters A, B, C, D, and X (Table 12.1). This category rating is now being phased out. The Pregnancy and Lactation Labeling (Drugs) Final Rule (PLLR) was published by the FDA in 2014.[2] This labeling

TABLE 12.1 PREGNANCY MEDICATION CATEGORIES

A = Controlled studies show no risk.

B = No evidence of risk in humans. The chance of fetal harm is remote but remains a possibility. Adequate, well-controlled studies in pregnancy women have not shown a risk of fetal abnormalities despite adverse findings in animals, or, in the absence of human studies, animal studies show no fetal risk.

C = Risk cannot be ruled out. Adequate, well-controlled human studies are lacking, and animal studies have shown a risk to the fetus or are lacking. There is a chance of fetal harm, but the potential benefits may outweigh the potential risk.

D = Positive evidence of risk. Studies in humans or investigational or post-marketing date, have demonstrated fetal risk. Only use if needed in a life-threatening situation for which alternative safer drugs are not available or are ineffective for condition.

X = Contraindicated in Pregnancy. Studies in animals or humans, or investigational or post-marketing reports, have demonstrated positive evidence of fetal abnormalities.

---

rule requires changes to both the content and format to better assist health-care providers in assessing the risk to benefit ratio for pregnant women and nursing mothers who need to take medication. The PLLR removes the pregnancy letter categories. The labeling change went into effect June 30, 2015, and new prescription drugs and biologics submitted after this date will use the new format, while labeling for medications approved on or after June 30, 2001, will be phased in gradually. Labeling for over-the-counter medicines will not change. However, as the package insert of many migraine prescription medications often still refers to the older letter rating, they will also be used.

A useful and comprehensive reference guide to refer to when making medication decisions during pregnancy is Drugs in Pregnancy and Lactation.[3] The most recent available edition is the 11th edition published in 2017.[4] This guide is a useful reference when counseling women trying to conceive or who have conceived and are struggling with migraines. Significantly, the authors removed the FDA's risk categories (A, B, C, D, X) in the ninth edition following the lead of the FDA, which had proposed new labeling as of 2008.

Treatment

Treatment during pregnancy is stratified based on the severity of the migraine attack. The route of administration needs to be taken into account especially if there is significant nausea or vomiting. Both acute and preventive medications that were effective prior to pregnancy should be reconsidered in terms of safety.

For acute treatment of migraine attacks during pregnancy, pharmacologic treatment should be given with the goal of being migraine free in 2 hours and back to full function with little to no side-effects on the medication and, importantly, with little to no risk to the fetus.

Acute Treatment

Acute oral treatment options

There are a number of safe oral medications that can be utilized in pregnancy and lactation for the acute relief of headache (Table 12.2). Additionally, The American Congress of Obstetricians and Gynecologists (ACOG) states that the recommendation of "taking B6 or Vitamin B6 plus doxylamine is safe and effective and should be considered as first-line treatment," based on consistent scientific evidence.[6] Although the combination of doxylamine/pyridoxine is indicated for the nausea and vomiting of pregnancy, it may also be useful for treating the nausea of migraine during pregnancy.

Non-oral rescue options

Non-oral medications are employed when a migraine attack is more severe or associated with nausea or vomiting. The majority of these are considered compatible with lactation.

- Magnesium (with fluids) IV; avoid long-term infusions
- Diphenhydramine IV
- Antiemetics IV (except ondansetron in the 1st trimester)
- Corticosteroids IV
- Sumatriptan injectable or nasal

Rescue procedure options in the office setting

- Occipital nerve blocks
- Transnasal sphenopalatine ganglion block
- Trigger point injections

TABLE 12.2 COMMON ORAL MEDICATIONS FOR TREATMENT OF HEADACHE

Medication	Pregnancy Category	Lactation	Comments
Memantine	B	Compatible	May be used in all 3 trimesters
Caffeine	B	Compatible in moderate doses	In moderation in all 3 trimesters
Doxylamine/Pyridoxine	A	Compatible in moderate doses	
Diphenhydramine	B	Compatible in moderate doses	
Ibuprofen	B- 1st/2nd Trimester D- 3rd Trimester	Compatible	
Metoclopramide	B	Compatible	
Ondansetron	B	Compatible- limited data	Avoid in 1st trimester
Promethazine	C	Compatible for occasional doses, concerns with chronic use	
Prochlorperazine	C	Compatible for occasional doses,	
Triptans[5]	C	Compatible- limited data	
Butalbital	C	No published data	D if used in high doses at term
Opioids	C	Concerns for potential infant CNS depression, limit dosage/observe	D if used in high doses at term

These office procedures often produce immediate relief with a variable duration of benefit. Lidocaine and ropivacaine are preferable (no pregnancy risk, category B) to bupivacaine (category C) in pregnant women due to shorter half-life (lidocaine) and less cardiac toxicity (bupivacaine). Locally acting nerve blocks without systemic levels should be compatible with lactation.

Non-invasive neuromodulation devices

- Supraorbital nerve stimulation (Cefaly™ Device)
- Transcranial magnetic stimulation (SpringTMS™)
- Non-invasive vagus nerve stimulator (gammaCore™)

Data are not available for the safety of using in neuromodulators during pregnancy and none of these devices are FDA-approved for use during pregnancy. However, they may be options for refractory migraine treatment during pregnancy and many women may already be using them prior to getting pregnant. The supraorbital nerve stimulator is FDA-approved for acute migraine treatment and migraine prevention. Non-invasive vagus nerve stimulation is FDA-approved for the acute treatment of migraine and episodic cluster headaches.

Other non-pharmacologic treatments

- Acupuncture and Acupressure
- Massage therapy
- Physical therapy

Acute migraine medications to avoid during pregnancy

- Ergotamines, including dihydroergotamine, are contraindicated (category X) during pregnancy because of vasoconstrictive effects on uterine blood vessels that may reduce placental and myometrial blood flow and contribute to fetal growth retardation based on observations in animals.
- Non-steroidal anti-inflammatory drugs (NSAIDs) increase the risk of miscarriage and malformations in early pregnancy and are associated with premature closure of the fetal ductus arteriosus and oligohydramnios after 30 weeks' gestation.

Preventive Migraine Treatment Options
Pre-pregnancy planning

Most pregnant women can taper off their preventive medications and do reasonably well given that

TABLE 12.3 COMMON HEADACHE MEDICATIONS THAT ARE NOT TYPICALLY
RECOMMENDED IN PREGNANCY

Divalproex sodium (Category X for migraine)
Topiramate (Category D)
Angiotensin receptor blockers (risk in 2nd & 3rd trimester causing severe fetal & neonatal toxicity similar to ACE
    inhibitors
Angiotensin converting enzyme (ACE) inhibitors (risk of fetal hypotension and decreased renal blood flow)
Paroxetine (risk of birth defects)

migraines generally lessen during pregnancy due to the high levels of estradiol. Some preventives should be tapered off before a woman is trying to get pregnant and are contraindicated during pregnancy (Table 12.3).

The decision of whether to continue or taper off anti-depressants, anti-psychotics, or anti-anxiety medication should be a collaborative decision with the woman's other treating providers including the psychiatrist as untreated depression or bipolar disorder could be devastating during a pregnancy and could lead to suicide or other unwanted outcomes.

If a preventive medication is felt necessary due to frequency of migraines during a woman's first trimester (see Table 12.4), it may often be tapered to a lower dose or even stopped by the second trimester. By the second trimester, estradiol levels are high and fairly steady; this can have a protective effect on migraine especially migraine without aura. A complete remission of attacks of migraine without aura can be induced during the third trimester with serum estradiol levels ranging from 13,000–15,000 pg/ml and progesterone levels ranging from 150–200 ng/ml.[7] The higher level of estradiol may also have a positive effect on depression and enable a woman to decrease the dose or taper off her anti-depressant if taking for migraine with coexisting depression.

TABLE 12.4 PREVENTIVE MIGRAINE TREATMENT OPTIONS

Medication	Pregnancy Category	Lactation	Comments
Memantine	B	No data	No clinical trials; may be beneficial for migraine and cluster headache
Beta blockers	C	Metaprolol preferred	Labetolol preferred, avoid atenolol [REF Briggs]
Selective serotonin reuptake inhibitors	C	Lactation consult needed to individualize treatment options	Avoid paroxetine
Serotonin norepinephrine reuptake inhibitors	C	Lactation consult needed to individualize treatment options	
Tricyclic antidepressants	C	Very limited data	
OnabotulinumtoxinA	C	Compatible	
Verapamil	C	Compatible	Most helpful for migraine with brainstem aura and cluster headache
Lamotrigine	C	Less compatible, consultation and close observation needed	No risk in pregnancy demonstrated to date. Most helpful for migraine with aura and hemiplegic migraine.

Complementary and Alternative Preventive Treatments

- Vitamin B2 (riboflavin)
- Magnesium
- Acupuncture
- Acupressure
- Biofeedback
- Stress-Rreduction
- Yoga
- Massage
- Physical terapy
- Adequate sleep, good nutrition, regular exercise

Pregnancy Registries

Health-care providers have a responsibility to report prescription medications that are purposefully or inadvertently taken during pregnancy. In some cases a woman may be taking medications not knowing she is pregnant. In other cases a woman may take a medication during pregnancy, as the risks of not taking the medication are deemed to be a worse potential consequence. By reporting and then following these women through pregnancy we can achieve higher numbers in pregnancy registries and be more informed when making treatment decisions. For some medications, registries are closed as there was no signal of increased risk of fetal malformation or increased risk of miscarriage after a number of years of reporting. Reporting is voluntary in the United States, so numbers reported do not likely reflect the total number of women exposed to a particular medication. A common misconception is that reporting a case will trigger countless hours of paperwork.

Nearing Delivery

As a woman is nearing the end of her third trimester extra caution needs to be taken with medication taken due to the risk of neonatal withdrawal symptoms or other health concerns that may occur in the neonate. Consultation with a neonatal specialist may be advisable to be better prepared to handle complications that could arise both during labor and delivery as well as after delivery.

Honest and open communication with the pregnant female is critical; some may be reluctant to admit alcohol or substance abuse during earlier stages of pregnancy but out of concern for their soon-to-born child may be more forthcoming closer to delivery.

Postpartum

The drop in estrogen and progesterone that occurs at delivery and the immediate postpartum can trigger a recurrence of severe migraine attacks. Triptans, NSAIDs, and narcotics can be used during this time for acute migraine management. Women who breastfeed often fare better with migraine than women who choose not to breastfeed. When making decisions about medications compatible with breastfeeding, several references can be useful, including the National Library of Medicine's Drugs and Lactation database (LactMed).[8] LactMed is a peer-reviewed, fully referenced database and is updated monthly. It can be accessed at http://toxnet.nlm.nih.gov. Other resources include a comprehensive manual *Medications and Mothers Milk* written by Thomas Hale, PhD, and *Drugs in Pregnancy and Lactation*.[3,9] Both are updated regularly. Hutchinson et al reviewed the topic in 2013 to provide background on migraine treatments while breastfeeding.[10] In general, the authors conclude that many of the commonly used migraine medications may be safely used in lactation, although data are often limited. Ibuprofen, diclofenac, and eletriptan have low breastmilk levels, making them good acute medications, although triptan data are limited. Aspirin and opiods are generally avoided in lactation. For prevention zonisamide, atenolol, and tizanidine are not recommended. (See also Section 5, Chapter 35 on breastfeeding.)

Summary

The majority of women with migraine experience improvement during pregnancy. For those who still suffer with migraines during pregnancy, there are many good treatment options including non-pharmacologic therpaies. As the data can change with regard to safety, it is prudent to stay up to date with the use of migraine medication and its effect on both the developing fetus and the newborn.

PSEUDOTUMOR CEREBRI SYNDROME

The syndrome of increased intracranial pressure without hydrocephalus, infection, inflammation, or mass lesion is termed the pseudotumor cerebri syndrome (PTCS). Causes include various medications (eg, tetracyclines, vitamin A and retinoids, corticosteroid withdrawal and others), increased cerebral venous pressure and an association with various systemic disorders (eg, Turner syndrome, Addison's disease, hyperparathyroidism, obstructive sleep apnea).[11] When no identifiable cause is found, the disorder is termed idiopathic intracranial hypertension (IIH). The terminology used in this section will refer to either the general syndrome (PTCS), which includes IIH, or specifically the idiopathic form (IIH).

IIH, the most common form of PTCS, typically affects obese women of childbearing age. Recent weight gain is also a risk factor.[12,13] Children with the syndrome generally have an underlying cause, but after menarche, girls with IIH resemble their adult counterparts.[14,15] The most common symptoms are headache, brief episodes of unilateral or bilateral visual loss, neck pain, pulsatile tinnitus, and diplopia. The hallmark sign is papilledema and some individuals have a unilateral or bilateral abducens nerve palsy. Prompt diagnosis and initiation of treatment are paramount to prevent permanent visual loss, including blindness in a small percentage of patients. The etiology of IIH and its propensity to affect women are uncertain.

There is no contraindication to a female with IIH becoming pregnant. IIH may develop during pregnancy, although given the amount and rate of weight gain during pregnancy and the associated fluid retention, it is puzzling that there is no increased risk of developing IIH during pregnancy compared to non-gravid control subjects.[16] There is no increased risk of spontaneous abortion.[17] The onset of PTCS during pregnancy or in the early postpartum period requires that cerebral venous sinus thrombosis be excluded as the etiology, as the presentation may be clinically indistinguishable from IIH.[18] Women with a history of previously treated IIH may have a recurrence during pregnancy, which tends to occur in the first 2 trimesters.[19] Additionally, females with active IIH may become pregnant.

PTCS is optimally management by a neurologist and ophthalmologist working together, with the neurologist coordinating the care (alternatively, a neuro-ophthalmologist may follow and manage the patient). During pregnancy, close communication with the obstetrician is critical to ensure the best patient outcome. A neurosurgeon or oculoplastic surgeon may be involved if the patient has a preexisting shunt or needs surgical therapy for visual loss during pregnancy.

Pre-Pregnancy Planning and Monitoring

The optimal management of patients with a history of IIH is to plan for the pregnancy in advance. Discontinue all medications that are contraindicated during pregnancy, such as topiramate and other medications used for headache prevention (see Migraine section), at least 1 to 2 months prior to attempted conception.

Diagnosis

The diagnosis of IIH during pregnancy and in the non-gravid state are similar. Medications are reviewed to exclude a secondary cause such as hypervitaminosis A or use of medications in the tetracycline family. Brain neuroimaging, preferably magnetic resonance imaging and magnetic resonance venography, is performed to exclude a secondary cause. Contrast agents, such as gadolinium, should be avoided during the first trimester if possible.[20] A lumbar puncture reveals an elevated opening pressure (at least 250 mm of water) with normal cerebrospinal fluid (CSF) contents.[21] If the opening pressure is elevated, enough CSF is removed to produce a closing pressure in the normal range (approximately 150 mm CSF). All patients should undergo a complete ophthalmological evaluation, including visual acuity, pupil examination, visual field assessment (automated perimetry), and a dilated ocular fundus examination.

Treatment and Monitoring

The treatment depends on the degree of visual loss that has occurred. The effectiveness of treatment of IIH patients with mild visual loss was studied in the Idiopathic Intracranial Hypertension Treatment Trial.[22,23] When combined with dietary management, acetazolamide given in doses up to 4 grams daily was superior to placebo in reversing visual field loss and improving papilledema at six months. Participants randomized to acetazolamide treatment also had significantly greater improvement in visual and general quality-of-life measures. (Women who were pregnant or had plans to become pregnant during the study were excluded from participation, and the few that became pregnant during their participation were taken off the study drug; there were no adverse pregnancy-related events.)

If the visual loss is mild, acetazolamide is initiated at a dosage of 500 mg twice daily. While isolated cases of birth defects have been reported, large series to date have not shown evidence of increased fetal or maternal complications using acetazolamide during pregnancy, even during the first trimester.[24,25] The dose may be increased if needed, although the lowest dose needed to control the symptoms and signs is recommended. Other diuretics, such as methazolamide, furosemide, hydrochlorothiazide, and spironolactone are often employed in non-gravid women if acetazolamide is not tolerated. The literature on diuretic use during pregnancy is inconsistent; the

European Guidelines do not recommend their use although the National Heart, Lung, Blood Institute (NHLBI) recommends them for second-line therapy of hypertension during pregnancy.[26,27] In general, diuretics should be used with caution during pregnancy because of the potential to reduce the maternal plasma volume.[26] However, there does not appear to be any increased risk to the fetus with diuretic use.[28,29] Acetazolamide is considered compatible with lactation as well.

Patients should follow a low sodium diet and limit weight gain to the minimum desired amount per obstetrical guidelines. Therapeutic lumbar punctures are employed during gestation as needed. If the vision deteriorates rapidly, a lumbar drain may be inserted to try and control the intracranial pressure in urgent situations. Corticosteroids are not recommended for routine treatment but are employed as a temporizing measure when the vision is rapidly failing.

Patients with visual acuity or severe visual field loss at presentation or those with rapidly progressive visual loss may require surgery to preserve their sight.[30] Optic nerve sheath fenestration has the advantage of avoiding hardware in the abdomen and requires the expertise of an experienced orbital surgeon. Ventriculoperitoneal shunting lowers the intracranial pressure, but there is a risk of the peritoneal catheter becoming obstructed with the expending uterus during pregnancy. Either procedure may fail over time. The role of venous sinus stenting, if significant venous sinus stenosis is uncertain but likely contraindicated in most cases because of the need for post-procedure antiplatelet therapy. In fulminant cases, more than one procedure may be needed.

There are no evidence-based guidelines for the management of IIH-associated headaches during pregnancy. If the headaches do not improve with measures to lower the CSF pressure, standard acute and preventive headache treatments are employed based on the patient's headache phenotype and general health. Acetaminophen (paracetamol) is often effective for tension-type headaches and may be employed for the treatment of mild to moderate pain.[31] The use of nonsteroidal anti-inflammatory drugs (NSAIDs) during pregnancy is controversial, and they should certainly be avoided after 30 weeks' gestation: use in late pregnancy increases the risk of premature closure of the ductus arteriosus, impaired renal function, neonatal intraventicular hemorrhage, persistent pulmonary hypertension of the newborn, necrotizing enterocolitis, and cerebral palsy.[31]

Accumulated data suggest that occasional use of triptans is probably safe during pregnancy, with the most data available for sumatriptan. Opioids are generally discouraged for headache treatment but sporadic use of codeine might be considered during pregnancy for rescue medication. Ergots are contraindicated but cause of their uterotonic effects and risk of low-birth-weight newborns.[32] Metoclopramide is currently the recommendation of choice if an antiemetic is needed.

Preventive treatment is considered for frequent headaches, particularly if acute treatment is required more than 2 days weekly. Migraine preventives to consider for use during pregnancy include tricyclic antidepressants, beta blockers, and calcium channel blockers. Beta blockers (propranolol and metoprolol) in the lowest effective dose are considered the first choice for prevention of migrainous headaches during pregnancy. Bradycardia, hypotension, and hypoglycemia from beta blockers may affect the fetus and newborn child.[31] A low dose of amitriptyline is considered second-line therapy and has the benefit of being useful for both migraine and tension-type headaches. Other medications, covered in the previous section, may also be considered, although antiepileptics (including topiramate) and flunarizine are contraindicated.[33] Limited data regarding onabotulinumtoxin during pregnancy from the Allergan Global Safety Database of 572 patients with pregnancy exposure over 24 years found a prevalence of fetal malformations consistent with background population rate.[34] However, many practitioners tend to err on the side of caution and avoid it during pregnancy. Conventional doses of riboflavin (vitamin B2), vitamin B2 and magnesium appear to be safe. Biofeedback, acupuncture, and pericranial nerve blocks using local anesthesia may be employed.[35]

Women with a history of IIH are followed closely during pregnancy for evidence of relapse. Patients with IIH who become pregnant may continue taking acetazolamide. Most of the time, medical management, limiting weight gain, and therapeutic lumbar punctures are successful in treating IIH during pregnancy. Therapeutic abortion is not advised unless there are extreme extenuating medical circumstances.

Delivery

Delivery for patients with IIH is no different than in the general population. IIH does not, in and of itself, require a cesarean section, and active labor does not pose an increased risk.[36] There is no contraindication to epidural or spinal anesthesia, although the presence of a lumboperitoneal shunt may pose an additional challenge to avoid puncturing the shunt tubing. Low forceps outlet may be used if there is concern for intracranial pressure during the second stage of labor.[30]

Postpartum

IIH developing in the postpartum period is managed using the methods described above after venous sinus thrombosis is excluded. The symptoms and signs may remit with weight loss. Patients should be followed for at least a year with interval ophthalmologic evaluation.

Conclusion

IIH may develop, recur or persist during pregnancy. Cerebral venous sinus thrombosis must be considered in women developing PTCS during pregnancy. The diagnosis and treatment are similar to non-gravid patients although topiramate may not be used. With prompt attention and a collaborative management, the outcome is favorable.

POSTNATAL HEADACHE

Headache commonly occurs in the postpartum period, and is one of the three most common reasons for acute care visits.[37] The reported incidence of postpartum headache ranges from 11% to 80% and may occur in approximately 40% of women in the first week after delivery.[38,39,40] Most headaches are benign and likely to improve with minimal intervention; however, life-threatening headaches can occur during this period, and a high index of suspicion for dangerous causes is appropriate.[40]

Although the differential diagnosis for postpartum headaches is extensive and includes all disorders that cause headache outside and during pregnancy, attention is directed at primary and secondary causes that are most common during this period.

Any headache that occurs for the first time during pregnancy requires a detailed history and physical examination with addition of radiographic or laboratory tests as appropriate to exclude secondary causes of headache.

Primary Causes

Primary headaches such as migraine, tension-type, and cluster headaches are the most common causes of postpartum headache. Approximately 50–75% of headaches during the postpartum period are due to primary headache disorders, particularly migraine and tension type headache.[37–39]

A history of previous headaches is a significant risk factor for the development of postpartum headaches.[40,42] Headaches that occur during pregnancy have also been associated with an increased risk of early postpartum headache. Turner et al reported that experiencing a headache before pregnancy is significantly associated with developing a headache 8 weeks after delivery while having headaches during pregnancy increases the risk of developing a headache within 72 hours after delivery.[37]

The abrupt estrogen withdrawal after delivery is a strong trigger for migraine attacks.[38,40,41,43] Approximately 55% of migraineurs experience a headache within a month after delivery, although the attacks are usually milder than the patient's typical migraines.[42, 43]

Comparing pre-pregnancy headache characteristics to the pattern of headache in pregnancy, and the postpartum period helps differentiate a primary headache. Any feature that is unusual or differs from the patient's typical headache history should be considered for further evaluation.

Secondary Causes

Given the possible obstetrical complications associated with pregnancy and the postpartum period, as well as the hypercoaguable state at these times, a secondary cause should be excluded in any postpartum woman presenting with headaches (Table 12.5).[41]

Secondary headaches include headaches due to regional anesthesia complications, obstetrical disease, or intracranial pathology.[40] Intracranial pathology from vascular causes includes cerebral venous sinus thrombosis, intracranial hemorrhage, and stroke (Chapters 14–17) and reversible cerebral vasoconstriction syndrome.

TABLE 12.5 SECONDARY CAUSES OF POSTPARTUM HEADACHE

Postdural puncture headache
Pre-eclampsia/eclampsia
Cerebral venous sinus thrombosis
Ruptured aneurysm or malformation
Subarachnoid hemorrhage
Stroke
Reversible cerebral vasoconstriction syndrome
Posterior reversible encephalopathy syndrome
Pituitary apoplexy

Reversible cerebral vasoconstriction syndrome

Reversible cerebral vasoconstriction syndrome (RCVS) is characterized by severe headaches and diffuse segmental vasoconstriction of cerebral arteries that resolve spontaneously.[44,45] Many terms have been used to describe this condition, but in the puerperium, the name postpartum angiopathy is often used.[38,41,44] The presentation of RCVS can mimic subarachnoid hemorrhage. The headache has a rapid onset and may be the only presenting symptom.[44] The headache, often described as thunderclap, may be occipital or diffuse and associated with photophobia and vomiting.[46] There may be other neurological deficits or seizures. The severe pain usually lasts a few hours but can recur over several weeks.[44] Angiography may reveal areas of stenosis ("string of beads") and dilation in multiple vessels but is normal in some cases.[41,46] Of postpartum cases, 70% are associated with the use of vasoconstrictive drugs, such as bromocriptine, ergots, pseudoephedrine, cannabis or SSRIs.[39,41,44]

Evaluation for RCVS includes a non-contrast CT scan of the head to rule out subarachnoid hemorrhage. A lumbar puncture may be performed to assess for subarachnoid hemorrhage not visible on CT, infection, or vasculitis; pleocytosis may be present in RCVS.[41] Magnetic resonance imaging (MRI), MRA, or CTA of the brain are used to evaluate for vasoconstriction, although catheter-based angiography is the gold standard.[46] It is treated with calcium channel blockers.

Posterior reversible encephalopathy syndrome

Posterior reversible encephalopathy syndrome (PRES) occurs in the setting of acute hypertension and is thus associated with pre-eclampsia and eclampsia. The typical features are headaches, seizures, and altered consciousness with prominent visual disturbances, including cortical blindness. Unlike RCVS, the PRES headache typically develops over several hours, is rarely thunderclap, and usually does not last more than 7 days.[39] Vasogenic edema is present in the subcortical white matter and may extend to the deep white matter or cortical surface, typically in the bilateral parieto-occipital regions.[39] Other areas of the brain may be affected and abnormalities are occasionally unilateral or infratentorial.[47] Small foci of intraparenchymal hemorrhage, subarachnoid hemorrhage, or intraparenchymal hematomas occur in up to two-thirds of patients and are unrelated to the degree of blood pressure elevation.

Stroke

Strokes (ischemic and hemorrhagic), subarachnoid hemorrhage, and cerebral venous sinus thrombosis can also be seen in the puerperium. Ischemic strokes tend to occur mainly in the third trimester and postpartum period, due to increased hypercoagulability as the pregnancy progresses, with its peak in the immediate puerperium.[48] About 17% to 34% of ischemic strokes are accompanied with headache, which is nonspecific in quality and moderate intensity.[49] Please refer to Chapters 14–17 for further discussion on stroke and vascular anomalies.

Post-dural puncture headache

Post-dural puncture headache (PDPH) commonly occurs in the postpartum period. Spinal fluid hypovolemia can be caused by unintended puncture of the dura in the setting of epidural or spinal anesthesia or from a dural tear from labor-related pushing.[50]

PDPH has a characteristic postural nature. Classically, the headache worsens in the upright posture and improves when the patient lies flat. Less commonly, the orthostatic component is minimal and patients may have progressively worsening pain throughout the day. Other features associated with the headache may include worsening with Valsalva maneuvers, such as coughing, sneezing, or bearing down, nausea, pain, or stiffness in the neck and shoulders—and less frequently, tinnitus, diplopia, or hyperacusia.

PDPH is a clinical diagnosis based on the history, postural component of the headache, and associated symptoms.[51] MRI of the brain may show diffuse pachymeningeal gadolinium enhancement, downward displacement of the brain and brain stem, subdural fluid collections, engorgement of the venous sinuses, and enlargement of the pituitary gland.[52]

PDPH is generally self-limited and >85% of headaches resolve without any treatment. Supportive treatment such as bedrest, rehydration, simple analgesics, anti-emetics, caffeine, and opioids are used for initial management.[53] If conservative measures fail, an epidural blood patch should be considered.[49] If PDPH is not recognized or is inadequately treated, chronic CSF hypovolemia may persist, often for years before being accurately diagnosed.

Pre-eclampsia and eclampsia

Pre-eclampsia is characterized by the clinical presence of hypertension and proteinuria or peripheral edema.[41,54] It can occur up to 6 weeks post-delivery.[55] Neurologic symptoms include severe persistent headache, visual defects, confusion, and seizures.[54] The term eclampsia is used when seizures occur in the setting of preeclampsia, not attributable to other causes.[41] Pre-eclampsia should be considered if a postpartum patient presents with hypertension and headache.[39]

Headaches associated with pre-eclampsia, anecdotally, are usually throbbing and either holocephalic or more posteriorly located.[41,55] The headache can be progressive and refractory to analgesics.[48] Several studies suggest that a history of migraine increases the likelihood of developing gestational hypertension and pre-eclampsia.[56] Given pre-eclampsia carries a higher risk of stroke, brain imaging should be considered.[55]

Pituitary apoplexy

Pituitary apoplexy is an uncommon cause of headache in the puerperium, and headache may be the only presenting symptom. Pituitary apoplexy is due to an acute ischemic infarction or hemorrhage of a preexisting pituitary tumor, which can be life threatening.[50] Patients may present with sudden severe headache, visual symptoms, hypotension, and altered mental status.[57] Pituitary apoplexy should be ruled out in any postpartum patient presenting with confusion and a sudden severe headache. Sheehan syndrome, in which there is necrosis of the pituitary gland (typically following postpartum hemorrhage or hypotensive shock) is a distinct condition resulting in slowly progressive panhypopituitarism sometimes accompanied by diabetes insipidus.[58] Patients with failure of lactogenesis (see also Section 5, Chapter 35) should be evaluated for this potential complication of delivery and referred to an endocrinologist and breastfeeding specialist for management as needed.

CONCLUSION

Tension-type headache and migraine account for the majority of headaches in the postpartum period. Although primary headache disorders are a common cause of postpartum headache, the diagnosis of benign headaches should not be assumed. A careful history and evaluation of the patient are needed to rule out secondary causes.

Any new-onset headache, change in prior headache, thunderclap headache, or headache with an abnormal neurological examination that occurs in the postpartum period requires further evaluation, such as laboratory testing and brain imaging, if necessary. Obstetrical complications are considered in the evaluation of a postpartum woman with headaches and include measurement of the blood pressure and urinary protein to rule out pre-eclampsia or eclampsia.

REFERENCES

1. Launer IJ, Terwindt GM, Ferrari MD. The prevalence and characteristics of migraine in a population-based cohort. *Neurology.* 1999; 53: 537–542.
2. US Food and Drug Administration. Labeling Pregnancy and Lactation Final Rule. http://www.fda.gov/Drugs/DevelopmentApprovalProcess/DevelopmentResources/Labeling/ucm093307.htm
3. Briggs GG, Freeman RK, Towers CV, Forinash AB, eds. *Drugs in Pregnancy and Lactation.* 11th ed. Philadelphia: Wolters Kluwer Health; 2017.
4. http://solution.lww.com/briggsdrugsinpregnancy
5. Loder E. The safety of sumatriptan in pregnancy: A review of the data so far. *CNS Drugs.* 2003; 17: 1–7.
6. American College of Obstetricians and Gynecologists (ACOG). Nausea and vomiting of pregnancy. Washington (DC): American College of Obstetricians and Gynecologists (ACOG). April 13, 2004.
7. Martin V, Behbehani. Ovarian hormones and migraine headache: Understanding mechanisms and pathogenesis—Part 2. *Headache.* 2006; 46(30): 365–386.
8. National Library of Medicine: LactMed Database. Available at http://toxnet.nlm.nih.gov
9. Hale T. *Medications and Mothers Milk.* New York, NY: Springer; 2017. Available at www.medsmilk.com
10. Hutchinson S, Marmura M, Calhoun A, et al. Use of common migraine treatments in breastfeeding women: A summary of recommendations. *Headache.* 2013; 53: 614–627.
11. Digre KB, Corbett JJ. Idiopathic intracranial hypertension (pseudotumor cerebri): A reappraisal. *The Neurologist.* 2001; 7: 2–67.
12. Ireland B, Corbett JJ. The search for causes of idiopathic intracranial hypertension. *Arch Neurol.* 1990; 47: 315–320.
13. Ko MW, Chang SC, Ridha MA, et al. Weight gain and recurrence in idiopathic intracranial hypertension: A case-control study. *Neurology.* 2011; 76(18): 1564–1567.
14. Balcer LJ, Liu GT, Forman S, et al. Idiopathic intracranial hypertension: Relationship of age and obesity in children. *Neurology.* 1999; 52: 870–872.

15. Rangwala LM, Liu GT. Pediatric idiopathic intracranial hypertension. *Surv Ophthalmol.* 2007; 52(6): 597–617.

16. Digre KB, Varner MW, Corbett JJ. Pseudotumor cerebri and pregnancy. *Neurology.* 1984; 34: 721–729.

17. Kesler A, Gadoth N. Pseudotumor cerebri (PTC—an update). *Harefuah* 2002; 141: 297–300.

18. Biousse V, Ameri A, Bousser MG. Isolated intracranial hypertension as the only sign of cerebral venous thrombosis. *Neurology.* 1999; 53: 1537–1542.

19. Huna-Baron R, Kupersmith MJ. Idiopathic intracranial hypertension in pregnancy. *J Neurol.* 2002; 249(8): 1078–1081.

20. Ray JG, Vermeulen MJ, Bharatha A, Montanera WJ, Park AL. Association between MRI exposure during pregnancy and fetal and childhood outcomes. *JAMA.* 2016; 316: 952–961.

21. Friedman DI, Liu GT, Digre KB. Revised diagnostic criteria for the pseudotumor cerebri syndrome in adults and children. *Neurology.* 2013; 81: 1159–1165.

22. Friedman DI, McDermott MP, Kieburtz K, et al. The Idiopathic Intracranial Hypertension Treatment Trial: Design considerations and methods. *J Neuro-Ophthalmol.* 2014; 34: 107–117.

23. Wall M, McDermott MP, Kieburtz KD, et al. Effect of acetazolamide on visual function in patients with idiopathic intracranial hypertension and mild visual loss. *JAMA Neurol.* 2014; 13(16): 1641–1651.

24. Falardeau J, Lobb BM, Golden S, Maxfield SD, Tanne E. The use of acetazolamide during pregnancy in intracranial hypertension patients. *J Neuro-Ophthalmol.* 2013; 33: 9–12.

25. Lee AG, Pless M, Falardeau J, Capazzoli T, Wall M, Kardon RH. The use of acetazolamide in idiopathic intracranial hypertension during pregnancy. *Am J Ophthalmol.* 2005; 139(5): 855–859.

26. Mancia G, Fagard R, Narkiewicz K, et al. 2013 ESH/ESC guidelines for the management of arterial hypertension: The task force for the management of arterial hypertension of the European Society of Hypertension (ESH) and of the European Society of Cardiology (ESC). *J Hypertens.* 2013; 31: 1281–1357.

27. Chobanian AV, Bakris GL, Black HR, et al. Joint National Committee on Prevention, Detection, Evaluation, and Treatment of High Blood Pressure. National Heart, Lung, and Blood Institute; National High Blood Pressure Education Program Coordinating Committee on Prevention, Detection, Evaluation, and Treatment of High Blood Pressure: The JNC 7—Complete report. *Hypertension,* 2003; 42: 1206–1252.

28. Pieper PG. Use of medication for cardiovascular disease during pregnancy. *Nat Rev Cardiol.* 2015; 12: 718–729.

29. Collins R, Yusuf S, Peto R. Overview of randomised trials of diuretics in pregnancy. *Br Med J.* 1985; 290: 17–23.

30. Evans RW, Friedman DI. Expert opinion: Management of pseudotumor cerebri during pregnancy. *Headache.* 2000; 40: 495–497.

31. Amundsen S, Nordeng H, Nezvlová-Hinriksen K, Stovner LJ, Spigset O. Pharmacological treatment of migraine during pregnancy and breastfeeding. *Nat Rev Neurol.* 2015; 11: 209–219.

32. Banhidy FN, Puho E, Czeizel AE. Ergotamine treatment during pregnancy and a higher rate of low birthweight and preterm birth. *Br J Pharmacol.* 2007; 64: 510–516.

33. Marmura MJ. Safety of topiramate for treating migraines. *Expert Opin Drug Saf.* 2014; 13: 1241–1247.

34. Brin MF, Kirby RS, Slavotinek A, et al. Pregnancy outcomes following exposure to onabotulinumtoxinA. *Pharmacoepidemiol Drug Saf.* 2016; 25: 179–187.

35. Airola G, Allais G, Castagnoli Gabellari I, Rolando S, Mana O, Benedetto C. Non-pharmacological management of migraine during pregnancy. *Neurol Sci.* 2010; 31(Suppl 1); S63–65.

36. Kassam SH, Hadi HA Fadel HE, Sims W, Jay WM. Benign intracranial hyperetension in pregnancy: Current diagnostic and therapeutic approach. *Obstetr Gyn Surv.* 1983; 38: 314–321.

37. Turner DP, Smitherman TA, Eisenach JC, Penzien DB, Houle TT. Predictors of headache before, during, and after pregnancy: A cohort study. *Headache.* 2012; 52(3): 348–362.

38. Stella CL, Jodick CD, How HY, Harkness UF, Sibai BM. Post-partum headache: Is your work up complete? *Am J Obstetr Gynecol.* 2007; 196(318): 1–7.

39. Wiles KS, Nortley R, Siddiqui A, Holmes P, Nelson-Piercy C. Reversible cerebral vasoconstriction syndrome: A rare cause of postpartum headache. *Pract Neurol.* 2015; 15(2): 41–144.

40. Goldszmidt E, Kern R, Chaput A, MacArthur A. The incidence and etiology of postpartum headaches: A prospective cohort study. *Can J Anaesth.* 2005; 52(9): 971–977.

41. Klein A, Loder E. Postpartum headache. *Intl J Obstet Anesth.* 2010; 19(4): 422–430.

42. Stein G, Morton J, Marsh A, et al. Headaches after childbirth. *Acta Neurol Scand.* 1984; 69(2): 74–79.

43. Sances G, Granella F, Nappi RE, et al. Course of migraine during pregnancy and postpartum: A

prospective study. *Cephalalgia,* 2003; 23(3): 197–205.

44. Ducros A. Reversible cerebral vasoconstriction syndrome. *Lancet Neurol.* 2012; 11(10): 906–917.

45. The International Classification of Headache Disorders. 3rd ed. (beta version). *Cephalalgia.* 2013; 33(9): 629–808.

46. Calabrese LH, Dodick DW, Schwedt TJ, Singhal AB. Narrative review: Reversible cerebral vasoconstriction syndromes. *Ann Int Med.* 2007; 146(1): 34–44.

47. Ollivier M, Bertrand A, Clarençon F, et al. Neuroimaging features in posterior reversible encephalopathy syndrome; A pictorial review. *J Neurol Sci.* 2017; 373: 188–200.

48. Wickstrom K, Edelstam G, Lowbeer CH, Hansson LO, Siegbahn A. Reference intervals for plasma levels of fibronectin, von Willebrand factor, free protein S and antithrombin during third-trimester pregnancy. *Scand J Clin Lab Invest.* 2004; 64(1): 31–40.

49. MacGregor EA. Headache in pregnancy. *Continuum,* 2014; 20: 128–147.

50. Spierings, EL, Sabin TD. De novo headache during pregnancy and puerperium. *Neurologist.* 2016; 21(1): 1–7.

51. Ahmed, SV, Jayawarna C, Jude E. Post lumbar puncture headache: Diagnosis and management. *Postgrad Med J.* 2006; 82(973): 713–716.

52. Mokri B. Spontaneous intracranial hypotension. *Curr Pain Headache Rep.* 2001; 5(3): 284–291.

53. Turnbull DK. Post-dural puncture headache: Pathogenesis, prevention and treatment. *Br J Anaesth.* 2003; 91(5): 718–729.

54. Assarzadegan F, Asadollahi M, Hesami O, Aryani O, Mansouri B, Beladi Moghadam N. Secondary headaches attributed to arterial hypertension. *Iran J Neurol.* 2013; 12(3): 106–110.

55. Cardona L, Klein A. Early postpartum headache: Case discussions. *Semin Neurol.* 2011; 31(4): 385–391.

56. Adeney LK, Williams MA. Migraine headaches and pre-eclampsia: An epidemiologic review. *Headache,* 2006; 46: 794–803.

57. Block HS, Biller J. Neurology of pregnancy. *Handb Clin Neurol* 2014; 121: 1595–1622.

58. Karaca Z, Laway BA, Bokmetas HS, Atmaca H, Kelestimur F. Sheehan syndrome. *Nat Rev Dis Primers.* December 2016; 22:2. doi 0.1038/nrdp.2016.92

13

Traumatic Brain Injury and Pregnancy

KARLA L. THOMPSON, WILLIAM FILER, MATTHEW HARRIS,
AND MICHAEL Y. LEE

INTRODUCTION

Traumatic brain injuries (TBI) are alterations in brain function caused by an external mechanical force. Acquired brain dysfunction due to congenital insults, disease, neurodegenerative disorders, and other causes (eg, stroke, anoxia/hypoxia) are excluded from this diagnosis,[1] even though symptoms of these disorders may sometimes overlap with those of TBI. TBIs are usually associated with a diminished or altered state of consciousness at the time of injury or soon after, and they typically result in impairments in physical and/or cognitive functioning and emotional/behavioral regulation that can be temporary or permanent.

TBI is a critical public health problem throughout the world. It is a major cause of death and disability, particularly in young adults,[2] but there are no readily available global data regarding the number of women of childbearing age who have had or are likely to sustain a TBI. In 2013, TBI contributed to the deaths of nearly 50,000 people and was a diagnosis in more than 282,000 hospitalizations and 2.5 million ED visits in the United States.[3] CDC data from 2001–2010 indicate that men were three times more likely than women to die from TBI,[4] but only about 1.5 times more to be seen in the ED[5] or hospitalized due to TBI.[4] In combination with CDC age-group data,[6,7] it can be estimated that more than 92,000 women of childbearing age are seen in the ED or hospitalized for TBI in the United States each year. These numbers do not include women treated in physicians' offices and other outpatient settings. In addition, an untold number of additional women—for example, victims of domestic violence—may never seek medical treatment at all.

Among survivors, the initial severity of TBI can be classified as mild, moderate, or severe, typically based upon early clinical presentation.[8] The vast majority of TBIs in developed countries (75–80%) are "mild." While there is a strong relationship between injury severity and the severity of post-TBI sequelae, outcomes can vary significantly. Mild TBIs can be a significant source of disability, particularly with respect to cognitive and emotional functioning, and those with moderate to severe injuries may experience more significant residual cognitive and physical impairments that may further complicate pregnancy, childbirth, and childrearing.

TBIs have the potential to disrupt almost any aspect of physical, cognitive, or emotional functioning[9] (see Table 13.1). A comprehensive review of the impact of all TBI-related functional impairments upon a woman's ability to conceive, carry, and deliver a healthy child is beyond the scope of this chapter, but issues that are most likely to impact pregnancy include mobility impairments, hormonal changes, post-traumatic seizures, cognitive dysfunction, and emotional and behavioral issues secondary to brain injury.

ACUTE TBI
IN PREGNANT WOMEN

Any discussion of pregnancy and TBI must examine both those instances of a woman who is pregnant and sustains a TBI and the woman with a history of TBI who becomes pregnant.

Motor vehicle accidents are one of the most common causes of brain injury in young adults in the United States.[10] TBI is therefore frequently associated with other orthopedic or visceral injuries that also require medical attention. Consequently, there is limited understanding of the effects of isolated brain trauma during pregnancy. However, isolated injuries may occur, such as in the case of blunt trauma, gunshot wounds, or assault.

TBI during pregnancy can be life threatening for both the mother and the fetus. Certain known factors that can add to risk of injury to the fetus include maternal high intracranial pressure,

---

TABLE 13.1 SYMPTOMS OF TBI

Physical
Headache
Vision changes
Disequilibrium
Sleep disturbance
Fatigue
Nausea/vomiting
Light/sound sensitivity
Tinnitus/hearing changes
Anosmia
Seizures
Weakness
Sensory changes
Muscle spasticity
Hormone changes
Fertility/sexual dysfunction

Cognitive
Poor attention
Difficulty concentrating
Memory problems
Slowed processing
Speech changes
Visuospatial/visuoperceptual changes
Impaired insight and judgment

Emotional and Behavioral
Depression
Anxiety and Post-Traumatic Stress Disorder
Irritability
Emotional lability
Impulsivity
Disinhibition

---

hypotension, anemia, and lesions with mass effect.[11] One small study suggested a link between traumatic brain injury in pregnant women and risk of cerebral palsy in the child, although more research is needed.[12]

Approaches to acute medical management of acute TBI vary with the nature and severity of injury.[13] Most mild injuries are associated with normal neurologic examinations and negative findings on imaging and do not require hospitalization, although ongoing monitoring of symptoms is recommended. Symptoms of emotional lability, mild cognitive impairment, and/or somatic symptoms (e.g., headaches or vestibular deficits) may merit treatment but are unlikely to significantly compromise pregnancy or delivery. Moderate to severe TBIs may require intracranial monitoring, surgical intervention, and/or prolonged hospitalization[14] and may be associated with decreased arousal, deficits in functional

mobility,[15] and other medical complications (e.g., seizures)[10,14] that can make prenatal and obstetric care more complicated. Severe cognitive impairment will also complicate pregnancy care.

As in other serious maternal trauma, stabilization of the mother is the first priority. During initial evaluation, the preferred imaging modality in acute TBI is head CT because it can detect skull fracture and intracranial bleeding that may require neurosurgical intervention. In the pregnant patient, head imaging should not be delayed because of concerns about fetal radiation exposure; current evidence suggests a head CT results in a minimal dose of fetal radiation.[16] The American College of Obstetricians and Gynecologists guidelines on the use of diagnostic imaging modalities during pregnancy state that MRI is not associated with known adverse fetal defects; however, they recommend avoiding use of contrast agents unless medically necessary for the mother.[17] Acute interventions emphasize maintenance of adequate oxygenation and cerebral perfusion. The secondary development of cerebral edema results in compensatory systemic blood pressure increases to maintain cerebral perfusion pressure, and intracranial pressure (ICP) monitoring is frequently required in the intensive care setting.[18]

Maternal brain death or persistent vegetative state caused by irreversible brain damage in pregnancy is rare, but successful prolongation of pregnancy to preserve the life of the fetus can be achieved. Chiossi and colleagues described two cases of successful delivery of neonates from mothers who were in persistent vegetative states after motor vehicle accidents.[19] Scheduled preterm or late preterm delivery is not always necessary.[20]

Once a pregnant woman is medically stable, functional recovery after TBI is optimized by provision of rehabilitation services. Physiatry (physical medicine and rehabilitation) is a medical specialty that focuses upon maximizing patient functioning after injury or illness. Consultation with physiatry is recommended during acute care for TBI and can guide later treatment. Many other physician specialists may also be involved in or manage post-acute TBI patient care, including neurologists, neurosurgeons, primary care providers, and in the case of pregnant women, OB-GYN specialists. As is the case with any complicated pregnancy, clear and consistent communication among specialists is essential.

Intensive TBI rehabilitation may be provided in an inpatient setting, where patients receive ongoing medical management and nursing care as well as rehabilitation therapies that may include physical

TABLE 13.2 INTERDISCIPLINARY
REHABILITATION TEAM

Physician
Physical therapist
Occupational therapist
Speech and language pathologist
Neuropsychologist, rehabilitation psychologist/
  counselor
Nurse
Social worker/case manager
Family/caregivers
Dietician
Prosthetist/orthotist
Chaplain

therapy (for deficits related to functional mobility), occupational therapy (for deficits related to self-care and independent living), speech therapy (for deficits in speech, swallowing, and cognition), recreation therapy (to support adaptive leisure and community reintegration), and/or psychological and neuropsychological services (see Table 13.2). Therapy may also be provided in nursing facilities, patients' homes, or in outpatient settings, with the setting, duration, nature, and intensity of therapies being determined by the patient's functional deficits. While rehabilitation is most effective when provided soon after injury, changes in a patient's functional status (eg, changes in mobility with pregnancy) may justify additional rehabilitation interventions.

ISSUES COMMON TO ACUTE AND CHRONIC TBI

Medications

To date, no medication has been shown to improve long-term neurological outcomes after brain injury.[21] However, many medications are prescribed to manage symptoms due to TBI during both the acute and post-acute stages of recovery. Commonly prescribed medications include antidepressants, mood-stabilizers, stimulants, cholinesterase inhibitors, and AEDs.[9] Physicians should carefully consider the indications for each medication, reference the US Food and Drug Administration guidelines for rating drug risk to mother and fetus during pregnancy,[22] and stop medications that are not clearly beneficial.

Post-traumatic Seizures

TBI is a known cause of seizures and accounts for 5% of all epilepsy. Post-traumatic seizures (PTS) are typically classified as early (<1 week after TBI) or late (>1 week after TBI). The incidence of late seizures in hospitalized patients is 4–7% in patients with non-penetrating injuries and 35%–65% in patients with injuries involving penetration of the dura. Early post-traumatic seizures are less likely to recur. Anti-epileptic drugs (AEDs) are often recommended for prophylaxis for the first 7 days after injury to prevent complications of seizure activity during the acute period, particularly in cases of penetrating trauma or depressed skull fracture.[8] However, animal and human studies have failed to provide evidence that AEDs prevent the later development of a PTS seizures focus,[23] and several AEDs have known or suspected teratogenic effects, most notably valproic acid.[24] Careful consideration should be given to the need for and potential benefits of AEDs for the mother as well as risks to the fetus or breastfeeding infant.

It is important to be aware that seizures may present with various manifestations, including cognitive, affective, and behavioral changes that may not be immediately attributed to an underlying epileptic disorder. Absence seizures, in particular, may go unrecognized as seizures due to their brevity and lack of motor involvement. Seizures with symptoms of auditory hallucination, fear or panic, and/or gustatory symptoms may be misdiagnosed. When physical, cognitive, or neuropsychiatric symptoms are intermittent and represent a marked departure from a previously established baseline, consideration should be given to the possibility of new-onset seizure activity.

Hormonal Changes and Fertility

Endocrine disorders are common in women after TBI,[25] but there has been little research regarding any relationship between persistence of postbrain injury endocrine dysfunction, fertility, and pregnancy in women. Hypopituitarism is a well-documented complication of TBI,[25] but the severity and permanence of such disturbances are variable. Disruptions of pituitary function often resolve spontaneously in the first year after injury. Other disruptions may become chronic and affect multiple hormones.[26,27] The gonadotropins, LH and FSH, relate directly to fertility and ovulation, and their levels may be suppressed due to brain injury. Likewise, insufficient TSH secretion (and subsequently, circulating thyroid hormone) may lead to clinical hypothyroidism and reduced fertility. Other known potential hormonal deficiencies include growth hormone, cortisol, and vasopressin. Prolactin levels are more often *increased* due to damage to descending inhibitory input from the hypothalamus. The effect of brain injury on oxytocin, a hormone important in lactation and for uterine contractions during labor, is largely unknown.

Menstrual system irregularities, including amenorrhea and more painful menses, have been documented in women with TBI.[28,29] One study found that women with a history of moderate-to-severe TBI did not report greater difficulties with conception or difficulties during pregnancy than non-injured age-matched controls, though they did report more fatigue, depression, mobility problems, decreased concentration, and lower extremity edema than non-injured controls. A pre-pregnancy history of TBI alone does not appear to affect a patient's ability to carry a child to term.[29]

Mobility Impairments

Mobility impairments resulting from TBI may result from muscle weakness and atrophy, joint contractures, heterotopic ossification, and/or deficits in sensation, balance, and coordination.[15] Limited mobility has the potential to make traditional approaches to intercourse challenging, increase a pregnant woman's risk for falls and DVTs, and complicate functional mobility during labor. For women with TBI whose mobility is limited, alternative positions for intercourse[30] or artificial insemination can increase the potential for conception. Physical therapy, including the prescription of assistive devices, may reduce deficits in strength, balance, and coordination and thereby the risk for falls and thrombogenesis during pregnancy. A 2013 Cochrane review found that increased mobility during first-stage labor was associated with shorter labors, better pain management, fewer cesarean births, and decreased risk for newborns requiring admission to a neonatal unit[31]; physical therapy during the later stages of pregnancy to maximize the mother's mobility could potentially benefit both mother and child. Consideration should also be made to maximize arm strength for holding, and a lactation consultant can assist breastfeeding mothers with positioning aids while nursing, if needed.

Cognitive Impairment

TBIs are frequently associated with changes in cognition, emotion, and behavior. While there may be significant recovery of function over time, many TBI survivors are left with some degree of persistent cognitive impairment. Impairments may include deficits in attention, processing speed, language, visuospatial abilities, memory, and/or executive functioning. When these deficits are relatively mild, external supports and compensatory strategies can limit their impact upon a woman's ability to care for herself and her child during and following pregnancy. External supports and compensatory strategies may include supervision, assistance with complex tasks, and utilization of external memory aids: for example, calendars, printed reminders, electronic alarms, and other organizational strategies. Occupational and speech therapies can provide interventions to ameliorate functional deficits in cognition as well as instruction in development and implementation of compensatory strategies.

Some patients with TBI lack the ability to fully appreciate the nature and severity of their cognitive and physical functional deficits. While sometimes interpreted as evidence of the psychological defense of "denial," this lack of awareness, or anosognosia, is often neurologically based. Patients' inability to recognize their functional limitations poses a significant safety risk and can be a significant barrier to effective rehabilitation and independent functioning, as patients may not be motivated to address deficits they do not recognize in themselves.[32] Failure to recognize the presence of cognitive deficits—or other functional deficits—may pose particular challenges for pregnant and breastfeeding women and those involved in their care.

Effect of Pregnancy on Cognition

Many resources available to the public, such as pregnancy guidebooks, mainstream media, and websites warn pregnant women of the possibility of cognitive issues (typically short-term memory problems) during pregnancy. This has been referred to as "baby brain" or "placenta brain." A systematic review found that pregnant women perform worse than non-pregnant women on memory and other cognitive tests,[33] and this has been shown in both cross-sectional[34] and longitudinal studies.[35] This research has been criticized on the grounds that the samples recruited in these studies were typically convenience samples, often recruiting volunteers from pregnancy groups who may already be concerned or anxious about the effects of pregnancy, including on cognition. These studies also were typically unable to control for factors related to pregnancy and motherhood such as fatigue and sleep deprivation. However, it seems reasonable to hypothesize that pregnancy might further exacerbate existing cognitive symptoms in a woman with a history of TBI.

Psychological and Behavioral Problems

Neuropsychiatric symptoms are also common following TBIs of all severity. Many studies have failed to demonstrate a relationship between injury severity and the severity of psychiatric symptoms post-injury, but it is widely accepted that a history of TBI increases risk for depression, anxiety, and substance abuse, and a previous history of psychiatric disturbance is associated with increased risk for poor outcomes following TBI. TBIs in pregnant women may also intensify preexisting emotional or psychological issues related to pregnancy/motherhood that are complicated by TBI.

Our review of the literature revealed no studies that have examined the impact of depression or other psychiatric disorders on reproductive health specifically in women with TBI. However, Colatonio (2010) noted that women with a history of TBI described poorer physical and mental health. They cited problems such as lack of emotional support and lower overall income, and compared to women without TBI, they were more likely to experience postpartum complications and depression.[29]

According to the American Congress of Obstetricians and Gynecologists (ACOG) between 14–23% of women will struggle with symptoms of depression during pregnancy. There is no reason to believe that rates of antepartum depression would be lower in women with a history of TBI. Untreated depression can lead to poor nutrition, substance abuse, and other self-harming behavior that can then cause premature birth, low birth weight, and developmental problems. A woman who is depressed may not have the strength or motivation to adequately care for herself or her developing baby prenatally, and postnatally she may additionally struggle to meet her breastfeeding goals as well as care for herself and her child. Screening for depression in pregnant women with TBI should be a routine part of prenatal and postpartum care. (For more information on post-partum depression, see Section 5, Chapter 34). Breastfeeding should be encouraged, as it been shown to decrease postpartum depression and improve bonding (see also breastfeeding, Section 5, Chapter 35).

Emotional and behavioral dysregulation—emotional lability, inappropriate or catastrophic emotional reactions, poor judgment, and impulsivity—are not uncommon, particularly following more significant TBIs. Deficits in these areas are often believed to be secondary to damage to the frontal executive system, and a woman's ability to appreciate the severity and consequences of her neuropsychiatric symptoms may also be compromised.

The most effective treatment options for anxiety and mood disorders are the same for pregnant women with a history of TBI as they are for non-pregnant women (i.e., cognitive-behavioral psychotherapy with or without the use of psychiatric medication). While cognitive impairment may limit the utility of some forms of psychotherapy, behaviorally based interventions can be effective even when attention, memory, and insight are significantly compromised.[36]

Capacity

Whether prior to or following conception, severe cognitive impairment and/or behavioral dysregulation due to TBI can raise complex medical, legal, and ethical issues. While mild or even moderate cognitive impairment may not significantly compromise a woman's capacity to make decisions regarding her health or that of her fetus, significant deficits in judgment, impulse control, reasoning, and/or memory may raise questions about the mother's ability to provide consent for medical care and the potential for risk to the child. For example, cognitive impairment may compromise a woman's ability to make decisions regarding whether to carry a child to term, consent to and follow through with recommendations regarding prenatal care, make specific decisions regarding the birthing process, or even breastfeed and care for an infant without assistance. Similarly, severe deficits in emotional regulation have the potential to raise concerns regarding a woman's ability to care appropriately for herself during pregnancy and to provide appropriate care for her child after delivery.

In some cases, treating physicians may feel that there is a need to formally evaluate a woman with TBI's capacity to make and communicate reasonable decisions regarding her care during pregnancy. Questions regarding a patient's capacity to provide informed consent are specific to the issues at hand. General intellectual impairment or severe cognitive deficits of other kinds do not, in and of themselves, necessarily mean than a woman lacks capacity to make medical decisions. Even a judicial ruling that someone is incompetent to the extent that a guardian is required does not automatically mean that the patient lacks capacity. For each significant decision which requires consent, the woman's capacity to provide consent should be addressed. If it is determined that a woman's decision-making capacity is absent or diminished, designated or surrogate decision makers (eg, partners, parents, immediate family members, or court-appointed representatives) should be involved in the process.

Neuropsychological Evaluation

Neuropsychological evaluation is an important tool for identifying and characterizing the severity of cognitive, emotional, and behavioral symptoms post-TBI. A thorough evaluation involves a clinical interview as well as up to several hours of cognitive and psychological testing. Interpretation of test data includes assessment of the validity of findings and analysis of patterns of performance, along with consideration of various factors that can affect neurobehavioral performance and functioning, for example, sleep, mood, neurological status, and premorbid functioning. Neuropsychological testing is useful for clinical decision making, planning, and monitoring treatment effects and can be particularly useful in addressing questions of capacity or the need for ongoing supports.

SUMMARY

This chapter has attempted to provide an overview of various patient-care issues related to the complicated intersection between traumatic brain injury (TBI) and pregnancy (Box 13.1). TBI is a global

---

BOX 13.1
CARE MAP FOR PREGNANCY IN THE TBI PATIENT

BEFORE PREGNANCY/PRE-PREGNANCY/NON-PREGNANT
Review prior obstetric and menstrual history
Assess TBI-specific maternal risk factors:
  Seizure disorder
  Post-traumatic hypopituitarism
  Muscle weakness, spasticity, deficits in balance or coordination
  Depression or other psychiatric comorbidities
  Cognitive deficits
Review medications:
  Counseling for potential teratogens
  Identify social support system

DURING PREGNANCY
Adjust medications for symptom management
Monitor for worsening of specific maternal risk factors
Consider physical medicine and rehabilitation consult
Practitioner to determine capacity in cases of cognitive impairment
  Consider neuropsychological evaluation
Monitor impact of physical changes on mobility
  Consider physical therapy

DELIVERY
Multidisciplinary discussion to plan best delivery route and location
Consider positioning difficulties
Anesthesia consultation

POSTPARTUM
Ensure ongoing social support to care for infant and mother
Physical or occupational therapy to address physical needs of caregiving
Monitor for postpartum depression

health crisis and can have an extremely wide range of effects on a person's life and functioning. While this variability can make it more difficult to understand and treat than other, more specific neurological problems, there are some specific considerations to make with TBI and pregnancy. These includes the effects of various injury factors (eg, intracranial pressure, bleeding) on both the mother and the fetus. Recommendations include stabilization of the mother first when possible, and careful monitoring and medical management of post-acute symptoms. Common sequelae that can affect pregnancy and pregnancy care include limited mobility, hormonal changes, seizures, and cognitive and neuropsychiatric symptoms. Neuropsychological evaluation can be useful in describing the nature and severity of cognitive, emotional, and behavioral dysfunction, identifying likely contributing factors, and generating treatment recommendations. Rehabilitation interventions can improve functional recovery after TBI and ameliorate the impact of residual impairments.

REFERENCES

1. Menon DK, Schwab K, Wright DW, Maas AI. Demographics and clinical assessment working group of the international and interagency initiative toward common data elements for research on traumatic brain injury and psychological health. Position statement: definition of traumatic brain injury. *Arch Phys Med Rehabil.* 2010; 91(11): 1637–1640. doi:10.1016/j.apmr.2010.05.017.

2. Roozenbeek B, Maas AIR, Menon DK. Changing patterns in the epidemiology of traumatic brain injury. *Nat Rev Neurol.* 2013; 9(4): 231–236. doi:10.1038/nrneurol.2013.22.

3. Taylor CA, Bell JM, Breiding MJ, Xu L. Traumatic brain injury-related emergency department visits, hospitalizations, and deaths—United States, 2007 and 2013. *MMWR Surveill Summ.* 2017; 66(9): 1–16. doi:10.15585/mmwr.ss6609a1.

4. Rates of TBI-related Deaths by Sex—United States, 2001–2010. Concussion, traumatic brain injury. CDC Injury Center. Available at https://www.cdc.gov/traumaticbraininjury/data/rates_deaths_bysex.html. Accessed March 13, 2017.

5. Rates of TBI-related Emergency Department Visits by Sex—United States, 2001–2010. Concussion, traumatic brain injury. CDC Injury Center. Available at: https://www.cdc.gov/traumaticbraininjury/data/rates_ed_bysex.html. Accessed March 13, 2017.

6. Rates of TBI-related emergency department visits by age group—United States, 2001–2010. Concussion, traumatic brain injury. CDC Injury Center. Available at https://www.cdc.gov/traumaticbraininjury/data/rates_ed_byage.html. Accessed April 5, 2017.

7. Rates of TBI-related hospitalizations by age group—United States, 2001–2010. Concussion, traumatic brain injury. CDC Injury Center. Available at https://www.cdc.gov/traumaticbraininjury/data/rates_hosp_byage.html. Accessed April 5, 2017.

8. Saatman KE, Duhaime A-C, Bullock R, et al. Classification of traumatic brain injury for targeted therapies. *J Neurotrauma.* 2008; 25(7): 719–738. doi:10.1089/neu.2008.0586.

9. Zasler ND, Katz DI, Zafonte RD, Arciniegas DB, Bullock MR, Kreutzer JS. *Brain Injury Medicine: Principles and Practices.* 2nd ed. New York, NY: Demos Medical; 2013.

10. NAMCS/NHAMCS—Ambulatory Health Care Data Homepage. Available at https://www.cdc.gov/nchs/ahcd/index.htm. Accessed March 29, 2017.

11. Vulkov I, Bozhinov P. Head injury during pregnancy. *Akush Ginekol (Sofiia)* 2016; 55(2): 22–26.

12. Leroy-Malherbe V, Bonnier C, Papiernik E, Groos E, Landrieu P. The association between developmental handicaps and traumatic brain injury during pregnancy: an issue that deserves more systematic evaluation. *Brain Inj.* 2006; 20(13–14): 1355–1365.

13. Sujit S, Gaddam K, Robertson CS. Critical Care. In: Zasler ND, Katz DI, Zafonte RD, Arciniegas DB, Bullock MR, Kreutzer JS, eds. *Brain Injury Medicine: Principles and Practices.* 2nd ed. New York, NY: Demos Medical; 2013: 343–356.

14. Sanchez JJ, Kahn DE, Bullock MR. Development of acute care guidelines and effect on outcome. In: Zasler ND, Katz DI, Zafonte RD, Arcinegas DB, Bullock MR, Kreutzer JS, eds. *Brain Injury Medicine: Principles and Practices.* New York, NY; 2013: 367–384.

15. Bell KR, Shenouda CN. Complications associated with immobility. In: Zasler ND, Katz DI, Zafonte RD, Arcinieags DB, Bullock MR, Kreutzer JS, eds. *Brain Injury Medicine: Principles and Practices.* 2nd ed. New York, NY: Demos Medical; 2013: 810–820.

16. Jain V, Chari R, Maslovitz S, et al. Guidelines for the management of a pregnant trauma patient. *J Obstet Gynaecol Can.* 2015; 37(6): 553–574.

17. ACOG Committee on Obstetric Practice. ACOG Committee Opinion. Number 299, September 2004 (replaces No. 158, September 1995). Guidelines for diagnostic imaging during pregnancy. *Obstet Gynecol.* 2004; 104(3): 647–651.

18. Aiolfi A, Benjamin E, Khor D, Inaba K, Lam L, Demetriades D. Brain trauma foundation guidelines for intracranial pressure monitoring: Compliance and effect on outcome.

World J Surg. 2017; 41(6): 1543–1549. doi:10.1007/s00268-017-3898-6.

19. Chiossi G, Novic K, Celebrezze JU, Thomas RL. Successful neonatal outcome in 2 cases of maternal persistent vegetative state treated in a labor and delivery suite. *Am J Obstet Gynecol.* 2006; 195(1): 316–322. doi:10.1016/j.ajog.2006.01.077.

20. Romagano MP, Scorza WE, Lammers SE, Dorr C, Smulian JC. Treatment of a pregnant patient in a persistent vegetative state. *Obstet Gynecol.* 2017; 129(1): 107–110. doi:10.1097/AOG.0000000000001759.

21. Stein DG. Embracing failure: What the Phase III progesterone studies can teach about TBI clinical trials. *Brain Inj.* 2015; 29(11): 1259–1272. doi:10.3109/02699052.2015.1065344.

22. Federal Register: Content and Format of Labeling for Human Prescription Drug and Biological Products; Requirements for Pregnancy and Lactation Labeling. Available at https://www.federalregister.gov/documents/2014/12/04/2014-28241/content-and-format-of-labeling-for-human-prescription-drug-and-biological-products-requirements-for. Accessed March 27, 2017.

23. Temkin NR, Jarell AD, Anderson GD. Antiepileptogenic agents: How close are we? *Drugs* 2001; 61(8): 1045–1055.

24. Tomson T, Battino D. Teratogenic effects of antiepileptic medications. *Neurol Clin.* 2009; 27(4): 993–1002. doi:10.1016/j.ncl.2009.06.006.

25. Urban RJ, Harris P, Masel B. Anterior hypopituitarism following traumatic brain injury. *Brain Inj.* 2005; 19(5): 349–358.

26. Krahulik D, Zapletalova J, Frysak Z, Vaverka M. Dysfunction of hypothalamic-hypophysial axis after traumatic brain injury in adults. *J Neurosurg.* 2010; 113(3): 581–584. doi:10.3171/2009.10.JNS09930.

27. Agha A, Thompson CJ. Anterior pituitary dysfunction following traumatic brain injury (TBI). *Clin Endocrinol (Oxf).* 2006; 64(5): 481–488. doi:10.1111/j.1365-2265.2006.02517.x.

28. Ripley DL, Harrison-Felix C, Sendroy-Terrill M, Cusick CP, Dannels-McClure A, Morey C. The impact of female reproductive function on outcomes after traumatic brain injury. *Arch Phys Med Rehabil.* 2008; 89(6): 1090–1096. doi:10.1016/j.apmr.2007.10.038.

29. Colantonio A, Mar W, Escobar M, et al. Women's health outcomes after traumatic brain injury. *J Womens Health (Larchmt).* 2010; 19(6): 1109–1116. doi:10.1089/jwh.2009.1740.

30. Kroll K, Klein EL. *Enabling Romance.* Horsham, PA: No Limits Communications; 2001.

31. Lawrence A, Lewis L, Hofmeyr GJ, Styles C. Maternal positions and mobility during first stage labour. *Cochrane Database Syst Rev.* 2013; (10): CD003934. doi:10.1002/14651858.CD003934.pub4.

32. Eslinger PJ, Zappala G, Chakara F, Barrett AM. Cognitive impairments. In: Zasler ND, Katz DI, Zafonte RD, Arciniegas DB, Bullock MR, Kreutzer JS, eds. *Brain Injury Medicine: Principles and Practices.* 2nd ed. New York, NY: Demos Medical; 2013: 990–1001.

33. Henry JD, Rendell PG. A review of the impact of pregnancy on memory function. *J Clin Exp Neuropsychol.* 2007; 29(8): 793–803. doi:10.1080/13803390701612209.

34. Swain AM, O'Hara MW, Starr KR, Gorman LL. A prospective study of sleep, mood, and cognitive function in postpartum and nonpostpartum women. *Obstet Gynecol.* 1997; 90(3): 381–386.

35. De Groot RHM, Vuurman EFPM, Hornstra G, Jolles J. Differences in cognitive performance during pregnancy and early motherhood. *Psychol Med.* 2006; 36(7): 1023–1032. doi:10.1017/S0033291706007380.

36. Cattelani R, Zettin M, Zoccolotti P. Rehabilitation treatments for adults with behavioral and psychosocial disorders following acquired brain injury: A systematic review. *Neuropsychol Rev.* 2010; 20(1): 52–85. doi:10.1007/s11065-009-9125-y.

14

Ischemic Stroke Management in Pregnancy

JODI DODDS, AARON I. LOOCHTAN, AND CHERYL D. BUSHNELL

INTRODUCTION

Ischemic stroke is a relatively uncommon but well-documented neurological complication of pregnancy and the postpartum state. A recent systematic review and meta-analysis estimated the pooled crude incidence rate of pregnancy-related stroke to be 30.0 per 100,000 pregnancies.[1] The stroke incidence by stages of pregnancy was estimated at 18.3 per 100,000 with antepartum/peripartum combined, and 14.7 per 100,000 postpartum.[1] One of the first studies to provide greater understanding of the timing of stroke during pregnancy came about with the publication of a retrospective population-based study in 1996, demonstrating that the risk of ischemic stroke during pregnancy is primarily during the first 6 weeks of the postpartum period (relative risk, or RR, 8.7 and RR 0.7 antepartum versus non-pregnant women, respectively).[2] The overall risk of stroke was not increased during pregnancy when combining women with ischemic stroke and intracerebral hemorrhage (RR 1.1, 95% CI 0.6–2.0) but was increased during the postpartum period (RR 7.9, 05% CI 6.0–12.7). Interestingly, no relative risk increase was found following abortion, further suggesting that cerebral infarction primarily arises from pathology occurring later in the pregnancy and during the postpartum period.[2] Another recent large retrospective population-based study found a decrease in the overall incidence of stroke in antepartum women when compared with their non-pregnant counterparts (10.7 per 100,000 person-years, 95% CI 7.6–15.1 versus 25 per 100,000 person-years, 95% CI 24.0–26.0, respectively), with a risk that significantly increased in postpartum period (161.1 per 100,000 person-years, 95% CI 80.6–322.1).[3]

ETIOLOGY

The explanation behind why stroke risk becomes more concerning later in pregnancy and in the puerperium is multifaceted. First, the pregnant body is preparing for blood loss as the time of delivery nears, and a number of physiological and coagulopathic changes occur to prevent catastrophic hemorrhage. As a normal pregnancy progresses, there are decreasing levels of coagulation inhibitors such as antithrombin III and protein S. Additionally, protein C resistance develops in approximately one-third of normal pregnancies, thus promoting a relative hypercoagulable state. This occurs concurrently with increased production of procoagulant factors, most notably in the third trimester as delivery is nearing.[4–5] The causes of ischemic stroke attributed to pregnancy, and are most common during pregnancy are listed in Table 14.1.

Cardioembolic Etiology

Given the hypercoagulable state present during pregnancy and the puerperium, venous thromboembolism with embolization in the presence of intracardiac shunting, such as a patent foramen ovale or atrial septal defect, is a potential etiology for ischemic stroke that should be considered. While the exact incidence in pregnancy is unknown, left common iliac vein compression with venous congestion and predisposition to deep venous thrombosis formation (May-Thurner syndrome) can present during pregnancy with the enlargement of the gravid uterus, and it can provide a source of paradoxical emboli to the brain in patients with interatrial shunts.[6] Evaluation with transthoracic or transesophageal echocardiography for patent foramen ovale or atrial septal defect should be sought, and if such a shunt is identified, lower extremity duplex evaluation for deep venous thrombosis and MR-venogram of the pelvic to assess for pelvic vein thrombosis should be undertaken.

While less common than in their older counterparts, paroxysmal atrial fibrillation should still be considered in pregnant and postpartum patients presenting with cryptogenic ischemic

TABLE 14.1 ETIOLOGIES OF ISCHEMIC STROKE ATTRIBUTED TO PREGNANCY OR ARE MOST COMMONLY ASSOCIATED WITH PREGNANCY

Vasculopathies
- Posterior reversible encephalopathy syndrome (PRES) associated with pre-eclampsia/eclampsia
- Reversible cerebral vasoconstriction syndrome (RCVS), which includes post-partum angiopathy

Cardiac or systemic source of emboli
- Post-partum cardiomyopathy
- Amniotic fluid embolus
- May-Thurner syndrome and paradoxical embolization via patent foramen ovale (PFO)

Hematologic
- Hemolysis, Elevated Liver enzymes, Low Platelets (HELLP syndrome)
- Antiphospholipid antibody syndrome
- Inherited thrombophilias (Factor V Leiden, prothrombin gene mutation)

strokes. Evaluation may include an electrocardiogram (ECG), telemetry monitoring while in the hospital and potentially outpatient prolonged cardiac monitoring with Holter, Loop, or implantable cardiac monitors.

Patients with congenital heart disease, cardiomyopathy, postpartum cardiomyopathy or mechanical heart valves who are already at an increased risk for stroke likely carry an even higher risk during this time of hypercoagulability.

Pre-eclampsia and Eclampsia

Strokes also occur later in pregnancy and in the puerperium because they frequently arise from disease states that tend to present as pregnancy progresses. Pre-eclampsia is defined as the new onset of hypertension during pregnancy with concurrent proteinuria.[7] Eclampsia is the term used to refer to pre-eclampsia once a seizure has occurred, likely due to cerebral edema. Approximately one-third of these strokes (ischemic and hemorrhagic combined) are associated with pre-eclampsia, a condition unique to pregnancy that typically develops after 20 weeks of gestation. It is estimated that the risk of stroke during pregnancy is approximately 4 times higher in women with pre-eclampsia.[8]

Pre-eclampsia and eclampsia are also associated with the development of posterior reversible encephalopathy syndrome (PRES). PRES is a disorder of cerebral autoregulation that results in

vasogenic edema, typically, but not always, in the posterior regions of the brain. While this differs from the traditional concept of arterial ischemic stroke in which an occlusion occurs and downstream infarction results, patients with PRES can sustain ischemic and hemorrhagic events if left untreated.[9] While the exact mechanism has not been fully elucidated, there are several hypotheses. Constriction and dilation of cerebral arterioles maintain consistent cerebral blood flow across a range of mean arterial pressures in a normal physiological state. However, many pregnant patients with PRES are not hypertensive in the non-pregnant state, but become hypertensive after pre-eclampsia develops. When arterioles have reached their maximum ability to constrict in this setting, fluid leakage from excessive cerebral blood flow and/or hemorrhage (rupture of an arteriole under strain) can occur. An alternative hypothesis is that endothelial dysfunction occurs, triggering a cascade which ultimately results in compromise of the blood-brain barrier.[10] Figure 14.1 demonstrates classic findings of PRES on MRI.

Reversible cerebrovascular vasoconstriction syndrome (RCVS) lies on the same continuum of cerebrovascular disorders as PRES, but rather than resulting in cerebral edema, idiopathic vasospasm occurs intracranially preceded by severe thunderclap headaches. RCVS has also been referred to as

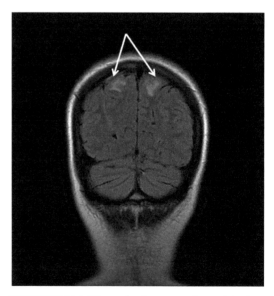

FIGURE 14.1 T2-weighted sequence from MRI of 24-year-old woman with acute onset of right-sided numbness, headache, and hypertension 10 days postpartum. The arrows point to two areas of intracerebral hemorrhage and vasogenic edema, consistent with posterior reversible encephalopathy syndrome (PRES).

postpartum cerebral angiopathy. This condition was discussed in detail previously in Chapter 13.

Antiphospholipid Antibody Syndrome

Antiphospholipid antibody syndrome (APS) is an autoimmune disorder that is associated with an increased risk of thrombosis, resulting in a number of clinical presentations: including DVT, recurrent pregnancy loss, intrauterine growth restriction, and stroke. International criteria for this diagnosis includes at least one thrombotic clinical manifestation in addition to at least one positive antiphospholipid (aPL) antibody lab (lupus anticoagulant [LA], anticardiolipin antibodies [ACL], anti-β2 glycoprotein I antibodies). These results must remain positive at least 12 weeks later.[11] One study found that, among 750 women with known primary APS who were pregnant, 630 (85.3%) were positive for one aPL antibody, while 90 (12.0%) were double positive and 20 (2.7%) were triple positive. Over half (54.5%) of women with more than one positive aPL antibody developed pre-eclampsia during pregnancy.[12] However, the study did not evaluate stroke risk among these patients. A critical literature review in 2013 found that among 31 full text papers about stroke, aPL antibodies were present in 13.5% of cases.[13]

Amniotic Fluid Embolism

Amniotic fluid embolism is a rare cause of stroke during pregnancy. In a systemic review of 121 typical cases of amniotic fluid embolism published in 2017, the mortality rate was 30.6%.[14] A study that retrospectively analyzed hospital discharge data in 5 nations found the incidence of amniotic fluid embolism to be 5.5 to 6.1 per 100,000.[15] This is most likely an underdiagnosed condition when severe sequelae or death does not occur. The incidence of amniotic fluid embolism resulting in stroke during pregnancy and the puerperium is unknown.

ACUTE ISCHEMIC STROKE IN PREGNANCY

When a patient is brought to the emergency department with symptoms concerning for acute stroke, a head CT scan without contrast should be obtained to determine whether an intracranial hemorrhage is the cause of these symptoms. If a patient is pregnant, there may be concern about the radiation exposure to her baby from such a test. The estimated effective dose of radiation associated with a head CT scan is around 2 millisieverts (mSv). Put into context, the average effective dose of background radiation naturally occurring in the United States is approximately 3 mSv/year.[17] If the abdomen and pelvis are properly shielded during the head CT scan, the amount of radiation reaching the fetus is low. Since most strokes will occur later in pregnancy (past organogenesis), the overall risk to the fetus is likely very low, when compared with the benefit of having the CT scan to guide management decisions in a woman who is experiencing an acute stroke.

Where available and able to be performed rapidly to avoid delays in treatment, brain MRI is another option that avoids exposing the fetus to radiation. In the subacute setting when urgent decision-making is not essential, MRI is a preferred imaging modality over CT because it will likely yield more detailed diagnostic information while avoiding the radiation exposure risk altogether. If stroke is large, defined as greater than one third of the middle cerebral artery (MCA) vascular territory or if ischemic stroke shows hemorrhagic conversion, transfer to a neurological ICU for closer monitoring should be considered.

In non-pregnant women and in men, multiple studies have clearly demonstrated benefit from IV recombinant tissue plasminogen activator (rt-PA) administration within the first 3 to 4.5 hours after the onset of ischemic stroke symptoms. While mortality rates are similar between patients receiving IV rt-PA and placebo in clinical trials, patients who receive IV rt-PA are more likely to return to functioning independently 3 months following stroke.[18-22] The hemorrhagic risk associated with IV rt-PA is around 6% in clinical trials. Out of concern for potential hemorrhagic complications during trial design, pregnancy was an exclusion criterion, and the decision about whether to administer IV rt-PA to a pregnant patient in the midst of a stroke remains somewhat controversial.

There is limited information published in the literature about the use of IV rt-PA during pregnancy, but what is present suggests that outcomes in pregnant patients appear to be similar to those seen in the nonpregnant stroke cohort and without evidence of teratogenicity in pregnant animal models.[22] One study retrospectively evaluated 40 pregnant and postpartum women with stroke who were treated with reperfusion therapy found a trend toward increased risk of intracerebral hemorrhage after IV rt-PA use, but their strokes were also of greater severity, for which there is a recognized association with intracerebral hemorrhage risk. There were no cases of in hospital mortality or major systemic bleeding, and rates of patients discharged to home were similar between pregnant/postpartum and their nonpregnant cohort.[23] Careful consideration should be given to each individual case of acute ischemic stroke who is eligible, weighing the potential benefits and risks, but IV rt-PA should not be withheld simply because the woman is pregnant.

Mechanical thrombectomy is an intra-arterial procedure during which an obstructive body (usually a clot) is physically extracted with a catheter. For nonpregnant patients with acute ischemic stroke, thrombectomy became a new standard of care (where available) for patients with middle cerebral artery occlusions suspected to be resulting in acute neurological deficits with moderate to severe symptoms in whom treatment could be initiated within six hours after symptom onset.[24] Two case reports have been published describing thrombectomy for stroke in pregnant women, demonstrating good outcomes.[25] Thrombectomy should be considered in patients with a large vessel occlusion (MCA territory) seen on intracranial vascular imaging. If neuro-interventional capabilities are not available, consideration of transfer to a facility with neuro-intervention, neurology, and obstetrical services is warranted.

Blood pressure management in the acute stroke period is unique to each case. If a patient has severe preeclampsia or cerebral edema associated with PRES, then carefully lowering the blood pressure is an indicated intervention. If a patient has a large artery occlusion secondary to hypercoagulable state, then permitting the patient to be hypertensive is appropriate. Careful collaboration between a maternal-fetal medicine obstetrician and a neurologist is an important part of optimizing care when a pregnant patient is experiencing an acute ischemic stroke.

Deep vein thrombosis (DVT) prophylaxis should be instituted immediately via sequential compression devices. If post-tPA, pharmacologic agents should be held for 24 hours. Pharmacologic DVT prophylaxis should be started by end of hospital day 2 unless a contraindication (eg, intracerebral hemorrhage) exists.

Secondary Stroke Prevention

Once a woman has had a stroke and neurological stability has been achieved, the focus then shifts to secondary stroke prevention. In the pregnant patient, this can be more complex, but in many ways, management may not be that different from the nonpregnant patient, depending on her risk factors.

If a specific etiology for stroke that is unique to pregnancy is present, further management depends on that particular mechanism and whether risk for another stroke may be ongoing. In the case of severe pre-eclampsia with or without PRES, consideration should be given to delivery if the patient is still pregnant and hemodynamically unstable. However, pre-eclampsia can persist beyond delivery, and in some cases, its initial onset can occur in the postpartum period.[16]

Risk factor modification is a mainstay of secondary stroke prevention in the general population and should also be a goal in the pregnant or postpartum patient, albeit with special mindfulness about benefit versus risk with certain medications. As is the case in the nonpregnant population, cigarette smoking cessation and abstention from illicit substance use should be emphasized and encouraged.

Antiplatelet therapy can be safely utilized for secondary stroke prevention in most cases. Aspirin 81mg daily has been used safely during pregnancy for women at risk for stroke, and current guidelines recommend its use even in women without history of stroke who are at high risk of developing preeclampsia.[26] However, the risk of bleeding complications during delivery exists, just as it would for a surgical procedure.[27] Aspirin 325mg daily when taken in the third trimester has been labeled as category D by the Food and Drug Administration out of concern for possible premature closure of the ductus arteriosus. Higher doses of aspirin (as high as 2000mg in one study) have been found to be associated with intracerebral hemorrhage, stillbirth, and other catastrophic abnormalities.[28]

The decision to start therapeutic anticoagulation in a pregnant patient is not without its risks as the time of delivery nears. The benefit of such therapy must be carefully weighed against the hemorrhagic risk, and an informed discussion should occur between the patient and her medical provider. Warfarin (pregnancy category X) has been demonstrated to result in a "Coumadin embryopathy" and abnormalities of central nervous system development. Low molecular weight heparin (Enoxaparin sodium) can be used safely in most patients with a need for anticoagulation during pregnancy, as it does not cross the placenta and does not appear to present significant hemorrhagic complications to the fetus. Data is currently lacking on the safety of direct thrombin inhibitors

BOX 14.1
CARE MAP FOR PREGNANCY IN THE ISCHEMIC STROKE PATIENT

BEFORE PREGNANCY/PRE-PREGNANCY/NON-PREGNANT

Review prior pregnancy complications

If history of previous clotting disorder, hypercoaguable state or history of ischemic stroke consider baseline laboratory testing (platelets, coagulation factors, CBC)

Assessment of disease specific maternal risk factors:
  Personal or family history of previous ischemic stroke
  Personal or family history of hypercoaguable states
  Personal history of eclampsia or preeclampsia
  Personal history of hypertension, hyperlipidemia, diabetes
  Personal history of tobacco, cocaine or other drugs of abuse

Medication adjustment, consolidation and review

DURING PREGNANCY

Monitor for acute focal neurologic deficits, seizures, headaches

If concern for ischemic stroke obtain a STAT non contrasted head CT

Determine if patient is a tPA candidate, administer if appropriate

After CT can consider acute vessel imaging (CT-A)

If intracranial clot found in MCA territory consult interventional team for thrombectomy evaluation

Consider transfer to a thrombectomy ready facility if no intervention team

Transfer to stroke unit or Neuro-ICU if large territory infarct (>1/3 MCA territory)

Maintain adequate blood pressure control based on clinical situation

Determine etiology with 2D ECHO, lipid panel, Hemoglobin

A1C, cardiac monitoring

Antiplatelet vs. anticoagulant based on clinical situation

DVT Prophylaxis by end of hospital Day #2

Secondary Stroke prevention: Anti-platelet, anti-coagulant, anti-hypertensive agents, cholesterol medications, control of diabetes, cessation of tobacco / drugs of abuse

DELIVERY

Multidisciplinary discussion to plan best delivery route and location

Anesthesia

POSTPARTUM

Monitor closely for signs of stroke in postpartum period

Continue frequent blood pressure and neurological checks

Continue secondary stroke prevention

PT/mobility consult/OT consult

Speech therapy consult

Outpatient neurology and PCP follow up

Continue to modify any risk factors (smoking, cocaine, stimulant use)

and factor Xa inhibitors ("NOACs") during pregnancy, and should not be used in place of low molecular weight heparin.

The deficiency of protein S during pregnancy is worth extra mention, as this can lead to the incorrect assumption that a woman has a long-standing intrinsic hypercoagulable state, and this conclusion may result in chronic prescribing of anticoagulation following pregnancy. However, protein S deficiency is a normal part of pregnancy, thus evaluation of protein S deficiency should be delayed until the postpartum period.[29] Additionally, an isolated protein S deficiency in a pregnant patient who has sustained an ischemic stroke should not preclude a more comprehensive evaluation to determine stroke etiology since this is a normal pregnancy lab result.

Statins should also be avoided during pregnancy. The drug class carries a category X label, and early published uncontrolled case series suggested statins were teratogenic. However, in the largest systematic review to date on the subject, 16 clinical studies were reviewed, and there was no identified association between statin use and major congenital malformations.[30] The authors concluded that statins should be avoided until more information is available.

Following delivery of the baby, it is worth reconsidering secondary preventative therapy options. Aspirin is present in small amounts in breast milk, and some rare adverse effects have been reported in nursing infants whose mothers are taking 325mg doses of aspirin or higher daily, but aspirin at the 81mg daily dose appears to be safe. If a woman requires anti-coagulation in the puerperium, warfarin is a reasonably safe option in patients who are breastfeeding. Low molecular weight heparin can be discontinued once the patient has a therapeutic INR on warfarin for ease of administration. As is the case in pregnancy with direct thrombin inhibitors and factor Xa inhibitors, evidence of their safety in breastfeeding is still lacking, and generally it is recommended that these medications be avoided while mothers are nursing their infants.

Lastly, smoking and drugs of abuse cessation counseling should be considered if either of these are implicated as a potential contributor to acute stroke in the pregnant population.

Other Treatment Considerations

While hospitalized, all pregnant women who have suffered an acute ischemic stroke should be evaluated by physical, occupational, and speech therapy. A treatment regimen utilizing all of these modalities should be instituted as soon as possible if there are no contra-indications from an obstetrical perspective. The continuation of these therapies as an outpatient should also be considered (Box 14.1).

Women are more likely to report depression after stroke than men.[31] It is important to screen for depression after a stroke occurs in pregnant women and consider initiation of cognitive behavioral therapy as well as pharmacologic agents. A team approach with the assistance of obstetrics and potentially psychiatry are important particularly if the patient manifests signs of depression prior to delivery. A screening for depression should also be done as an outpatient in clinic during a post-stroke follow-up appointment.

Women who have suffered a stroke in the puerperium or postpartum period represent a unique patient population. Multiple considerations for these patients need to be taken into account with regard to hormonal issues and future pregnancies. A recent consensus statement provides guidance on these topics specifically with regard to future pregnancies, type of delivery, labor induction, and secondary prevention during future pregnancy and lactation.[32] Women with previous stroke during child bearing should be followed throughout their lifetime to help manage lifelong vascular risk factors that may arise. Additionally, following these patients may lead to development of an international registry that could help answer questions about this disease state as randomized controlled trials are unlikely to exist in the near future.[32]

REFERENCES

1. Swartz RH, Cayley ML, Foley N. The incidence of pregnancy-related stroke: A Systematic review and meta-analysis. *Int J Stroke*. 2017; 12(7): 687–697.
2. Kittner SJ, Stern BJ, Feeser BR, et al. Pregnancy and the risk of stroke. *N Engl J Med*. 1996; 335: 768–774.
3. Ban L, Sprigg N, Abdul Sultan A, et al. Incidence of first stroke in pregnant and nonpregnant women of childbearing age: A population-based cohort study from England. *J Am Heart Assoc*. 2017; 6(4): published online April 21, pii: e004601. doi:10.1161/JAHA.116.004601
4. Wickström K, Edelstam G, Löwbeer CH, Hansson LO, Siegbahn A. Reference intervals for plasma levels of fibronectin, von Willebrand factor, free

protein S and antithrombin during third-trimester pregnancy. *Scand J Clin Lab Invest*. 2004; 64: 31–40.

5. Clark P, Brennand J, Conkie JA, McCall F, Greer IA, Walker ID. Activated protein C sensitivity, protein C, protein S and coagulation in normal pregnancy. *Thromb Haemost*. 1998; 79: 1166–1170.

6. Wax JR, Pinette MG, Rausch D, Cartin A. May-Thurner syndrome complicating pregnancy: A report of four cases. *J Reprod Med*. 2014; 59(5–6): 333–336.

7. Crovetto F, Somigliana E, Peguero A, Figueras F. Stroke during pregnancy and pre-eclampsia. *Curr Opin Obstet Gynecol*. 2013; 25: 425–432.

8. James AH, Bushnell CD, Jamison MG, Myers ER. Incidence and risk factors for stroke in pregnancy and the puerperium. *Obstet Gynecol*. 2005; 106: 509–516.

9. Lee VH, Wijdicks EF, Manno EM, Rabinstein AA. Clinical spectrum of reversible posterior leukoencephalopathy syndrome. *Arch Neurol*. 2008; 65:205–210.

10. Marra A, Vargas M, Striano P, Del Guercio L, Buonanno P, Servillo G. Posterior reversible encephalopathy syndrome: The endothelial hypotheses. *Med Hypotheses*. 2014; 82: 619–622.

11. Miyakis S, Lockshin MD, Atsumi T, et al. International consensus statement on an update of the classification criteria for definite antiphospholipid syndrome (APS). *Thromb Haemost*. 2006; 4: 295–306.

12. Saccone G, Berghella V, Maruotti GM, et al. on behalf of PREGNANTS working group. Antiphospholipid antibody profile based obstetric outcomes of primary antiphospholipid syndrome: The PREGNANTS study. *Am J Obstet Geyncol*. 2017; 216(5): 525.e1–525.e12.

13. Andreoli L, Chighizola CB, Banzato A, et al. on behalf of APS ACTION. Estimated frequency of antiphospholipid antibodies in patients with pregnancy morbidity, stroke, myocardial infarction, and deep vein thrombosis: a critical review of the literature. *Arthritis Care Res*. 2013; 65: 1869–1875.

14. Indraccolo U, Battistoni C, Mastrantonio I, Di Iorio R, Pantaleo G, Indraccolo R. Risk factors for fatality in amniotic fluid embolism: A systematic review and analysis of a data pool. *J Maternal-Fetal and Neonatal Med*. 2018 Mar; 31(5): 661–665.

15. Knight M, Berg C, Brocklehurst P, et al. Amniotic fluid embolism incidence, risk factors and outcomes: a review and recommendations. *BMC Pregnancy Childbirth*. 2012; 12(7): 1–11.

16. Bushnell C, Chireau M. Preeclampsia and stroke: Risks during and after pregnancy. *Stroke*

Res Treat. 2011; 2011: 1–9. doi:10.4061/2011/858134

17. McCollough CH, Bushberg JT, Fletcher JG, Eckel LJ. Answers to common questions about the use and safety of CT scans. *Mayo Clinical Proceedings*. 2015; 90(10): 1380–1392.

18. The National Institute of Neurological Disorders and Stroke rt-PA Stroke Study Group. Tissue plasminogen activator for acute ischemic stroke. *N Engl J Med*. 1995; 333(24): 1581–1587.

19. Hacke W, Kaste M, Fieschi C, et al. Intravenous thrombolysis with recombinant tissue plasminogen activator for acute hemispheric stroke: The European Cooperative Acute Stroke Study (ECASS). *JAMA*. 1995J; 274(13): 1017.

20. Hacke W, Kast M, Fieschi C, et al. Randomised double-blind placebo-controlled trial of thrombolytic therapy with intravenous alteplase in acute ischaemic stroke (ECASS II). Second European-Australian Acute Stroke Study Investigators. *Lancet*. 1998; 352(9136): 1245–1251.

21. Hacke W, Kaste M, Bluhmki E, et al. Thrombolysis with alteplase 3 to 4.5 hours after acute ischemic stroke. *N Engl J Med*. 2008; 359(13): 1317–1329.

22. De Keyser J, Gdovinovà Z, Uyttenboogaart M, Vroomen PC, Luijckx GJ. Intravenous alteplase for stroke beyond the guidelines and in particular clinical situations. *Stroke*. 2007; 38; 2612–2618.

23. Leffert LR, Clancy CR, Bateman BT, et al. Treatment patterns and short-term outcomes in ischemic stroke in pregnancy or postpartum period. *AM J Obstet Gynecol*. 2015; 214(6): 723, e1–723.e11.

24. Powers WJ, Derdeyn CP, Biller J, et al. 2015 AHA/ASA focused update of the 2013 guidelines for the early management of patients with acute ischemic stroke regarding endovascular treatment. *Stroke*. 2015; 46(11): 1–51.

25. Sanjith A, Shyamkumar NK, Sunithi A, et al. Mechanical thrombectomy for acute ischemic stroke in pregnancy using the penumbra system. *Ann Indian Acad Neurol*. 2016; 19(2): 261–263.

26. Henderson JT, O'Connor E, Whitlock EP. Low dose aspirin for the prevention of morbidity and mortality from preeclampsia. *Ann Intern Med*. 2014; 161(8): 613–614.

27. Parazzini F, Bortolus R, Chatenoud L, Restelli S, Benedetto C. Follow-up of children in the Italian study of aspirin in pregnancy. *Lancet*. 1994; 343(897): 1235.

28. Schoenfeld A, Bar Y, Merlob P, Ovadia Y. NSAIDs: Maternal and fetal considerations. *Am J Reprod Immunol*. 1992; 28(3–4):141–147.

29. Faught W, Garner P, Jones G, Ivey B. Changes in protein C and protein S levels in normal pregnancy. *Am J Obstet Gynecol.* 1995; 172: 147–150.
30. Karalis DG, Hill AN, Clifton S, Wild RA. The risks of statin use in pregnancy: A systematic review. *J Clin Lipidol.* 2016; 10(5): 1081–1090.
31. Persky RW, Turtzo LC, McCullough LD. Stroke in women: Disparities and outcomes. *Curr Cardiol Rep.* 2010; 12(1): 6–13.
32. Caso V, Falorni A, Bushnell CD, et al. Pregnancy, hormonal treatments for infertility, contraception, and menopause in women after ischemic stroke: A consensus document. *Stroke.* 2017; 48(2): 501–506.

15

Hemorrhagic Stroke Management in Pregnancy

AARON I. LOOCHTAN, JODI DODDS, AND CHERYL D. BUSHNELL

INTRODUCTION

Intracerebral hemorrhage (ICH) is the second most common cause of stroke worldwide, estimated at a rate of 10–20% of all strokes.[1] While rare, ICH during pregnancy can be devastating with significant morbidity and mortality.[2] The mortality rate varies globally and has a range reported from 13%–50%.[3-4] Data from adminstrative sources in the United States list the in-hospital mortality rate for pregnancy-related ICH at 10.1%–20.3%.[5,6]

Globally, the incidence of pregnancy-related ICH varies. In the United States pregnancy-related ICH has been reported at 6.1/100,000 deliveries.[7] A Canadian study listed the incidence at 8/100,000 deliveries[2]; European studies reported an incidence of 0.6/100,000 deliveries in the UK[8] and 4.6 in 100,000 deliveries in France.[9] Asian countries generally have higher incidences of pregnancy-related ICH. A Taiwanese study reported an incidence of 25.4 in 100,000 pregnancies (Table 15.1).[10] Other studies of general populations report 2 times higher incidence of hemorrhagic stroke in Japan as compared to Western countries, while a Chinese study revealed a higher proportion of ICH in Chinese versus white populations.[11,12] Over the past 20 years there has been an increase in pregnancy-related hospitalizations with regard to stroke in the United States.[13]

ETIOLOGY AND RISK FACTORS

It is important to consider the timing at which ICH occurs in the course of pregnancy and the puerperium. While ICH during pregnancy can occur at any age, being older than 35 during pregnancy portends a higher likelihood of pregnancy-related ICH.[7,14] The third trimester and the postpartum period are when the mother is at highest risk of ICH and stroke.[15,16]

As with ischemic stroke, the etiology and risk factors of ICH during pregnancy and the puerperium period are similar as compared to the non-pregnant female population. Risk factors for pregnancy-related ICH are: age > 35, eclampsia, pre-eclampsia, substance abuse (cocaine/tobacco/alcohol), coagulopathy, thrombocytopenia, African American race, and undiagnosed cerebrovascular malformations.[7,8,14]

In terms of etiology, cerebrovascular malformations specifically, arteriovenous malformations (AVMs) and aneurysms are relatively common causes of ICH. Multiple studies have demonstrated that undiagnosed vascular malformations can be the inciting cause of ICH in 21.4%–55.7% of cases. AVMs generally cause pregnancy-related ICH at a higher frequency than unruptured aneurysms.[8,9,15,17] In one study, the detection rate of baseline cerebrovascular disorders before the 32nd week of gestation was significantly higher than that after the 32nd week of gestation.[17] Other vascular causes include moyamoya disease, reversible cerebrovascular vasoconstriction syndrome (RCVS), posterior reversible encephalopathy syndrome (PRES), and cavernous angiomas.[18]

Other structural abnormalities that can lead to pregnancy-related ICH are primary CNS neoplasms or metastatic lesions. Primary CNS neoplasms that are most likely to bleed in general are pilocytic astrocytomas or other gliomas, while the most prone metastatic lesions to bleed include: melanoma, renal cell carcinoma, choriocarcinoma, bronchogenic carcinoma, thyroid papillary carcinomas, hepatocellular carcinomas, and breast cancers.[19-21] However, most of these malignancies are rare in women of childbearing age.

Non-structural lesions are also a common cause of primary ICH in pregnant patients. Uncontrolled hypertension in the setting of pre-eclampsia and eclampsia are common causes.[7-9]

TABLE 15.1 INCIDENCE RANGE OF PREGNANCY-RELATED ICH BASED ON COUNTRY OF ORIGIN

Country	Incidence (per 100,000 deliveries)	95% Confidence Interval (if available)
United States	6.1	
Canada	8.0	
United Kingdom	0.6	0.3–1.0
France	4.6	2.6–7.5
Taiwan	25.4	

Elevated blood pressure in the setting of cocaine or other stimulant use are also plausible mechanisms for uncontrolled hypertension leading to ICH. Lastly, HELLP syndrome has also been implicated as a cause of pregnancy-related ICH.[18]

CLINICAL PRESENTATION

The presenting complaints of pregnancy-related ICH vary depending on the location of the lesion. Cortical insults can present with language deficits (aphasia), visual field deficits, seizures, sensory disturbances, and/or motor symptoms, among other manifestations. Infratentorial lesions can present with coma, diplopia, nausea, vomiting, posturing, ophthalmoplegias or other cranial nerve palsies.[21] Acute severe headache in the pregnant patient should warrant further neurological investigation.

PHYSIOLOGY

While a detailed account of physiological changes during pregnancy is out of the scope of this chapter, a brief mention of basic physiological principles is warranted. Vascular remodeling from the placenta and increased cardiac filling and output can create a hypercoaguable state leading to ischemic stroke. Hypocoaguability in the postpartum state may also occur, which may lead to an increased risk of hemorrhagic stroke.[16,22,23] With regard to hypertension in preeclampsia/eclampsia, systemic vascular resistance increases, which results in hypertension as well as decreased cardiac output and plasma volume.[24] Additionally, excess catecholamine release during pregnancy is also a proposed mechanism of increased hypertension during pregnancy.[25] After ICH, blood becomes intermixed with normal brain tissue, leading to the accumulation of metabolites, thrombin, and hemoglobin,

which leads to molecular disturbances, inflammation, and disruption of the blood brain barrier and subsequent edema.[21] It has been postulated that at approximately 24 hours post-delivery physiological changes return to pre-pregnancy baseline.[24]

EVALUATION AND NON-SURGICAL MANAGEMENT

ICH is a medical emergency. Primary evaluation of the airway, breathing, and circulation should be the first step in stabilization. Intubation should be considered if the ICH is infratentorial or if the Glasgow Coma Scale (GCS), is <8.[21]

For diagnosis, a non-contrasted head CT scan is the first step. There is a relatively low risk of adverse effects to the fetus given fetal malformations occur around a level of 100mgY and a non-contrast head CT exposes one to <0.005 mgY.[70] Precautions should be taken to properly shield the abdomen and pelvis during radiation exposure. After identification of ICH, evaluation for an underlying vascular malformation may be warranted. One option is CT angiography (CT-A) of the brain, which has a small risk of neonatal hypothyroidism as iodinated contrast crosses the placenta.[24] Another diagnostic option is MR-angiography (MR-A). MRI in pregnant patients is indicated after analysis of the risk-benefit ratio, but gadolinium contrast should probably be avoided in most cases as it crosses the placenta and risks to the fetus are unknown (see also Section 1, Chapter 7).[26] Imaging of intracranial vessels with a CT-A/MR-A or CT-venography (CT-V)/MR-venography (MR-V) may also be necessary to evaluate for other underlying vascular etiologies but should not delay initial evaluation for parenchymal lesions. CT and MRI can both be utilized with contrast without interruption in the postpartum lactating patient.

During the initial evaluation it is also reasonable to obtain basic labs, including a complete blood count and coagulation labs to assess for an underlying thrombophilia or hematological abnormality. Deep venous thrombosis (DVT) prophylaxis should also be initiated immediately with sequential compression devices (SCDs), as DVT occurs in 1.6% of all ICH patients.[27] After cessation of bleeding, low-dose subcutaneous low molecular weight heparin (LMWH) or unfractionated heparin may be considered for prevention of DVT in patients with impaired mobility 1 to 4 days from the onset of hemorrhage.[28] Lastly, as with any stroke, we recommend physical, occupational, and speech therapy services during and after hospitalization as indicated.

Blood Pressure Management

Much debate exists with regard to blood pressure parameters in acute hemorrhagic stroke. At the time of this publication, no randomized controlled trial studies have evaluated the pregnant and puerperium population. Thus, management is guided by current guidelines for the non-pregnant ICH population.

The most recent American Heart Association guidelines state that for ICH patients presenting with systolic blood pressures (SBP) of 150 to 220mmHg without contraindication to blood pressure treatment, acute lowering to SBP <140 is safe (Class 1 Level A evidence).[28] Multiple recent studies and meta-analyses have evaluated this topic and have revealed trends in reduction in mortality and dependency at 90 days and decreased hematoma expansion size in intensive BP treated groups, however, these results have not been statistically significant.[29-32] Additionally, according to ATACH-2, aggressive blood pressure lowering did not improve outcomes, and patients in the aggressive blood pressure lowering group had more renal dysfunction than patients whose BP was not aggressively lowered.[32] It is important to note that the average age of individuals in most of these studies were much older than the age of most pregnant women. Additionally, pregnant women and women in the immediate postpartum period were largely excluded. Lastly, many of these studies have a predominately male sample population.

Acute blood pressure management in the setting of ICH in pregnant women or in the postpartum period should be determined on a case by case basis. It is important to keep in mind physiological effects to the fetus in pregnant women, such as decreased placental perfusion pressures.[24] Suggested pregnancy class C agents for the treatment of HTN acutely in pregnant women include: methyldopa, labetalol, and nifedepine. Agents that are contraindicated include atenolol, angiotensin receptor blockers and direct renin inhibitors, as they cause a variety of fetopathies.[16]

Edema Management

Cerebral edema is a common consequence of large vessel ischemic strokes and ICH. Increased edema can lead to multiple types of herniation with brainstem herniation being incompatible with life. Preventing herniation with proper edema management is essential.

Cerebral edema occurs most rapidly in the first 72 hours after ICH, but may persist for up to 7 days after the initial event. If intubated, hyperventilation for a goal PaCO2 to 25–35 mmHG can be an initial temporizing measure to help treat edema.[21] Raising the head of the bed to 30 degrees is often done to help decrease intracranial pressures (ICP). ICP monitoring should also be considered if GCS <9. Maintaining normothermia and normoglycemia is also pertinent as elevated blood sugars and temperatures can increase metabolic demand and result in higher ICP. Treating pain, anxiety, and/or discomfort is also of utility as this can decrease ICP.[33]

Hyperosmolar therapy remains controversial. Mannitol is sometimes used but may result in fetal hypoxia as well as acid-base shifts.[34] Mannitol is dosed initially as a 0.5 to 1.5 g/kg bolus, followed by 0.25 to 0.5 g/kg every 4 to 6 hours, then titrated to a goal of serum sodium between 145–155 mmol/L or goal serum osmolality 310–320 mOsm/kg.[21,27,33] Hypertonic saline is another agent generally given as a 23% 250-ml bolus followed by a continuous infusion for a targeted goal of serum sodium of 145–155 mmol/L.[21] Less is known about this medication in pregnant patients so this should be used with caution. Both of these agents are known to decrease intracranial pressures, however, they do not have evidence supporting improved clinical outcomes.[27] The use of barbiturates is another option for refractory cerebral edema; however, its use in pregnancy is limited to case reports.[35,36]

Other non-medical treatments include external ventricular device (EVD) placement if hydrocephalus occurs, or if there is extensive intraventricular blood. Hemicraniectomy is indicated based on the severity of swelling, the clinical exam, and early signs of herniation on imaging.[21] If possible, pregnant women with ICH should be monitored in a stroke unit.[8] If a stroke unit does not exist, transfer to a tertiary care center with neurology, neurosurgery, neuroradiology, and maternal fetal medicine services is recommended.[24]

DELIVERY AND SURGICAL OPTIONS

Surgery and delivery during ICH are controversial topics. Premature delivery prior to term should be avoided. However, some instances warrant consideration for pre-term delivery. If the cause of ICH is refractory hypertension in the setting of severe pre-eclampsia, then expedited delivery may be helpful. This may also be the case if an underlying vascular abnormality is present, such as an AVM or ruptured intracranial aneurysm. Decreasing the Valsalva and provocative maneuvers in untreated AVMs may be beneficial, but data are not robust to support this view.[24] One study found that the route of delivery (C-section versus vaginal) does not affect outcomes in patients with an underlying vascular anomaly.[37] There is less evidence that surgical excision of AVMs, even with a high risk of rebleeding, is beneficial during pregnancy, but surgical management of ruptured aneurysms during pregnancy is associated with lower maternal and fetal mortality rates.[4]

For surgical candidates, it is not unreasonable to consider emergent C-section if near term prior to attempting correction of ruptured aneurysms or vascular malformations.[38] Other surgical options include: microsurgical excision, pre-surgical embolization, and endovascular embolization with coiling. An individualized approach with consideration of multimodal therapies should be considered for each patient.[39]

For parenchymal ICH not due to an underlying vascular lesion, observational data has suggested that patients with cerebellar hemorrhages who undergo surgical treatment versus medical management have better outcomes in terms of National Institutes of Health Stroke Scale (NIHSS) or Japan Stroke Scale (JSS) score after surgery.[40] This has also been supported in another study in those with cerebellar ICH volumes of >40mL or GCS <14.[41] For supratentorial ICH, randomized control trials have shown no overall benefit from early surgery as compared to initial conservative management at 24 hours, and no significant difference in outcome exists when evaluating surgical intervention versus surgery plus medical management.[42,43] It is not recommended that hypothermia protocols be used for neurosurgical procedures, as there is no clear benefit, and in some cases of cardiothoracic procedures there are reports of increased rates of fetal mortality.[44,45]

Newer technologies have created management options for those with intraventricular hemorrhage as a consequence of primary ICH.[46] Administration of intraventricular thrombolytic therapy (recombinant tissue plasminogen activator, rt-PA) via an EVD has shown accelerated resolution of intraventricular hemorrhage.[47] Analyses of clot removal using this system did not substantially improve functional outcomes in a randomized trial but did show an association between the amount of clot removed and improved odds of attaining a modified Rankin scale (mRS) of ≤3, raising the possibility of some functional benefit to this therapeutic regimen.[48]

ADJUNCTIVE THERAPIES

Seizures and AED Prophylaxis

Eclampsia is a well-known cause of seizures in the pregnant patient. In patients with ICH they have a nidus for seizure activity in addition to their potential underlying propensity to develop eclampsia. In non-pregnant ICH patients, seizures occur at a frequency of 10–15%.[21] It is not unreasonable to place a pregnant patient with ICH on an anti-epileptic drug (AED) for seizure prophylaxis[27]; however, this is usually not necessary if the location of insult is in the basal ganglia or infratentorial region.[49] AED prophylaxis can generally be discontinued in the absence of seizures at 2–4 weeks after inciting event.[50] AED choice needs to be tailored to the clinical situation, with benzodiazepines given acutely for generalized convulsive status epilepticus as a first-line agent. There are many maintenance therapies available, and side-effect profile, teratogenicity risk, and acceptability for breastfeeding all need to be considered once starting a maintenance therapy. Magnesium sulfate can also be added to patients with pre-eclampsia or eclampsia. The general loading dose is 4 to 6g intravenously followed by a maintenance infusion dose between 1–3g/hr.[51,52]

Blood Products and Reversal Agents

Special circumstances arise in those with acute ICH in which consideration of addition of blood products and or reversal agents for antiplatelet or anticoagulant medications need to be discussed. It is important to keep in mind each patient's wishes prior to administration of any of these agents, as certain cultures and religions do not support the routine use of donor blood products.

Platelets

Platelet transfusions may be considered if platelet counts are <100,000 and there is evidence of ongoing active bleeding. If patients are at risk for CNS bleeding or are undergoing a neurosurgical procedure, it is optimal to keep platelet counts >100,000 per cubic millimetre.[53] One trial demonstrated that those who were given platelets for antiplatelet use within one week of ICH had higher odds of death or dependence at 3 months and/or an increase risk of serious adverse events as compared to those not given platelets (Odds ratio 2.05).[54] It is important to communicate with neurosurgery colleagues with regard to the need for blood products and potential neurosurgical procedures.

Heparin and vitamin-K dependent oral anticoagulation

The indication for anticoagulation needs to be considered in the setting of an active ICH prior to reversal. If reversal is indicated, the first step would be to stop the offending agent. For those on heparin or low molecular weight heparin products, the only reversal agent is protamine sulfate (pregnancy category: class C).[28] Protamine sulfate is administered as 1mg per 100 units of heparin, and at a rate no faster than 50mg/min to avoid hypotension.[55]

The vitamin K dependent oral anticoagulants (Coumadin and warfarin) work by inhibiting the vitamin K dependent co-factors: II, VII, IX, X as well as protein C and S.[56] Generally speaking, vitamin-K dependent anticoagulants are avoided in the first trimester of pregnancy secondary to the increased risk of fetal anomalies during this time.[57] While women may not be using warfarin during pregnancy it may be encountered in postpartum women who are breastfeeding.

Direct oral anticoagulants

Presently, there are many more oral anticoagulant options. Specifically the direct oral anti-coagulants are: dabigatran (direct thrombin inhibitor) and rivaroxaban, apixaban, edoxaban, and betrixaban (factor Xa inhibitors; Table 15.2).[56] These medications are preferred in many instances as no requirement for serial monitoring exists.[58] Placental transfer of some of these agents is unknown. Their use postpartum while breastfeeding is not generally recommended because of the potential transfer to breast milk. Current recommendations for reversal of these medications are guided by supportive care, blood transfusions as needed, and monitoring kidney function. If renal function is normal most of these medications are largely metabolized within 24–48 hours. Activated charcoal may be used in those who have taken dabigatran, apixaban, or rivaroxaban if taken within 2 hours of ingestion.[28,59] In rare instances, hemodialysis is used to reverse dabigatran if taken within a few hours and if impaired renal function exists. The factor Xa inhibitors are more protein-bound, making hemodialysis less useful.[59] Currently, the only commercially available reversal agent for DOACs is idarucizumab, a monoclonal antibody fragment that reverses dabigatran's coagulant effects within minutes without any major safety concerns.[60] An investigational recombinant modified human factor Xa decoy protein also exists that binds to factor Xa inhibitors with high affinity, removing factor Xa inhibitors and enhancing endogenous activity of Xa.[61,62] There is much active research in this area with multiple studies underway to establish new agents to help reverse DOACs.[63–68] Breastfeeding does not need to be interrupted for blood transfusions, hemodialysis, or activated charcoal administration. Though there is no data on breastfeeding with idarucizumab, its large molecular weight makes it highly unlikely to enter breastmilk, after which it is likely denatured in the infant's gastrointestinal tract. Therefore breastfeeding during its use is generally considered safe.

PROGNOSIS AND ETHICAL CONSIDERATIONS

While relatively uncommon, ICH in pregnancy can be devastating, with a mortality rate cited as high as 50%.[4] Pregnant women with ICH tend to be younger and have less risk factors upon admission, which may portend a better outcome.[6] For instances where the stroke affects the patient's pituitary, lactational failure may occur. If irreversible brain death occurs as a consequence of hemorrhage, many decisions must be made, usually through a surrogate decision maker. It is important to keep the patient's wishes at the forefront of any discussions; however, one must also keep in mind the viability of the unborn fetus. Approaches such as maintaining physiologic parameters until term, organ donation, and other end-of-life decisions are difficult but must be made in rare instances.[69] The care map for counselling and treating pregnant women with ICH is found in Box 15.1.

TABLE 15.2 CHARACTERISTICS OF DIRECT ORAL ANTICOAGULANTS

Drug	Mechanism of Action	Reversal Agent	Pregnancy Category	Breast Feeding Safety
Dabigatran	Direct Thrombin inhibitor (IIa)	Idarucizumab	C	Alternative anticoagulation preferred
Apixaban	Factor Xa inhibitor	Investigational	B	Avoid
Edoxaban	Factor Xa inhibitor	Investigational	C	Alternative anticoagulation preferred
Rivaroxaban	Factor Xa inhibitor	Investigational	C	Alternative anticoagulation preferred

BOX 15.1
CARE MAP FOR PREGNANCY IN THE INTRACEREBRAL HEMORRHAGE PATIENT

BEFORE PREGNANCY/PRE-PREGNANCY/NON-PREGNANT

Review prior pregnancy complications
If history of previous bleeding disorder or ICH consider baseline
laboratory testing (platelets, coagulation factors, CBC)
Assessment of disease specific maternal risk factors:
  Personal or family history of previous ICH
  Personal or family history of aneurysms or vascular malformations
  Personal history of eclampsia or preeclampsia
  Personal history of hypertension
  Personal history of tobacco, cocaine or other stimulant use
  Personal use of anticoagulant or antiplatelet
Medication adjustment, consolidation and review

DURING PREGNANCY

Monitor for acute headache, vision changes, focal neurologic deficits, seizures
If concern for ICH obtain a STAT non contrasted head CT
After CT can consider vessel imaging (MR-A or CT-A)
Maintain adequate blood pressure control (Goal SBP <160)
Consider AED prophylaxis for cortical lesion
Consult neurosurgery for potential surgical intervention
Consider blood product administration if on anti-platelet
Consider anticoagulation reversal if on anti-coagulation
Transfer to stroke unit or Neuro-ICU

DELIVERY

Multidisciplinary discussion to plan best delivery route and location
Anesthesia and potentially neurosurgical consultation

POSTPARTUM

Continue frequent blood pressure and neurological checks
Cerebral edema management if needed
DVT Prophylaxis at 1–4 days post ICH
Consider cessation of AED after 1–4 weeks if no seizures
PT/mobility consult
OT consult
Speech therapy consult
Discuss future anticoagulation if on anticoagulation prior to bleed
Out patient neurology and PCP follow up to ensure adequate blood pressure
  management
Modify any risk factors (smoking, cocaine, stimulant use)

REFERENCES

1. Feigin VL, Lawes CMM, Bennett DA, Barker-Collo SL, Parag V. Worldwide stroke incidence and early case fatality reported in 56 population-based studies: a systematic review. *Lancet Neurol.* 2009; 8(4): 355–369.
2. Jaigobin C, Silver FL. Stroke and pregnancy. *Stroke* 2000; 31: 2948–2951.
3. Minematsu K, Yamaguchi T. Management of intracerebral hemorrhage. In: Fisher M, ed. *Stroke Therapy.* 2nd ed. Boston: Butterworth Heinemann; 2001: 287–299.
4. Dias MS, Sekhar LN. Intracranial hemorrhage from aneurysms and arteriovenous malformations during pregnancy and the puerperium. *Neurosurgery,* 1990; 27: 855–866.
5. Tate J, Bushnell C. Pregnancy and stroke risk in women. *Womens Health (Lond)* 2011; 7(3): 363–374.
6. Leffert LR, Clancy CR, Bateman BT, et al. Patient characteristics and outcomes after hemorrhagic stroke in pregnancy. *Circ Cardiovasc Qual Outcomes.* 2015; 8(6 Suppl 3): S170–179.
7. Bateman BT, Schumacher HC, Bushnell CD, et al. Intracerebral hemorrhage in pregnancy: Frequency, risk factors, and outcome. *Neurology.* 2006; 67: 424–429.
8. Scott CA, Bewley S, Rudd A, et al. Incidence, risk factors, management, and outcomes of stroke in pregnancy. *Obstet Gynecol.* 2012; 120: 318–324.
9. Sharshar T, Lamy C, Mas JL. Incidence and causes of strokes associated with pregnancy and puerperium. A study in public hospitals of Ile de France. Stroke in Pregnancy Study Group. *Stroke* 1995; 26: 930–936.
10. Liang CC, Chang SD, Lai SL, Hsieh CC, Chueh HY, Lee TH. Stroke complicating pregnancy and the puerperium. *Eur J Neurol.* 2006; 13: 1256–1260.
11. Suzuki K, Izumi M. The incidence of hemorrhagic stroke in Japan is twice compared with western countries: The Akita stroke registry. *Neurol Sci.* 2015; 36: 155–160.
12. Tsai CF, Thomas B, Sudlow CL. Epidemiology of stroke and its subtypes in Chinese vs white populations: a systematic review. *Neurology.* 2013; 81: 264–272.
13. Kuklina EV, Tong X, Bansil P, George MG, Callaghan WM. Trends in pregnancy hospitalizations that included a stroke in the United States from 1994 to 2007: Reasons for concern? *Stroke.* 2011; 42: 2564–2570.
14. James AH, Bushnell CD, Jamison MG, Myers ER. Incidence and risk factors for stroke in pregnancy and the puerperium. *Obstet Gynecol.* 2005; 106: 509–16.
15. Kittner SJ, Stern BJ, Feeser BR, et al. Pregnancy and the risk of stroke. *N Engl J Med* 1996; 335: 768–774.
16. Bushnell CD, McCullough LD, Awad IA, et al. American Heart Association Stroke Council; Council on Cardiovascular and Stroke Nursing; Council on Clinical Cardiology; Council on Epidemiology and Prevention; Council for High Blood Pressure Research. Guidelines for the prevention of stroke in women: A statement for healthcare professionals from the American Heart Association/American Stroke Association. *Stroke.* 2014; 45: 1545–1588.
17. Takahashi JC, Iihara K, Ishii A, Watanabe E, Ikeda T, Miyamoto S. Pregnancy-associated intracranial hemorrhage: Results of a survey of neurosurgical institutes across Japan. *J Stroke Cerebrovasc Dis.* 2014; 23: e65–e71.
18. Yoshida K, Takahashi JC, Takenobu Y, Suzuki N, Ogawa A, Miyamoto S. Strokes associated with pregnancy and puerperium a nationwide study by the Japan Stroke Society. *Stroke.* 2017; 48: 276–282.
19. Lieu AS, Hwang SL, Howng SL, Chai CY. Brain tumors with hemorrhage. *J Formos Med Assoc.* 1999; 98 (5): 365–367.
20. Mandybur TI. Intracranial hemorrhage caused by metastatic tumors. *Neurology.* 1977; 27 (7): 650–655.
21. Nyquist P. Management of acute intracranial and intraventricular hemorrhage. *Crit Care Med.* 2010; 38(3): 946–953.
22. Grear KE, Bushnell CD. Stroke and pregnancy: Clinical presentation, evaluation, treatment, and epidemiology. *Clin Obstet Gynecol.* 2013; 56: 350–359.
23. Razmara A, Bakhadirov K, Batra A, Feske SK. Cerebrovascular complications of pregnancy and the postpartum period. *Curr Cardiol Rep.* 2014; 16: 532.
24. Fairhall JM, Stoodley MA. Intracranial haemorrhage in pregnancy. *Obstet Med.* 2009; 2(4): 142–148.
25. Hamann GF, Strittmatter M, Hoffmann KH, et al. Pattern of elevation of urine catecholamines in intracerebral haemorrhage. *Acta Neurochir (Wien).* 1995; 132: 42–47.
26. Kanal E, Barkovich A, Bell C, et al. ACR guidance document for safe MR practices: 2007. *Am. J.Roentgenol.* 2007; 188: 1447–1474.
27. Broderick J, Connolly S, Feldmann E, et al. Guidelines for the management of spontaneous intracerebral hemorrhage in adults:2007 update: A guideline from the American Heart Association/American Stroke Association Stroke Council, High Blood Pressure Research Council, and the Quality of Care and Outcomes in Research Interdisciplinary Working Group. *Circulation.* 2007; 116: e391–e413.
28. Hemphill JC III, Greenberg SM, Anderson CS, et al. Guidelines for the management of spontaneous

intracerebral hemorrhage: A guideline for health-care professionals from the American Heart Association/American Stroke Association. *Stroke.* July 2015; 46(7): 2032–2060.

29. Zhang Y, Liu Y, Hang J, et al. Intensive or standard: A meta-analysis of blood pressure lowering for cerebral haemorrhage. *Neurol Res.* 2017; 39(1): 83–89.

30. Tsivgoulis G, Katsanos AH, Butcher KS, et al. Intensive blood pressure reduction in acute intracerebral hemorrhage: A meta-analysis. *Neurology.* 2014; 83(17): 1523–1529.

31. Anderson CS, Heeley E, Huang Y, et al. Rapid blood-pressure lowering in patients with acute intracerebral hemorrhage. *NEJM.* 2015; 368(25): 2355–2365.

32. Qureshi A, Palesch YY, Barsan WG, et al. Intensive blood-pressure lowering inpatients with acute cerebral hemorrhage. *NEJM.* 2016; 375(11): 1033–1043.

33. Rabinstein AA. Treatment of cerebral edema. *Neurologist.* 2006; 12(2): 59–73.

34. Wilterdink JL, Feldmann E. Intracranial hemor-rhage. *Adv Neurol.* 2002; 90: 63–74.

35. Montiela V, Grandin C, Goffette P, Fomekong E, Hantson P. Refractory high intracranial pressure following intraventricular hemorrhage due to Moyamoya Disease in a pregnant Caucasian woman. *Case Rep Neurol.* 2009; 1: 1–7.

36. Williams DL, Martin IL, Gully RM. Intracerebral hemorrhage and Moyamoya disease in pregnancy. *Can J Anaesth.* 2000; 47(10): 996–1000.

37. Treadwell S, Thanvi B, Robinson T. Stroke in preg-nancy and the puerperium. *Postgrad Med J* 2008; 84: 238–245.

38. Roman H, Descargues G, Lopes M, et al. Subarachnoid hemorrhage due to cerebral an-eurysmal rupture during pregnancy. *Acta Obstet Gynecol Scand.* 2004; 83: 330–334.

39. Agarwal N, Guerra JC, Gala N, et al. Current treatment options for cerebral arteriovenous malformations in pregnancy: A review of the lit-erature. *World Neurosurg.* 2014; 81: 83e90.

40. Morioka J, Fujii M, Kato S, et al: Surgery for spon-taneous intracerebral hemorrhage has greater remedial value than conservative therapy. *Surg Neurol.* 2006; 65: 67–72.

41. Wijdicks EF, St Louis EK, Atkinson JD, Li H. Clinician's biases toward surgery in cerebellar hematomas: An analysis of decision making in 94 patients. *Cerebrovasc Dis.* 2000; 10: 93–96.

42. Mendelow AD, Gregson BA, Fernandes HM, et al. Early surgery versus initial conservative treatment in patients with spontaneous supratentorial intracerebral haematomas in the International

Surgical Trial in Intracerebral Haemorrhage (STICH): A randomized trial. *Lancet.* 2005; 365: 387–397.

43. Mendelow AD, Gregson BA, Rowan EN, et al. Early surgery versus initial conserva-tive treatment in patients with spontaneous supratentorial lobar intracerebral haematomas (STICH II): A randomised trial. *Lancet.* 2013; 382(9890): 397–408.

44. Pomini F, Mercogliano D, Cavalletti C, Caruso A, Pomini P. Cardiopulmonary bypass in pregnancy. *Ann Thorac Surg.* 1996; 61: 259–268.

45. Todd MM, Hindman BJ, Clarke WR, Torner JC, IHAST Investigators et al. Mild intraoperative hy-pothermia during surgery for intracranial aneu-rysm. *N Engl J Med.* 2005; 352: 135–45.

46. Nyquist P, Hanley DF. The use of intraventricular thrombolytics in intraventricular hemorrhage. *J Neurol Sci.* 2007; 261: 84–88.

47. Webb AJ, Ullman NL, Mann S, et al. Resolution of intraventricular hemorrhage varies by ven-tricular region and dose of intraventricular thrombolytic: The Clot Lysis: Evaluating Accelerated Resolution of IVH (CLEAR IVH) program. *Stroke.* 2012; 43(6): 1666–1668.

48. Hanley DF, Lane K, McBee N. Thrombolytic removal of intraventricular haemorrhage in treatment of severe stroke: results of the randomised, multicentre, multiregion, placebo-controlled CLEAR III trial. *Lancet.* 2017; 389(10069): 603–611.

49. Messe SR, Sansing LH, Cucchiara BL, et al: Prophylactic antiepileptic drug use is associ-ated with poor outcome following ICH. *Neurocrit Care.* 2009; 11: 38–44.

50. Silverman IE, Restrepo L, Mathews GC. Poststroke seizures. *Arch Neurol.* 2002; 59: 195–201.

51. Sibai BM. Magnesium sulfate prophylaxis in pree-clampsia: Lessons learned from recent trials. *Am J Obstet Gynecol.* 2004; 190(6): 1520.

52. Sibai BM, Lipshitz J, Anderson GD et. Al. Reassessment of intravenous MgSO4 therapy in preeclampsia-eclampsia. *Obstet Gynecol.* 1981; 57(2): 199.

53. Hunt BJ. Bleeding and coagulopathies in critical care. *N Engl J Med.* 2014; 370(9): 847–859.

54. Baharoglu MI, Cordonnier C, Al-Shahi Salman R, et al. Platelet transfusion versus standard care after acute stroke due to spontaneous cerebral haemorrhage associated with antiplatelet therapy (PATCH): A randomised, open-label, phase 3 trial. *Lancet.* 2016; 387(10038): 2605–2613.

55. Aguilar MI, Freeman WD. Treatment of coagulopathy in intracranial hemorrhage. *Curr Treat Options Neurol.* 2010; 12(2): 113–28.

56. Barnes GD, Ageno W, Ansell J, Kaatz S. Recommendation on the nomenclature for oral anticoagulants: Communication from the SSC of the ISTH. *J Thromb Haemost.* 2015; 13(6): 1154–6.

57. Bates SM, Greer IA, Middeldorp S, et al. VTE, thrombophilia, antithrombotic therapy, and pregnancy: Antithrombotic therapy and prevention of thrombosis, 9th ed. American College of Chest Physicians Evidence-Based Clinical Practice Guidelines. *Chest.* 2012; 141(2 suppl): e691S–736S.

58. Baglin T, Hillarp A, Tripodi A, Elalamy I, Buller H, Ageno W. Measuring oral direct inhibitors (ODIs) of thrombin and factor Xa: A recommendation from the Subcommittee on Control of Anticoagulation of the Scientific and Standardization Committee of the International Society on Thrombosis and Haemostasis. *J Thromb Haemost.* 2013; 11: 756–760.

59. Kaatz S, Kouides PA, Garcia DA, et al. Guidance on the emergent reversal of oral thrombin and factor Xa inhibitors. *Am J Hematol.* 2012; 87(Suppl 1): 141–145.

50. Pollack CV, Reilly PA, Eikelboom J, et al. Idarucizumab for dabigatran reversal. *N Engl J Med.* 2015; 373(6): 511–520.

61. Lu G, DeGuzman FR, Hollenbach, SJ, et al. A specific antidote for reversal of anticoagulation by direct and indirect inhibitors of coagulation factor Xa, *Nat Med.* 2013; 19(4): 446–451.

62. Nafee T, Aslam A, Chi G, et al. Andexanet alfa for the reversal of anticoagulant activity in patients treated with direct and indirect factor Xa inhibitors. *Expert Rev Cardiovasc Ther.* 2017; 15(4): 237–245.

63. Tummala R, Kavtaradze A., Gupta A, Gosh RK. Specific antidotes against direct oral anticoagulants: A comprehensive review of clinical trials data. *Int J Cardiol.* 2016; 214: 292–298.

64. Crowther M, Lu G, Conley PB, et al. Reversal of factor Xa inhibitors-induced anticoagulation in healthy subjects by and exanet alfa. *Crit Care Med.* 2014; 42(12): A1469–A1469.

65. Siegal DM, Curnutte JT, Connolly SJ, et al. Andexanet Alfa for the reversal of factor xa inhibitor activity. *N Engl J Med.* 2015; 373: 2413–2424.

66. Laulicht B, Bakhru S, Jiang X, et al. Antidote for new oral anticoagulants: Mechanism of action and binding specificity of PER977. Presented at the 24th Congress of the International Society on Thrombosis and Haemostasis, Amsterdam, June 29–July 4, 2013.

67. Ruff CT, Giugliano RP, Braunwald E, et al. Association between edoxaban dose, concentration, anti-factor Xa activity, and outcomes: an analysis of data from the randomised, double-blind ENGAGE AF-TIMI 48 trial. *Lancet.* 2015; 385(9984): 2288–2295.

68. Ansell JE, Bakhru SH, Laulicht BE, et al. Use of PER977 to reverse the anticoagulant effect of edoxaban. *N Engl J Med.* 2014; 371: 2141–2142.

69. Feldman DM, Borgida AF, Rodis JF, Campbell WA. Irreversible Maternal Brain Injury During Pregnancy: A Case Report and Review of the Literature. *Obstet Gynecol Surv.* 2000; 55(11): 708–714.

70. ICRP. Pregnancy and medical radiation. Ann ICRP. 2000; 30: ii–viii, 1–43.

16

Management of Intracranial Vascular Lesions During Pregnancy

JACLYN J. RENFROW, AQIB H. ZEHRI, KYLE M. FARGEN,
JASMEET SINGH, JOHN A. WILSON, AND STACEY Q. WOLFE

INTRODUCTION

The management of intracranial vascular lesions during pregnancy and the postpartum period poses a significant challenge due to the physiologic changes of pregnancy, morbidity of intracranial hemorrhage, and unclear natural history of these lesions. Symptoms of intracranial lesions such as headache, seizures, or hypertension can be confused with pre-eclampsia and eclampsia.[1] Cohort studies investigating the natural history of intracranial vascular lesions exist, but translation to individual patients remains a challenge. Furthermore, there is inherent risk of conventional diagnostic and treatment modalities, including ionizing radiation, which may affect both mother and fetus. Usually, such decisions involve an in-depth discussion with the patient and their family regarding the risk-benefit ratio of intervention versus conservative management and optimal timing. This chapter will discuss key physiologic alterations found during pregnancy that influence clinical treatment, as well as management of the most common intracranial vascular abnormalities during pregnancy, including cerebral aneurysms, arteriovenous malformations (AVMs), and cavernous malformations (CMs) (Box 16.1).

PHYSIOLOGIC CHANGES OF PREGNANCY

Many cardiovascular, hemodynamic, and hormonal changes occur during pregnancy. These physiologic changes support the growing fetus and uterus and enable the parturient to withstand labor and the postpartum course.[2] These factors may modify the natural history of intracranial vascular lesions during pregnancy.

Maternal blood volume increases due to expansion of both plasma and red blood cell volume during pregnancy to allow sufficient perfusion to the placenta and fetus and prepare the mother for blood loss associated with parturition.[2] Cardiovascular changes begin in the first trimester of pregnancy when cardiac output increases 30–50% from the early first trimester and reaches its peak at 25–30 weeks of gestation.[2] This increase has been attributed to increased rates of hemorrhage from arteriovenous malformations during pregnancy.[3,4]

Blood pressure in pregnancy tends to be approximately 20% lower than pre-pregnancy values due to progesterone-driven vasodilation in response to increased blood volume.[2,5] Systemic vascular resistance reaches a nadir in the second trimester, followed by a gradual increase until term.

Hormonal signaling, including VEGF, bFGF, placental growth factor, estrogen, and progesterone, increase during pregnancy to promote the vascular proliferation and expansion for placental development.[6,7] These same angiogenic factors, however, may also promote growth, thrombosis, and hemorrhage of vascular lesions such as AVMs, moyamoya disease, and cavernomas.[6,7] The impact of hormonal changes on intracranial vascular lesions requires further investigation.

TREATMENT CONSIDERATIONS DURING PREGNANCY

Radiation Risks

Imaging during pregnancy, especially that using ionizing radiation, raises concern for teratogenic effects to the fetus and increased carcinogenic risk during childhood. The threshold radiation dose (for which there is believed to be no teratogenic risk) is

---

BOX 16.1

CARE MAP FOR PREGNANCY IN THE NEUROVASCULAR PATIENT

BEFORE PREGNANCY/PRE-PREGNANCY/NON-PREGNANT

Review of prior pregnancy complications

Confirmation of neurological diagnosis with appropriate imaging

Assessment of disease specific maternal risk factors:

    Coagulation abnormalities

    Hypertension, autonomic dysfunction

Contraceptive counseling

Medications adjustment, consolidation and review

Pre-conception MFM consult If known AVM consider definitive treatment

If known aneurysm > 6mm consider definitive treatment

DURING PREGNANCY

Adjust medications for symptoms

Monitor for worsening of specific maternal risk factors

Monitor BP

Early anesthesia consult

In event of rupture: airway evaluation and possible intubation, clot stabilization, blood pressure reduction, cerebral edema management, and control of seizures

If known aneurysm careful control of risk factors and monitoring for development of neurologic symptoms

DELIVERY

Multidisciplinary discussion to plan best delivery route and location

Anesthesia consultation

Pain management

Alert Neonatologist/NICU team; Notify pediatrician if anticipated fetal involvement

POSTPARTUM

Consider consultation with specialists as needed prior to discharge

Plan for social support to care for infant and mother

Schedule Neurosurgery follow-up

Medication adjustments

Venous thromboembolism prophylaxis

---

between 5 to 15 rad (50 to 150 mGy).[8] Childhood cancer risk after radiation exposure in utero may be increased to an excess risk of 1 in 2000 after 5 rad exposure.[9] The American College of Obstetricians and Gynecologists discusses carcinogenic risk of radiation during pregnancy as "very small" and conclude "abortion should not be recommended."[10]

Intracranial imaging exposes mothers to 0.17 rad for a head CT and 0.47 rad for a CTA head/neck.[11] Fetal radiation exposure from a head CT is 0 rad.[12] Fetal radiation exposure from a CTA head/neck is not reported; however, it can be compared to the radiation exposure during a CT angiogram of the aorta (chest through pelvis) at 3.4 rad, which is still below the reported teratogenic doses. Shielding of the fetus may serve to further minimize radiation exposure.

CT vascular imaging also raises the safety of iodinated contrast in the pregnant patient. In vivo experiments with iodinated contrast show no teratogenic effect[13]; however, there is a theoretical risk of neonatal hypothyroidism.

MRIs are believed to be safe,[14] yet gadolinium contrast has a risk of teratogenicity, though most vascular imaging may be done without gadolinium. Small human studies of gadolinium use during pregnancy have shown safety, but it remains a category C FDA drug (to be administered "if the potential benefit justifies the potential risk to the fetus").[15] Recent FDA investigations into the deposition of gadolinium in neural tissues show nothing measurable with doses <100mL (or approximately 5 contrasted MRIs), which would be highly unlikely in 9 months of pregnancy.[16]

Of note, iodinated and gadolinium contrast can be given without interrupting breast feeding.[17,18]

Endovascular Considerations

As a key diagnostic and treatment modality for vascular lesions, strategies to reduce radiation during angiography include shielding the fetus, using low-dose radiation algorithms, tight collimation, and a low pulse rate. Radiation to the pelvis can be minimized by foregoing use of a femoral closure device. In this case, low femoral access is achieved without fluoroscopic assistance to localize a puncture site above the bifurcation, no femoral angiography is performed, and manual compression is used for hemostasis after sheath removal.

Further limitation of abdominal radiation can be achieved by using a J-wire to navigate the aorta, thereby avoiding the need for fluoroscopy to monitor potential migration into the renal arteries or aortic branches.

Anesthesia Considerations

Surgical emergencies may often be treated without significant fetal risk with modern anesthetic techniques[1]; however, waiting until the third trimester or one month post-partum for semi-elective conditions is optimal. Anesthesia modifications include fetal monitoring and close availability of an obstetrical anesthesiologist. Maintaining normotension is advantageous to fetal physiology. Use of nitroprusside and nimodipine raise potential concern for fetal perfusion.[1] Certain neurosurgical drugs such as mannitol should be avoided due to dehydrating effects and anti-convulsants only used in times of absolute necessity. Older anti-epileptics such as valproate are definitively associated with birth defects, including neural tube defects. Levetiracetam is most common chosen when anti-epileptics are necessary in our practice.

Positioning during surgical procedures require the left lateral decubitus position to prevent IVC compression, most important after 24 weeks of pregnancy because of the expanding size of the uterus.[6] This position can be accomplished by placing a wedge under the patient's right hip.[2,6]

The nasal and respiratory tract mucosa become edematous and hyperemic with the increased estrogen and blood volume of pregnancy, predisposing to bleeding with airway manipulation.[2] Airway edema, breast engorgement, and the expected weight gain of pregnancy may also contribute to airway obstruction and reduced glottic opening.[6] Intubation should be performed with care, using sufficient lubricant and smaller endotracheal tubes to minimize bleeding and airway compromise.[6]

Delivery via cesarean section may be chosen for close blood pressure control in the setting of a known intracranial vascular malformation. Vaginal delivery remains an option in cases of cerebral aneurysm or cavernoma, with some physicians advocating for the use of an epidural anesthetic to shorten the second stage of labor.[19]

For repairs in the postpartum period, consideration should be made for breastfeeding mothers to avoid engorgement in prolonged procedures or surgeries. With appropriate consent, expression of breastmilk by pumping for a mother during anesthesia may be necessary.

THE EPIDEMIOLOGY OF CEREBRAL ANEURYSMS

Approximately 0.8–6% of the population have an intracranial aneurysm.[20–24] They are more prevalent in females over the age of 30 of Japanese, Finnish, Korean, and Chinese descent.[25] Other known risk factors include hypertension, family history, smoking, and alcohol use. Diseases associated with intracerebral aneurysms include polycystic kidney disease, Marfan's, and Ehlers-Danlos. The natural history of cerebral aneurysms has been extensively studied, and factors associated with increased risk of rupture include irregular morphology (daughter sac), growth, location (anterior communicating artery and posterior circulation), smoking, previous rupture, and aneurysm size. The International Study of Unruptured Intracranial Aneurysms (ISUIA) study, including over 4,000 patients, show negligible 5-year rupture risks for anterior circulation aneurysms <7mm[26]. Aneurysm size positively correlated with rupture rates with 2.6% 5-year risk for 7–12mm aneurysms, 14.5% for 13–24mm, and 40% for > 25mm for anterior circulation aneurysms, whereas posterior circulation 5-year rupture rates were 2.5% for <7mm, 14.5% for 7–12mm, 18.4% for 13–24mm, and 50% for >25mm. The Japanese Unruptured Aneurysm study followed over 6000 patients with annual rupture rates 0.36% for 3–4mm aneurysms, 0.5% for

5–6mm, 1.69% for 7–9mm, 4.37% for 10–24mm, and 33.4% for > 25mm.[27] In 2015, the American Heart Association published guidelines for the management of unruptured aneurysms based on the best evidence for risk of rupture.[28]

While the overall rate of hemorrhage is low, aneurysm rupture morbidity and mortality rates are 20–30%.[29,30] Rupture may be further complicated by hydrocephalus, subdural, or intraparenchymal hematoma, seizure, cardiomyopathy, vasospasm, and delayed ischemic events, among others. For this reason, treatment is usually recommended for aneurysms measuring ≥7mm or larger, or 5–6mm with one of the aforementioned risk factors.

TREATMENT OF CEREBRAL ANEURYSMS IN PREGNANCY

Unruptured Cerebral Aneurysms

In a Nationwide Inpatient Sample study, 1.8% of women between the ages of 16 to 44 (childbearing age) carried a diagnosis of cerebral aneurysm.[31] Fortunately, aneurysm rupture during pregnancy appears to be a rare event, estimated to occur in approximately 1–10 per 100,000 pregnancies (0.001–0.01%).[3] Cases of rupture occur antepartum in the vast majority (92%) as opposed to postpartum (8%)[32], most often in the third trimester (80%), with only 10% rupturing in each the first and second trimesters.[33] Only 2 of the 28 ruptured aneurysms (7%) bled during the childbirth.[34] Vaginal delivery does not appear to increase the risk of aneurysm rupture.[31]

Asymptomatic, stable aneurysms typically do not require treatment in pregnancy.[35] However, hemodynamic changes during the third trimester, including rising blood pressure, may increase the incidence of aneurysmal enlargement and be responsible for the higher rate of rupture observed during this time. An analysis of 50 aneurysms that did rupture during pregnancy found that 91% were 6 mm or larger, suggesting this cutoff may be more appropriate than the rate of rupture in the general population (7 mm).[34] Aneurysms between 3–6mm in pregnant women had a 62% rupture rate, which may be retrospective study bias; however, it demonstrates the importance of close monitoring. Further, the development of symptoms necessitates repeat evaluation to ensure the aneurysm is not enlarging. Given this, treatment for known 3–6mm aneurysms in women planning a pregnancy may be warranted (Figure 16.1).

Ruptured Cerebral Aneurysms

Pregnant patients with aneurysmal subarachnoid hemorrhage represent a different patient population than the traditional cerebral aneurysm patient. Pregnant patients are usually younger, and may therefore make more substantial neurologic recoveries. However, younger patients have more brain volume and less ability to accommodate intracranial mass lesions, making the need for surgical hematoma evacuation or craniectomy more likely. Maternal mortality rates from ruptured aneurysms range from 3.0–6.7%.[34] Survival of the fetus is predicated on survival of the mother, and definitive treatment of the mother's ruptured aneurysm improves fetal outcomes.[36] As in the general population, >90% of pregnant patients with ruptured aneurysms are treated to secure the ruptured aneurysm to prevent rebleeding.[34]

Endovascular treatment for ruptured aneurysms in pregnant patients has been found to result in a lower complication rate when compared to surgical clipping (9.5% vs. 23%),[34] yet this is dependent on individual characteristics of the aneurysm and patient. For example, a 32-year-old in the late second trimester with a ruptured wide-neck ophthalmic artery aneurysm would usually be treated with endovascular flow diversion or stent-assisted coiling; however, these therapies require the use of dual antiplatelet agents (usually aspirin and clopidogrel), which may be harmful during pregnancy. As the second trimester is too early to deliver a fetus, open surgical clipping may be preferable in this case with continuous fetal monitoring during the general anesthetic. In contradistinction, a 32-year-old in the third trimester harboring a ruptured narrow neck small posterior communicating artery aneurysm may best be treated with endovascular coiling, as this can be done quickly with minimal radiation without the need for general anesthesia. Such an example is presented in Figure 16.2 with a case of a ruptured cerebral aneurysm presenting with subarachnoid hemorrhage and hydrocephalus (Figure 16.2A) with an identified ophthalmic aneurysm (Figure 16.2B) which was treated with endovascular coiling (Figure 16.2C).

A combined neurosurgical-obstetrical approach was used in many of these patients, with cesarean delivery either immediately before or after the neurosurgical procedure, if the patient is close to term, due to the prolonged severity of maternal illness and hemodynamic

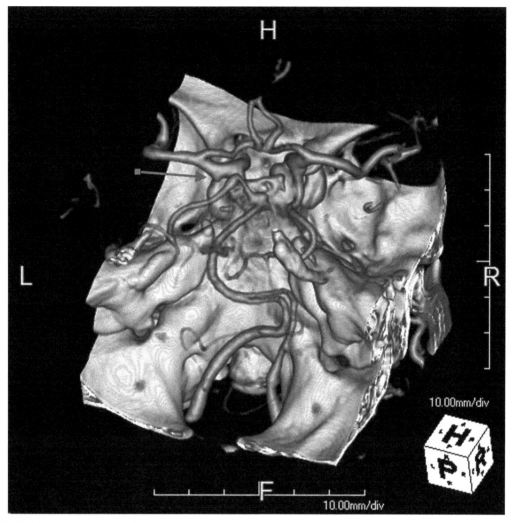

FIGURE 16.1 Reconstructed CTA images in 3D rendering demonstrating a focal out pouching from at the origin of the left posterior communicating artery, potentially representative of a small aneurysm verses an infundibulum.

shifts seen with vasospasm following subarachnoid hemorrhage.[34]

Other Causes of Subarachnoid Hemorrhage

Subarachnoid hemorrhage (SAH) can occur from etiologies other than aneurysms and overall is responsible for 5–12% of maternal deaths.[32] Consideration in these circumstances should be given to perimesencephalic subarachnoid hemorrhage and reversible cerebral vasoconstriction syndrome, which can be differentiated based on the pattern of the hemorrhage.

Benign pretruncal (perimesencephalic) SAH has been reported during pregnancy[37] and is characterized by SAH primarily confined to the cisterns around the midbrain with no extension to the lateral Sylvian fissures, as it is usually due to venous hemorrhage (Figure 16.3 A/B).[38,39] This accounts for approximately 10% of SAH and angiography is normal. When compared to aneurysmal SAH, clinical outcomes are better, rebleeding is rare, and life expectancy is not altered, though there does remain a small risk of vasospasm, hyponatremia, and hydrocephalus.[38,40]

Convexity SAH is characterized by hemorrhage over the hemispheres but not in the basal cisterns, and can have many vascular causes, including trauma, hypertension, arteriovenous malformations, cerebral venous thrombosis, and can be associated with reversible cerebral vasoconstriction syndrome in younger patients (RCVS).[41,42] Venous thrombosis and RCVS are most concerning in the postpartum

CASE 1

A 29-year-old female was the passenger in a motor vehicle accident and presented to the emergency room. She was hemodynamically stable and subsequently underwent routine trauma radiographic studies. An incidentally discovered 2–3mm out pouching, concerning for a potential aneurysm, was discovered at the origin of the left posterior communicating artery (Figure 16.1). The morphology was round without irregularities. She was without other injuries. Her hematologic evaluation studies returned with a positive pregnancy result, which was a new diagnosis. Neurologically, she was without clinical symptoms and had no family history of aneurysms. She did smoke cigarettes, 1 pack per day for 10 years. A discussion was held with the patient regarding the natural history and risks/benefits of treatment. She was counseled on smoking cessation. The patient decided to monitor the aneurysm during the course of her pregnancy. She followed up closely with neurosurgery, remained abstinent from cigarettes, and monitored her blood pressure closely. She was also referred for Ob-Gyn for management. As her pregnancy progressed a collaborative discussion decided for elective delivery via Cesarean section for optimal blood pressure control. She progressed well and delivered a baby girl successfully. Annual imaging follow-up of her aneurysm remains stable to date.

period, due to the hormonal and angiogenic fluctuations, and there must be a high clinical suspicion in this demographic presenting with convexity SAH (Figure 16.4A). Cerebral venous thrombosis appears as subarachnoid and intraparenchymal hemorrhage around the occluded sinus due to venous congestion and must be treated with heparinization with possible endovascular thrombectomy. Heparin does not cross the placenta and passes in only small amounts into breast milk and can be used in the pregnant and postpartum breastfeeding mother. RCVS is characterized by acute onset of headache, with or without neurological deficits, and prolonged but reversible vasoconstriction of the cerebral arteries that usually resolve in 3 months (Figure 16.4B).[43,44] Imaging may demonstrate convexity subarachnoid hemorrhage in approximately one-third of patients.[45] It is often seen in the early postpartum period, up to 6 weeks, following an uncomplicated pregnancy,[43] likely due to increased serotoninergic tone and arterial vasoconstriction.[44] RCVS is usually a self-limiting disease, thus supportive care and observation are the mainstays of treatment, although severe

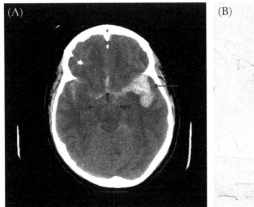 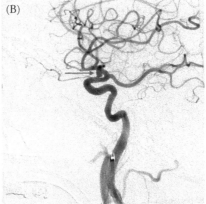 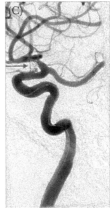

FIGURE 16.2 A) Unenhanced CT demonstrating subarachnoid hemorrhage in the basal cisterns encircling the midbrain and extending into the bilateral Sylvian fissures, left greater than right, and interhemispheric fissure. B) Lateral view left internal carotid arteriogram demonstrating the superiorly directed 6.5 x 4mm ophthalmic aneurysm with a daughter sac on the superior aspect. C) Oblique view left internal carotid after completion of coil embolization of the aneurysm.

CASE 2

A 36-year-old G4P3 at 37 weeks gestation presented to the emergency room with nausea, vomiting, and sudden onset of the worst headache of her life. Neurologically she was drowsy without focal deficit. CT head with fetal shielding demonstrating subarachnoid hemorrhage in the basal cisterns consistent with aneurysmal SAH and hydrocephalus (Figure 16.2A). Her blood pressure was 200/120 and was treated to SBP < 140 with a cardene drip. An external ventricular drain was emergently placed to treat the hydrocephalus and Ob/Gyn was consulted for co-management.

Angiography was performed under general anesthesia due to patient condition with special attention to minimizing contrast and radiation. The fetus was shielded, the femoral artery was accessed with ultrasound (rather than fluoroscopic) guidance and a J-wire used to navigate into the aortic arch, at which time we used 2 frames per second with tight collimation to minimize radiation. An irregular, superiorly projecting 6.5mm ophthalmic aneurysm was identified with a daughter sac (Figure 16.2B). The aneurysm was completely coiled (Figure 16.2C). Given the potential risks associated with a ruptured aneurysm over the next several weeks, including fluid shifts, vasospasm, hyponatremia and hydrocephalus, Ob/Gyn took the patient for delivery via C-section since she was at term while still under anesthesia and a healthy boy was delivered.

The patient was monitored in the neuro ICU with daily transcranial doppler, and regular neurologic assessments to monitor for development of vasospasm, in addition to scheduled oral nimodipine. She was kept euvolemic with intravenous fluids and treated with 3% hypertonic saline for hyponatremia, which developed post-bleed day 5 to 129. On post-bleed day 7, she developed right-sided weakness and aphasia. Her blood pressure was augmented with vasopressors to systolics 180 without symptom resolution. She was emergently taken for angiography, which demonstrated severe left middle cerebral artery (MCA) vasospasm for which she underwent angioplasty. The patient returned to the intensive care unit (ICU) with a normal neurologic exam. She was treated with vasopressors over the next two days after which the vasospasm began to resolve. She required a ventriculoperiotoneal shunt after 10 days due to the hydrocephalus. She was discharged home to her healthy baby boy in normal neurologic condition on post-bleed day 17.

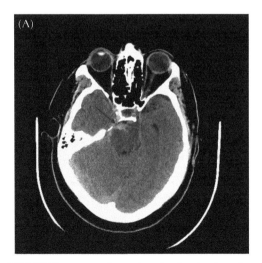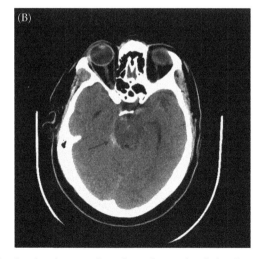

FIGURE 16.3 Unenhanced CT head with subarachnoid blood in the A) interpeduncular, right crural and B) ambient cisterns, consistent with a perimesencephalic hemorrhage pattern. Diagnostic cerebral angiogram was negative for vascular malformations.

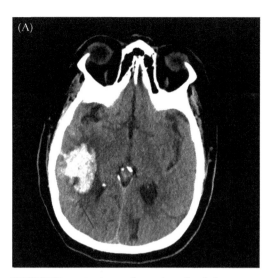
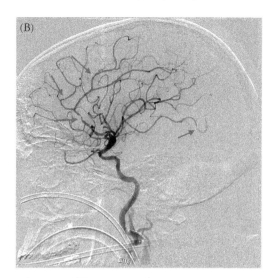

FIGURE 16.4 A) Unenhanced CT head demonstrating a right temporal hematoma with surrounding edema and subarachnoid hemorrhage extending to the convexity surface, consistent with a nonaneurysmal pattern of SAH. B) Right carotid injection, lateral view cerebral angiogram demonstrating multiple arterial irregularities suggestive of arteriopathy associated with diffuse cerebral vasculitis.

RCVS may need to be treated with medications and angioplasty.[46]

ARTERIOVENOUS MALFORMATIONS

In the general population the prevalence of AVMs is 18 per 100,000.[47] Natural history studies demonstrate an annual AVM rupture risk between 2–4%, with meta-analysis of 3923 patients showing unruptured AVMs to carry a 2.2% risk of rupture per year.[44] Ruptured AVMs have a 4.5% annual rupture risk after a transiently increased rebleeding risk within the first 6–12 months of 6–15%.[48] AVMs can be pial or dural based, and both carry potential for hemorrhage.

AVMs are the most common cause of major intracerebral hemorrhage in the expectant patient,[32,49] with a trend toward higher rupture rates during pregnancy. A review of 154 spontaneous cerebral hemorrhages during pregnancy revealed AVM to be the underlying etiology in 23%.[32] In 1974 the first series of 24 AVMs in pregnant patients was published, with 11 ruptures during pregnancy (45.8%).[3] Gross et al reported five hemorrhages in four patients during 62 pregnancies, yielding a rupture risk of 8% per pregnancy.[50] Two radiosurgery-only cohorts of women with AVMs report a baseline annual rupture risk which increased during pregnancy (3.1% to 3.5%[51] and 4.5% to 9.3%,[52] respectively).

CASE 3

A 29-year-old G2P1 female at 17 weeks pregnancy was incidentally discovered to have a 4mm left posterior communicating artery after a rollover MVC. The morphology was round without irregularities. She was without other injuries and neurologically intact. She had no family history of aneurysms but did smoke cigarettes. She was counseled on smoking cessation and her blood pressure and symptoms closely monitored. The aneurysm was monitored with MRA without contrast in the 3rd trimester, prior to delivery. As the aneurysm had not grown in size, a collaborative decision with the patient, OB and neurosurgery was made to proceed with vaginal delivery with an epidural and close blood pressure monitoring. The delivery progressed without complication and she delivered a healthy baby girl. Annual radiographic follow-up of her aneurysm remains stable to date.

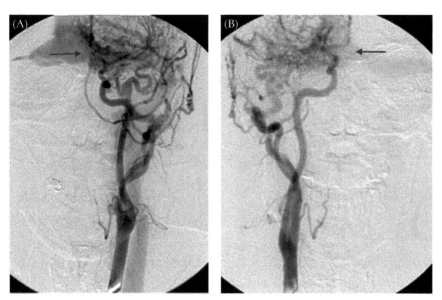

FIGURE 16.5 A) Pre-embolization left common carotid injection—there are numerous small arteries flowing into the left transverse sinus with early opacification of the left transverse sinus, consistent with the presence of a left transverse sinus dural arteriovenous fistula (AVF). This portion of the bilateral transverse sinus dural AVF is fed by branches of a markedly enlarged left occipital artery as well as distal pial branches of the left posterior cerebral artery. The torcula is noted to be markedly enlarged. B) Pre-embolization right common carotid injection—the right transverse sinus is occluded with numerous small feeding arteries reconstituting it are demonstrated, consistent with the presence of a complex right transverse sinus dural arteriovenous malformation. This is fed by the markedly enlarged and tortuous right occipital artery, an enlarged right posterior middle meningeal artery, and through pial dural parasitization of vessels off the distal right posterior cerebral artery. The right meningohypophyseal trunk is enlarged and appears to connect to a branch of the right posterior cerebral artery.

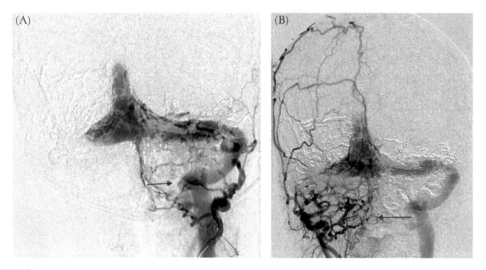

FIGURE 16.6 A) Post-embolization left common carotid injection with demonstrated early opacification of the enlarged torcula and left transverse sinus fed predominately by fistulous branches of the enlarged left distal occipital artery. The dural AVM also appears to be fed by distal branches of the left middle meningeal. Both appear slightly increased in caliber. B) Post-embolization right common carotid injection continues to demonstrate early opacification of the enlarged torcula and left transverse sinus fed predominately by enlarged branches of the right occipital artery and middle meningeal artery, however, there has been overall a decrease in size of the middle meningeal artery, superficial temporal artery, and occipital artery supplying the AVM. There is also decreased retrograde flow from the enlarged torcula into the superior sagittal sinus.

CASE 4

A 36-year-old G3P1 developed headaches and visual changes in her left eye with papilledema at 16 weeks into her pregnancy. A Brain MRI/MRA/MRV demonstrating bilateral transverse sinus thrombosis and prominent occipital arteries bilaterally, found to be an occipital dural arteriovenous fistula. The patient was supported during the remainder of her pregnancy with acetazolamide and a therapeutic spinal tap (opening pressure 29 cm H_2O). Formal visual exams were performed every two weeks until delivery at 34 weeks via C-section with spinal anesthesia. Following delivery, her vision and papilledema rapidly improved and an angiogram was performed, showing a large dural AVM centered at the torcula and fed from both internal and external carotid arteries (occipital, middle meningeal, posterior cerebral, and superior cerebellar arteries) and vertebral arteries bilaterally. Reflux was noted into the superior sagittal sinus, straight sinus, vein of Galen, and basal vein of Rosenthal (Figure 16.5). She underwent multiple embolization procedures (Figure 16.6) with improvement in venous reflux and recanalization of the left transverse sinus. She remained neurologically stable at 7 years follow-up.

Given this documented increased risk of hemorrhage, if a woman has a known AVM and is planning a pregnancy, particularly if her AVM has previously bled, elective treatment of the AVM is recommended.[50] AVMs can be treated by surgical resection, radiosurgery, embolization, or a combination. Figure 16.5A/B demonstrates a case of a posterior fossa arteriovenous fistula and Figure 16.6A/B demonstrates post-embolization treatment. However, in order to ensure protection from hemorrhage, treatment must result in complete removal of the AVM. Therefore, radiosurgery may not be the best choice given the lag time of 2 to 5 years until obliteration, depending on the dose and size.

AVMs tend to rupture earlier in the course of pregnancy than aneurysms, peaking during the 20th to 24th weeks of gestation with a second wave occurring in the peripartum period.[53] In the case of rupture, goals of care are the same as for any patient, including airway management, blood pressure reduction (Systolic BP<140), management of cerebral edema, and seizure control. Rates of rebleeding after AVM rupture during pregnancy vary in the literature, and range from 7.3%[50] to as high as 27%.[49] Reports of mortality also vary, with older reports up to 28%,[3] though a more recent cohort reports 4.6%.[33] Limited data suggests that surgical resection may result in improved mortality for both mother and fetus. In one study, surgically treated women (N = 13) had a 23% mortality rate (0% fetal mortality rate) and observed women (N = 22) had a 32% mortality rate (23% fetal mortality rate).[32] Yet, in practice there remain patients who are medically supported until after delivery for definitive treatment unless they develop acute clinical deterioration.[1,50]

If the AVM has been definitely treated, vaginal delivery does not increase maternal or fetal risk.[31] For those with AVMs in pregnancy, strong consideration is recommended for delivery via cesarean section for improved blood pressure control and to prevent rupture.[50]

CAVERNOUS MALFORMATIONS

Cavernous malformations, also known as cavernous hemangiomas, cavernomas, and cavernous angiomas, are benign, slow growing vascular anomalies made of dysplastic capillaries.[54] Cavernous malformations (CM) can be found throughout the central nervous system, predominantly in the brain and less commonly in the spine.[54,55] CM can be divided into a sporadic form, characterized by isolated lesions, and a familial form, characterized by multiple lesions with autosomal dominant inheritance.[56] Symptomatic lesions occur in all age groups and both sexes.[7] Based on a meta-analysis of 11 natural history studies representing 837 patients, the overall male to female ratio is 1:1 with mean age at presentation of 30.6 years.[57] The most recent data show a 0.42% prevalence, ranging from 0.4 to.0,8%. Accordingly, approximately half a million women will have a cavernoma during their pregnancy.[58] While these lesions carry a similar rupture rate to AVMs, the morbidity is usually much less as they are not arterial lesions.

CM have a highly variable presentation depending on the size, multiplicity, and location of the lesion. Many are asymptomatic and found incidentally, or upon screening relatives of patients with familial CM.[56,59] CM can present during pregnancy with hemorrhage-related neurological symptoms, such as headaches, focal neurological deficit, and most commonly seizures.[57,58,60] Thus, CM should remain as a differential diagnosis for newly diagnosed seizures in pregnancy.[6,60] Symptomatic CM can occur in any trimester of pregnancy and at any age.[61] The annual hemorrhage rate of CM is calculated to be 2.4% per patient-year but can range from 0.7% to 5%.[6,57] Prior hemorrhage, age, female gender, location, and size of the lesion are all associated with higher risk of rupture.[6,57]

The literature is mixed regarding whether pregnancy is associated with more aggressive behavior of cavernomas. Some studies show increased de novo formation, growth, propensity to hemorrhage, and exacerbation of symptoms.[6,7,62,63] In a case series of brainstem CM, 11% of the 62 women suffered a hemorrhage during pregnancy.[64] Proposed mechanisms include fluctuation of progesterone and estrogen during pregnancy, along with an increase in vascular and fibroblast growth during pregnancy that can induce angiogenesis and growth of CM.[6] However, more recent studies show no increased risk during pregnancy, delivery, or the peripartum period, and failed to demonstrate receptors for progesterone and estrogens in CM.[58,61] In a retrospective series of 168 pregnancies among 64 patients with CM (28 sporadic, and 36 familial), they were only 5 symptomatic hemorrhages, with an overall risk of a symptomatic hemorrhage of 3% per pregnancy (1.8% in the sporadic group and 3.6% in the familial group).[58] This percentage is well within the reported natural history of this disease. Another series of 349 pregnancies in 186 patients showed only three hemorrhages.[59] These studies concluded that there is no evidence to support the recommendation to avoid pregnancy or to opt for termination of pregnancy to reduce the hemorrhage risk in women with CM.[61]

Treatment strategies during pregnancy have been based on limited clinical data. If a cavernoma is asymptomatic or clinically stable with minor symptoms, conservative treatment with clinical follow-up is appropriate.[61,63] Treatment of seizures with anti-epileptics must be done carefully due to the effect of some antiepileptics on the developing fetus. Most symptomatic cases of CM during pregnancy, even those that occur early in pregnancy, have been treated after the pregnancy (by either vaginal or cesarean delivery) without apparent risk of adverse outcomes.[7,61] If the symptoms are severe, rebleeding occurs, or there is risk to maternal or fetal life, treatment may precede delivery, though the need for this is rare, and usually occurs only in patients with hemorrhagic brainstem CM.[61,65] Reported emergent cases showed no obstetric complications and patients subsequently delivered at term.[61]

With regard to the mode of delivery, several studies have reported that vaginal delivery may increase the risk of hemorrhage and therefore cesarean section is the preferred mode of delivery. Nevertheless, recent data suggest that management of labor in an asymptomatic woman should be based on obstetrical indications.[58,61] In a large series, there were no documented episodes of hemorrhage in the 149 pregnancies with vaginal delivery.[58] In cases of symptomatic CM, C-section seems to be preferred among obstetricians, however again, there are no reported complications with vaginal delivery after a symptomatic CM has been discovered.[6,61,65]

REFERENCES

1. Qaiser R, Black P. Neurosurgery in pregnancy. *Semin Neurol.* 2007; 27(5): 476–481.
2. Hill CC, Pickinpaugh J. Physiologic changes in pregnancy. *Surg Clin North Am.* 2008; 88(2): 391–401, vii.
3. Robinson JL, Hall CS, Sedzimir CB. Arteriovenous malformations, aneurysms, and pregnancy. *J Neurosurg.* 1974; 41(1): 63–70.
4. Liu XJ, Wang S, Zhao YL, et al. Risk of cerebral arteriovenous malformation rupture during pregnancy and puerperium. *Neurology.* 2014; 82(20): 1798–1803.
5. Chang J, Streitman D. Physiologic adaptations to pregnancy. *Neurol Clin.* 2012; 30(3): 781–789.
6. Yamada S, Nakase H, Nakagawa I, Nishimura F, Motoyama Y, Park YS. Cavernous malformations in pregnancy. *Neurol Med Chir (Tokyo).* 2013; 53(8): 555–560.
7. Safavi-Abbasi S, Feiz-Erfan I, Spetzler RF, et al. Hemorrhage of cavernous malformations during pregnancy and in the peripartum period: Causal or coincidence? Case report and review of the literature. *Neurosurg Focus.* 2006; 21(1): e12.
8. Berlin L. Radiation exposure and the pregnant patient. *AJR Am J Roentgenol.* 1996; 167(6): 1377–1379.
9. Ginsberg JS, Hirsh J, Rainbow AJ, Coates G. Risks to the fetus of radiologic procedures used in the diagnosis of maternal venous thromboembolic disease. *Thromb Haemost.* 1989; 61(2): 189–196.
10. Practice ACoO. ACOG Committee Opinion. Number 299, September 2004 (replaces No. 158, September 1995). Guidelines for diagnostic imaging during pregnancy. *Obstet Gynecol.* 2004; 104(3): 647–651.

11. Cohnen M, Wittsack HJ, Assadi S, et al. Radiation exposure of patients in comprehensive computed tomography of the head in acute stroke. *AJNR Am J Neuroradiol*. 2006; 27(8): 1741–1745.

12. McCollough CH, Schueler BA, Atwell TD, et al. Radiation exposure and pregnancy: When should we be concerned? *Radiographics*. 2007; 27(4): 909–917; 917–908.

13. Morisetti A, Tirone P, Luzzani F, de Haën C. Toxicological safety assessment of iomeprol, a new X-ray contrast agent. *Eur J Radiol*. 1994;18(Suppl 1): S21–31.

14. Schwartz JL, Crooks LE. NMR imaging produces no observable mutations or cytotoxicity in mammalian cells. *AJR Am J Roentgenol*. 1982; 139(3): 583–585.

15. Kanal E, Barkovich AJ, Bell C, et al. ACR guidance document for safe MR practices: 2007. *AJR Am J Roentgenol*. 2007; 188(6): 1447–1474.

16. McDonald RJ, McDonald JS, Kallmes DF, et al. Intracranial Gadolinium Deposition after Contrast-enhanced MR Imaging. *Radiology*. 2015; 275(3): 772–782.

17. Webb JA, Thomsen HS, Morcos SK, (ESUR) MoCMSCoESoUR. The use of iodinated and gadolinium contrast media during pregnancy and lactation. *Eur Radiol*. 2005; 15(6): 1234–1240.

18. Ito S. Drug therapy for breast-feeding women. *N Engl J Med*. 2000; 343(2): 118–126.

19. Greenberg MS. *Handbook of neurosurgery*. 8th ed. New York: Thieme; 2016.

20. Chason JL, Hindman WM. Berry aneurysms of the circle of Willis; results of a planned autopsy study. *Neurology*. 1958; 8(1): 41–44.

21. De la Monte SM, Moore GW, Monk MA, Hutchins GM. Risk factors for the development and rupture of intracranial berry aneurysms. *Am J Med*. 1985; 78(6 Pt 1): 957–964.

22. Horikoshi T, Akiyama I, Yamagata Z, Nukui H. Retrospective analysis of the prevalence of asymptomatic cerebral aneurysm in 4518 patients undergoing magnetic resonance angiography—when does cerebral aneurysm develop? *Neurol Med Chir (Tokyo)*. 2002; 42(3): 105–112, 113.

23. Winn HR, Jane JA, Taylor J, Kaiser D, Britz GW. Prevalence of asymptomatic incidental aneurysms: review of 4568 arteriograms. *J Neurosurg*. 2002; 96(1): 43–49.

24. Agarwal N, Guerra JC, Gala NB, et al. Current treatment options for cerebral arteriovenous malformations in pregnancy: a review of the literature. *World Neurosurg*. 2014; 81(1): 83–90.

25. Winn HR. *Youmans and Winn neurological surgery*. 7thth ed Philadelphia: Elsevier; 2017.

26. Wiebers DO, Whisnant JP, Huston J, et al. Unruptured intracranial aneurysms: natural history, clinical outcome, and risks of surgical and endovascular treatment. *Lancet*. 2003; 362(9378): 103–110.

27. Morita A, Kirino T, Hashi K, et al. The natural course of unruptured cerebral aneurysms in a Japanese cohort. *N Engl J Med*. 2012; 366(26): 2474–2482.

28. Thompson BG, Brown RD, Amin-Hanjani S, et al. Guidelines for the management of patients with unruptured intracranial aneurysms: A guideline for healthcare professionals from the American Heart Association/American Stroke Association. *Stroke*. 2015; 46(8): 2368–2400.

29. Molyneux AJ, Kerr RS, Yu LM, et al. International subarachnoid aneurysm trial (ISAT) of neurosurgical clipping versus endovascular coiling in 2143 patients with ruptured intracranial aneurysms: A randomised comparison of effects on survival, dependency, seizures, rebleeding, subgroups, and aneurysm occlusion. *Lancet*. 2005; 366(9488): 809–817.

30. McDougall CG, Spetzler RF, Zabramski JM, et al. The Barrow ruptured aneurysm trial. *J Neurosurg*. 2012; 116(1): 135–144.

31. Kim YW, Neal D, Hoh BL. Cerebral aneurysms in pregnancy and delivery: Pregnancy and delivery do not increase the risk of aneurysm rupture. *Neurosurgery*. 2013; 72(2): 143–149, 150.

32. Dias MS, Sekhar LN. Intracranial hemorrhage from aneurysms and arteriovenous malformations during pregnancy and the puerperium. *Neurosurgery*. 1990; 27(6): 855–865, 865–856.

33. Lv X, Liu P, Li Y. Pre-existing, incidental and hemorrhagic AVMs in pregnancy and postpartum: Gestational age, morbidity and mortality, management and risk to the fetus. *Interv Neuroradiol*. 2016; 22(2): 206–211.

34. Barbarite E, Hussain S, Dellarole A, Elhammady MS, Peterson E. The management of intracranial aneurysms during pregnancy: A systematic review. *Turk Neurosurg*. 2016; 26(4): 465–474.

35. Sloan MA, Stern BJ. Cerebrovascular disease in pregnancy. *Curr Treat Options Neurol*. 2003; 5(5): 391–407.

36. Tarnaris A, Haliasos N, Watkins LD. Endovascular treatment of ruptured intracranial aneurysms during pregnancy: Is this the best way forward? Case report and review of the literature. *Clin Neurol Neurosurg*. 2012; 114(6): 703–706.

37. Hirsch KG, Froehler MT, Huang J, Ziai WC. Occurrence of perimesencephalic subarachnoid hemorrhage during pregnancy. *Neurocrit Care*. 2009; 10(3): 339–343.

38. van Gijn J, Rinkel GJ. Subarachnoid haemorrhage: diagnosis, causes and management. *Brain*. 2001; 124(Pt. 2): 249–278.

39. Herrmann LL, Zabramski JM. Nonaneurysmal subarachnoid hemorrhage: A review of clinical

course and outcome in two hemorrhage patterns. *J Neurosci Nurs*. 2007; 39(3): 135–142.

40. Greebe P, Rinkel GJ. Life expectancy after perimesencephalic subarachnoid hemorrhage. *Stroke*. 2007; 38(4): 1222–1224.

41. Geraldes R, Sousa PR, Fonseca AC, Falcão F, Canhão P, Pinho e Melo T. Nontraumatic convexity subarachnoid hemorrhage: Different etiologies and outcomes. *J Stroke Cerebrovasc Dis*. 2014; 23(1): e23–30.

42. Khurram A, Kleinig T, Leyden J. Clinical associations and causes of convexity subarachnoid hemorrhage. *Stroke*. 2014; 45(4): 1151–1153.

43. Miller TR, Shivashankar R, Mossa-Basha M, Gandhi D. Reversible cerebral vasoconstriction syndrome, part 1: Epidemiology, pathogenesis, and clinical course. *AJNR Am J Neuroradiol*. 2015; 36(8): 1392–1399.

44. Albano B, Del Sette M, Roccatagliata L, Gandolfo C, Primavera A. Cortical subarachnoid hemorrhage associated with reversible cerebral vasoconstriction syndrome after elective triplet cesarean delivery. *Neurol Sci*. 2011; 32(3): 497–501.

45. Singhal AB, Hajj-Ali RA, Topcuoglu MA, et al. Reversible cerebral vasoconstriction syndromes: Analysis of 139 cases. *Arch Neurol*. 2011; 68(8): 1005–1012.

46. Skeik N, Porten BR, Kadkhodayan Y, McDonald W, Lahham F. Postpartum reversible cerebral vasoconstriction syndrome: Review and analysis of the current data. *Vasc Med*. 2015; 20(3): 256–265.

47. Al-Shahi R, Fang JS, Lewis SC, Warlow CP. Prevalence of adults with brain arteriovenous malformations: A community based study in Scotland using capture-recapture analysis. *J Neurol Neurosurg Psychiatry*. 2002; 73(5): 547–551.

48. Gross BA, Du R. Natural history of cerebral arteriovenous malformations: A meta-analysis. *J Neurosurg*. 2013; 118(2): 437–443.

49. Sadasivan B, Malik GM, Lee C, Ausman JI. Vascular malformations and pregnancy. *Surg Neurol*. 1990; 33(5): 305–313.

50. Gross BA, Du R. Hemorrhage from arteriovenous malformations during pregnancy. *Neurosurgery*. 2012; 71(2): 349–355, 355–346.

51. Horton JC, Chambers WA, Lyons SL, Adams RD, Kjellberg RN. Pregnancy and the risk of hemorrhage from cerebral arteriovenous malformations. *Neurosurgery*. 1990; 27(6): 867–871, 871–862.

52. Forster DM, Kunkler IH, Hartland P. Risk of cerebral bleeding from arteriovenous malformations

in pregnancy: the Sheffield experience. *Stereotact Funct Neurosurg*. 1993; 61 (Suppl 1):v20–22.

53. Winn HR, Youmans JR. Youmans neurological surgery. 2004; 5th:4 v. (lxiv, 5296, cviii) ill. (some col.) 5228 cm. + 5291 CD-ROM (5294 5293/5294 in.).

54. Haber JS, Kesavabhotla K, Ottenhausen M, et al. Conservative management of cavernous sinus cavernous hemangioma in pregnancy. *J Neurosurg*. 2014; 120(6): 1309–1312.

55. Pars K, Garde N, Conzen J, et al. Intraspinal cavernous bleeding during early pregnancy. *J Neurol*. 2016; 263(10): 2127–2129.

56. Zabramski JM, Wascher TM, Spetzler RF, et al. The natural history of familial cavernous malformations: results of an ongoing study. *J Neurosurg*. 1994; 80(3): 422–432.

57. Gross BA, Lin N, Du R, Day AL. The natural history of intracranial cavernous malformations. *Neurosurg Focus*. 2011; 30(6): E24.

58. Kalani MY, Zabramski JM. Risk for symptomatic hemorrhage of cerebral cavernous malformations during pregnancy. *J Neurosurg*. 2013; 118(1): 50–55.

59. Witiw CD, Abou-Hamden A, Kulkarni AV, Silvaggio JA, Schneider C, Wallace MC. Cerebral cavernous malformations and pregnancy: hemorrhage risk and influence on obstetrical management. *Neurosurgery*. 2012; 71(3): 626–630, 631.

60. Awada A, Watson T, Obeid T. Cavernous angioma presenting as pregnancy-related seizures. *Epilepsia*. 1997; 38(7): 844–846.

61. Simonazzi G, Curti A, Rapacchia G, et al. Symptomatic cerebral cavernomas in pregnancy: A series of 6 cases and review of the literature. *J Matern Fetal Neonatal Med*. 2014; 27(3): 261–264.

62. Pozzati E, Acciarri N, Tognetti F, Marliani F, Giangaspero F. Growth, subsequent bleeding, and de novo appearance of cerebral cavernous angiomas. *Neurosurgery*. 1996; 38(4): 662–669, 669–670.

63. Burkhardt JK, Bozinov O, Nürnberg J, et al. Neurosurgical considerations on highly eloquent brainstem cavernomas during pregnancy. *Clin Neurol Neurosurg*. 2012; 114(8): 1172–1176.

64. Porter RW, Detwiler PW, Spetzler RF, et al. Cavernous malformations of the brainstem: experience with 100 patients. *J Neurosurg*. 1999; 90(1): 50–58.

65. Flemming KD, Goodman BP, Meyer FB. Successful brainstem cavernous malformation resection after repeated hemorrhages during pregnancy. *Surg Neurol*. 2003; 60(6): 545–547, 547–548.

17

Cerebral Venous Thrombosis

MICHAEL R. PICHLER AND ROBERT D. BROWN JR.

ABSTRACT

Thrombosis of cortical veins and/or dural venous sinuses (CVT) is a rare but potentially devastating condition. CVT is more common in women and is strongly associated with pregnancy and the postpartum period, likely due to numerous procoagulant changes during this time. CVT can cause a wide range of symptoms depending on location of thrombosis. Clinical manifestations can include headache, cranial nerve deficits, seizures, and venous infarction with associated focal neurologic deficits. Severe cases may progress to coma and death, emphasizing the importance of early diagnosis and treatment. The approach to management of CVT during pregnancy and the postpartum period must be tailored to prevent complications to the mother and child. This chapter addresses the pathogenesis, clinical manifestations, diagnosis, and treatment of CVT in pregnancy and the postpartum period.

EPIDEMIOLOGY AND PATHOGENESIS

Cerebral venous thrombosis (CVT) refers to thrombosis of cortical veins and/or dural venous sinuses. This rare and potentially devastating condition tends to affect young adults, particularly women. CVT in the general population affects around 5 people per million and accounts for less than one percent of all strokes.[1] While relatively rare in the general population, CVT is 3 times more common in women, reflecting an increased risk associated with pregnancy and hormonal contraceptive use. Because of the association with pregnancy, the incidence of CVT is higher than in the general population, approximately 12 per 100,000 deliveries in the United States.[2] In developed countries, up to 20% of CVT occurs during pregnancy or postpartum, with an even higher occurrence in less developed countries.[3-5]

The clinical manifestations, natural history, risk factors, and prognosis of CVT were assessed in the International Study on Cerebral Vein and Dural Sinus Thrombosis (ISCVT). This prospective, multicenter study of symptomatic CVT included 624 consecutive patients. An identifiable risk factor was found in 85% of patients, with exogenous hormone use being the most common (54%). Additionally, 20% of patients were pregnant or postpartum, emphasizing the effects that hormonal changes can have on thrombosis.[3] Numerous procoagulant changes have been noted during pregnancy, including a progressive increase in certain coagulation factors, fibrinogen, and von Willebrand factor, as well as increased resistance to activated protein C.[6] The greatest risk for CVT during pregnancy extends from the third trimester to 1-month postpartum, with a majority of cases occurring shortly after delivery.[5,7,8]

While pregnancy or postpartum state is a commonly recognized provoking factor for CVT, screening for additional prothrombotic conditions is recommended, as nearly half of patients with CVT have multiple risk factors. Inherited thrombophilias are seen in up to 34% of cases and include Factor V Leiden mutation (resistance to activated protein C), prothrombin G20210A mutation, hyperhomocysteinemia, and deficiencies in antithrombin III, protein C, or protein S.[3,9] Additional risk factors include Cesarean section or traumatic delivery, infection, dehydration, and CSF leak related to epidural anesthesia. Chronic conditions that persist during pregnancy may also contribute to CVT, such as cancer, antiphospholipid syndrome, and autoimmune disorders. Numerous medications have been linked to an increased risk of thrombosis, including CVT. Table 17.1 lists associated risk factors for CVT during pregnancy.

Regardless of the cause of thrombosis, the pathogenesis of CVT progresses in a similar and predictable way based on anatomical structures. The venous system contains approximately 70% of the cerebral blood volume and can be divided into cerebral veins (deep and superficial) and dural venous sinuses. The cerebral veins drain the brain parenchyma and empty into the dural venous sinuses, located at the edges of the falx cerebri and

TABLE 17.1 RISK FACTORS
FOR CEREBRAL VENOUS THROMBOSIS
DURING PREGNANCY[2,9,32]

Prothrombotic conditions
 Deficiencies of antithrombin, protein C, or protein S
 Antiphospholipid syndrome
 Factor V Leiden mutation (resistance to activated
  protein C)
 Prothrombin G20210A mutation
 Hyperhomocysteinemia
Excessive vomiting and dehydration
Mechanical precipitants
 Head injury or direct trauma to venous sinuses or
  jugular veins
 CSF hypotension following lumbar puncture or epi-
  dural anesthesia
 Traumatic vaginal delivery or Cesarean section
Chronic systemic or inflammatory diseases
 Thyroid disease
 Irritable bowel disease
 Systemic lupus erythematosus
 Behçet disease
 Sarcoidosis
Infection
 Localized (otitis, mastoiditis, sinusitis) or systemic
  (sepsis)
 Meningitis
Medications
 Fertility treatments at time of conception
 Medications used to treat coexisting conditions
  (corticosteroids, L-asparaginase, erythropoietin, etc.)
Hematologic disorders
 Anemia
 Sickle cell disease
 Polycythemia, thrombocythemia
 Paroxysmal nocturnal hemoglobinuria
Cancer
Nephrotic syndrome

tentorium cerebelli. In contrast to cerebral veins, venous sinuses are formed by dura mater and lined by endothelial cells. The sinuses in turn empty into the jugular veins in the neck and return blood to the superior vena cava.[10] The venous system also plays an important role in reabsorption of cerebrospinal fluid (CSF) into the superior sagittal sinus via arachnoid granulations. Occlusion at any point in the venous drainage system may affect hemodynamics upstream. The anatomy of the cerebral venous system is summarized in Figure 17.1.

Thrombosis of the cerebral veins may cause localized edema and venous infarction in the distribution of tissue drained by the thrombosed vein. Petechial hemorrhage and hemorrhagic

transformation of infarct may also occur, leading to hematoma formation with characteristic appearance on computed tomography (CT) scan. Thrombosis involving the venous sinuses may lead to intracranial hypertension due to increased venous pressure as well as impaired reabsorption of CSF.[11] Thrombosis of cerebral veins and venous sinuses often coexist, leading to a wide range of clinical manifestations depending on the location and extent of venous structures involved.

CLINICAL MANIFESTATIONS
Headache is the most common symptom of CVT and occurs in around 90% of cases.[3] Pain typically progresses over a number of days, but can uncommonly present as a thunderclap headache or with migrainous character. When venous sinuses are involved, coexisting papilledema and diplopia (from abducens nerve palsy) may become apparent due to increased intracranial pressure. In a minority of patients, headache may be the only presenting symptom.[12,13] New onset atypical or progressive headache in a pregnant or postpartum patient should therefore lead to consideration of CVT as a possible cause.

Headache may occur slightly more frequently in women, but other clinical manifestations of CVT are similar regardless of gender or underlying etiology.[14] Thrombosis of the deep venous system (straight sinus and its tributaries) may lead to bilateral thalamic lesions, causing behavioral changes or decreased consciousness. CVT involving the deep venous system (11%) is less common than involvement of the superior sagittal (62%) or transverse sinuses (45%) but is associated with a nearly three-fold increased occurrence of death or disability.[3] Thrombosis of superficial cortical veins may occur in isolation or result from propagation of dural sinus thrombosis. Any localized venous infarct can lead to focal neurologic deficits (aphasia, hemiparesis, etc.) based on infarct localization. These lesions may also serve as a nidus for seizure activity, which is seen in up to 40% of patients.[3] The common clinical manifestations based on location of CVT are highlighted in Table 17.2.

DIAGNOSIS
Neuroimaging is needed to diagnose CVT. However, imaging options are limited in the setting of pregnancy. Non-contrast head CT is often the first test in evaluating a patient with acute neurologic symptoms, but is abnormal in only 30% of patients with CVT. Hyperdensity of a cortical vein or dural sinus may be a clue to the diagnosis. Head CT during pregnancy scatters attenuated radiation throughout the mother's body, exposing the fetus to

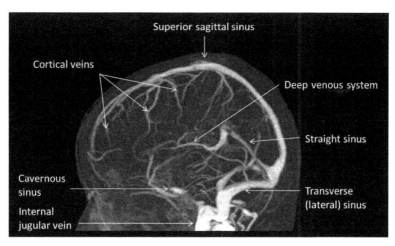

FIGURE 17.1 Cerebral venous anatomy. Magnetic resonance venogram showing the cerebral venous system. Venous blood flows from the cortical veins and deep venous system into the larger dural venous sinuses and ultimately drains via the paired internal jugular veins.

a very low amount of indirect radiation (< 0.01 rad). Radiation exposure less than five rad does not carry an increased risk of fetal complications (spontaneous abortion, developmental malformations, or mental retardation). However, there is a small increase in rate of childhood malignancy linked to radiation exposure, and fetal-absorbed doses greater than 5 rad may also carry a small increased risk of congenital defects.[15] Because of these potential complications, CT is avoided during pregnancy if possible.

TABLE 17.2 POTENTIAL CLINICAL FEATURES OF THE MOST COMMON SITES OF VENOUS THROMBOSIS, AS REPORTED IN THE INTERNATIONAL STUDY ON CEREBRAL VENOUS AND DURAL SINUSES THROMBOSIS (N = 624)[3]

Site of Venous Thrombosis	Clinical Features*
Superior sagittal sinus (62%)	Motor and/or sensory deficits Seizures
Transverse (lateral) sinus (41-45%)	Isolated headache or intracranial hypertension Focal motor and/or sensory deficits Aphasia if dominant transverse sinus Pulsatile tinnitus
Straight sinus (18%)	Encephalopathy Motor deficits
Cortical veins (17%)	Focal motor and/or sensory deficits Seizures
Jugular vein (12%)	Pulsatile tinnitus Neck pain and swelling Jugular foramen syndrome
Deep venous system (11%)	Decreased level of consciousness Motor and/or sensory deficits
Cavernous sinus (1%)	Orbital pain Chemosis Proptosis Oculomotor palsies

*Headache is the most common symptom associated with cerebral venous thrombosis and can be associated with any site of venous occlusion.

CT venography uses an iodinated contrast dye to directly visualize the venous system and is very effective in diagnosing CVT. Although prior studies raised concern for possible fetal hypothyroidism following administration of fat-soluble dyes, there have been no such reports with newer water-soluble agents. The contrast dye has not shown a risk to the fetus in animal studies, and there are no well-controlled studies in pregnant women (pregnancy category B by the US Food and Drug Administration). Given the lack of data to suggest harm to the fetus, the American College of Radiology does not recommend extra precautions during pregnancy with the use of iodinated contrast agents.[16] However, with the associated risk of radiation exposure from CT and theoretical risk of complications from contrast dye, CT venogram during pregnancy is generally avoided in clinical practice.

Because of the potential risks associated with CT and CT venography, magnetic resonance imaging (MRI) is the preferred imaging modality to diagnose CVT in pregnancy. Non-contrast head MRI provides higher sensitivity than CT and may show absent flow voids or abnormal signal intensity in the venous sinuses. Supportive evidence of CVT, such as focal edema or venous infarct, is also better visualized on MRI.[9] MR venography, when performed with two-dimensional time-of-flight sequences, can assess the patency of cerebral veins and dural sinuses without exposure to contrast dye. Although studies in humans are lacking, contrast-enhanced MRI or MR venography with use of gadolinium is typically avoided unless absolutely necessary during pregnancy, due to potential fetal risk. Iodinated contrast and gadolinium administration are not contraindicated during lactation, and CT and MR venography may be performed in the postpartum setting.[15–17]

Imaging may be difficult to interpret based on age of clot as well as normal anatomic variants such as dural sinus hypoplasia and asymmetric flow. If the diagnosis remains unclear after CT or MR venography, catheter cerebral angiogram may be used if clinical suspicion for CVT remains high. However, this is an invasive diagnostic procedure and is rarely required due to current sensitivity of other imaging modalities.

Once a diagnosis of CVT is confirmed, workup should include a search for additional contributing factors. Routine blood work is indicated in all cases of suspected CVT and should include screening for infectious, inflammatory, and hypercoagulable conditions. At a minimum, a complete blood count, chemistry panel, sedimentation rate, prothrombin time, and partial thromboplastin time should be obtained.[9] Additional workup should

be tailored to patient specific risk factors based on history.

Elevated D-dimer, a fibrin degradation product, is a sensitive but nonspecific marker of thrombosis in otherwise healthy adults. Normal D-dimer values, when used with other clinical assessments, have a high negative predictive value useful in ruling out deep vein thrombosis and pulmonary emboli.[18] However, D-dimer levels may increase during normal pregnancy, making them a less reliable indicator of thrombosis in this setting.[19,20] The role of D-dimer in pregnancy-associated CVT is even less certain because in addition to the variations that may occur with pregnancy, D-dimer values are influenced by acuity and extent of CVT.[21] Thus, D-dimer should not be used to guide management in pregnant patients with concern for CVT.

Lumbar puncture is not helpful in diagnosis of CVT and should only be done to rule out alternative causes, such as meningitis, depending on the clinical picture. There are no specific CSF abnormalities in CVT, though frequent findings include elevated opening pressure (>80% of cases), cell counts (~50% of cases), and protein (~35% of cases).[9]

MANAGEMENT

Upon diagnosis of CVT, patients should be admitted to a stroke unit with initiation of treatment as soon as possible. Anti-coagulation is the preferred treatment for CVT, even in patients with intracerebral hemorrhage. While counterintuitive at first glance, this recommendation is based on the underlying pathophysiology of CVT. If hemorrhage stems from venous thrombosis and elevated venous pressure, only treatment of thrombosis will address the underlying cause. Improved functional outcome and mortality with anticoagulation has been confirmed in numerous randomized and non-randomized studies.[9]

Low-molecular weight heparin (LMWH) is the anticoagulant of choice during pregnancy because it is not associated with the teratogenicity or risk of fetal bleeding seen with unfractionated heparin (UFH) or vitamin K antagonists (such as warfarin). Guidelines published by the American College of Chest Physicians recommend pregnant women with acute venous thromboembolism receive LMWH throughout pregnancy.[22] Due to concern for bleeding complications if regional anesthesia is pursued during delivery, LMWH may be held at onset of spontaneous labor or at least 24 hours prior to labor induction or cesarean section.[23] Following delivery, anticoagulation with LMWH or an oral vitamin K antagonist is continued for at least 6 weeks postpartum. Both LMWH and warfarin are acceptable for use during breastfeeding. These recommendations have been adopted by the American Heart Association/American Stroke Association to apply to CVT in pregnant women, with additional recommendation for a total minimum duration of 3 to 6 months of treatment unless laboratory testing suggests the presence of a significant thrombophilia which requires longer-term anti-coagulation, as outlined below.[9]

Successful direct endovascular thrombolysis and mechanical thrombectomy has also been demonstrated in management of CVT. However, there are limited data regarding these procedures in CVT and even less evidence guiding their use in the setting of pregnancy.[9,24] Currently, these procedures are reserved for patients who deteriorate despite systemic anti-coagulation.

In patients with recurrent CVT, subsequent venous thromboembolism, or severe thrombophilia, indefinite anticoagulation may be necessary. Severe thrombophilias have been defined based on the risk of recurrent thrombosis and include homozygous prothrombin G20210A; homozygous factor V Leiden; deficiencies of protein C, protein S, or antithrombin; combined thrombophilia defects; or antiphospholipid syndrome.[9,25] Assays testing protein C, protein S, and antithrombin activity are unreliable in the setting of acute CVT or in patients taking warfarin, and testing is generally indicated at least two weeks after completion of anticoagulation. Hematology consultation may be warranted to guide testing and management of underlying thrombophilia.[9] Novel oral anticoagulants such as direct thrombin inhibitors (dabigatran) and direct factor Xa inhibitors (rivaroxaban, apixaban, and edoxaban) are not used during pregnancy or lactation due to a lack of information on efficacy and fetal/infant safety. There is also limited information regarding their efficacy in CVT, which is not an FDA approved indication.

The high risk of seizures associated with CVT becomes especially worrisome in the setting of pregnancy, where convulsive activity could potentially cause fetal harm. There are no randomized trials to guide treatment in this situation. Data from the ICVST and expert consensus recommend that anticonvulsant therapy be considered even after a single seizure in the setting of CVT, with the strongest evidence of benefit in patients with supratentorial lesions (venous infarct or intracerebral hemorrhage) on initial imaging. Prophylactic antiepileptic use is not recommended in CVT.[9,26]

Follow-up imaging with CT or MR venography is typically performed 3 to 6 months after diagnosis of CVT to assess for venous recanalization,

which occurs in approximately 85% of cases. However, recanalization does not affect outcome, and failure to recanalize after an appropriate duration of anticoagulation does not necessitate ongoing treatment.[9]

Women with CVT in the setting of pregnancy should subsequently avoid all estrogen-based contraception, regardless of route of administration. Several large studies have failed to show an increased risk of venous thromboembolism or stroke in women taking progestin-only medications.[27,28] However, there are limited data regarding recurrent risk in CVT, and some observational studies suggest that the risk of CVT is higher with any form of hormonal contraception compared to non-exposed women.[29] Barrier contraception or copper intrauterine device is thus preferred to minimize risk of recurrent CVT.

PATIENT OUTCOMES

Outcomes in CVT have improved significantly due to advances in diagnosis and treatment. Widely available neuroimaging modalities allow earlier diagnosis of CVT, preventing late complications in many cases. Widespread use of anticoagulation has also improved outcomes. Mortality in contemporary cases ranges from 3 to 15%. Herniation from a large intracranial hemorrhage, a direct result of CVT, is the most common cause of death in the acute setting. Delayed mortality is typically secondary to the underlying cause of CVT, most commonly cancer.[9] CVT associated with pregnancy and the postpartum period tends to have a better prognosis than CVT due to other factors.[5,14] This may be influenced by the younger age of these patients or perhaps more regular medical care in the setting of pregnancy and earlier diagnosis. Fortunately, complete recovery is seen in over 80% of women.[14] Isolated intracranial hypertension is a predictor of good outcome, emphasizing the importance of early diagnosis.[30] Predictors of poor outcome include thrombosis of the deep venous system, coma, intracranial hemorrhage, posterior fossa lesions, and cancer.[3]

Data from multiple studies suggest low risk of recurrent CVT (0–3%) or of other complications during subsequent pregnancies.[24] However, voluntary or spontaneous abortion may be more common in these patients, with rates as high as 12%.[9] Given the low risk of complications, past CVT is not a contraindication to future pregnancy. Prophylaxis with LMWH during pregnancy and the postpartum period may be beneficial in women with prior CVT, though prospective clinical trials are needed to better define the risks and benefits.[9,31] A management summary for CVT in pregnancy is provided in Box 17.1.

BOX 17.1
CARE MAP FOR PREGNANCY IN THE CEREBRAL VENOUS THROMBOSIS (CVT) PATIENT

BEFORE PREGNANCY

Review prior pregnancy complications

If history of venous thromboembolism or CVT, check for underlying thrombophilia

Assessment of disease specific maternal risk factors:

    Personal or family history of venous thromboembolism or miscarriage

    Use of exogenous hormones (fertility treatment)

Medication adjustment, consolidation and review

DURING PREGNANCY

Monitor for headache, vision changes, focal neurologic deficits, seizures

If concern for CVT, obtain magnetic resonance venography with time-of-flight (non-contrast) imaging

Once diagnosis of CVT is confirmed, assess for coexisting infectious, inflammatory, and hypercoagulable conditions based on history and patient specific risk factors

Workup for thrombophilia should include antiphospholipid and anticardiolipin antibodies, homocysteine levels, prothrombin and factor V Leiden mutations, and activity of antithrombin, protein C, and protein S

Initiate treatment with therapeutic low-molecular weight heparin (LMWH) and continue throughout pregnancy

DELIVERY

Multidisciplinary discussion to plan best delivery route and location

Anesthesia consultation

LMWH may be held at onset of spontaneous labor or at least 24 hours prior to labor induction or Cesarean section to prevent hemorrhagic complications

POSTPARTUM

Continue anticoagulation with LMWH or vitamin K antagonist such as warfarin (goal INR 2-3) for at least 6 weeks, with a total minimum duration of 3 to 6 months of therapy

If precipitating cause of CVT remains unclear, consult hematology for further recommendations regarding repeat thrombophilia testing and need for indefinite anticoagulation

Follow-up imaging to assess for recanalization 3–6 months after diagnosis

Contraception counseling:

    Avoid estrogen and hormonal contraception indefinitely

    Recommend barrier method or copper intrauterine device

Discuss risks associated with future pregnancy:

    Future pregnancy is not contraindicated

    There is low risk of recurrent CVT with subsequent pregnancies (0–3%), but there may be a higher rate of spontaneous abortion

    Consider prophylactic LMWH during future pregnancies and the postpartum period

REFERENCES

1. Bousser MG, Ferro JM. Cerebral venous thrombosis: An update. *Lancet Neurol.* 2007; 6: 162–170.
2. Lanska DJ, Kryscio RJ. Risk factors for peripartum and postpartum stroke and intracranial venous thrombosis. *Stroke.* 2000; 31: 1274–1282.
3. Ferro JM, Canhao P, Stam J, Bousser MG, Barinagarrementeria F. Prognosis of cerebral vein and dural sinus thrombosis: Results of the International Study on Cerebral Vein and Dural Sinus Thrombosis (ISCVT). *Stroke.* 2004; 35: 664–670.
4. Bousser MG, Crassard I. Cerebral venous thrombosis, pregnancy and oral contraceptives. *Thromb Res.* 2012; 130(Suppl 1): S19–22.
5. Cantu C, Barinagarrementeria F. Cerebral venous thrombosis associated with pregnancy and puerperium. Review of 67 cases. *Stroke.* 1993; 24: 1880–1884.
6. Trigg DE, Wood MG, Kouides PA, Kadir RA. Hormonal influences on hemostasis in women. *Semin Thromb Hemost.* 2011; 37: 77–86.
7. Jeng JS, Tang SC, Yip PK. Incidence and etiologies of stroke during pregnancy and puerperium as evidenced in Taiwanese women. *Cerebrovasc Dis.* 2004; 18: 290–295.
8. Jaigobin C, Silver FL. Stroke and pregnancy. *Stroke.* 2000; 31: 2948–2951.
9. Saposnik G, Barinagarrementeria F, Brown RD, Jr., et al. Diagnosis and management of cerebral venous thrombosis: a statement for healthcare professionals from the American Heart Association/American Stroke Association. *Stroke.* 2011; 42: 1158–1192.
10. Caplan LR. *Caplan's Stroke: A Clinical Approach.* 4th ed. Philadelphia: Elsevier/Saunders, 2009.
11. Stam J. Thrombosis of the cerebral veins and sinuses. *N Engl J Med.* 2005; 352: 1791–1798.
12. Biousse V, Ameri A, Bousser MG. Isolated intracranial hypertension as the only sign of cerebral venous thrombosis. *Neurology.* 1999; 53: 1537–1542.
13. Cumurciuc R, Crassard I, Sarov M, Valade D, Bousser MG. Headache as the only neurological sign of cerebral venous thrombosis: A series of 17 cases. *J Neurol Neurosurg Psychiatry.* 2005; 76: 1084–1087.
14. Coutinho JM, Ferro JM, Canhao P, et al. Cerebral venous and sinus thrombosis in women. *Stroke.* 2009; 40: 2356–2361.
15. Bove RM, Klein JP. Neuroradiology in women of childbearing age. Continuum (Minneap Minn) 2014; 20: 23–41.
16. Radiology ACo. ACR Manual on Contrast Media, Version 10.2. 2016. Available at https://www.acr.org/~/media/37D84428BF1D4E1B9A3A2918DA9E27A3.pdf. Accessed December 10, 2016.
17. Webb JA, Thomsen HS, Morcos SK, Members of contrast media safety committee of European Society of Urogenital R. The use of iodinated and gadolinium contrast media during pregnancy and lactation. *Eur Radiol.* 2005; 15: 1234–1240.
18. Stein PD, Hull RD, Patel KC, et al. D-dimer for the exclusion of acute venous thrombosis and pulmonary embolism: a systematic review. *Ann Intern Med.* 2004; 140: 589–602.
19. Nishii A, Noda Y, Nemoto R, et al. Evaluation of D-dimer during pregnancy. *J Obstet Gynaecol Res.* 2009; 35: 689–693.
20. Reger B, Peterfalvi A, Litter I, et al. Challenges in the evaluation of D-dimer and fibrinogen levels in pregnant women. *Thromb Res.* 2013; 131: e183–187.
21. Kosinski CM, Mull M, Schwarz M, et al. Do normal D-dimer levels reliably exclude cerebral sinus thrombosis? *Stroke.* 2004; 35: 2820–2825.
22. Bates SM, Greer IA, Middeldorp S, et al. VTE, thrombophilia, antithrombotic therapy, and pregnancy: Antithrombotic therapy and prevention of thrombosis. 9th ed. American College of Chest Physicians Evidence-Based Clinical Practice Guidelines. *Chest.* 2012; 141: e691S–736S.
23. James A. Committee on practice B-O. Practice bulletin no. 123: Thromboembolism in pregnancy. *Obstet Gynecol.* 2011; 118: 718–729.
24. Niwa J, Ohyama H, Mastumura S, Sasaki T. Successful treatment of superior sagittal sinus thrombosis. Direct thrombolysis with local infusion of t-PA via venography in the acute phase. *Interv Neuroradiol.* 1997; 3(Suppl 2): 198–200.
25. Lijfering WM, Brouwer JL, Veeger NJ, et al. Selective testing for thrombophilia in patients with first venous thrombosis: Results from a retrospective family cohort study on absolute thrombotic risk for currently known thrombophilic defects in 2479 relatives. *Blood.* 2009; 113: 5314–5322.
26. Ferro JM, Canhao P, Bousser MG, Stam J, Barinagarrementeria F, Investigators I. Early seizures in cerebral vein and dural sinus thrombosis—Risk factors and role of antiepileptics. *Stroke.* 2008; 39: 1152–1158.
27. Bergendal A, Persson I, Odeberg J, et al. Association of venous thromboembolism with hormonal contraception and thrombophilic genotypes. *Obstet Gynecol.* 2014; 124: 600–609.
28. Chakhtoura Z, Canonico M, Gompel A, Thalabard JC, Scarabin PY, Plu-Bureau G. Progestogen-only contraceptives and the risk of stroke: A meta-analysis. *Stroke,* 2009; 40: 1059–1062.
29. Jick SS, Jick H. Cerebral venous sinus thrombosis in users of four hormonal contraceptives: Levonorgestrel-containing oral contraceptives,

norgestimate-containing oral contraceptives, desogestrel-containing oral contraceptives and the contraceptive patch. *Contraception.* 2006; 74: 290–292.

30. Dentali F, Gianni M, Crowther MA, Ageno W. Natural history of cerebral vein thrombosis: A systematic review. *Blood.* 2006; 108: 1129–1134.

31. Aguiar de Sousa D, Canhao P, Ferro JM. Safety of pregnancy after cerebral venous thrombosis: A systematic review. *Stroke.* 2016; 47: 713–718.

32. Ou YC, Kao YL, Lai SL, et al. Thromboembolism after ovarian stimulation: Successful management of a woman with superior sagittal sinus thrombosis after IVF and embryo transfer: Case report. *Hum Reprod.* 2003; 18: 2375–2381.

18

Brain Tumors in Pregnancy

CHINAZOM IBEGBU AND NIMISH A. MOHILE

ABSTRACT

Approximately 79,000 people are diagnosed with a central nervous system (CNS) tumor each year, but only a few of these patients are pregnant women. There is no evidence that pregnancy confers an increased risk of developing a brain tumor and incidence during child-bearing years is estimated to be 12.24 per 100,000 women. The care and management of all patients with primary brain tumors can be challenging and requires a multidisciplinary team that includes neurologists, medical neuro-oncologists, neurosurgeons, radiation-oncologists, and palliative care physicians. In a pregnant patient, this multidisciplinary team should also include a high-risk obstetrician. This chapter provides a detailed care map for pregnant patients with brain tumors. All management decisions regarding the neoplasm must consider the health of the expectant mother, the health of the fetus, the neurological and medical complications due to the brain tumor, and the potential effect that the brain tumor has on the patient's survival.

CLINICAL PRESENTATION

Tumor location, size, and surrounding edema dictate a patient's presenting signs and symptoms. During pregnancy, these signs and symptoms may be unmasked due to neuronal dysfunction caused by volume expansion normally seen in pregnancy.[1] This is most common in the late second trimester and third trimester when fluid shifts are at their highest.[2] Any new unexplained focal neurologic symptom during pregnancy should be evaluated with a neurological examination and if symptoms and signs localize to the brain, neuroimaging should be pursued.

Seizures are the most common presenting symptoms of a brain tumor[3] but may also be a complication of pregnancy itself. A seizure due to eclampsia usually occurs in the second or third trimesters and rarely, in the postpartum period. These seizures are usually generalized. Seizures due to brain tumors are focal in onset and therefore any focal features based on semiology, abnormal neurological examination, or localized dysfunction on electroencephalography should be evaluated for a structural abnormality. Seizures due to brain tumors are not associated with hypertension, proteinuria, diffuse hyperreflexia, and other findings commonly seen in patients with eclampsia.

Headaches, especially with nausea and vomiting, can be a symptom of increased intracranial pressure (ICP), seen when a tumor exerts mass effect. Headaches also occur more frequently during normal pregnancy due to hormonal changes, physical stressors, and psychological stressors. A new headache should be evaluated with a thorough history and neurological examination. Headaches that change with position, worsen with coughing or Valsalva, or become more intense overnight and result in early morning awakenings suggest increased ICP. Venous sinus thrombosis and idiopathic intracranial hypertension are common in pregnancy and often present with similar headaches. Nausea and vomiting due to increased intracranial pressure may be confused with symptoms expected during normal pregnancy such as morning sickness. Morning sickness typically consists of relatively mild nausea and vomiting and is most prominent during the first trimester. More severe symptoms with other signs of increased intracranial pressure need to be evaluated with a detailed neurological examination.

DIAGNOSTIC IMAGING

MRI with gadolinium contrast is the imaging modality of choice in the non-emergent setting for patients with brain tumors. MRI provides a greater level of detail than CT and it allows better delineation of the tumor for operative and radiation planning. MRI is considered safe during pregnancy,[4] but the safety of gadolinium-based contrast agents is controversial. The American College of Obstetricians and Gynecologists recommends caution with the use of gadolinium-based contrast

TABLE 18.1 PRIMARY BRAIN TUMORS, RADIOLOGIC FEATURES AND TREATMENT IN WOMEN OF CHILD-BEARING AGE

Tumor Type	MRI Imaging Features	Treatment
Benign		
Meningioma	Dural-based lesion; T1-hypointense, T2-hyperintense, homogenous enhancement pattern	Total surgical resection is curative, can be followed if asymptomatic
Pituitary Tumors	Sellar mass, isointense on T1 and T2, variable enhancement	Total surgical resection is curative Medical treatment with dopamine agonists for prolactinoma
Nerve Sheath Tumors	Predilection for cranial nerve V and VIII, T1 isointense, T2 hyperintense, variable contrast enhancement	Total surgical resection is curative, can be followed if asymptomatic
Low-Grade		
Diffuse oligodendroglioma Diffuse astrocytoma	T1 hypo/isointense, T2 hyperintense, usually zero or minimal contrast enhancement, some vasogenic edema	Surgical resection followed by upfront RT and/or chemo vs. close surveillance and treatment when there is growth
High-Grade		
Anaplastic oligodendroglioma Anaplastic astrocytoma Glioblastoma	T1 hypo/isointense, T2 hyperintense, ring-enhancement contrast pattern is common but variable, significant vasogenic edema	Urgent surgical resection followed by upfront RT and chemo

Abbreviations: MRI = magnetic resonance imaging, RT = radiotherapy.

agents due to inadequate safety data and possible teratogenicity.[5] Gadolinium administration allows the MRI to elucidate any areas where there is blood-brain barrier breakdown; this can help distinguish higher-grade gliomas from low-grade gliomas. We recommend its use for the first MRI in order to better evaluate tumor extent and predict tumor grade. Follow up MRIs, if needed, can typically done without gadolinium. Table 18.1 describes common brain tumor types during pregnancy and imaging features. CT may be indicated in emergent settings and is particularly helpful for excluding intracranial hemorrhage. CT, MRI and contrast agents may be used safely during breastfeeding.

ANTI-NEOPLASTIC THERAPY

Once a pregnant woman is found to have a brain tumor, her team of providers must approach her care with consideration of both mother and fetus. Box 18.1 provides a detailed pregnancy care map for patients with primary brain tumors. Treatment will often involve a combination of surgery, chemotherapy, and radiotherapy (Figure 18.1). Benign tumors such as meningiomas, pituitary adenomas, or nerve sheath tumors will rarely require any intervention during pregnancy unless they are symptomatic. This can involve surgical resection or medical management of pituitary hormone abnormalities. In women with non-contrast-enhancing tumors who are suspected of having a low-grade glioma, surgical resection and cancer treatment can be safely delayed until the pregnancy is over. These tumors are slow-growing and deferral of therapy is unlikely to result in tumor growth or increased neurologic morbidity. In patients with evidence of contrast enhancement and a suspected high-grade glioma, treatment should be initiated as soon as possible, and a tissue sample is needed to finalize diagnosis. Early initiation of therapy, especially surgical resection, is critically important to prevent tumor growth and is likely associated with improved maternal survival.[6] We recommend initiating therapy with the same modalities indicated for a non-pregnant patient

---

BOX 18.1
CARE MAP FOR PREGNANT PATIENTS WITH BRAIN TUMORS

BEFORE PREGNANCY

- Contraception counseling
- Complete treatment of brain tumor with continued multidisciplinary follow-up (neuro-oncology, radiation-oncology, neurosurgery)
- Pre-conception MFM consult
- Pre-conception infertility consultation

DURING PREGNANCY

- MFM consultation
- Multidisciplinary neuro-oncology team involvement including medical neuro-oncology, neurosurgery, radiation-oncology, and palliative care
  - Decisions about imaging modality and surveillance
  - Seizure management
  - Corticosteroid management
  - Development of a multi-disciplinary treatment plan
  - Surgical and radiotherapy planning, if indicated
  - Psychosocial support

DELIVERY

- Multidisciplinary discussion about best delivery route and timing
- Anesthesia consultation
- Pain management

POSTPARTUM

- VTE prophylaxis, early mobilization
- Lactation consultation
- Follow up with all neuro-oncology providers
- Contraception counseling

MFM = maternal fetal medicine, VTE = venous thrombo-embolism.

---

and then tailoring these therapies, if possible, to minimize risk to the fetus.[7] Should surgery/resection be needed, there is the possibility that the woman will no longer be able to successfully breastfeed. Discussion and referral to a lactation specialist to optimize her case and support is recommended (see also Section 5, Chapter 32).

Imaging alone is never sufficient for making an oncologic diagnosis. A biopsy or resection is necessary to determine the pathologic diagnosis and should be done in all but rare cases prior to initiating therapy. Maximal safe surgical resection is associated with improved overall survival and neurologic function compared to biopsy alone.[8] It

is critical to obtain sufficient tissue to accurately describe molecular and genetic characteristics of a tumor to make the correct diagnosis, estimate prognosis, tailor treatments, and predict response to therapy.

The safest time to perform a biopsy or resection of a brain tumor in a pregnant woman may be early in the second trimester. Surgery in the first trimester is associated with an increased risk of miscarriage. In the late second and third trimester, there is an increased risk for intracranial hemorrhage as maternal intravascular volumes increase during this time.[9] The timing of surgery needs to be a collaborative decision based on the mother's neurologic disability from the tumor, goals of

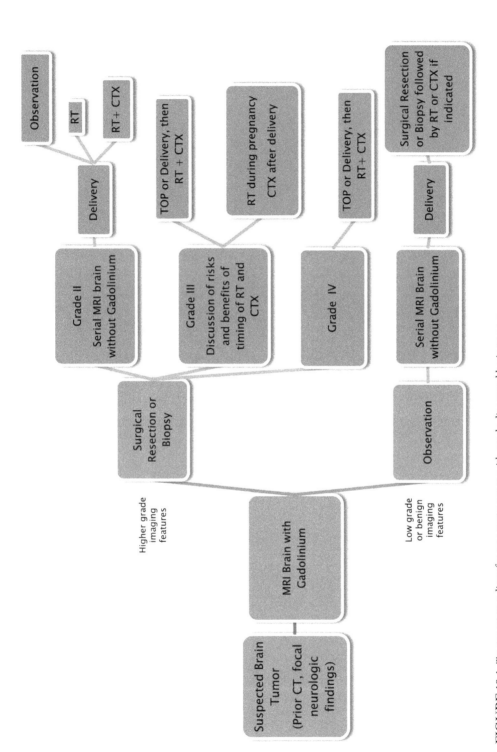

FIGURE 18.1 Treatment paradigm for pregnant women with newly diagnosed brain tumors.

CT= Computed Axial Tomography; MRI = Magnetic Resonance Imaging; RT = Radiotherapy; CTX= Chemotherpay; TOP =Termination of Pregnancy.

surgery, and presumed tumor type. Surgical resections are often performed on patients in the prone position. This may be difficult to do in a gravid patient and neurosurgeons may decide to perform these operations with patients in the sitting or lateral decubitus position if it does not compromise the safety and effectiveness of the procedure.[10] Fetal monitoring, especially after the age of viability, should occur during these operations in conjunction with the obstetrics team.[11]

Following surgery, high grade gliomas are most commonly treated with intensity-modulated radiation therapy or 3D conformal radiation therapy. Exposure to ionizing radiation can result in minor and major fetal malformations with risk highest in the first trimester. If it is necessary to start radiation therapy during pregnancy, the fetus can be shielded to minimize exposure. Delays in starting radiation therapy in a patient with an aggressive brain tumor such as glioblastoma may lead to worse prognosis.

Chemotherapeutics are cytotoxic to tumor cells but also injure healthy and rapidly dividing cells, thereby placing a fetus at particular risk. Almost all cytotoxic chemotherapies are contraindicated during pregnancy and will result in major malformations or fetal death. The most common chemotherapy regimens for brain tumors include alkylating chemotherapies that cross the blood-brain barrier such as temozolomide and nitrosurea drugs. Biologic therapies such as bevacizumab, a monoclonal antibody to VEGF-A (vascular endothelial growth factor), have been incorporated into regimens for recurrent tumor and for many patients, experimental therapies given via clinical trials are an important aspect of treatment. Timing of therapy depends on the patient's post-surgical neurologic function and tumor type. In low-grade gliomas and some anaplastic gliomas, waiting to complete the pregnancy is a feasible option as the exact timing of chemotherapy is not definitively known to affect survival. In patients with glioblastoma, data suggests that treatment should be initiated within 4 to 6 weeks of surgery and delays beyond that are associated with clinically meaningful tumor progression and poor prognosis.[12] In these cases, molecular biomarkers that predict sensitivity to chemotherapy can help the patient and clinicians decide whether chemotherapy can be deferred. If it cannot be safely deferred, then the patient will need to consider a termination of pregnancy prior to chemotherapy.

Carmustine wafers are polymers impregnated with an alkylating chemotherapy that can be embedded into surgical cavity walls after resection and serves as a form of local chemotherapy. There is no systemic absorption of chemotherapy. A few trials support its use in malignant gliomas.[13] It can be given safely during pregnancy and may represent a possible option allowing for deferral of systemic chemotherapy for a few months.

Supportive Care

Seizures occur in most patients with brain tumors.[14] In patients who have not had seizures, there is no evidence to support the use of prophylactic therapy.[15] For patients with seizures, enzyme-inducing anti-epileptic drugs should be avoided due to interactions with chemotherapy and corticosteroids.

Vasogenic edema represents capillary leakage of fluid from disruption of the blood-brain barrier. This is more prominent in higher grade brain tumors and for many patients, the neurologic dysfunction from the tumor can cause more symptoms than the brain tumor itself. In rare cases, edema can be significant enough to lead to brain herniation and death. Corticosteroids can help reduce edema and are commonly used in brain tumor patients. While corticosteroids are generally safe during pregnancy, chronic use can contribute to maternal weight gain, peripheral edema, myopathy, mood disturbance, and predisposition to infections. At all times, patients should be on the lowest effective dose. Dosing should be dictated by the patient's neurologic symptoms and not based on the neuroimaging. Although it is rare, corticosteroid use can cause adrenal insufficiency in the neonate.[16]

Patients with brain tumors have a high risk of venous thromboembolism (VTE) due to procoagulant factors secreted by the tumor, immobility, and surgical resection.[17] Pregnant women are already at a higher risk of VTE and pulmonary embolism is the leading cause of maternal death in the developed world.[18] Symptomatic VTE can occur in up to 30% of brain tumor patients and is most common in the post-operative period.[19] The diagnosis of VTE can be complicated because symptoms such as leg swelling, tachypnea, dyspnea, and tachycardia may occur in normal pregnancy. These symptoms should be evaluated carefully given the high risk. Lower extremity ultrasound can be safely performed during pregnancy and may be the test of choice even in patients with pulmonary symptoms to minimize exposure to CT or radionuclide scans.

There is data to support the use of chemical thromboprophylaxis with low molecular weight heparin (LMWH) in the peri-operative period but not later in the disease course in patients with brain tumors.[20] In patients who develop VTE, LMWH is the treatment of choice and is considered superior to warfarin in clot prevention for cancer patients.[21] The risk of intracranial hemorrhage is low and is outweighed by the morbidity and mortality associated with untreated VTE. Warfarin should be avoided due to teratogenicity and the safety and efficacy of the newer oral anticoagulants has not been established. Inferior vena cava filters are associated with higher complication rates than LMWH and when used in conjunction with LMWH are associated with a higher incidence of breakthrough events.[22] An inferior vena cava filter should only be placed when there are contraindications to LMWH.

Obstetric and Gynecologic Care

Women with brain tumors who are interested in becoming pregnant should undergo all antineoplastic therapy before trying to conceive. They should be specifically counseled about the teratogenicity of chemotherapy and its potential long-term effects on fertility. Following chemotherapy, the optimal timing of conception is not known, but it may take 6–12 months before menstrual periods return to normal. Consultation with an infertility specialist prior to treatment is suggested to discuss options such as freezing eggs or embryos.

Optimal timing and method of delivery should be determined by obstetrics. In patients with elevated intracranial pressure, cesarean section is generally favored over vaginal delivery due to exacerbation of ICP when a woman bears down during labor and with uterine contractions.[23] These elevations in intracranial pressure are normally safe during labor, but in women with brain tumors they can compound preexisting elevations in ICP leading to neurologic dysfunction, herniation or in severe cases, death. In patients who have undergone complete resections, ICP may return to normal and vaginal delivery is feasible. Intracranial pressures reach their apex during the second stage of labor[24] and in cases of vaginal delivery, this stage can be shortened using a low or outlet forceps application.[25] Spinal or epidural anesthesia should be used with caution in patients with tumors causing asymmetric mass effect or compression of the fourth ventricle. If there is a large pressure gradient between the intracranial and lumbar compartments, a lumbar puncture can lead to cerebral herniation.

In the postpartum period, VTE prophylaxis may be necessary for patients with prolonged immobility. Sleep deprivation and fatigue can exacerbate neurologic symptoms and sometimes lower a patient's threshold for seizures. All antineoplastic treatments can be safely administered to the mother during this period except bevacizumab which can delay wound healing. However, patients should be aware of which of their medications may enter breast milk and have an informed discussion about any potential risks with consideration given to bottle feeding instead of breastfeeding.

Lactation

Women undergoing treatment for cancer may desire to breastfeed. However, the long half-lives and high toxicity of many chemotherapeutic regimens make breastfeeding a difficult, if not impossible, choice. Depending on the timing of chemotherapy and surgeries, a mother can sometimes be offered a window in which she can breastfeed or provide breastmilk for her baby. Other times, mothers may desire to pump and discard their milk until it is safe to use. Sometimes, neither of these are possible, and a mother may require additional support for the loss of this expectation. Her choices are best supported by pre or perinatal consultation with a breastfeeding specialist.

CONCLUSION

The diagnosis of a brain tumor in a woman that is pregnant can be both emotionally difficult and medically complex with potentially fatal implications for the mother or child. Patients and families will require psychosocial support in addition to multidisciplinary care at the time of diagnosis and throughout the pregnancy. A combined knowledge of the obstetric, neurosurgical, and oncologic issues involved will inform a treatment plan that can best improve function and survival for the mother and preserve the health of the fetus.

REFERENCES

1. Tewari KS, Cappuccini F, Asrat T, et al. Obstetric emergencies precipitated by malignant brain tumors. *Am J ObstetGynecol.* 2000; 182(5): 1215–1221. doi:10.1016/s0002-9378(00)70188-8.
2. Hytten F. Blood volume changes in normal pregnancy. Clin Haematol. 1985; 14(3): 601–612.

3. Breemen MSV, Wilms EB, Vecht CJ. Epilepsy in patients with brain tumours: Epidemiology, mechanisms, and management. Lancet Neurol 2007; 6(5): 421–430. doi:10.1016/s1474-4422(07)70103-5.

4. Tremblay E, Thérasse E, Thomassin-Naggara I, Trop I. Quality initiatives: Guidelines for use of medical imaging during pregnancy and lactation. *Radiographics.* 2012; 32(3): 897–911. doi:10.1148/rg.323115120.

5. Committee on Obstetric Practice. Guidelines for diagnostic imaging during pregnancy and lactation. *Obstet Gynecol.* 2016; 127(2): 418. doi:10.1097/aog.0000000000001309.

6. Terry AR, Barker FG, Leffert L, Bateman BT, Souter I, Plotkin SR. Outcomes of hospitalization in pregnant women with CNS neoplasms: A population-based study. *Neuro Oncol.* 2012; 14(6): 768–776. doi:10.1093/neuonc/nos078.

7. Bonfield CM, Engh JA. Pregnancy and brain tumors. *Neurol Clin.* 2012; 30(3): 937–946. doi:10.1016/j.ncl.2012.04.003.

8. Kılıç TCBC, Özduman K, Elmacı I, Sav A, Pamir MN. Effect of surgery on tumor progression and malignant degeneration in hemispheric diffuse low-grade astrocytomas. *J Clin Neurosci.* 2002; 9(5): 549–552. doi:10.1054/jocn.2002.1136.

9. Jayasekera BAP, Bacon AD, Whitfield PC. Management of glioblastoma multiforme in pregnancy. *J Neurosurg.* 2012; 116(6): 1187–1194. doi:10.3171/2012.2.jns112077.

10. Giannini A, Bricchi M. Posterior fossa surgery in the sitting position in a pregnant patient with cerebellopontine angle meningioma. *Br J Anaesth.* 1999; 82(6): 941–944. doi:10.1093/bja/82.6.941.

11. Cohen-Gadol AA, Friedman JA, Friedman JD, Tubbs RS, Munis JR, Meyer FB. Neurosurgical management of intracranial lesions in the pregnant patient: A 36-year institutional experience and review of the literature.*J Neurosurg.* 2009; 111(6): 1150–1157. doi:10.3171/2009.3.jns081160.

12. Spratt DE, Folkert M, Zumsteg ZS, et al. Temporal relationship of post-operative radiotherapy with temozolomide and oncologic outcome for glioblastoma. *J Neurooncol.* 2013; 116(2): 357–363. doi:10.1007/s11060-013-1302-1304.

13. Perry J. Gliadel® wafers in the treatment of malignant glioma: A systematic review. *Current Oncol.* 2007; 14(5): 189–194. doi:10.3747/co.2007.147.

14. Breemen MSV, Wilms EB, Vecht CJ. Epilepsy in patients with brain tumours: Epidemiology, mechanisms, and management. *Lancet Neurol.* 2007; 6(5): 421–430. doi:10.1016/s1474-4422(07)70103-5.

15. Glantz MJ, Cole BF, Forsyth PA, et al. Practice parameter: Anticonvulsant prophylaxis in patients with newly diagnosed brain tumors: Report of the Quality Standards Subcommittee of the American Academy of Neurology. *Neurology.* 2000; 54(10): 1886–1893. doi:10.1212/wnl.54.10.1886.

16. Trainer PJ. Corticosteroids and pregnancy. Semin reprod med. 2002; 20(4): 375–380. doi:10.1055/s-2002-36710.

17. Cote DJ, Smith TR. Venous thromboembolism in brain tumor patients. *J Clin Neurosci.* 2016; 25: 13–18. doi:10.1016/j.jocn.2015.05.053.

18. Marik PE, Plante LA. Venous thromboembolic disease and pregnancy. *N EngJMed.* 2008; 359(19): 2025–2033. doi:10.1056/nejmra0707993.

19. Gerber DE. Management of venous thromboembolism in patients with primary and metastatic brain tumors. *J Clin Oncol.* 2006; 24(8): 1310–1318. doi:10.1200/jco.2005.04.6656.

20. Alshehri N, Cote DJ, Hulou MM, et al. Venous thromboembolism prophylaxis in brain tumor patients undergoing craniotomy: A meta-analysis. *JNeurooncol.* 2016; 130(3): 561–570. doi:10.1007/s11060-016-2259-x.

21. Lee AY, Levine MN, Baker RI, et al. Low-molecular-weight heparin versus a coumarin for the prevention of recurrent venous thromboembolism in patients with cancer. *N Eng J Med.* 2003; 349(2): 146–153. doi:10.1056/nejmoa025313.

22. Levin JM, Schiff D, Loeffler JS, Fine HA, Black PM, Wen PY. Complications of therapy for venous thromboembolic disease in patients with brain tumors. *Neurology.* 1993; 43(6): 1111–1111. doi:10.1212/wnl.43.6.1111.

23. Ravindra V, Braca J, Jensen R, Duckworth EM. Management of intracranial pathology during pregnancy: Case example and review of management strategies. *Surg Neurol Int.* 2015; 6(1): 43. doi:10.4103/2152-7806.153845.

24. Girault A, Dommergues M, Nizard J. Impact of maternal brain tumours on perinatal and maternal management and outcome: a single referral centre retrospective study. *Eur J Obstet Gynecol Reprod Biol.* 2014; 183: 132–136. doi:10.1016/j.ejogrb.2014.10.027.

25. Kempers RD, Miller RH. Management of pregnancy associated with brain tumors. *Am J Obstet Gynecol.* 1963; 87(7): 858–864. doi:10.1016/0002-9378(63)90283-7.

19

Movement Disorders in Pregnancy

JAMIE L. ADAMS AND CHRISTOPHER G. TAROLLI

ABSTRACT

Movement disorders occurring in women of childbearing age or arising during pregnancy are uncommon. However, advancing maternal age increases the likelihood for a pregnant women to have a preexisting movement disorder. Studies are limited regarding the effects of movement disorders and their treatment on pregnancy or the effects of pregnancy on preexisting movement disorders. More research is needed to provide better evidence-based guidelines. Still, there are special considerations when encountering movement disorders in this population, particularly with regard to diagnostic investigation and the safety of medications.

RESTLESS LEG SYNDROME

Restless leg syndrome (RLS) is the most common movement disorder of pregnancy, estimated to affect between 10–26% of pregnant women.[2,3] It is characterized by a distressing urge to move the legs while at rest often described as tension, aching, or "creepy-crawly" sensation, with associated relief with movement. Symptoms occur most commonly in the evening or at other times of rest.[3]

The majority of women experiencing RLS in pregnancy have de novo disease.[2] Onset is most commonly in the second and third trimesters, and symptoms tend to worsen over the course of the pregnancy. In the majority of individuals with new RLS during pregnancy, symptoms resolve within 1 month of delivery. However, symptoms can persist beyond 6 months in up to 5% of cases.[2,4] Women with new onset RLS during pregnancy have a 36% chance of developing RLS in subsequent pregnancies and a fourfold increase in risk of developing non-pregnancy RLS.[5]

Most women with preexisting RLS will experience a worsening of symptoms during pregnancy, though up to 11% may experience improvement.[2]

The pathophysiology of RLS is thought to be related to family history, brain dopamine levels, and low brain iron. Low serum ferritin and folate levels have also been associated with increased risk of RLS.[6] These vitamin deficiencies are more common in pregnancy, postulated to mediate the increased prevalence of RLS in pregnancy; no other pregnancy-specific features have been identified as risk factors.[7]

A diagnostic and therapeutic algorithm for RLS in pregnancy and lactation is presented in (Figure 19.1). Serum hemoglobin, ferritin, and iron levels should be evaluated in any pregnant woman with RLS. Iron supplementation is recommended for those with serum ferritin levels <75mcg/L. Non-pharmacological interventions are recommended for those with mild to moderate symptoms and include increasing physical activity and avoiding exacerbating factors (caffeine, nicotine, serotonergic medications, and dopamine blocking agents).[8]

For women with severe or refractory RLS in pregnancy, carbidopa/levodopa or low dose clonazepam are first-line therapy, though both are category C in pregnancy. Dopamine agonists are generally considered unsafe in pregnancy and should be avoided.[8] There is no evidence on the use of dopamine agonists in breastfeeding. However, due to their low molecular weight and biphasic elimination pattern resulting in a 5–7 hour half life, it is conceivable that these medications could pass into breastmilk. They are also known to lower serum prolactin and therefore may impact milk supply. Their use in breastfeeding should therefore be discouraged (also see Box 19.1).

CHOREA

Chorea is a hyperkinetic movement disorder characterized by involuntary, non-rhythmic, irregular, and unpredictable movements that may appear to flow from one muscle to the next. It can affect the face, trunk or limbs. The movements can be partially suppressed and patients may incorporate them into more purposeful movements.[9]

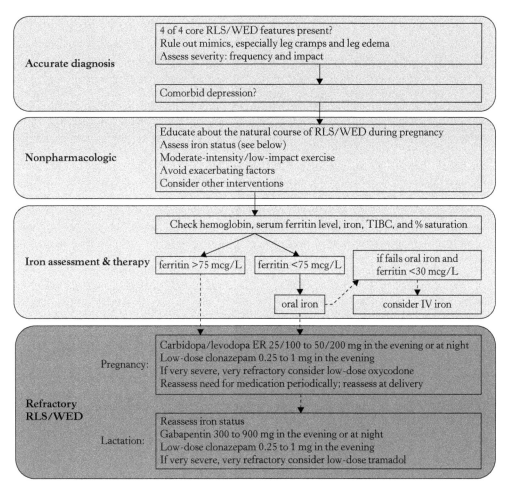

FIGURE 19.1 Diagnostic and treatment algorithm for restless leg syndrome during pregnancy and lactation.

Reprinted from Picchietti DL, Hensley JG, Bainbridge JL, et al., Sleep Medicine Reviews. © 2015, with permission from Elsevier.

BOX 19.1
RESTLESS LEG SYNDROME CARE MAP

BEFORE PREGNANCY
No disease specific concerns

DURING PREGNANCY
Counseling on potential worsening of symptoms
Evaluate serum hemoglobin, ferritin, iron
Eliminate exacerbating factors
Initiate non-pharmacologic interventions
Consider iron supplementation
Medication initiation, review, and adjustment—avoid dopamine agonists

DELIVERY
No disease specific concerns

POST-PARTUM
Reassess iron status
Medication review and adjustment—avoid dopamine agonists during lactation
Schedule neurology follow-up

Chorea Gravidarum

Chorea that arises during pregnancy was first associated with rheumatic fever and labeled chorea gravidarum. Other causes of chorea gravidarum have emerged including systemic lupus erythematosus, antiphospholipid antibody syndrome, syphilis, and encephalitis.[10] The condition may result from hormonal changes unmasking preexisting basal ganglia dysfunction.[11] Abnormal movements typically begin in the first or early second trimester and resolve prior to delivery in one-third of cases and shortly after delivery in the remainder.[1] About 20% of women have recurrence in subsequent pregnancies.[10]

Several drugs can cause chorea including opiates, amphetamines, cocaine, neuroleptics, antihistamines, and anti-epileptics. Therefore, a careful review of illicit and prescription drug use is important when evaluating pregnant women with chorea. Additional causes of chorea that should be considered include Huntington's disease, Wilson disease, neuroacanthocytosis, thyrotoxicosis, and basal ganglia infarctions.[12] Investigations to determine the cause of chorea arising during pregnancy can include a variety of blood tests (Table 19.1). Neuroimaging can be considered, but unless urgent, should be delayed until after delivery.

Treatment should be aimed at the underlying cause of chorea. Symptomatic treatment should be reserved for disabling cases and is often unnecessary.[12] Chorea is most often treated with dopamine receptor-blocking agents such as haloperidol or dopamine depleting agents such as tetrabenazine. Both are considered pregnancy category C and should be avoided in the first trimester. Haloperidol may be safe in low doses during pregnancy, and is preferred over other dopamine receptor blocking agents given less maternal anticholinergic, antihistaminergic, and hypotensive effects.[13]

Huntington's Disease

Huntington's disease (HD) is an autosomal dominant inherited neurodegenerative disorder

TABLE 19.1 CHOREA AND PREGNANCY: DIFFERENTIAL DIAGNOSIS AND EVALUATION

Differential Diagnosis	Evaluation
Huntington disease	Genetic testing (Huntington gene mutation, $\geq$ 36 CAG repeats)
Wilson disease	Serum ceruloplasmin (low) 24-hour urine copper excretion (elevated) Ophthalmologic examination for Kayser-fleischer rings Liver biopsy Genetic testing (ATP7B gene mutation)
Neuroacanthocytosis	Peripheral blood smear for RBC morphology (looking for acanthocytes)
Autoimmune disorders: antiphospholipid antibody syndrome, lupus	Anti-phospholipid antibodies (lupus anti-coagulant, anti-cardiolipin antibody, anti-beta-2 glycoprotein I) Anti-nuclear antibody (ANA) Anti-double stranded DNA antibody Anti-smith antibody
Rheumatic fever	Electrocardiogram (ECG) Echocardiogram Blood cultures Anti-streptococcal antibody (past infection)
Thyrotoxicosis	Thyroid-stimulating hormone Free T3 Free T4
Vascular disease: basal ganglia stroke	Head imaging
Drug-induced	Check medication list Serum and/or urine toxicology screen

Adapted from Miyasaki JM, Aldakheel A. Movement disorders in pregnancy. *Continuum (Minneapolis, Minn)*. 2014; 20(1 Neurology of Pregnancy):148–161.

characterized by movement disorders (chorea, dystonia, parkinsonism), cognitive impairment and psychiatric disease. HD is caused by a cytosine, adenosine, and guanine (CAG) trinucleotide repeat expansion in the Huntingtin gene, with at least 36 CAG repeats on one allele required for manifest disease. Symptom onset is typically after childbearing years, though symptoms can emerge earlier in some and may be present during pregnancy, particularly with advancing maternal age.

Treatment of chorea should be reserved for disabling cases as noted above. Treatment of the psychiatric aspects of the disease should be managed by a psychiatrist and maternal health specialist and the risks and benefits of using psychiatric medications must be considered.[14]

Pre-symptomatic genetic testing is an option for individuals with a family history of HD with some individuals aware of genetic status prior to family planning. However, less than 20% of at-risk individuals pursue genetic testing.[15] Genetic and prenatal counseling should therefore be provided for any at-risk individual, particularly regarding the ability to care for children as the disease progresses.

Pre-implantation genetic testing of embryos using in vitro fertilization is now possible, with implantation of only unaffected embryos. This technique avoids revealing HD gene status to at-risk individuals, if desired. Extensive counseling and multidisciplinary care teams are required.[16]

Chorea should not interfere with vaginal delivery in most cases. There are no reported contraindications to general anesthesia for patients with chorea who require cesarean section (also see Box 19.2).

DYSTONIA

Dystonia is characterized by persistent or intermittent muscle contractions that result in abnormal postures or twisting or repetitive movements. It may be genetic or idiopathic in etiology, or it may be secondary to other neurologic diseases or drugs. Dystonia can be focal, multifocal, segmental, or generalized in distribution and may affect the neck, trunk, limbs, face, or vocal cords.[9] The average age of onset for all forms of dystonia

---

BOX 19.2
CHOREA CARE MAP

BEFORE PREGNANCY
Genetic counseling and testing in those at risk for Huntington's disease (HD)
Discuss pre-implantation genetic testing with IVF in women or partners with known HD
Medication adjustment, consolidation, and review
Psychiatry consult for patients with HD and psychiatric disease—review psychiatric medications

DURING PREGNANCY
Review of medications to rule out medication-induced chorea
Additional blood work may be required to determine etiology of chorea (see Table 19.1)
Neuroimaging if vascular etiology is suspected
Reserve symptomatic treatment for disabling cases and avoid treatment in the first trimester—low dose haloperidol can be considered in severe cases after the first trimester
Psychiatry involvement for patients with HD and psychiatric disease

DELIVERY
No disease specific concerns

POSTPARTUM
Medication review and adjustment
Monitor for postpartum depression, particularly in patients with HD
Schedule neurology follow-up

is 27 years with peaks during childhood and the fifth decade.[1,10]

Dystonia Arising during Pregnancy

Nausea and vomiting during pregnancy is common, occurring in 70–80% of women.[17] Drug-induced dystonic reactions may occur during pregnancy, particularly with the use of anti-dopaminergic anti-emetics such as metoclopramide, promethazine, and prochlorperazine for pregnancy-associated nausea or hyperemesis gravidarum.[17] These medications are known to be associated with acute dystonic reactions including torticollis, opisthotonus, oculogyric crises, and orofacial movements. The reaction may occur after the first dose and happens within 5 days of starting the medication in 90% of cases.[9] Most cases of acute dystonia resolve without treatment within 12 to 48 hours after stopping the offending agent. However, symptoms can resolve within minutes if treated with parenteral antihistamines or anticholinergics such as diphenhydramine and benztropine, respectively. Diphenhydramine is pregnancy category B,[18] while benztropine is pregnancy category C. Thus, if treatment is desired, IV diphenhydramine 50mg can be considered.

A few cases of dystonia arising during pregnancy without an identifiable cause have been reported in the literature. This entity has been labeled "dystonia gravidarum." Two cases were treated with low-dose clonazepam with clinical improvement. Dystonia in each case resolved before or shortly after delivery.[19-21]

Pregnancy in Women with Dystonia

Genetic and idiopathic forms of dystonia as well as dystonia related to Wilson disease or Parkinson's disease may affect women of childbearing age. Overall, pregnancy does not appear to have a significant effect on dystonia symptoms. In one survey of 62 women with dystonia, 27 had at least one pregnancy since dystonia onset, and only 4 reported changes in dystonia symptoms during pregnancy.[22] Another study of 10 women who became pregnant after developing dystonia reported that 3 women had partial or complete remission of dystonia, 2 women had exacerbations of symptoms, and 5 women had no change.[23] There are limited data regarding the effects of dystonia on pregnancy—while focal dystonia may not have any harmful consequences, severe generalized dystonia may interfere with vaginal delivery in some cases. However, there are cases reports of uneventful labor and vaginal delivery in patients

with generalized dystonia with adequate symptom control from medications and/or deep brain stimulation. Appropriate delivery route should be discussed by the patient's obstetrician and neurologist. There are no reported contraindications to general anesthesia for dystonia patients who require cesarean section.

Several genetic forms of dystonia are autosomal dominant and affected women considering pregnancy should be offered prenatal genetic counseling. DYT5 or dopamine responsive dystonia usually starts in childhood or early adulthood and is characterized by a dramatic response to low-dose levodopa therapy, typically up to 300mg/day. Levodopa monotherapy has not been shown to have an adverse effect on pregnancy and can be continued in these patients to avoid worsening dystonia symptoms.[24] DYT1 is a generalized dystonia that typically begins in childhood, usually requiring treatment with lifelong medication or deep brain stimulation.[25]

Botulinum toxin injections, trihexyphenidyl, baclofen, and clonazepam are often used in the treatment of dystonia outside of pregnancy. While avoiding or reducing medications is typically preferred during pregnancy, dystonia symptoms may increase without treatment, particularly in those with genetic forms of dystonia where symptoms can become disabling. Appropriate counseling about the safety of these therapies during pregnancy is important.

Botulinum toxin injections are pregnancy category C and the product monogram recommends that it not be administered during pregnancy.[10] Still, there have been several cases of continued use of botulinum toxin A during pregnancy without complications (up to 300 units).[26,27] Trihexyphenidyl is an anticholinergic medication that is pregnancy category C. Anticholinergic medications have been linked to eclamptic seizures.[28] However, there are case reports of high dose trihexyphenidyl and uneventful pregnancies.[29] Baclofen is pregnancy category C. Oral baclofen has been associated with neonatal withdrawal seizures.[30] There is one case report showing safety of an intrathecal baclofen pump during pregnancy in a patient with generalized dystonia[31] and several reports showing successful use of this therapy for spasticity during pregnancy.[32] Clonazepam is a benzodiazepine that is pregnancy category D. It has been successfully used during pregnancy, but in rare cases has caused neonatal withdrawal symptoms, hypotonia, and respiratory depression.[33] If use is necessary, low doses are recommended.

BOX 19.3
DYSTONIA CARE MAP

BEFORE PREGNANCY
Genetic counseling and testing for those with genetic forms of dystonia
Review of prior pregnancy complications
Medication adjustment, consolidation, and review

DURING PREGNANCY
Review and elimination of medications that can cause dystonia, particularly in patients with
pregnancy-associated nausea/vomiting
Counseling on potential worsening of symptoms
Adjust medications for symptoms

DELIVERY
Severe generalized dystonia may interfere with vaginal delivery

POSTPARTUM
Medication review and adjustment
Schedule neurology follow-up

Deep brain stimulation is effective for medically-refractory dystonia. Case reports and case series have demonstrated that deep brain stimulation in dystonia patients is safe during pregnancy, labor and delivery, and breastfeeding (also see Box 19.3).[34,35]

WILSON DISEASE

Wilson disease (WD) is an autosomal recessive disorder caused by a mutation of the *ATP7B* gene resulting in reduced copper excretion and the accumulation of copper in the liver and brain, most prominently in the basal ganglia. This results in a combination of liver dysfunction, neuropsychiatric features, and abnormal movements including dystonia, tremor, gait dysfunction, parkinsonism, and chorea.[36]

Most women with WD have symptom onset before or during childbearing age, with typical age of onset between 5–35 years.[36] Untreated WD is associated with impaired fertility and increased risk of spontaneous abortion.[37] However, since the advent of chelating therapy, a normal reproductive life can be achieved in most affected women.[38] D-penicillamine is the most commonly used chelating therapy in WD. The medication is category D in pregnancy due to a potential risk of connective tissue disorders in the offspring of individuals treated with D-penicillamine for cystinuria. However, lower doses are used for

the treatment of WD, and numerous case series have documented safety during pregnancy for those already receiving therapy.[39] Zinc sulfate and trientene are alternative chelating agents that may be considered; both are category C in pregnancy, and multiple case series document the safety of use during pregnancy.[40] Given the risk of fetal, hepatic, and neurotoxicity without chelating therapy, continuation of prenatal chelation therapy at the lowest possible dose is recommended.[41]

Historic reports of the effect of pregnancy on WD symptoms suggest that movement disorders improve in most women during pregnancy.[37] Close follow-up with hepatology is recommended throughout pregnancy for women with hepatic manifestations of WD due to an increased risk of complications.[38]

Similar to other inherited neurological conditions, prenatal genetic counseling is recommended for family planning in any individual with WD (also see Box 19.4).

TICS/TOURETTE SYNDROME

Tics are intermittent, non-rhythmic, repetitive movements or vocalizations that are briefly suppressible and characterized by a premonitory urge and sense of relief following the movement.

BOX 19.4
WILSON DISEASE CARE MAP

BEFORE PREGNANCY

Genetic counseling and testing
Review of prior pregnancy complications
Initiation of copper chelating therapy

DURING PREGNANCY

Genetic counseling and testing if not done before
Medication adjustment—reduction of prenatal chelating therapy to lowest tolerated dose
Dedicated referral to hepatology for co-management of hepatic manifestations

DELIVERY

Multidisciplinary planning discussion with hepatology and obstetrics

POSTPARTUM

Medication adjustment
Schedule neurology follow-up

Tourette syndrome (TS) is a chronic tic disorder with onset in childhood characterized by multiple motor tics and one or more vocal tics lasting longer than a year.[42] Tic phenomenology and severity varies over time; up to 50% of children will have resolution of tics by age 18.[43]

TS is about 4 times more common in males than females and most individuals have a significant reduction or resolution of tics by the time of pregnancy. As such, limited data exist on the effect of pregnancy on TS symptoms. A single case series of eight women with TS found 45% of pregnancies resulted in improved tic severity, 27% of pregnancies resulted in worsened tic severity, and 27% of pregnancies resulted in no change in tic severity.[44] Given the fluctuating nature of tics over time, the authors concluded that there was no consistent effect of pregnancy on tic severity.

Increasing evidence now supports Comprehensive Behavioral Intervention for Tics (CBIT), a habit reversal therapy, for the treatment of bothersome tics; given the low risk, this is considered first line for the treatment of tics in pregnancy.[45] Neuroleptics are the only FDA-approved medications for the treatment of tics, though dopamine depleting agents (eg, tetrabenazine or haloperidol) and alpha adrenergic agents (eg, clonidine or guanfacine) are also commonly used.[46] All are category C in pregnancy and should be used with caution.

Botulinum toxin injections are occasionally used for disabling focal tics in the non-pregnant population but limited data exist on safety in pregnancy.[10] Deep brain stimulation has emerged as a treatment for refractory tic disorders and has demonstrated efficacy and safety during pregnancy, delivery, and lactation (also see Box 19.5).[47]

ATAXIA

Ataxia arising during pregnancy should first prompt an evaluation for structural causes such as stroke or neoplasm. Another possible cause of ataxia arising during pregnancy is Wernicke's encephalopathy resulting from thiamine deficiency, which should be suspected in pregnant women with hyperemesis gravidarum. The classic triad is ataxia, confusion and oculomotor abnormalities, though all three signs occur in less than 20% of cases.[48] Symptoms typically appear within 2–8 weeks of severe vomiting.[49] The diagnosis is clinical, though MRI brain may reveal T2 FLAIR hyperintensities in the bilateral medial thalamus, mammillary bodies and/or periadqueductal gray matter.[50] Prompt treatment with high dose intravenous (IV) thiamine should be initiated in any individual with a suspicion of Wernicke's encephalopathy to avoid maternal and fetal morbidity and mortality. Ideal dosing has not yet been determined, but a possible regimen is 500mg IV

BOX 19.5
TICS/TOURETTE SYNDROME CARE MAP

BEFORE PREGNANCY
No disease specific concerns

DURING PREGNANCY
Medication adjustment—reduction/elimination of symptomatic therapy as able
Initiation of Comprehensive Behavioral Intervention for Tics (CBIT) for bothersome tics

DELIVERY
No disease specific concerns

POSTPARTUM
No disease specific concerns

---

thiamine every 8 hours for 2–3 days followed by 250mg IV thiamine daily for 5 days and then 100mg oral thiamine daily for at least 3 months.[51] Thiamine should be administered before glucose. Symptoms usually improve with treatment, though complete resolution is not always achieved.

Friedreich ataxia (FRDA) is an autosomal recessive, neurodegenerative disorder characterized by ataxia, dysarthria, weakness, neuropathy, scoliosis, diabetes, and cardiomyopathy. Onset is usually in late childhood, and life expectancy is typically 1–2 decades after diagnosis. Affected women may contemplate pregnancy, and a retrospective study of 31 women with FRDA showed that these women were capable of successful pregnancy with low complication rates. In the same study, equal numbers of women reported improvement, worsening, or no change in FRDA symptoms during pregnancy.[52] Given cardiac and endocrine co-morbidities, patients should

---

BOX 19.6
ATAXIA CARE MAP

BEFORE PREGNANCY
Genetic counseling and testing for those with genetic ataxias (Friedreich ataxia, spinocerebellar ataxias)

DURING PREGNANCY
Neuroimaging for possible structural causes in women with ataxia arising during pregnancy
Prompt treatment with IV thiamine in those with concern for Wernicke's encephalopathy
Counseling on potential worsening of symptoms in those with preexisting ataxia
Cardiology follow up and close glucose monitoring in women with Friedreich ataxia

DELIVERY
No disease specific concerns

POSTPARTUM
Medication review and adjustment
Schedule neurology follow-up

have cardiology follow-up and close glucose level monitoring. Case reports have not revealed any worsening of these conditions during pregnancy. There are no guidelines for cardiac monitoring of patients with FRDA during pregnancy, though a cardiovascular examination and an electrocardiogram should be performed in all patients. Any patient with known left ventricular hypertrophy or symptoms such as shortness of breath or palpitations should also have an echocardiogram during pregnancy and electrocardiographic monitoring throughout labor.[53]

Over 30 types of autosomal dominant spinocerebellar ataxia (SCA) syndromes have been described.[9] Symptoms may include ataxia, dysarthria, oculomotor abnormalities, or abnormal movements. Genetic testing is available for diagnosis. In couples with known SCA, in-vitro fertilization (IVF) with preimplantation testing has been performed resulting in unaffected infants (also see Box 19.6).[54,55]

TREMOR

Tremor is a rhythmic, oscillatory movement of one or more parts of the body. Essential tremor (ET) is the most common cause of tremor in the United States. ET is characterized by a postural limb, vocal, and/or head/neck tremor, and affects men and women equally. The condition is more common in later life, but individuals may develop tremor by the second decade.[56] There is limited literature on the effect of pregnancy on the severity of tremor in individuals with ET.

In women with new onset or worsening tremor in pregnancy, an evaluation for causative or exacerbating factors should be undertaken. This includes evaluation for hyperthyroidism, excessive adrenergic activity, illicit or prescription sympathomimetic use, and various medications including corticosteroids, lithium, and sodium valproate.[27]

Pharmacotherapy for ET in pregnancy should be reserved for individuals with disabling tremor. Propranolol and gabapentin are both pregnancy category C and should be used with caution; primidone and topiramate are pregnancy category D and should be avoided or discontinued for the duration of the pregnancy and during lactation. Sotalol for ET is supported by lower level evidence than propranolol, but is pregnancy category B and can be considered for women with severe tremor (also see Box 19.7).[57]

PARKINSONISM

Parkinson's disease (PD) is the prototypic hypokinetic movement disorder and is characterized by four cardinal motor features: tremor, rigidity, bradykinesia, and postural instability. PD is a neurodegenerative condition, typically with mid- to late-life onset, making it relatively uncommon in women of childbearing age; however, onset in the third and fourth decades can occur, and cases are more likely with advancing maternal age.[58]

The largest reported case series examining the effect of pregnancy on PD symptoms found that around 60% of pregnancies resulted in a mild but

---

BOX 19.7
TREMOR CARE MAP

BEFORE PREGNANCY

No disease specific concerns

DURING PREGNANCY

Evaluation for and elimination of causative or exacerbating factors
Medication adjustment—discontinuation of primidone and topiramate

DELIVERY

No disease specific concerns

POSTPARTUM

Medication adjustment—avoidance of primidone and topiramate during lactation

---

BOX 19.8

PARKINSONISM CARE MAP

BEFORE PREGNANCY

No disease specific concerns

DURING PREGNANCY

Medication adjustment—transition to carbidopa/levodopa monotherapy

DELIVERY

No disease specific concerns

POSTPARTUM

Medication adjustment—avoid dopamine agonists during lactation

---

durable worsening of PD motor symptoms or rate of decline.[59] However, other data in the literature (mostly case reports) presents conflicting evidence on the effect of pregnancy on PD and the duration of effect.[60] While limited data exist, there is currently no evidence that PD has an impact on fertility, pregnancy, or delivery.

Carbidopa/levodopa is considered category C in pregnancy; however, numerous case reports citing the safety of levodopa in pregnant women with PD up to doses of 1000mg/day make it first line therapy for the symptomatic management of PD in pregnancy.[61] Non-ergot dopamine agonists, anti-cholinergics, and amantadine are all category C in pregnancy. Similar to other movement disorders, pre-implanted DBS is considered safe and effective in pregnancy.[47]

Limited data exists for the long-term use of levodopa during breastfeeding. However, the limited data available suggests that it is poorly excreted in breastmilk. It may lower serum prolactin, which could affect breastfeeding women, particularly those without a well-established milk supply.[62] As stated above in the discussion on restless-leg treatments, dopamine agonist use is discouraged in breastfeeding. Amantadine is discouraged while breastfeeding for similar reasons—it decreases prolactin levels and its combination of a low molecular weight, long half life and high oral bioavailability make it more likely to pass into breastmilk.[63] Though no studies support the safety of anticholinergics while breastfeeding, trihexyphinidyl has the shortest half-life of available agents and in one case report of 3 pregnancies, a mother was able to breastfeed successfully without measureable developmental effects on the children out to 8 years of life (also see Box 19.8).[64]

REFERENCES

1. Kranick SM, Mowry EM, Colcher A, Horn S, Golbe LI. Movement disorders and pregnancy: a review of the literature. *Movement Disorders: Official Journal of the Movement Disorder Society.* 2010; 25(6): 665–671.
2. Manconi M, Govoni V, De Vito A, et al. Restless legs syndrome and pregnancy. *Neurology.* 2004; 63(6): 1065–1069.
3. Earley CJ. Clinical practice. Restless legs syndrome. *New England Journal of Medicine.* 2003; 348(21): 2103–2109.
4. Goodman JD, Brodie C, Ayida GA. Restless leg syndrome in pregnancy. *BMJ (Clinical research ed).* 1988; 297(6656): 1101–1102.
5. Cesnik E, Casetta I, Turri M, et al. Transient RLS during pregnancy is a risk factor for the chronic idiopathic form. *Neurology.* 2010;75(23): 2117–2120.
6. Sun ER, Chen CA, Ho G, Earley CJ, Allen RP. Iron and the restless legs syndrome. *Sleep.* 1998; 21(4): 371–377.
7. Sikandar R, Khealani BA, Wasay M. Predictors of restless legs syndrome in pregnancy: A hospital based cross sectional survey from Pakistan. *Sleep Medicine.* 2009; 10(6): 676–678.
8. Picchietti DL, Hensley JG, Bainbridge JL, et al. Consensus clinical practice guidelines for the diagnosis and treatment of restless legs syndrome/ Willis-Ekbom disease during pregnancy and lactation. *Sleep Medicine Reviews.* 2015; 22: 64–77.
9. Fahn S, Jankovic J, Hallett M. *Principles and Practice of Movement Disorders.* 2nd ed. Edinburgh: W. B. Saunders; 2011.

10. Miyasaki JM, Aldakheel A. Movement disorders in pregnancy. *Continuum (Minneapolis, Minn).* 2014; 20(1 Neurology of Pregnancy): 148–161.

11. Maia DP, Fonseca PG, Camargos ST, Pfannes C, Cunningham MC, Cardoso F. Pregnancy in patients with Sydenham's Chorea. *Parkinsonism & Related Disorders.* 2012; 18(5): 458–461.

12. Robottom BJ, Weiner WJ. Chorea gravidarum. *Handbook of Clinical Neurology.* 2011; 100: 231–235.

13. Use of psychoactive medication during pregnancy and possible effects on the fetus and newborn. Committee on Drugs. American Academy of Pediatrics. *Pediatrics.* 2000; 105(4 Pt. 1): 880–887.

14. Byatt N, Deligiannidis KM, Freeman MP. Antidepressant use in pregnancy: A critical review focused on risks and controversies. *Acta Psychiatrica Scandinavica.* 2013; 127(2): 94–114.

15. Harper PS, Lim C, Craufurd D. Ten years of presymptomatic testing for Huntington's disease: the experience of the UK Huntington's Disease Prediction Consortium. *Journal of medical genetics.* 2000;37(8):567–571.

16. Sermon K, De Rijcke M, Lissens W, et al. Preimplantation genetic diagnosis for Huntington's disease with exclusion testing. *European Journal of Human Genetics: EJHG.* 2002; 10(10): 591–598.

17. Bustos M, Venkataramanan R, Caritis S. Nausea and vomiting of pregnancy—What's new? *Autonomic Neuroscience: Basic & Clinical.* 2017 Jan; 202: 62–72.

18. Etwel F, Faught LH, Rieder MJ, Koren G. The risk of adverse pregnancy outcome after first trimester exposure to H1 antihistamines: A systematic review and meta-analysis. *Drug Safety.* 2017 Feb; 40(2): 121–132.

19. Buccoliero R, Palmeri S, Malandrini A, Dotti MT, Federico A. A case of dystonia with onset during pregnancy. *Journal of the Neurological Sciences.* 2007; 260(1–2): 265–266.

20. Fasano A, Elia AE, Guidubaldi A, Tonali PA, Bentivoglio AR. Dystonia gravidarum: A new case with a long follow-up. *Movement Disorders: Official Journal of the Movement Disorder Society.* 2007; 22(4): 564–566.

21. Lim EC, Seet RC, Wilder-Smith EP, Ong BK. Dystonia gravidarum: a new entity? *Movement Disorders: Official Journal of the Movement Disorder Society.* 2006; 21(1): 69–70.

22. Gwinn-Hardy KA, Adler CH, Weaver AL, Fish NM, Newman SJ. Effect of hormone variations and other factors on symptom severity in women with dystonia. *Mayo Clinic Proceedings.* 2000; 75(3): 235–240.

23. Rogers JD, Fahn S. Movement disorders and pregnancy. *Advances in neurology.* 1994; 64: 163–178.

24. Nomoto M, Kaseda S, Iwata S, Osame M, Fukuda T. Levodopa in pregnancy. *Movement disorders: Official Journal of the Movement Disorder Society.* 1997; 12(2): 261.

25. Nageshwaran S, Nageshwaran S, Edwards MJ, Morcos M. Management of DYT1 dystonia throughout pregnancy. *BMJ Case Reports.* 2011 Sep 4; 2011.

26. Newman WJ, Davis TL, Padaliya BB, et al. Botulinum toxin type A therapy during pregnancy. *Movement Disorders: Official Journal of the Movement Disorder Society.* 2004; 19(11): 1384–1385.

27. Morgan JC, Iyer SS, Moser ET, Singer C, Sethi KD. Botulinum toxin A during pregnancy: A survey of treating physicians. *Journal of Neurology, Neurosurgery, and Psychiatry.* 2006; 77(1): 117–119.

28. Kobayashi T, Sugimura M, Tokunaga N, et al. Anticholinergics induce eclamptic seizures. *Seminars in Thrombosis and Hemostasis.* 2002; 28(6): 511–514.

29. Robottom BJ, Reich SG. Exposure to high dosage trihexyphenidyl during pregnancy for treatment of generalized dystonia: Case report and literature review. *The Neurologist.* 2011; 17(6): 340–341.

30. Ratnayaka BD, Dhaliwal H, Watkin S. Drug points: Neonatal convulsions after withdrawal of baclofen. *BMJ Clinical Research Ed.* 2001; 323(7304): 85.

31. Mendez-Lucena C, Chacon Pena J, Garcia-Moreno JM. Intrathecal baclofen for dystonia treatment during pregnancy: A case report. *Neurologia (Barcelona, Spain).* 2016; 31(2): 131–132.

32. Dalton CM, Keenan E, Jarrett L, Buckley L, Stevenson VL. The safety of baclofen in pregnancy: Intrathecal therapy in multiple sclerosis. *Multiple Sclerosis (Houndmills, Basingstoke, England).* 2008; 14(4): 571–572.

33. Weinstock L, Cohen LS, Bailey JW, Blatman R, Rosenbaum JF. Obstetrical and neonatal outcome following clonazepam use during pregnancy: A case series. *Psychotherapy and Psychosomatics.* 2001; 70(3): 158–162.

34. Ziman N, Coleman RR, Starr PA, et al. Pregnancy in a series of dystonia patients treated with deep brain stimulation: Outcomes and management recommendations. *Stereotactic and Functional Neurosurgery.* 2016; 94(1): 60–65.

35. Paluzzi A, Bain PG, Liu X, Yianni J, Kumarendran K, Aziz TZ. Pregnancy in dystonic women with in situ deep brain stimulators. *Movement*

Disorders: *Official Journal of the Movement Disorder Society.* 2006; 21(5): 695–698.

36. Stremmel W, Meyerrose KW, Niederau C, Hefter H, Kreuzpaintner G, Strohmeyer G. Wilson disease: Clinical presentation, treatment, and survival. *Annals of Internal Medicine.* 1991; 115(9): 720–726.

37. Dreifuss FE, McKinney WM. Wilson's disease (hepatolenticular degeneration) and pregnancy. *JAMA.* 1966; 195(11): 960–962.

38. Scheinberg IH, Sternlieb I. Pregnancy in penicillamine-treated patients with Wilson's disease. *New England Journal of Medicine.* 1975; 293(25): 1300–1302.

39. Mjolnerod OK, Dommerud SA, Rasmussen K, Gjeruldsen ST. Congenital connective-tissue defect probably due to D-penicillamine treatment in pregnancy. *Lancet (London, England).* 1971; 1(7701): 673–675.

40. Malik A, Khawaja A, Sheikh L. Wilson's disease in pregnancy: Case series and review of literature. *BMC Research Notes.* 2013; 6: 421.

41. Weiss KH. Wilson disease. In: Pagon RA, Adam MP, Ardinger HH, et al., eds. *GeneReviews(R).* Seattle: University of Washington, 1993.

42. Sanger TD, Chen D, Fehlings DL, et al. Definition and classification of hyperkinetic movements in childhood. *Movement Disorders: Official Journal of the Movement Disorder Society.* 2010; 25(11): 1538–1549.

43. Robertson MM. The Gilles de la Tourette syndrome: The current status. *Archives of Disease in Childhood Education and Practice Edition.* 2012; 97(5): 166–175.

44. Salarian A, Zampieri C, Horak FB, Carlson-Kuhta P, Nutt JG, Aminian K. Analyzing 180 degrees turns using an inertial system reveals early signs of progression of Parkinson's disease. *Conference Proceedings: Annual International Conference of the IEEE Engineering in Medicine and Biology Society IEEE Engineering in Medicine and Biology Society Annual Conference.* 2009; 2009: 224–227.

45. Scahill L, Woods DW, Himle MB, et al. Current controversies on the role of behavior therapy in Tourette syndrome. *Movement disorders: official journal of the Movement Disorder Society.* 2013; 28(9): 1179–1183.

46. Kurlan R. Clinical practice. Tourette's Syndrome. *New England Journal of Medicine.* 2010; 363(24): 2332–2338.

47. Scelzo E, Mehrkens JH, Botzel K, et al. Deep brain stimulation during pregnancy and delivery: Experience from a series of "DBS Babies." *Frontiers in Neurology.* 2015; 6: 191.

48. Harper CG, Giles M, Finlay-Jones R. Clinical signs in the Wernicke-Korsakoff complex: A retrospective analysis of 131 cases diagnosed at necropsy. *Journal of Neurology, Neurosurgery, and Psychiatry.* 1986; 49(4): 341–345.

49. Ashraf VV, Prijesh J, Praveenkumar R, Saifudheen K. Wernicke's encephalopathy due to hyperemesis gravidarum: Clinical and magnetic resonance imaging characteristics. *Journal of Postgraduate Medicine.* 2016; 62(4): 260–263.

50. Yahia M, Najeh H, Zied H, et al. Wernicke's encephalopathy: A rare complication of hyperemesis gravidarum. *Anaesthesia, Critical Care & Pain Medicine.* 2015; 34(3): 173–177.

51. Cook CC, Hallwood PM, Thomson AD. B Vitamin deficiency and neuropsychiatric syndromes in alcohol misuse. *Alcohol and Alcoholism (Oxford, Oxfordshire).* 1998; 33(4): 317–336.

52. Friedman LS, Paulsen EK, Schadt KA, et al. Pregnancy with Friedreich ataxia: A retrospective review of medical risks and psychosocial implications. *American Journal of Obstetrics and Gynecology.* 2010; 203(3): 224, e221–225.

53. MacKenzie WE. Pregnancy in women with Friedreich's ataxia. *British medical journal (Clinical research ed).* 1986; 293(6542): 308.

54. Moutou C, Nicod JC, Gardes N, Viville S. Birth after pre-implantation genetic diagnosis (PGD) of spinocerebellar ataxia 2 (Sca2). *Prenatal Diagnosis.* 2008; 28(2): 126–130.

55. Drusedau M, Dreesen JC, De Die-Smulders C, et al. Preimplantation genetic diagnosis of spinocerebellar ataxia 3 by (CAG)(n) repeat detection. *Molecular Human Reproduction.* 2004; 10(1): 71–75.

56. Jankovic J, Fahn S. Physiologic and pathologic tremors. Diagnosis, mechanism, and management. *Annals of Internal Medicine.* 1980; 93(3): 460–465.

57. Zesiewicz TA, Elble RJ, Louis ED, et al. Evidence-based guideline update: treatment of essential tremor: Report of the Quality Standards subcommittee of the American Academy of Neurology. *Neurology.* 2011; 77(19): 1752–1755.

58. Mayeux R, Marder K, Cote LJ, et al. The frequency of idiopathic Parkinson's disease by age, ethnic group, and sex in northern Manhattan, 1988-1993. *American Journal of Epidemiology.* 1995; 142(8): 820–827.

59. Golbe LI. Parkinson's disease and pregnancy. *Neurology.* 1987; 37(7): 1245–1249.

60. Scott M, Chowdhury M. Pregnancy in Parkinson's disease: Unique case report and review of the literature. *Movement Disorders: Official*

Journal of the Movement Disorder Society. 2005; 20(8): 1078–1079.

61. Shulman LM, Minagar A, Weiner WJ. The effect of pregnancy in Parkinson's disease. *Movement Disorders: Official Journal of the Movement Disorder Society.* 2000; 15(1): 132–135.

62. Thulin PC, Woodward WR, Carter JH, Nutt JG.Levodopa in human breast milk: clinical implications. *Neurology.* 1998; 50: 1920–1921.

63. Lactmed: Amantadine Accessed Oct 10, 2017. http://toxnet.nlm.nih.gov/cgi-bin/sis/search2/r?dbs+lactmed:@term+@DOCNO+434

64. Lactmed: TRIHEXYPHENIDYL   Accessed Oct 10, 2017. http://toxnet.nlm.nih.gov/cgi-bin/sis/search2/r?dbs+lactmed:@term+@DOCNO+769

SECTION 3

Epilepsy, Seizure, and Sleep Disorders

20

Pregnancy and Epilepsy

TRENTON TOLLEFSON AND LYNN LIU

ABSTRACT

Epilepsy is the fourth most common neurologic disorder behind migraine, stroke, and Alzheimer's disease. The Center for Disease Control (CDC) data estimates about 3.4 million people in the United States have active epilepsy. Approximately 1 million women of childbearing age in the United States have epilepsy, and about 2 to 5 infants of 1000 pregnancies are born to mothers with epilepsy. Therefore, providers should consider additional aspects of epilepsy care unique to women with epilepsy (WWE) of childbearing age such as planning for and care during pregnancy; concern how epilepsy may affect pregnancy and how pregnancy may impact seizure control. Fortunately, more than 90% of pregnant WWE will give birth to healthy infants. Providers should maintain these important items in mind when caring for a WWE of child-bearing age. This chapter focuses on the effects of pregnancy on seizures and the effects of seizures on pregnancy in pregnant WWE.

THE EFFECTS OF PREGNANCY ON SEIZURES

Sex hormones interact with the central nervous system in various ways. In neurons they bind to intracellular steroid receptors that modulate transcription through various mechanisms including direct interaction with the genome and with transcription factors.[11,12] Sex hormones also bind to cell membrane receptors that further modulate activity at the G-Protein Coupled Receptors and ionotropic receptors including the N-methyl-D-aspartate (NMDA) receptor and gamma-aminobutyric acid (GABA) receptor.[11,12] Estradiol contributes to lowering the seizure threshold through multiple mechanisms, most notably through an augmentation of glutamate activity at the NMDA receptor. Progesterone and its metabolites act to raise the seizure threshold also through multiple mechanisms, most notably through potentiation of activity at the $GABA_A$ receptor.[14] In fact, hormone-mediated (catamenial) epilepsy may affect up to one-third of women with intractable complex partial seizures.[13] Through these mechanisms, hormonal effects can play a significant role in the frequency of seizures during pregnancy specifically.

The fluctuations of these sex hormone levels have a significant impact on the evolving physiology of the pregnant woman and can impact peripartum seizure frequency. Based on prospective case control data, between 54 and 80% of women will experience no change in seizure frequency during pregnancy compared to baseline, and approximately 15–32% of women will experience an increase in seizure frequency.[15,16] Planning a pregnancy and taking anti-epileptic drug (AED) therapy have been associated with lower seizure frequency during pregnancy.[17,18] Women with catamenial epilepsy note a higher rate of seizure freedom and seizure reduction during pregnancy compared to women without catamenial epilepsy.[19] One possible explanation for this phenomenon is the absence of monthly cyclical hormonal fluctuations as well as the rise of serum progesterone over the course of the pregnancy.[19] Since women with catamenial epilepsy may have epileptic networks that are more sensitive to the effects of sex hormones at baseline, the changes in these hormones during pregnancy influence their seizure frequency more than in women without catamenial epilepsy. Additional proposed mechanisms for this improvement in seizure frequency during pregnancy in women with catamenial epilepsy include fluctuation in fluid and electrolyte balance and AED serum levels during pregnancy.[20,21] Ultimately, women with epilepsy can be counseled that they will most likely experience no significant increase in seizure frequency, particularly if their epilepsy has a prominent catamenial component at baseline.

While the complex interplay between sex hormone levels (estradiol and progesterone) and seizure frequency has been partially elucidated, the interaction between sex hormones and antiepileptic medications (AEDs) has not been clearly determined. Estrogen induces hepatic isoenzyme glucuronidation and increases hepatic metabolism of AEDs, lowering circulating levels of certain AEDs.[22-24] Comparison of valproate and lamotrigine levels between the follicular and the luteal phases of the menstrual cycle showed a minor reduction in the levels of both medications, but neither result reached statistical significance.[25] However, levels of lamotrigine, valproate, and oxcarbazepine are significantly reduced with concurrent use of estrogen-containing hormonal contraception.[24-26] Thus, levels of these medications should be monitored when starting this form of contraception. (See also C|hapter 3.) Further data regarding the interaction between sex hormones and AEDs in the setting of pregnancy is limited.

In addition to hormonal effects on AED metabolism, other aspects of pregnancy physiology can decrease the serum concentration of certain AEDs. Enteral absorption of medications can be decreased due to decreased gastric pH, decreased rate of gastric emptying, and decreased small intestine motility.[27,28] The volume of distribution increases during pregnancy due to increased blood volume, water, and fat stores.[27] In addition, AEDs that are highly protein-bound may undergo an apparent decrease in total serum concentration; however, due to lower levels of serum albumin during pregnancy, the unbound or free AED level may not change in concentration. Increased protein binding of endogenous compounds may displace the AED resulting in a higher percentage of unbound drug.[27] For this reason, free levels of AEDs with significant protein binding (including phenytoin, carbamazepine, and valproate) should be followed during pregnancy. Metabolism of many AEDs is increased due to increased activity of some hepatic cytochrome P450 enzymes leading to more rapid AED metabolism.[22,27] Lastly, increased glomerular filtration rate causes increased renal clearance of renally excreted AEDs such as levetiracetam, topiramate, lacosamide, gabapentin, pregabalin, and oxcarbazepine resulting in lower levels and increased risk of seizures.[27,29] Following key AED levels over the course of the pregnancy and adjusting the doses accordingly may minimize the risk of seizures during pregnancy.

Lamotrigine is perhaps the most dramatic example of alterations in AED concentration during pregnancy. Lamotrigine serum concentrations decrease throughout pregnancy, with nadir during the third trimester often leading to a maintenance dose of twice the pre-pregnancy dose.[30] This is largely due to increased levels of estrogen inducing the UDP-glucuronosyl-transferase (UGT) enzyme system.[27,31] When lamotrigine level decreases to 65% of the target level, seizure frequency increases.[32] A smaller degree of reduction in serum drug concentration was found for carbamazepine, phenytoin, and oxcarbazepine.[32] Levetiracetam is a commonly used AED in women of childbearing age due to its perceived low risk of associated fetal malformations.[33] The serum concentration of levetiracetam has been found to drop up to 50% during pregnancy.[34] This is felt to be most likely due to enhanced elimination of the drug during pregnancy.[35]

Significant variability in reduction of AED serum concentration occurs between individuals during pregnancy. The American Academy of Neurology (AAN) released Practice Parameters in 2009 recommending that AED level monitoring be individualized for each patient.[27] If a woman has reasonable control of her seizures, serum AED concentrations prior to conception serve as a target to maintain this control.[32] The guidelines specifically address monitoring serum lamotrigine, carbamazepine, and phenytoin levels although the frequency of monitoring was not specified.[32] In addition, monitoring levetiracetam and oxcarbazepine levels may be considered. The guideline committee did not feel sufficient evidence existed to support or refute any pregnancy-related concentration change of phenobarbital, valproate, primadone or ethosuximide, but recommends that this lack of evidence should not discourage monitoring levels of these medications.[32] In practice, serum AED levels should be followed monthly, especially for women on lamotrigine.[22,36] The AED dose can then be adjusted in order to maintain similar levels to those prior to pregnancy. Data regarding the timing of return to baseline AED dosing postpartum is somewhat limited, as no clear data exist to shape practice parameters. The level of lamotrigine quickly returns to pre-pregnancy levels, so the dose should be reduced to the pre-pregnancy dose within about 2–3 weeks to avoid symptoms of toxicity.[31] Consideration may be given to keeping the patient on an AED dose slightly higher than pre-pregnancy for 1–3 months post-partum in order to provide additional protection in the setting of sleep deprivation.[36] Patients should be provided with a post-pregnancy taper schedule prior to delivery. For a discussion regarding the potential adverse effects of AED on the fetus, see Section 3, Chapter 21.

THE EFFECTS OF SEIZURES ON PREGNANCY

Additional aspects of how epilepsy will impact their pregnancy must also be considered as part of pre-pregnancy counseling. WWE should know they have a similar likelihood of achieving pregnancy, time to achieve pregnancy, and pregnancy outcomes compared to a group of healthy peers.[37] However, WWE have a slightly increased risk for adverse outcomes compared to women without epilepsy.[38]

One common concern that arises during pre-pregnancy counseling is the risk of neural tube defects. The neural tube is formed prior to when many women find out they are pregnant. Deficiencies in folic acid have been associated with increased rates of fetal neural tube defects. Many AEDs interfere with folic acid metabolism, prompting the need for folic acid supplementation.[39] The AAN Practice Parameters recommend that WWE of child-bearing age be on folic acid supplementation prior to pregnancy. However, insufficient evidence exists as to the optimal dose of folic acid with recommended doses between 0.4–5 mg daily.[22,32,40] Women who take valproate during pregnancy are up to 9.7 times more likely to have a child with a neural tube defect[41]; therefore, women who take valproate should be on a higher dose (4–5 mg daily) of folic acid. Another concern involves the injury that could be sustained due to fall as a result of a seizure. These falls could potentially result in injury to the WWE, injury to the fetus, bleeding, placental abruption, and rupture of membranes with pre-term labor.[42] A recent systematic review and meta-analysis found that women with epilepsy had slightly increased odds of antepartum hemorrhage and induction of labor. However, there was no difference in the odds of WWE experiencing early pre-term birth (<34 weeks), fetal death or stillbirth, perinatal death, or admission to neonatal intensive care unit compared to women without epilepsy.[38] Thus, the risk of injury to the fetus sustained by trauma during a seizure is probably low. It is reasonable to have women with epilepsy take the same seizure precautions during pregnancy that they should take during all other times in their lives.

Tonic-clonic seizures specifically can potentially expose the fetus to anoxia, prolonged uterine contractions, and heart rate deceleration.[36,42] Furthermore, seizure-induced alterations in physiology including electrolyte alterations and increased blood pressure could potentially harm the fetus.[43] Even complex partial seizures have been associated with increased uterine contractions, heart rate alterations, and hypoxia.[36,43] Seizures during pregnancy may also increase the risk for small-for-gestational-age infants.[44] Thus, the risk of injury to the fetus as a result of a seizure likely far outweighs the risks associated with exposure to an AED, especially when the lower-risk AEDs (lamotrigine, levetiracetam) are used. However, more data is needed on this subject. Other obstetric outcomes indicate that WWE have a higher risk of maternal hemorrhage, induction of labor, birth via cesarean section, hypertensive disorders, and birth before 37 weeks gestation.[38,45] Reviewing all WWE did not identify an increased risk of intrauterine death or still birth.[38,46] However, current data suggest a slightly higher risk of intrauterine death in the setting of AED polytherapy or in the setting of one of the parents having a major congenital malformation.[46] Providers should not recommend tapering seizure medications once they find out that their patients are pregnant due to the risk of seizures during pregnancy.

Enzyme-inducing AEDs have been thought to cross the placenta and cause increased turnover of vitamin K.[47] Due to the concern of higher risk of intracranial hemorrhage in the setting of enzyme-inducing AED usage, vitamin K supplementation has been considered during the third trimester of pregnancy in WWE. A recent retrospective cohort study showed no significant increased risk of neonatal hemorrhage in babies born to WWE including women on enzyme-inducing AEDs.[48] At present, there is insufficient evidence to support an increased risk of intracranial hemorrhage and the benefit of third trimester vitamin K supplementation.[32] Thus, the infant receiving standard Vitamin K supplementation at delivery is felt to be sufficient.[32,36]

Pregnant WWE have different concerns as delivery nears. They worry about labor and delivery and having a seizure, as well as possible complications of delivery. If a woman experiences a seizure during labor, routine seizure first aid such as protecting the patient from harm, clearing the airway, and putting them on their side should be followed. If the patient is on oral AEDs and cannot take medications by mouth, consider changing to an IV formulation; oral absorption during labor may be lower than baseline anyway.[39] Workup for eclampsia should be considered, as it can be difficult to ascertain whether the seizure was secondary to the underlying epilepsy or to eclampsia. WWE have been noted to have higher risk of hypertensive disorders during pregnancy.[38] Magnesium sulfate should be administered if there is any concern for eclampsia.

WWE also have higher odds of undergoing cesarean section as a method of delivery.[38] Unless an obstetric indication for cesarean section exists, WWE are capable of undergoing a normal vaginal delivery.[36,39,43] Reported maternal death rate during labor and delivery in women with epilepsy is 80 out of 100,000 deliveries compared to 6 out of 100,000 deliveries in women without epilepsy.[49] This increase in maternal mortality could be due to the increased risk of obstetric complications described earlier and the complications related to seizures during labor and delivery. These slightly increased risks should be included during counseling of WWE before and during pregnancy and warrants close specialized prenatal care.

For a first-time seizure during pregnancy, an expanded differential diagnosis should be considered during the evaluation. For anyone with a first time seizure, evaluation should include electroencephalography (EEG) and magnetic resonance imaging of the brain (MRI). The etiology in non-pregnant women such as various anatomic brain lesions, metabolic derangement, genetic disorder, or toxic/medication-related should also be considered. For a pregnant woman with a seizure, eclampsia should be considered at the top of the differential diagnosis. Additional concerns include Posterior Reversible Encephalopathy Syndrome (PRES), cerebral venous sinus thrombosis, Reversible Cerebral Vasoconstriction Syndrome (RCVS), Thrombotic Thrombocytopenic Purpura (TTP), amniotic fluid embolism, or air embolism.[50]

Overall, WWE should be counseled prior to pregnancy and be informed that most women with epilepsy have uncomplicated pregnancy and produce normal, healthy infants (see Table 20.1). Some women have slightly higher risk of complications during pregnancy and delivery, risks related to

---

TABLE 20.1 PREGNANCY CARE MAP IN EPILEPSY

- At Diagnosis
  - Ensure that appropriate diagnostic work-up is done to support or refute the diagnosis of epilepsy. Diagnostic work-up may include labwork, EEG, MRI, or admission for video-EEG monitoring
  - Start the AED that is most appropriate for treatment of the patient's epilepsy. If more than one option is available, choose the one with the lowest risk of teratogenicity
  - Counsel patient on risk of AED-related teratogenesis and possible interaction between AED and contraceptives
  - Start folic acid 1–4 mg daily
- Preconception
  - Aim for lowest dose of AED that provides adequate seizure control
  - Obtain serum AED concentration during period of seizure control, preferably more than once
  - In appropriate patients who have been seizure free for at least 2 years, consideration may be given to taper of AED
  - Continue folic acid
- Patient Planning Pregnancy
  - Discuss risks and benefits of continued use of AED regimen
  - Ensure baseline AED serum concentration during period of seizure control has been obtained to serve as target level to use during pregnancy
  - Avoid changes in AEDs used unless patient is taking valproate.
  - Discuss genetic counseling if appropriate
  - Continue folic acid, start pre-natal vitamin
  - Discuss breastfeeding
  - Discuss slightly increased risk of maternal hemorrhage, induction of labor, hypertensive disorders, birth before 37 weeks gestation, small for gestational age infants, and maternal mortality.
  - If patient becomes pregnant, she should immediately inform her care team
- During Pregnancy
  - Increase folic acid to 4-5 mg daily, continue prenatal vitamin

AED exposure and seizures, and require close monitoring of AED doses. Pregnant WWE should be followed carefully by both their obstetrician and neurologist. In cases where seizures are difficult to control or AED serum concentrations are difficult to maintain, consultation with an epileptologist should be considered.

REFERENCES

1. Hirtz D, Thurman DJ, Gwinn-Hardy K, Mohamed M, Chaudhuri AR, Zalutsky R. How common are the 'common' neurologic disorders? *Neurology.* 2007; 68: 326–337.
2. https://www.cdc.gov/epilepsy/basics/fast-facts.htm
3. Kobau R, Luo Y, Zack M, Helmers S, Thurman D. Epilepsy in adults and access to care—United States, 2012. *MMWR.* 2012; 61: 909–913.
4. US Census Bureau, Population Division. Annual estimates of the resident population by sex, age, race, and Hispanic origin for the United States, States, and Counties: April 1, 2010, to July 1, 2013. Release Date: June 2014. https://factfinder.census.gov/faces/tableservices/jsf/pages/productview.xhtml?src=bkmk. Accessed 1/8/2018.
5. Russ SA, Larson K, Halfon N. A national profile of childhood epilepsy and seizure disorder. *Pediatrics* 2012; 129: 256–64.
6. Olafsson E, Hallgrimsson JT, Hauser WA, Ludvigsson P, Gudmundsson G. Pregnancies of women with epilepsy: A population-based study in Iceland. *Epilepsia* 1998; 39: 887–892.
7. Katz O, Levy A, Wiznitzer A, Sheiner E, Pregnancy and perinatal outcome in epileptic women: a population-based study. *J Matern Fetal Neonatal Med.* 2006; 19: 21–25.
8. Yerby MS. Quality of life, epilepsy advances, and the evolving role of anticonvulsants in women with epilepsy. *Neurology.* 2000; 55: S21–31.
9. Putta S, Pennell PB. Management of epilepsy during pregnancy: Evidence-based strategies *Future Neurol.* 2015; 10:161–176.
10. Morrow J, Russell A, Guthrie E, et al. Malformation risks of antiepileptic drugs in pregnancy: A prospective study from the UK Epilepsy and Pregnancy Register. *J Neurol Neurosurg Psychiatry.* 2006; 77: 193–198.
11. Cersosimo MG, Benarroch, EE. Estrogen actions in the nervous system: Complexity and clinical implications. *Neurology.* 2015; 85:263–273.
12. Velíšková J, DeSantis, KA. Sex and hormonal influences on seizures and epilepsy. *Hormones and Behavior.* 2013; 63: 267–277.
13. Herzog AG. Menstrual disorders in women with epilepsy. *Neurology.* 2006; 66: S23–28.
14. Herzog AG. Catamenial epilepsy: Definition, prevalence, pathophysiology and treatment. *Seizure.* 2008; 17: 151–159.
15. Borgelt LM, Hart FM, Bainbridge JL. Epilepsy during pregnancy: Focus on management strategies. *International Journal of Women's Health.* 2016; 8: 505–517.
16. La Neve A, Boero G, Francavilla T, Plantamura M, De Agazio G, Specchio LM. Prospective, case–control study on the effect of pregnancy on seizure frequency in women with epilepsy. *Neurol Sci.* 2015; 36: 79–83.
17. Abe K, Hamada H, Yamada T, Obata-Yasuoka M, Minakami H, Yoshikawa H. Impact of planning of pregnancy in women with epilepsy on seizure control during pregnancy and on maternal and neonatal outcomes. *Seizure.* 2014; 23: 112–116.
18. Vajda FJE, O'Brien TJ, Graham J, Lander CM, Eadie MJ. The outcomes of pregnancy in women with untreated epilepsy. *Seizure.* 2015; 24: 77–81.
19. Cagnetti C, Lattanzi S, Foschi N, Provinciali L, Silvestrini M. Seizure course during pregnancy in catamenial epilepsy. *Neurology.* 2014; 83: 339–344.
20. Reddy DS. Perimenstrual catamenial epilepsy. *Womens Health (Lond)* 2007; 3: 195–206.
21. Foldvary-Schaefer N, Falcone T. Catamenial epilepsy: Pathophysiology, diagnosis, and management. *Neurology.* 2003; 61: S2–S15.
22. Velez-Ruiz NJ, Pennell PB. Issues for women with epilepsy. *Neurol Clin.* 2016; 34: 411–425.
23. Christensen J, Petrenaite V, Atterman J, et al. Oral contraceptives induce lamotrigine metabolism: Evidence from a double-blind, placebo-controlled trial. *Epilepsia.* 2007; 48: 484–489.
24. Sabers A. Pharmacokinetic interactions between contraceptives and antiepileptic drugs. *Seizure.* 2008; 17: 141–144.
25. Herzog AG, Blum AS, Farina EL, et al. Valproate and lamotrigine level variation with menstrual cycle phase and oral contraceptive use. *Neurology.* 2009; 72: 911–914.
26. Herzog AG. Differential impact of antiepileptic drugs on the effects of contraceptive methods on seizures: Interim findings of the epilepsy birth control registry. *Seizure.* 2015; 28: 71–75.
27. Tomson T, Landmark CJ, Battino D. Antiepileptic drug treatment in pregnancy: Changes in drug disposition and their clinical implications. *Epilepsia.* 2013; 54: 405–414.
28. Pennell PB. Antiepileptic drug pharmacokinetics during pregnancy and lactation. *Neurology.* 2003; 61: S35–S42.
29. Reisinger TL, Newman M, Loring DW, Pennell PB, Meador KJ. Antiepileptic drug clearance and

seizure frequency during pregnancy in women with epilepsy. *Epilepsy & Behavior.* 2013; 29: 13–18.

30. Harden CL. Pregnancy effects on lamotrigine levels. *Epilepsy Currents.* 2002; 2: 183.

31. Polepally AR, Pennell PB, Brundage RC, et al. Model-based lamotrigine clearance changes during pregnancy: Clinical implication. *Annals of Clinical and Translational Neurology.* 2014; 1: 99–106.

32. Harden CL, Pennell PB, Koppel BS, et al. Practice parameter update: Management issues for women with epilepsy—focus on pregnancy (an evidence-based review): Vitamin K, folic acid, blood levels, and breastfeeding. *Neurology.* 2009; 73: 142–149.

33. Koubeissi M. Levetiracetam: More evidence of safety in pregnancy. *Epilepsy Currents.* 2013; 13: 279–281.

34. Westin AA, Reimers A, Helde G, Nakken KO, Brodtkorb E. Serum concentration/dose ratio of levetiracetam before, during and after pregnancy. *Seizure.* 2008; 17: 192–198.

35. Tomson T, Palm R, Kallen K, et al. Pharmacokinetics of levetiracetam during pregnancy, delivery, in the neonatal period and lactation. *Epilepsia.* 2007; 48: 1111–1116.

36. Gerard EE, Meador KJ. Managing epilepsy in women. *Continuum (Minneap Minn).* 2016; 22: 204–226.

37. French J, Harden C, Pennell P, et al. A prospective study of pregnancy in women with epilepsy seeking conception (The WEPOD Study). *Neurology.* 2016 86: 16(Suppl I5.001). http://n.neurology.org/content/86/16_Supplement/I5.001.abstract

38. Viale L, Allotey J, Cheong-See F, et al. Epilepsy in pregnancy and reproductive outcomes: A systematic review and meta-analysis. *Lancet.* 2015; 386: 1845–1852.

39. Ruth DJ, Barnett J. Epilepsy in pregnancy. *J Perinat Neonat Nurs.* 2013; 27: 217–224.

40. Patel SI, Pennell PB. Management of epilepsy during pregnancy: An update. *Ther Adv Neurol Disord.* 2016; 9: 118–129.

41. Werler MM, Ahrens KA, Bosco JLF, et al. The National Birth Defects Prevention Study. Use of antiepileptic medications in pregnancy in relation to risks of birth defects. *Ann Epidemiol.* 2011; 21: 842–850.

42. Bangar S, Shastri A, El-Sayeh H, Cavanna AE. Women with epilepsy: Clinically relevant issues. *Functional Neurology.* 2016; 31: 127–134.

43. Sveberg L, Svalheim S, Taubøll E. The impact of seizures on pregnancy and delivery. *Seizure.* 2015; 28: 35–38.

44. Chen Y, Chiou H, Lin H, Lin H. Affect of seizures during gestation on pregnancy outcomes in women with epilepsy. *Arch Neurol.* 2009; 66: 979–984.

45. Borthen I, Gilhus NE. Pregnancy complications in patients with epilepsy. *Curr Opin Obstet Gynecol.* 2012; 24: 78–83.

46. Tomson T, Battino D, Bonizzoni E, et al. Antiepileptic drugs and intrauterine death. A prospective observational study from EURAP. *Neurology.* 2015; 85: 580–588.

47. Thorp JA, Gaston I, Caspers DR, Pai ML. Current concepts and controversies in the use of vitamin K. *Drugs* 1995; 49:376–387.

48. Sveberg L, Vik K, Henriksen T, Taubøll E. Women with epilepsy and post partum bleeding—Is there a role for vitamin K supplementation? *Seizure.* 2015; 28: 85–87.

49. MacDonald SC, Bateman BT, McElrath TF, Hernández-Díaz S. Mortality and morbidity during delivery hospitalization among pregnant women with epilepsy in the United States. *JAMA Neurol.* 2015; 72: 981–988.

50. Aya AG, Ondze B, Ripart J, Cuvillon P. Seizures in the peripartum period: Epidemiology, diagnosis and management. *Anaesth Crit Care Pain Med.* 2016; 35S: S13–S21.

21

Seizure Medications Effects on Fetus, Neonate, and Lactation

TARA A. LYNCH AND J. CHRISTOPHER GLANTZ

INTRODUCTION

Treatment of any chronic disease in pregnancy requires balancing the benefits of maternal symptom control with the risks of adverse fetal effects. If a pregnant woman can maintain health without a medication, then even small risks to the fetus may outweigh maternal benefits. If maternal health would be significantly compromised without the medication, however, then by extension, so would fetal health. Epilepsy is generally accepted as an example of the latter. In addition to maternal trauma, hypoxia, and even death from uncontrolled seizures, maternal convulsions have been associated with fetal hypoxia and acidosis, rupture of membranes, placental abruption, and fetal demise.[1] The drugs used to prevent maternal seizures are not without risk to the fetus. Compared with a general rate of major congenital malformations of approximately 2% (those requiring postnatal intervention or adversely affecting function, health, or development), the rate is increased to 4-to-9% by various antiepileptic drugs (AED). The precise degree to which this anomaly risk is driven by AED exposure is difficult to discern because untreated epilepsy may also be associated with increased fetal anomaly risk.[2] Adding to the uncertainty is that different studies, done with different methodologies, on different populations of women with different types of epilepsy—using different drugs, different drug doses, and different combinations of drugs—often report different results, ranging from dramatic risks to little to no effect.

Despite potential untoward AED effects on the fetus, prevention of seizure activity is considered central to the management of epilepsy. Unless the woman has been seizure-free for long enough that her neurologist decides it is safe to discontinue her medications, the benefits of maternal treatment typically outweigh the risk of fetal anomalies. As such, treatment rarely should be withheld, and the decision becomes what medication works best for maternal seizure control versus what medication is safest for the fetus. Unfortunately, the answers to these two questions often conflict. A detailed understanding of AED efficacy and potential fetal adverse effects is required to guide treatment options because medication selection is influenced by a patient's responsiveness to the medication, its dose, need for polytherapy, and gestational age. Regardless, epilepsy management during pregnancy requires multidisciplinary collaboration between obstetrics and neurology. Of note, some combination oral contraceptives may interfere with the metabolism of AEDs, making failure of contraception more common, and/or necessitating dose adjustments of AED (See Chapter 3 for further discussion.) Therefore, for the women with epilepsy who do not want to get pregnant, discussion of ideal therapy options and/or dose adjustments may be necessary.

ADVERSE PERINATAL EFFECTS OF ANTI-EPILEPTIC DRUGS

The majority of adverse fetal effects observed with AEDs are attributed to first trimester exposure (Table 21.1). Selecting an optimal regimen during pregnancy should be based on a balance between seizure control and known fetal effects, and ideally, this discussion should take place *before* conception. There are several medications with minimal or no known increased risk for major fetal malformations, such as levetiracetam, although these may be less effective in controlling seizures in some patients.[3] In contrast, medications such as valproate may be more effective but have significantly greater malformation risks. Higher doses and concurrent use of multiple AEDs have been shown to increase malformation risk.[4,5] If multiple

TABLE 21.1 MAJOR CONGENITAL MALFORMATIONS ASSOCIATED WITH AEDS[31]

System	Malformation
Cardiovascular	Atrial Septal Defect
	Ventricular Septal Defect
	Patent Ductus Arteriosus
	Pulmonary Stenosis
	Coarctation of the Aorta
	Tetralogy of Fallot
Urogenital	Glandular Hypospadias
Neural Tube Defects	Lower Neural Tube Defects
	Hydrocephaly
Face	Cleft Lip
	Cleft Palate

antiepileptic agents are needed for symptom control, there is evidence that certain combinations such as lamotrigine and carbamazepine have lower rates of major congenital malformations.[6] In short, if a woman's seizures can be controlled with a single, low-dose, less-teratogenic medication, then consideration should be given to this alternative regimen. Of course, unless this was addressed before conception, a woman presenting during the first trimester may already have placed her fetus at risk through early exposure during organogenesis. Changing medications at that point may be too late and simply expose the fetus to a second AED that may or may not be the most effective for the pregnant woman.

Fetal effects other than structural anomalies may extend beyond the first trimester. There is evidence that exposure to any AED has been associated with growth restriction, and the use of certain antiepileptic medications at any gestational age has been associated with a decreased intelligence quotient (IQ).[7] One study on the cognitive and language development of children exposed to AEDs demonstrated that outcomes for children exposed to in utero levetiracetam were similar to unexposed children. In contrast, children exposed to valproate during gestation had a statistically significant decrease in motor skills and language capabilities.[8] This was again demonstrated in a recent prospective study in which children exposed to a higher dose of valproate had an eight-fold increased need for educational support at 6 years of age.[9] Numerous other studies, including a 2014 Cochrane review, have further confirmed the association between valproate exposure and reduced IQ.[10] In contrast, exposure to other AEDs

such as lamotrigine and carbamazepine has not demonstrated neurocognitive effects.[9] Therefore, the fetal effects of exposure to certain antiepileptic medications can extend beyond embryogenesis and may have long-term neurocognitive implications.

The physiologic changes that occur in pregnancy further complicate the balance between seizure control and fetal exposure because AED levels and pharmacokinetics are altered throughout gestation. Cardiovascular changes include a 50% expansion of plasma volume and increases in cardiac output and renal perfusion, which increase renal clearance of medications and decrease drug availability.[11] Total drug concentration also is altered by changes in plasma proteins and glycoproteins that affect drug binding.[1] Many AEDs are highly bound to serum proteins, and lower concentrations of these proteins may lower total drug concentrations. Because it is the free fraction of a drug that is active, and this may or may not change in concert with the protein-bound fraction, it usually is preferable to measure free AED rather than total concentration. Alterations in gastric absorption and emptying can decrease serum drug concentrations, and early pregnancy nausea may decrease compliance or tolerance of medications.[11] Furthermore, seizures may be effected by hormones. Progesterone tends to increase the seizure threshold while estrogen lowers it.[1] Based on these changes, current recommendations include monitoring of AED concentration (Table 21.2) at least every trimester, with increased frequency if there is evidence of suboptimal seizure control.[1]

The treatment of epilepsy in pregnancy can be complex, with the goal of maximizing maternal seizure control while minimizing fetal risks. Knowledge of AED medications and their specific associations will help obstetric providers and neurologists select optimal AED regimens. Throughout this chapter we will review common medications used in the treatment of epilepsy, their mechanisms of action, and drug specific considerations in pregnancy. There are other newer drugs that have not been studied in pregnancy, and as such will not be reviewed. When considering the effect of these medications on pregnancy, one also should bear in mind which will be most compatible with breastfeeding.

ANTI-EPILEPTIC DRUGS

Fetal effects from AEDs have been reported since the late 1960s.[12] Classic AEDs include phenobarbital, phenytoin, carbamazepine, and valproate. When the older AEDs were being developed, there

TABLE 21.2 THERAPEUTIC DRUG REFERENCE RANGES
FOR ANTIEPILEPTIC MEDICATIONS[56-61]

Drug	Concentration Reference Range (mg/l)	Change in Pregnancy
Zonisamide	10–40	Unknown
Levetiracetam	12–46	↓40-60%
Topiramate	5–20	↓30%
Lamotrigine	2.5–15	Unpredictable
Gabapentin	12–20	No change
Valproate	50–100	↓50%
Oxcarbazepine	12–35	↓36-50%
Phenobarbital	15–40	↓55%
Phenytoin	10–20	↓20%
Carbamazepine	4–12	↓25%

was a tendency every time a new medication came out to think it would be safer than the previous ones. Women often would be switched from one to another during pregnancy (even after the period of organogenesis had ended, or when the alternative AED was not necessarily as effective for that patient's seizure control). In most cases, however, the newer "classic" AEDs did not prove safer (and in the case of valproic acid, sometimes were more teratogenic than its predecessors). Newer generation AEDs include oxcarbazepine, lamotrigine, gabapentin, levetiracetam, and zonisamide (Table 21.3). True to form, these currently are thought to be safer than the classic AEDs. At present there is evidence supporting this contention, although by virtue of being newer, they are not as well studied as the older medications.

In 2015, the classic categorizations of medication use in pregnancy and lactation (Tables 21.4 and 21.5) were transitioned to a new labeling system by the Food and Drug Administration (FDA). This new Pregnancy and Lactation Labeling Rule (PLLR) consists of mandated narrative descriptive sections on the risks of medications in pregnancy, lactation and reproduction (refer to the following for details: https://www.fda.gov/Drugs/DevelopmentApprovalProcess/DevelopmentResources/Labeling/ucm093307.htm).[13] In the following sections we will use both the new PLLR labeling system and the old classification for reference.

Phenobarbital (Luminal®)

Phenobarbital is a barbiturate that was one of the first AEDs used during pregnancy. It acts on γ-aminobutyric acid (GABA) receptors that modulate chloride channels and inhibit seizure activity. Phenobarbital is metabolized in the liver, partially excreted in urine, and primarily used for the treatment of seizure disorders. It has a long half-life and several known side effects including sedation, neurotoxicity, and behavioral and cognitive effects.[14] During pregnancy, phenobarbital levels decline by as much as 55%, with the greatest decline observed in the first trimester.[15]

The risk of major congenital malformations associated with phenobarbital is estimated to be about 5.5%.[3] This risk appears to be dose dependent: doses <150 mg/day were associated with a malformation rate of 4.2%, whereas doses >150 mg/day were associated with a 13.7% rate of malformations.[4] Associated anomalies include cardiac defects (up to 8% with high doses), oral clefts, cardiac malformations, and urogenital anomalies.[3,16] Historically, it is classified as pregnancy category D, and rarely is used during pregnancy today. Phenobarbital is considered high risk (L4) during breastfeeding because it has been associated with apnea, sedation, and neonatal addiction.[17]

Phenytoin (Dilantin®)

Phenytoin, also known as hydantoin, has been used widely for epilepsy for many years. The mechanism of action is inhibition of neurotransmitters and modulation of GABA receptors.[18] Phenytoin is well absorbed (although absorption is decreased by antacids) and undergoes hepatic metabolism with formation of a reactive epoxide intermediate that, if not quickly broken down by the enzyme epoxide hydrolase, oxidatively damages surrounding molecules and cells. In experimental

TABLE 21.3 SPECIFIC ANTIEPILEPTIC DRUGS AND ASSOCIATED RATES
OF MAJOR MALFORMATIONS

Medication	Rate of Major Malformations	Associated Major Malformations
Valproate	6.7%[2] to 9.3%[3] RR 5.69 (95% CI 3.33 to 9.73)*	**Neural Tube Defect (1.1%)** Facial Cleft (1.1%) Cardiac (1.1%) Genitourinary (1.2%) Gastrointestinal (0.6%) Skeletal (0.8%)
Phenobarbital	5.5%[3] RR 2.84 (95% CI 1.57-5.13)*	**Cardiac Defects (2.5%)** Oral Clefts (2.0%) Urogenital anomalies (<1%)
Phenytoin	2.9%[3] to 5.4%[16] RR 2.38 (95% CI 1.12 to 5.03)*	Cardiac Defects (<1%) Oral Clefts (0.5%) Urogenital Anomalies Skeletal Anomalies **Fetal Hydantoin Syndrome**
Topiramate	4.2%[3] RR 3.69 (95% CI 1.36 to 10.07)*	**Cleft lip (1.4%)**
Carbamazepine	2.6% to 3.0%[3] RR 2.01 (95% CI 1.20 to 3.36)*	Neural Tube Defect (0.2%) Facial Cleft (0.2%) Cardiac (0.8%) Genitourinary (0.3%) Gastrointestinal (0.3%) Skeletal (0.2%)
Lamotrigine	2.0%[3] to 2.3%[2]	Neural Tube Defect (0.1%) Facial Cleft (0.1%) Cardiac (0.4%) Genitourinary (0.5%) Gastrointestinal (0.4%) Skeletal (0.1%)
Levetiracetam	2.4%[3]	No increased risk
Oxcarbazepine	2.2%[5]	No increased risk
Gabapentin	0.7%[5] to 1.7%[40]	No increased risk
Zonisamide	0%[5]	No increased risk

* relative risk compared to women without epilepsy.[16]

TABLE 21.4 LACTATION SAFETY CATEGORIES[62]

Category	Description
L1	Safest—A large number of studies have been performed which do not demonstrate any increased risk or the possibility of neonatal harm is remote.
L2	Safer—A limited number of studies have been performed without any observed increased risk.
L3	Moderately Safe—Controlled studies have been performed and demonstrate a potential for minimal non-adverse effects.
L4	Hazardous—There is evidence of neonatal effects with breastfeeding.
L5	Contraindicated—There is significant documented harm in breast fed neonates.

TABLE 21.5 CLASSIC PREGNANCY MEDICATION SAFETY CATEGORIES

Category	Description
A	Adequate and well-controlled studies have failed to demonstrate a risk to the fetus
B	Animal reproduction studies have failed to demonstrate a risk in the fetus. There are no adequate well-controlled studies in pregnant women.
C	Animal reproduction studies have shown an adverse effect on the fetus and there are no adequate well-controlled studies in pregnancy women.
D	There is evidence of human risk based on data from investigational or marketing experience of studies in humans, but benefits of use may outweigh the risks.
X	Studies have demonstrated fetal abnormalities and there is evidence of human fetal risk. Risks clearly outweigh the benefits.

studies, fetuses with low levels of epoxide hydrolase as measured in amniocytes are at higher risk of adverse effects of phenytoin, including fetal anomalies.[19] However, the clinical utility of this enzyme levels is limited to research protocols. Levels of phenytoin can decline by 20% during pregnancy with a maximum change observed in the first trimester. There is a return to pre-pregnancy levels by 12 weeks postpartum.[1,15]

Much of the teratogenicity of phenytoin is theorized to occur secondary to oxidative stress resulting in cell death.[20] Overall, phenytoin is associated with a 5.4% malformation risk, including cardiovascular anomalies, urogenital anomalies, and oral clefts.[3,16] Fetal hydantoin syndrome is a constellation of structural, behavioral, and developmental defects characteristic of fetal phenytoin exposure, thought to occur in approximately 10% of exposed pregnancies. Associated malformations include, finger nail hypoplasia, growth disturbances, rib abnormalities, hirsutism, and abnormal palmar creases.[21] As with many AEDs, data on the association with fetal anomalies are conflicting, however, with a recent metaanalysis reporting no increased risk of oro-facial clefting, skeletal malformations, or cardiac malformations in patients using phenytoin when compared to women without epilepsy.[16] This may be due to differences in methodologies, populations, and dosing between studies. Historically, phenytoin is classified as pregnancy category D. During lactation, phenytoin is considered a low risk AED (L2).[17]

Carbamazepine (Tegretol®), Oxcarbazepine (Trileptal®), and Eslicarbazepine (Aptiom®)

Carbamazepine is an antiepileptic drug that inhibits seizure activity by effecting voltage-gated sodium channels. The newer oxcarbazepine and eslicarbazepine are related to carbamazepine, and

in fact, eslicarbazepine is the main active metabolite of both carbamazepine and oxcarbazepine. Although the structures of these medications are similar, the metabolic pathways differ, which may impact the side-effect profile and teratogenicity.[22] These newer formulations have improved the known side-effect profile of gastrointestinal upset, drowsiness, and dizziness that is associated with carbamazepine, and all three are used for treatment of epilepsy.[23] Carbamazepine is metabolized in the liver, also with a reactive epoxide intermediary. It is 75% protein-bound and serum levels decline during pregnancy, mostly in the third trimester.[24]

Carbamazepine's association with fetal malformations has been well studied, whereas there is less data on oxcarbazepine and eslicarbazepine. One study of 1718 patients with carbamazepine monotherapy reported a rate of major congenital malformations of 2.6% that was increased to 5.3% with dosages greater than 1000 mg (p = 0.01).[2] Other studies have observed a rate as high as 5.6%.[4] This dose-dependent relationship was reconfirmed in a subsequent study that observed a rate of malformations of 1.3%, 3.2% and 7.7% at doses less than 400 mg, 400 mg to 1000 mg, and greater than 1000 mg, respectively.[4] Fetal anomalies that have been associated with carbamazepine include spina bifida, facial clefts, genitourinary, gastrointestinal, skeletal, and possibly cardac anomalies.[25] A carbamazepine syndrome consisting of craniofacial, fingernail, and developmental abnormalities has been described, but not all studies have confirmed this. There is evidence of transplacental transmission of oxcarbazepine but with minimal accumulation in the neonate (7–10% of maternal serum levels).[26]

A pregnancy registry reported no significant increase in the rate of major malformations associated with oxcarbazepine use in pregnancy.[3] However, there have not been studies on rates of specific malformations such as neural tube defects, cardiac malformations, or on a dose dependent malformation rate with oxcarbazepine.[16] Finally, there have been no studies on eslicarbazepine use in pregnancy.[27] Historically, carbamazepine is classified as pregnancy category D and oxcarbazepine and eslicarbazepine are classified as category C. Postpartum these drugs are considered low risk (L2) and are compatible with lactation, although this is based on limited data.[17]

Valproate (Depakote®/Depakene®)

Valproic acid, converted in the gut to valproate, is a first-line AED and mood-stabilizer used for the treatment of epilepsy, migraines, and bipolar disease.[28] Theorized mechanisms of action include pathways involved with GABA, N-methyl-d-aspartate (NMDA), and calcium channels.[29] Valproate is highly protein-bound, hepatically metabolized, and inactive forms are excreted in the urine. Concentrations of available drug are influenced by gestational age, with studies demonstrating a maximum decrease of drug availability by about 50% in the third trimester. After delivery, concentrations can increase by as much as 25%, and therefore levels should be monitored postpartum with appropriate dose adjustments.[30,31]

Valproate has been studied extensively and is known to be associated with fetal congenital anomalies, particularly neural tube defects (up to 2%).[32] Other anomalies include cardiac, craniofacial, and skeletal malformations.[16,33] One study of 1290 women exposed to valproate monotherapy demonstrated a 6.7% risk of major congenital malformations. This risk was further increased with larger doses: valproate doses greater than 1500 mg daily were associated with a 9.7% rate of malformations.[2] The International Registry of Antiepileptic Drugs and Pregnancy (EURAP) study observed that the doses of valproate <700 mg, 700 mg to 1500 mg, and >1500 mg were associated with a 4.2%, 9.0%, and 23.2% risk of malformations, respectively.[4] Compared to lamotrigine and carbamazepine, valproate is associated with a higher rate of all defects. Furthermore, valproate use in multi-agent regimens is associated with a much higher rate of fetal malformations. In one study of 159 patients, the rate of malformations was as high as 31% when valproate at doses greater than 1500 mg was used with lamotrigine.[6]

The effect of valproate on pregnancy outcomes is not limited to the first trimester. Prenatal exposure at any gestation has been associated with neurocognitive delay and a lower intelligence quotient.[3,8–10] Historically, valproate is classified as

pregnancy X for the treatment of migraines and D for all other indications. Postpartum, valproate appears to be present at low levels in breast milk, although no definitive neonatal reactions have been reported in the literature. The half-life is 4 times as long as in adults, and there is the potential for accumulation in the neonate over time.[34] For this reason it is categorized as a high-risk drug during lactation (L4).[17] As with any medication, combination therapy may increase the risk of sedation and poor growth.

Lamotrigine (Lamictal®)

Lamotrigine is a new generation anticonvulsant that inhibits calcium channels and is commonly used for the treatment of epilepsy and mood disorders.[35] Lamotrigine is hepatically metabolized, 55% protein bound, and renally excreted.[11] There is a wide variation in serum levels throughout pregnancy with a rapid return to prepregnancy concentrations 2 weeks postpartum.[36] Drug metabolism is also influenced by polytherapy with other AEDs. For example, when lamotrigine is used with carbamazepine or phenytoin, its clearance is increased by 62% to 160%, respectively.[37] Use with valproic acid is associated with a two-fold decrease in drug concentration.[38] Maximum clearance of lamotrigine occurs at about 32 weeks. Individual clearance rates can be unpredictable and therefore serum lamotrigine levels may need to be monitored every month during pregnancy.[39]

When compared to valproate and carbamazepine, lamotrigine has the lowest rate of major congenital malformations. One study of 2198 patients demonstrated a 2.3% rate of major congenital malformations with lamotrigine monotherapy.[2] There is conflicting evidence of an increased risk of malformations with higher lamotrigine doses. Some studies have observed an increased risk, whereas others have not.[2,4] Historically, lamotrigine is classified as pregnancy category C. Postpartum, lamotrigine is present in breast milk in concentrations about 30% of the maternal serum concentration, although neonate's abilty to metabolize the drug is limited. Withdrawal has been reported with abrupt cessation of breastfeeding. Use of lamotrigine is not a reason to discontinue breastfeeding, though infants should be monitored for central nervous system depression.[1,17]

Newer Antiepileptic Drugs With Limited Data in Human Pregnancy

Gabapentin (Neurontin*) is used for the treatment of seizures but has also been used for the treatment of pain, restless leg syndrome, and nausea and vomiting during pregnancy.[40] The rate of malformations associated with gabapentin is estimated to be around 0.7 to 1.7%, similar to the general population.[5,40] Gabapentin is classically classified as pregnancy category C. There is evidence that gabapentin is transmitted to the neonate via breast milk, with concentrations between 6–12% of maternal concentrations, but no adverse neonatal reactions have been reported and it is considered compatible with breastfeeding.[41]

Levetiracetam (Keppra®) is well-known AED without evidence of teratogenicity based on limited human use. The estimated rate of major malformations is 1.8%, and there is no evidence of increased risk with increasing doses.[16] Concentrations decrease by about 40–60% during pregnancy and clearance increases by 243%. Following delivery levels typically return to pre-pregnancy values in about 1 week.[42] Historically, levetiracetam is classified as pregnancy category C.[31] Levetiracetam is transmitted into breast milk but neonates are able to rapidly eliminate this drug. It generally is considered compatible with breastfeeding.[43]

Zonisamide (Zonegran®) is another newer AED. As such, there has not been as much research on its use and associated effects pregnancy. To date, one study of 90 pregnancies did not demonstrate any increased risk of major congenital abnormalities.[44] During pregnancy, case reports suggest that there likely is a decrease in serum concentrations.[45] Based on the old FDA classification system zonisamide is considered pregnancy category C. Furthermore, there is limited data regarding zonisamide and breastfeeding. There is evidence of transmission in breast milk, but no adverse neonatal effects have been documented.[45]

Topiramate (Topamax®) is a newer generation AED used for the treatment of epilepsy, migraines, appetite suppression and psychiatric disorders.[46] The exact mechanism of action is unknown but is theorized to act on voltage-gated sodium channels, GABA receptors, and glutamate receptors.[28] It is associated with a ten-fold increased risk of cleft lip with first trimester exposure[3,5] and a 4.3% rate of major congenital malformations in general.[16] As such, it is classified as pregnancy category D. Although there is evidence of transmission to the neonate via breast milk, there have been no adverse effects, and infant serum concentrations are exceedingly low.[45] Topiramate generally is avoided during pregnancy but is considered safe with breastfeeding.

OTHER ISSUES WITH ANTI-EPILEPTIC DRUG USE DURING PREGNANCY

Folate Supplementation

Possibly due to interference with folate absorption or to increased catabolism, older AEDs are associated with lower serum folate concentrations, which themselves are associated with increased risk of neural tube defects (NTD). Because folate supplementation has been shown to lower the risk of recurrent NTD in women with spina bifida or who have given birth to a previous infant with an NTD, a common recommendation to women taking first-generation AEDs is to empirically increase their folate intake in an attempt to lower the risk of an AED-associated NTD.[47] Although there is a plausible biologic mechanism behind this, the mechanism through which AEDs interfere with neural tube to closure may not be folate-dependent, and folate supplementation has not been shown to lower AED-related NTD risk.[48,49] As such, recommendations to supplement folate in women taking "classic" AEDs, while commonly made, are based on plausibility and lack of harm, not on evidence of efficacy.[48,50,51]

Vitamin K Supplementation

Neonatal vitamin K levels are normally low, and it is routine for neonates to receive vitamin K shortly after birth to prevent bleeding. Because of older AEDs' enzyme-inducing properties that increase fetal vitamin K catabolism, older AEDs are associated with even lower serum levels of vitamin K. As a result, recommendations have been made for pregnant women using AEDs to take vitamin K supplements at the end of their pregnancy because their infants might be at increased risk of perinatal hemorrhage. Despite demonstrable laboratory increases in neonatal vitamin K levels after maternal supplementation, there is no evidence that perinatal hemorrhage is more common in infants born to women taking AEDs than to controls, nor that maternal vitamin K supplementation improves clinical outcome.[52]

Fetal Echocardiography

Several older AEDs are associated with increased risk of cardiac malformations,[53] and the question arises whether fetal echocardiography should be done routinely in such mothers. This particular practice is somewhat controversial. Current recommendations from the American Heart Association include first trimester AED exposure

---

BOX 21.1
CARE MAP FOR PREGNANCY: MANAGEMENT OF MEDICATIONS

BEFORE PREGNANCY/PRE-PREGNANCY/NON-PREGNANT
- Maternal confirmation of the diagnosis of epilepsy
- Preconception control of seizure disorder (if possible) with goals for medical therapy of:
  - Monotherapy
  - Lowest dose possible
  - Least teratogenic medication
    - Avoid: valproate, phenobarbital, phenytoin, topiramate
    - Consider: lamotrigine, carbamazepine, levetiracetam, oxcarbazepine, gabapentin, zonisamide
- Preconception Maternal Fetal Medicine consult

DURING PREGNANCY
- Early initiation of prenatal care
- Serum monitoring of antiepileptic serum levels every trimester (increased frequency as clinically indicated)
- Lactation consultation

DELIVERY
- Continue antiepileptic medications

POSTPARTUM
- Post-delivery decrease antiepileptic medication to pre-pregnancy dose
- Contraception counseling
- Neurologic follow up for medication adjustments as needed (individualized)
- Lactation consultation

---

as a potential indication for fetal echocardiogram, although the yield is likely to be very low.[54] The extent to which a fetal echocardiogram is indicated has not been fully elucidated, and individual assessment of the patient's risk for fetal cardiac defects therefore should guide the recommendation for fetal echocardiogram.[55]

CONCLUSIONS

Medication selection when pregnancy is complicated by maternal epilepsy is complex and should balance the risks of fetal effects with the benefits of maternal seizure control. Optimal anti-epileptic selection ideally would occur prior to conception. Equally important, preconception control of seizure disorder should be directed toward the patient's reproductive goals. If a woman is planning on pursuing pregnancy, then optimization of her regimen would

involve seizure control with a single agent, at lowest dose possible, with the least teratogenic potential. Consultation with Maternal-Fetal Medicine should be considered to review the effects of the patient's specific AED and any pregnancy related risks. Once pregnancy is achieved, the patient should establish early obstetric care in addition to close neurology follow-up to allow for monitoring of AED efficacy. Post-delivery the antiepileptic medication should be decreased to pre-pregnancy dose in collaboration with the patient's neurologist (Box 21.1).

Overall, the physiologic changes of pregnancy, coupled with provider and patient hesitancy to continue medications, can make the pharmacologic management of epilepsy complex. Additionally, it is important to recognize that some medications can have effects far beyond the first trimester. As treatment requires careful balance between the risks of fetal effects and the benefits of maternal seizure control, informed consent and shared decision making with the patient and her care team providers is paramount to providing optimal care for the patient and her pregnancy.

REFERENCES

1. Pennell PB. Antiepileptic drug pharmacokinetics during pregnancy and lactation. *Neurology.* 2003; 61(6 Suppl 2): S35–42.
2. Campbell E, Kennedy F, Russell A, et al. Malformation risks of antiepileptic drug monotherapies in pregnancy: Updated results from the UK and Ireland Epilepsy and Pregnancy Registers. *Journal of Neurology, Neurosurgery, and Psychiatry.* 2014; 85(9): 1029–1034.
3. Hernandez-Diaz S, Smith CR, Shen A, et al. Comparative safety of antiepileptic drugs during pregnancy. *Neurology.* 2012; 78(21): 1692–1699.
4. Tomson T, Battino D, Bonizzoni E, et al. Dose-dependent risk of malformations with antiepileptic drugs: an analysis of data from the EURAP epilepsy and pregnancy registry. *The Lancet Neurology.* 2011; 10(7): 609–617.
5. Velez-Ruiz NJ, Pennell PB. Issues for women with epilepsy. *Neurologic Clinics.* 2016; 34(2): 411–425, ix.
6. Tomson T, Battino D, Bonizzoni E, et al. Dose-dependent teratogenicity of valproate in mono- and polytherapy: An observational study. *Neurology.* 2015; 85(10): 866–872.
7. Veiby G, Daltveit AK, Engelsen BA, Gilhus NE. Fetal growth restriction and birth defects with newer and older antiepileptic drugs during pregnancy. *Journal of Neurology.* 2014; 261(3): 579–588.
8. Shallcross R, Bromley RL, Cheyne CP, et al. In utero exposure to levetiracetam vs valproate: Development and language at 3 years of age. *Neurology.* 2014; 82(3): 213–221.
9. Baker GA, Bromley RL, Briggs M, et al. IQ at 6 years after in utero exposure to antiepileptic drugs: A controlled cohort study. *Neurology.* 2015; 84(4): 382–390.
10. Bromley R, Weston J, Adab N, et al. Treatment for epilepsy in pregnancy: neurodevelopmental outcomes in the child. *The Cochrane Database of Systematic Reviews.* 2014; (10): Cd010236.
11. Tomson T, Landmark CJ, Battino D. Antiepileptic drug treatment in pregnancy: Changes in drug disposition and their clinical implications. *Epilepsia.* 2013; 54(3): 405–414.
12. Meadow SR. Anticonvulsant drugs and congenital abnormalities. *Lancet (London, England).* 1968; 2(7581): 1296.
13. Ramoz LL, Patel-Shori NM. Recent changes in pregnancy and lactation labeling: Retirement of risk categories. *Pharmacotherapy.* 2014; 34(4): 389–395.
14. Meador KJ, Loring DW, Moore EE, et al. Comparative cognitive effects of phenobarbital, phenytoin, and valproate in healthy adults. *Neurology.* 1995; 45(8): 1494–1499.
15. Yerby MS, Friel PN, McCormick K, et al. Pharmacokinetics of anticonvulsants in pregnancy: Alterations in plasma protein binding. *Epilepsy Research.* 1990; 5(3): 223–228.
16. Weston J, Bromley R, Jackson CF, et al. Monotherapy treatment of epilepsy in pregnancy: Congenital malformation outcomes in the child. *The Cochrane Database of Systematic Reviews.* 2016; 11: Cd010224.
17. Newton ER, Hale TW. Drugs in breast milk. *Clinical Obstetrics and Gynecology.* 2015; 58(4): 868–884.
18. Nolan SJ, Marson AG, Weston J, Tudur Smith C. Carbamazepine versus phenytoin monotherapy for epilepsy: An individual participant data review. *The Cochrane Database of Systematic Reviews.* 2015(8): Cd001911.
19. Buehler BA, Delimont D, van Waes M, Finnell RH. Prenatal prediction of risk of the fetal hydantoin syndrome. *New England Journal of Medicine.* 1990; 322(22): 1567–1572.
20. Alexander PG, Clark KL, Tuan RS. Prenatal exposure to environmental factors and congenital limb defects. *Birth Defects Research Part C, Embryo Today: Reviews.* 2016; 108(3): 243–273.
21. Scheinfeld N. Phenytoin in cutaneous medicine: its uses, mechanisms and side effects. *Dermatology Online Journal.* 2003; 9(3): 6.
22. Kalis MM, Huff NA. Oxcarbazepine, an antiepileptic agent. *Clinical therapeutics.* 2001;23(5):680–700; discussion 645.
23. Gierbolini J, Giarratano M, Benbadis SR. Carbamazepine-related antiepileptic drugs for the treatment of epilepsy—a comparative review. *Expert opinion on pharmacotherapy.* 2016; 17(7): 885–888.
24. Perucca E, Crema A. Plasma protein binding of drugs in pregnancy. *Clinical Pharmacokinetics.* 1982; 7(4): 336–352.
25. Jentink J, Dolk H, Loane MA, et al. Intrauterine exposure to carbamazepine and specific congenital malformations: Systematic review and case-control study. *BMJ (Clinical Research Ed).* 2010; 341: c6581.
26. Bulau P, Paar WD, von Unruh GE. Pharmacokinetics of oxcarbazepine and 10-hydroxy-carbazepine in the newborn child of an oxcarbazepine-treated mother. *European Journal of Clinical Pharmacology.* 1988; 34(3): 311–313.

27. de Jong J, Garne E, de Jong-van den Berg LT, Wang H. The risk of specific congenital anomalies in relation to newer antiepileptic drugs: A literature review. *Drugs—Real World Outcomes.* 2016; 3(2): 131–143.

28. Goldenberg MM. Overview of drugs used for epilepsy and seizures: Etiology, diagnosis, and treatment. *P & T: A Peer-reviewed Journal for Formulary Management.* 2010; 35(7): 392–415.

29. Schmidt D. Starting, choosing, changing, and discontinuing drug treatment for epilepsy patients. *Neurologic Clinics.* 2016; 34(2): 363–381,viii.

30. Yerby MS, Friel PN, McCormick K. Antiepileptic drug disposition during pregnancy. *Neurology.* 1992; 42(4 Suppl 5): 12–16.

31. Pennell PB. Antiepileptic drugs during pregnancy: What is known and which AEDs seem to be safest? *Epilepsia.* 2008; 49(Suppl 9): 43–55.

32. Harden CL, Meador KJ, Pennell PB, et al. Practice parameter update: management issues for women with epilepsy—focus on pregnancy (an evidence-based review). Teratogenesis and perinatal outcomes: Report of the Quality Standards Subcommittee and Therapeutics and Technology Assessment Subcommittee of the American Academy of Neurology and American Epilepsy Society. *Neurology.* 2009; 73(2): 133–141.

33. Veroniki AA, Rios P, Cogo E, et al. Comparative safety of antiepileptic drugs for neurological development in children exposed during pregnancy and breast feeding: A systematic review and network meta-analysis. *BMJ open.* 2017; 7(7): e017248.

34. Nau H, Rating D, Koch S, Hauser I, Helge H. Valproic acid and its metabolites: Placental transfer, neonatal pharmacokinetics, transfer via mother's milk and clinical status in neonates of epileptic mothers. *Journal of Pharmacology and Experimental Therapeutics.* 1981; 219(3): 768–777.

35. Ramaratnam S, Panebianco M, Marson AG. Lamotrigine add-on for drug-resistant partial epilepsy. *Cochrane Database of Systematic Reviews.* 2016; (6): Cd001909.

36. Pennell PB, Peng L, Newport DJ, et al. Lamotrigine in pregnancy: clearance, therapeutic drug monitoring, and seizure frequency. *Neurology.* 2008; 70(22 Pt. 2): 2130–2136.

37. Anderson GD, Gidal BE, Messenheimer JA, Gilliam FG. Time course of lamotrigine de-induction: impact of step-wise withdrawal of carbamazepine or phenytoin. *Epilepsy Research.* 2002; 49(3): 211–217.

38. Kanner AM, Frey M. Adding valproate to lamotrigine: A study of their pharmacokinetic interaction. *Neurology.* 2000; 55(4): 588–591.

39. Tran TA, Leppik IE, Blesi K, Sathanandan ST, Remmel R. Lamotrigine clearance during pregnancy. *Neurology.* 2002; 59(2): 251–255.

40. Guttuso T, Jr., Shaman M, Thornburg LL. Potential maternal symptomatic benefit of gabapentin and review of its safety in pregnancy. *European Journal of Obstetrics, Gynecology, and Reproductive Biology.* 2014; 181: 280–283.

41. Kristensen JH, Ilett KF, Hackett LP, Kohan R. Gabapentin and breastfeeding: A case report. *Journal of Human Lactation: Official Journal of International Lactation Consultant Association.* 2006; 22(4): 426–428.

42. Westin AA, Reimers A, Helde G, Nakken KO, Brodtkorb E. Serum concentration/dose ratio of levetiracetam before, during and after pregnancy. *Seizure.* 2008; 17(2): 192–198.

43. Johannessen SI, Helde G, Brodtkorb E. Levetiracetam concentrations in serum and in breast milk at birth and during lactation. *Epilepsia.* 2005; 46(5): 775–777.

44. Bokhari A, Coull BA, Holmes LB. Effect of prenatal exposure to anticonvulsant drugs on dermal ridge patterns of fingers. *Teratology.* 2002; 66(1): 19–23.

45. Reimers A. New antiepileptic drugs and women. *Seizure.* 2014; 23(8): 585–591.

46. Alsaad AM, Chaudhry SA, Koren G. First trimester exposure to topiramate and the risk of oral clefts in the offspring: A systematic review and meta-analysis. *Reproductive Toxicology (Elmsford, NY).* 2015; 53: 45–50.

47. Harden CL, Pennell PB, Koppel BS, et al. Management issues for women with epilepsy—focus on pregnancy (an evidence-based review): III. Vitamin K, folic acid, blood levels, and breast-feeding: Report of the Quality Standards Subcommittee and Therapeutics and Technology Assessment Subcommittee of the American Academy of Neurology and the American Epilepsy Society. *Epilepsia.* 2009; 50(5): 1247–1255.

48. Kjaer D, Horvath-Puho E, Christensen J, et al. Antiepileptic drug use, folic acid supplementation, and congenital abnormalities: A population-based case-control study. *BJOG: An International Journal of Obstetrics and Gynaecology.* 2008; 115(1): 98–103.

49. Pittschieler S, Brezinka C, Jahn B, et al. Spontaneous abortion and the prophylactic effect of folic acid supplementation in epileptic women undergoing antiepileptic therapy. *Journal of Neurology.* 2008; 255(12): 1926–1931.

50. Hernandez-Diaz S, Werler MM, Walker AM, Mitchell AA. Folic acid antagonists during pregnancy and the risk of birth defects. *New England Journal of Medicine.* 2000; 343(22): 1608–1614.

51. Meijer WM, de Walle HE, Kerstjens-Frederikse WS, de Jong-van den Berg LT. Folic acid sensitive birth defects in association with intrauterine exposure to folic acid antagonists. *Reproductive Toxicology (Elmsford, NY)*. 2005; 20(2): 203–207.

52. Kaaja E, Kaaja R, Matila R, Hiilesmaa V. Enzyme-inducing antiepileptic drugs in pregnancy and the risk of bleeding in the neonate. *Neurology*. 2002; 58(4): 549–553.

53. Matalon S, Schechtman S, Goldzweig G, Ornoy A. The teratogenic effect of carbamazepine: A meta-analysis of 1255 exposures. *Reproductive Toxicology (Elmsford, NY)*. 2002; 16(1): 9–17.

54. Donofrio MT, Moon-Grady AJ, Hornberger LK, et al. Diagnosis and treatment of fetal cardiac disease: A scientific statement from the American Heart Association. *Circulation*. 2014; 129(21): 2183–2242.

55. Jenkins KJ, Correa A, Feinstein JA, et al. Noninherited risk factors and congenital cardiovascular defects: current knowledge: A scientific statement from the American Heart Association Council on Cardiovascular Disease in the Young: endorsed by the American Academy of Pediatrics. *Circulation*. 2007; 115(23): 2995–3014.

56. Jacob S, Nair AB. An updated overview on therapeutic drug monitoring of recent antiepileptic drugs. *Drugs R & D*. 2016; 16(4): 303–316.

57. Johannessen SI, Tomson T. Pharmacokinetic variability of newer antiepileptic drugs: when is monitoring needed? *Clinical Pharmacokinetics*. 2006; 45(11): 1061–1075.

58. Greenberg RG, Melloni C, Wu H, et al. Therapeutic index estimation of antiepileptic drugs: A systematic literature review approach. *Clinical Neuropharmacology*. 2016; 39(5): 232–240.

59. Westin AA, Nakken KO, Johannessen SI, Reimers A, Lillestolen KM, Brodtkorb E. Serum concentration/dose ratio of topiramate during pregnancy. *Epilepsia*. 2009; 50(3): 480–485.

60. Tomson T, Battino D. Pharmacokinetics and therapeutic drug monitoring of newer antiepileptic drugs during pregnancy and the puerperium. *Clinical Pharmacokinetics*. 2007; 46(3): 209–219.

61. Sabers A, Tomson T. Managing antiepileptic drugs during pregnancy and lactation. *Current Opinion in Neurology*. 2009; 22(2): 157–161.

62. McCarter-Spaulding DE. Medications in pregnancy and lactation. *MCN The American Journal of Maternal Child Nursing*. 2005; 30(1): 10–17, 18–19.

22

Postpartum Care for Women with Epilepsy

ELIZABETH FOUNTAINE, PATRICIA ROGERS, AND LYNN LIU

INTRODUCTION

The care for women with epilepsy (WWE) is often concentrated on the ante- and peripartum period. Most clinic visits focus on seizure control; however, WWE should also have annual discussions about fertility and contraception, counseling regarding teratogenic effects of medications and monitoring medication levels during pregnancy. Important health-care discussions for WWE included in this chapter include the care of WWE during the postpartum period—a time that WWE may feel abandoned without additional medical guidance.[1] An essential component of caring for WWE is to prepare women prior to delivery regarding potential postpartum challenges.

PERIPARTUM CARE

WWE often worry about having a seizure during labor or delivery, which is fortunately rare[2]. (See also Chapter 20.) WWE should continue regularly scheduled medications throughout the labor and delivery process as missing medications may increase the risk of seizure. All WWE should be placed on seizure precautions (padded side rails, bed on lowest position) for protection in the event of a seizure. Suction equipment should be available at the bedside for assistance in preventing aspiration of posterior pharyngeal secretions. Staff should be trained on patient care in the event of a seizure, which includes remaining calm and reassuring. (See Figure 22.1) The patient should not be restrained but must be confirmed to be in a safe location. Any potentially harmful objects including any loose or restraining items should be removed. The woman's head should be protected and they should be ideally turned to their left side to increase blood supply to the fetus[2] and prevent aspiration. Oxygen saturation should be monitored especially during the recovery period of a prolonged seizure for optimization of maternal and fetal status. A short acting

benzodiazepam, such as intravenous lorazepam, should be administered if the seizure does not resolve within two minutes.[2]

POSTPARTUM CARE

Every woman has a period of adjustment after delivery; however, WWE have additional concerns. Recovery from delivery, hormonal fluctuations, caring for a newborn, and sleep deprivation all put WWE at higher risk for seizures. Preparing WWE prior to delivery is essential to ensure the safety of both the mother and the infant. The physiological changes which occur immediately postpartum should be discussed with WWE so that they can anticipate these adjustments. These women may need additional social supports to allow them to attend to self-care and ensure sufficient sleep. All WWE should receive instruction on parental modifications to maintain safety for not only themselves but also their infant (see Figure 22.2).

The relatively rapid shifts of estrogen and progesterone, both of which have neuroactive properties, may alter a woman's seizure threshold. Additionally, these hormones interact with medications used to treat seizures. Over the course of the pregnancy, medication doses often must be titrated up to maintain adequate drug levels for seizure prevention. Providers should keep in mind that resolution of pregnancy physiology in the postpartum period will result in altered protein binding, hepatic glucuronidation, and altered excretion of medications. Without adjustments of drug doses, a WWE on seizure medications could potentially get toxic quickly. Individualized care plans regarding dose tapers and follow up laboratory studies should be made prior to delivery to guarantee patient safety as medications are brought back to pre-pregnancy levels. This plan should be available to the entire treatment team to ensure the new mother with epilepsy receives a consistent message. The patient should be instructed to put

1.	**Time:**	Note the start **time** of the seizure
	Protect from injury:	**Remove** any hard objects that could cause injury. Protect the head as best you can- place something soft under the head.
	DO NOT:	**DO NOT** attempt to restrain or to stop the jerking. **DO NOT** put anything in their mouth.
2.	**Gently roll:**	**Roll** person onto one side to keep the airway clear.
	Stay:	**Stay** with the person until the seizure ends naturally.
	Time:	**Note** the end **time** of the seizure.
3.	**Recover:**	**Calmly talk** to the person until they regain consciousness. Let them know where they are, that they are safe and that you are there.

FIGURE 22.1 Acute seizure care

Adapted from: Epilepsy Australia

http://www.epilepsyaustralia.net/seizure-first-aid/

copies of this plan in her delivery bag and in a highly visible place in her home. These schedules, where doses often change every few days to weeks, can be complicated to follow especially when a WWE is fatigued and her daily routine is interrupted by a newborn.

Providers should address reducing stressors in the home by ensuring that the significant other, family, or friends are available to help during this transition period. Sleep deprivation is frequently cited as a trigger for seizures. Mothers of newborns can easily become sleep deprived due to frequently interrupted sleep patterns. A plan should be implemented to ensure prolonged periods of nocturnal sleep. If the mother is struggling with loss of sleep due to breastfeeding, she may need to consider pumping to allow at least one overnight

feeding to be done by a support person. This will permit for one longer period of uninterrupted sleep. Allowing another person to provide a bottle at night or potentially supplementing with formula may be additional options. Assistance with other children and/or with household responsibilities can allow strategic napping while the baby sleeps during the day to aid in preventing fatigue. A support network at home can also promote the maintenance of other basic needs such as nutrition, hygiene, and exercise.

Despite the fact that WWE with need extra help and support, the social stigmatization of an epilepsy diagnosis often leaves WWE without the necessary social network. The Norwegian Maternal and Child Cohort Study[3] showed that WWE were more likely to have unplanned pregnancies and

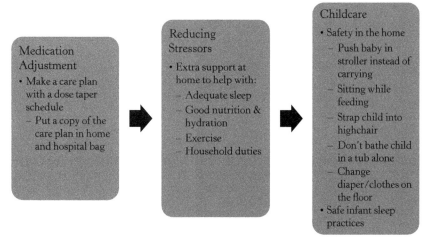

FIGURE 22.2 Care planning for WWE prior to delivery

were less likely to be in a relationship with the father of the baby. As a result, they often have the additional challenges of being a socially isolated single mother. Promoting accessible contraception and prioritizing family planning for WWE can help reduce unplanned pregnancies which in turn will allow WWE to defer pregnancy to a time in their lives when they feel supported and ready to parent.

Child Care

When a WWE is responsible for an infant, she should take additional precautions. Child-care courses do not typically address modifications for a parent with epilepsy. Furthermore, some WWE may not have the knowledge to care for an infant or know to ask for instruction. For example, a study in India examined if WWE would benefit from additional resources but implementation and acceptance were difficult in this culture.[4,5]

Modifications in routine care can allow WWE to remain responsible and participate in the care of infant(s). The Epilepsy Foundation recommends establishing parenting plans[6] (see Figure 22.2). WWE should not carry their baby long distances without supervision. Alternatively, the use an infant car seat or similarly reinforced baby carrier to ensure additional physical protection for the infant is recommended. If a WWE tends to fall with her seizures, then she may opt for a small umbrella stroller to move the infant from one area to another. When in the kitchen, the baby should not be placed near hot or sharp items. WWE should never hold a baby when cooking on the stove or when taking hot objects out of the microwave. She should not feed the baby while standing, instead she should sit where she can be supported: a chair, bed, or the floor. Like all children, the child should be strapped in when using a high chair or a booster seat. If a WWE does breastfeed during the night, she should keep the crib/bassinet at bedside to minimize night time arousals but should not sleep in bed with her infant.

It is recommended that a WWE never bathe their infant in a tub alone because the baby could be at risk of drowning if she were to lose awareness. If she needs to bathe her infant and no other adult is present, recommendations suggest giving a sponge bath instead of utilizing a tub. Changing diapers on the floor (rather than an elevated table) is the safest recommendation. If a changing table is used, then the baby should be strapped in to prevent falls. Additionally, keeping infant supplies on every floor minimizes the need to go up and down stairs. Having an enclosed area to prevent the child from wandering if a mother loses awareness during

a seizure provides an additional safety measure. Even young children can be taught to call an adult for help in the event of a seizure.

Most children of WWE are neurodevelopmentally normal. However, women who suffer from epilepsy do have an increased risk of having a child with a physical malformation or long-term cognitive issue. Based on the Neurodevelopmental Effects of Antiepileptic Drugs (NEAD) Study Group, the use of valproic acid during pregnancy can lead to lower cognitive function that endures beyond 6 years of age.[7–10] Caring for a child with developmental challenges adds additional difficulties that can overwhelm any new mother, but especially one with her own medical concerns. Without social support these women are at risk of losing the ability to independently care for their children.

Postpartum Depression

Women with epilepsy have higher rates of depression and anxiety and thus are at higher risk for depression in the postpartum period. Based on the Norwegian Maternal and Child Cohort Study,[3] these mothers report lower global life satisfaction and self-esteem. They have lower general self-efficacy, quality of somatic health, and relationship satisfaction. These women also have added work strain at the 18-month mark, noting that in Norway maternity leave lasts 10–12 months. WWE should be screened for depression readily and offered support as well as treatment options from behavioral therapy to medications (see also Chapter 34).

Breastfeeding

There are numerous neonatal and maternal advantages to breast feeding. WWE need to be aware that all seizure medications are found in breast milk but typically in concentrations lower than what the fetus was exposed to in utero. The drug concentrations in breast milk vary depending on the molecule size, protein binding properties, half-life, milk-to-plasma ratio, and oral bioavailability.[11] Breast feeding may benefit infants suffering from neonatal withdrawal syndrome secondary to exposure to phenobarbital, primidone, or benzodiazepines. Mothers choosing to breastfeed on anti-epileptic medications should be educated on the signs of infant toxicity including excessive sedation, irritability, or failure to thrive. Strategies to minimize exposures and toxicity risks include feeding immediately prior to dose administration (when medications are at trough), and timing doses to the longest period between feeds such as nighttime. The exact recommendations regarding breastfeeding will depend on the dosage and medications that a WWE is utilizing as well as any other prescriptions she is taking (see also Chapter 21). The NEAD group and the Norwegian Maternal and Child Cohort Study have shown no negative effect of breast feeding on intelligence quotient (IQ) of infants exposed to certain antiepileptic drugs (AED). In fact, the IQs of breastfed babies were found to be higher than the IQs of infants who were not breastfed.[12–14] Given the paucity of data and the conflicting reports, utilizing a national well-established breastfeeding service (OTIS or Lactation Study Center) to determine risk can help to individualize a plan for WWE (see also Chapter 35 for resources). A lactation consultation prior to delivery to establish a breastfeeding plan can also be helpful, both to assure that the mother is comfortable with initiating breastfeeding, as well as to optimize medication dosage and to develop a plan for infant assessment and monitoring.

Contraception

Assuring that women with epilepsy disorders do not become pregnant unexpectedly and have appropriately timed and spaced pregnancies requires that physicians discuss contraception. Given the challenges faced by WWE in the peripartum and postpartum period, contraception is pivotal for WWE so that they may have a planned pregnancy. Adjusting contraceptive plans with change or initiation of AEDs is essential (see Chapter 3 for full discussion of AED and contraceptive counseling).

Preventative health

Both pregnancy and breastfeeding states are strong utilizers of calcium and calcium stores. WWE are at increased risk of accelerated osteoporosis due to the prolonged use of medications used to treat seizures which alter bone metabolism. Therefore, WWE should take 1200 mg Calcium and 600 IU of Vitamin D daily to maximize bone density. Any women pregnant, breastfeeding, or contemplating pregnancy should take a daily vitamin with folate supplementation. (See Chapter 21 for risks/benefits of different AEDs in pregnancy).

CONCLUSION

During the postpartum period, WWE should be prepared for the changes in their bodies and new responsibilities (see Figure 22.3). Attending to changes in medication doses, established social supports for self and infant care and education about feeding choices are some of the things they may not know to ask and the treatment team should be prepared to provide. It is not too soon to anticipate future reproductive and bone health issues as well.

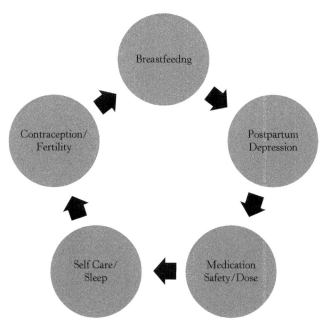

FIGURE 22.3 WWE postpartum care map

PROVIDER RESOURCES

Epilepsy Society
www.epilepsysociety.org.uk/pregnancy-and-parenting

UK Women with Epilepsy:
http://www.womenwithepilepsy.co.uk/

American Epilepsy Society:
https://www.aesnet.org/clinical_resources/women_with_epilepsy/reproductive_aged_women_with_epilepsy

World Health Organization
http://www.who.int/mental_health/mhgap/evidence/epilepsy/q11/en/

REFERENCES

1. Rousseau JB. Meeting the needs of the postpartum woman with epilepsy. MCN *Am J Matern Child Nurs*. 2008; 33: 84–89.
2. Gerard, E. & Samuels, P. Neurologic disorders in pregnancy. In: Gabbe, S., Nyebyl, J., Galan, H., et al. *Obstetrics: Normal and Problem Pregnancies*. 6th ed. Philadelphia: Saunders; 2006: 1030–1056.
3. Reiter SF, Bjørk MH, Daltveit AK, Veiby G, Kolstad E, Engelsen BA, Gilhus NE. Life satisfaction in women with epilepsy during and after pregnancy. *Epilepsy Behav*. 2016; 62: 251–257.
4. Saramma PP, Sarma PS, Thomas SV. Women with epilepsy have poorer knowledge and skills in child rearing than women without epilepsy. *Seizure*. 2011; 20: 575–579.
5. Saramma PP, Sarma PS, Thomas SV.Effect of a self-instructional module on the child rearing knowledge and practice of women with epilepsy. *Seizure*. 2014; 23: 424–428.
6. http://www.epilepsy.com/information/women/epilepsy-and-pregnancy/after-baby-born Accessed January 13, 2017.
7. Meador, KJ, Baker, GA, Browning, N, et al. Effects of fetal antiepileptic drug exposure Outcomes at age 4.5 years. *Neurology*. 2012; 78: 1207–1214.
8. Meador, KJ, Baker, GA, Browning, N, et al. Cognitive function at 3 years of age after fetal exposure to antiepileptic drugs. *New England Journal of Medicine*. 2009; 360: 1597–1605.
9. Meador, KJ, Baker, GA, Browning, N, et al. Effects of fetal antiepileptic drug exposure Outcomes at age 4.5 years. *Neurology*. 2012; 78: 1207–1214.
10. Meador KJ, Baker GA, Browning N, et al. Fetal antiepileptic drug exposure and cognitive outcomes at age 6 years (NEAD study): A prospective observational study. *Lancet Neurology*. 2013; 12: 244–252.
11. Davanzo R, Dal Bo S, Bua J, Copertino M, Zanelli E, Matarazzo L. Antiepileptic drugs and breastfeeding. *Italian Journal of Pediatrics*. 2013; 39: 50.
12. McVearry KM, Gaillard WD, VanMeter J, Meador KJ. A prospective study of cognitive fluency and originality in children exposed in utero to carbamazepine, lamotrigine, or valproate monotherapy. *Epilepsy Behav*. 2009; 16: 609–616.
13. Meador KJ, Baker GA, Browning N., et al. NEAD Study Group. Effects of breastfeeding in children of women taking antiepileptic drugs. *Neurology*. 2010; 75: 1954–1960.
14. Veiby G, Engelsen BA, Gilhus NE. Early child development and exposure to antiepileptic drugs prenatally and through breastfeeding: A prospective cohort study on children of women with epilepsy. *JAMA Neurol*. 2013; 70: 1367–1374.

23

Sleep Disorders and Pregnancy

LYNN LIU

INTRODUCTION

Sleep is an essential function to maintain health and wellness. Disruption and lack of sleep alters mood, reduces daytime functioning, and decreases quality of life. Furthermore, poor sleep affects physiological properties such as endocrine levels, immune function, and metabolic parameters resulting in increased morbidity and mortality. Sleep disorders are common in the general population, but the dynamic nature of pregnancy can put women in an increasingly vulnerable situation. Based on the National Sleep Foundation Poll in 2007,[1] 30% of pregnant women reported that they rarely or never got a good night's sleep and that 54% napped at least twice a week.

With the hormonal changes during the first trimester, women describe hypersomnia and increased sleep duration. By the third trimester, the increasingly gravid uterus, alterations in maternal physiology, and the anxiety related to pregnancy all affect the quality of sleep. Other physical changes such as fetal movements, nocturia, heartburn, cramps, and shortness of breath can further disrupt the continuity of sleep. The rapid physical and physiological changes that occur during pregnancy can result in the development or exacerbate underlying sleep disorders, with potential adverse consequences to both the mother and developing fetus. Some studies suggest increased obstetric complications such as pre-eclampsia, small for gestational age infants and increased use of cesarean sections in women who have unrecognized or under treated sleep disorders.

The International Sleep Disorders Classification-3[2] categorizes sleep disorders into several categories: insomnia, sleep-related breathing disorders, central disorders of hypersomnolence, circadian rhythm sleep-wake disorders, parasomnias, and sleep-related movement disorders. The most common disorders that can be influenced by pregnancy include: obstructive sleep apnea (OSA), restless legs syndrome (RLS), insomnia, and narcolepsy. At least 84% of pregnant women responded to the National Sleep Foundation in 2007[1] that they had insomnia a few days each week and 40% reported snoring, sleep apnea or RLS.

The presence of a multidisciplinary team aware of and screening for such disorders during prenatal care facilitates earlier recognition and treatment that should improve outcomes. Some disorders may be limited to pregnancy and resolve after delivery. Once identified, they should be referred to sleep medicine professionals for co-management since treatment options may be limited by teratogenicity of medications, feasibility of use, or potential to cross into breast milk. Informed management strategies can potentially change the overall quality of life for the mother, the outcome of the fetus, and the obstetric and anesthetic management during delivery.

OBSTRUCTIVE SLEEP APNEA SYNDROME

Definition: Obstructive sleep apnea (OSA), the most common form of sleep-related breathing disorder, is characterized by repeated narrowing of the upper airway resulting in apneas or hypopneas lasting more than 10 seconds.[2] Respiratory events can be associated with desaturations and/or arousals from sleep that disrupt the continuity of sleep and result in daytime sleepiness, fatigue, or insomnia symptoms. People with OSA will describe waking while choking or gasping, while their bed partners witness snoring and periods of apnea. OSA has been shown to affect 24% of adult men. Despite being considered a disorder of middle-aged men, it also affects 9% of adult women especially after menopause.[3] Women with OSA present with daytime sleepiness, morning headache, and unrefreshing sleep. Risk factors for OSA include obesity, large neck circumference, and narrowed upper airway anatomy. Repeated apneas triggers a cascade of both inflammatory and oxidative stress pathways that have been associated with hypertension, heart disease, stroke, diabetes mellitus type 2, and cognitive or mood disorders.[4] Diagnosis is made by overnight polysomnograms either at home or in the sleep laboratory.

Treatment typically targets the airway preventing obstruction due to reduced tone during sleep. Positional therapy, avoiding the supine position, prevents the posterior pharynx from dropping back and obstructing the airway. Weight loss is the most enduring treatment option but harder for most people to achieve. Continuous positive airway pressure (CPAP) therapy provides a pneumatic splint for the upper airway. Manipulations of the tongue and palate with devices and surgery are recommended for those who cannot tolerate the first line treatment options.

Issues related to pregnancy: Increasing levels of progesterone increase minute ventilation by modulating the central drive for breathing but can also enhance nasopharyngeal edema that narrows the upper airway predisposing to OSA. Weight gain and the gravid uterus limit the functional reserve capacity. Although a third of pregnant women snore, outcome studies suggest that isolated snoring may not lead to medical complications reported in OSA, so these two conditions should be distinguished.[5,6] These changes over the course of a pregnancy can result in new onset OSA but also increase the risk of hypertension, gestational diabetes, and pre-term labor among women who already have OSA.[7] Those who were considered obese prior to pregnancy have been shown to be at highest risk of having, developing, or exacerbating OSA over the course of the pregnancy.[8,9] They are also at higher risks of complications including gestational hypertension and pre-eclampsia.

Screening questionnaires such as the Berlin questionnaire, STOP, and STOP-BANG have been validated in the non-pregnant population, but they have had variable sensitivity and specificity in the pregnant population and may change over the course of the pregnancy.[10–12] In laboratory polysomnography (PSG) needs to be timely, and pregnant women find them cumbersome. Unattended studies can be considered as alternatives, and several portable devices such as the watch-PAT and the Apnea Risk Evaluation System (ARES) have been compared to in laboratory PSG with reasonable results.[13,14]

Since weight loss is not an option, pregnant women with OSA should avoid exacerbating factors such as sedatives and alcohol. Positional therapy by sleeping on their side or a seated position may be of benefit. CPAP has been recommended, but automated CPAP may be the best option given the potentially evolving nature of the disorder.

Management during delivery: Women with OSA should be considered at higher risk to anesthesia because they are more vulnerable to sedatives leading to apneas that cause hypoxemia and hypercapnia. One survey suggested only a minority of obstetric anesthesiologists screened for OSA. They screened only if the woman was obese or had essential hypertension.[15] When pregnant women with OSA deliver, obstetric anesthesiologists should be prepared to have a regional anesthetic plan minimizing the use of systemic sedatives since these women are more likely to require an urgent cesarean section. Post-operatively, these women should be screened for respiratory parameters and CPAP should be available if they are still sedated or fall asleep.

Maternal outcomes: Women diagnosed with OSA during the course of their pregnancy have higher rates of pre-eclampsia, gestational diabetes, and cesarean sections. Obese pregnant women who have OSA also have higher rates of pulmonary embolism and maternal mortality than those with obesity alone.[16] For some women, OSA is temporary and resolves after delivery. Sleep providers should continue to monitor weight loss, adjust the use of CPAP, and confirm resolution of OSA. If they continue to have OSA postpartum, they could be at risk for long-term cardiovascular complications, persistent daytime sleepiness, and lower quality of life.

Infant health outcomes: Review of the Taiwanese National Health Insurance Database suggested pregnant women with OSA are more likely to have cesarean sections[17] and have babies that are preterm, low birth weight, small for gestational age or have lower Apgars scores. Another study noted that neonates of mother's with OSA have more admissions to the neonatal intensive care unit for respiratory issues.[18] Due to the retrospective nature of these studies, these data may be biased and this area has been understudied.

Identifying and treating women with OSA has potential to improve the well-being of the mother and likely will positively influence the progress of the pregnancy and the development of the fetus (also see Box 23.1).

RESTLESS LEGS SYNDROME

Definition: Restless legs syndrome (RLS) is a sensorimotor disorder characterized by the urge

---

BOX 23.1
CARE MAP FOR PREGNANCY IN THE WOMEN WITH SLEEP-RELATED BREATHING DISORDERS

BEFORE PREGNANCY/PRE-PREGNANCY/NON-PREGNANT
Vital signs
  Height
  Weight
  Body mass index (BMI)
  Blood pressure
Screen for obstructive sleep apnea
  Sleepiness
    Epworth Sleepiness Scale
  Witnessed apneas
  Neck circumference
  OSA questionnaires
    STOP-BANG
    Berlin
    Wisconsin Sleep Questionnaire

DURING PREGNANCY
Weight monitoring
Blood pressure
Screen for gestational diabetes
Continue to screen for obstructive sleep apnea (as above)
If positive, test for sleep apnea (polysomnogram or home sleep testing)
If positive, treatment for sleep apnea
  Positional treatment
  Continuous positive airway pressure (CPAP)

DELIVERY
Weight monitoring
Blood pressure
Anesthesia consultation
Venous thromboembolism prophylaxis

POSTPARTUM
Schedule sleep medicine follow-up
Monitor for postpartum depression

---

to move the legs often due to uncomfortable or unpleasant sensations that are exacerbated by the seated or reclined position, improved with movement such as walking or stretching, and has a diurnal variation tending to be worse in the evening or at night disrupting sleep.[2] This clinical diagnosis is based on standardized criteria established by the International Restless Legs Syndrome Study Group (IRLSSG).[19] The pathophysiology is thought to be related to CNS iron deficiency and dopamine regulation. Iron and folate are co-factors for tyrosine hydroxylase, which is essential for the synthesis of dopamine. Early onset idiopathic RLS has been associated with an autosomal dominant inheritance pattern.[2] It affects 5–10% of Europeans and North Americans, but clinically significant symptoms that impair psychosocial, mental health, and sleep functions[19] affect only 2–3%. Secondary etiologies for RLS include iron deficiency, ESRD, peripheral neuropathy, and pregnancy.

In 2016 the American Academy of Neurology (AAN) released practice guidelines for the treatment of non-pregnant people with RLS.[20] Targets for treatment include iron supplementation, modulating the dopaminergic system, and pain control. They recommend assessing iron stores with hemoglobin, serum ferritin level, iron, TIBC, and percent saturation. Those with a serum ferritin less than 75 mg/L should be supplemented with ferrous sulfate with vitamin C. Dopaminergic agonists, ropinirole and pramipexole, improve the symptoms of RLS, and ropinirole could possibly improve anxiety associated with this condition. However, there is concern that treatment leads to augmentation of symptoms with symptoms presenting earlier in the day. Levodopa, does not have an FDA indication and clinically is not used much because of augmentation. Ergots were used in the past but not used currently due to risk of fibrotic reactions. If sleep complaints or anxiety are the primary issue, gabapentin, and pregabalin improve symptoms. Opioids are held in reserve for refractory severity RLS. No clear evidence supports non-pharmacological treatments such as near infra-red spectroscopy, pneumatic compression and vibrating pads, but transcranial direct current stimulation should be avoided.

Issues Related to Pregnancy

Nulliparous women have the same prevalence of RLS as men. Women over 35 years experience RLS twice as often as men, but this observation may be related to their parity. Women who have a history of gestational RLS have a fourfold increased risk of developing chronic RLS.[19] RLS is 2–3 times more prevalent during pregnancy than in the general population affecting 2.9–32% of pregnant women[21] and is more severe if there was a prior history of RLS. The incidence increases over the course of the pregnancy, peaks during the third trimester, and typically resolves within a month of delivery. The diagnosis should exclude mimics common during pregnancy including leg cramps, venous stasis, leg edema, compression/stretch neuropathies, sore leg muscles, ligament sprain/

tendon strain, and positional ischemia resulting in numbness.

During pregnancy estrogen and progesterone levels both increase peaking during the third trimester and falling postpartum. Both hormones are neuroactive steroids that interact in the dopaminergic system, though the exact mechanism remains unclear. Human chorionic gonadotropin stimulates the thyroid to release thyroid hormone early in pregnancy. Diminished dopamine increases thyroid hormone, but it is not clear if the reciprocal effect and the timing impact RLS.[22] The AAN practice guidelines do not address treatment options for pregnant women with RLS. The IRLSSG convened an expert panel to address this specific population.[23] Based on consensus opinion, iron status should be assessed, since iron stores become depleted during pregnancy. Oral replacement is recommended if serum ferritin levels are less than 75 mg/L but above 30 mg/L. If oral iron fails or the ferritin level falls below 30 mg/L then intravenous iron should be considered. In contrast to non-pregnant patients, the panel recommends avoiding exacerbating factors and nonpharmacological options despite the lack of data; pneumatic compression and massage may provide counter stimulation. Near-infrared spectroscopy utilizing light therapy alters nitrous oxide levels in the local vasculature thus increasing circulation and relieving symptoms.

There are no data on teratogenic effects of dopaminergic agents or infant outcomes. The panel could not recommend these as treatment options. If symptoms remained refractory and clinically significant, then low doses of carbidopa/levodopa could be considered based on small case reports of 18 parkinsonian women and 38 cases of RLS.[24] Alternatively, gabapentin is included as a variety of anti-epileptic drug registries that have shown a relative risk of 1.2 of fetal malformations in women with epilepsy.[25] If symptoms are very refractory, then clonazepam or opioids could be used despite the concerns of postnatal withdrawal.

Management during delivery: If the use of clonazepam or opioids is recommended, increased sedation or increased apneas should be taken into consideration with the anesthetic plan.

Maternal outcomes: For women who develop gestational RLS, the symptoms typically resolve within one month postpartum. For women who had the diagnosis prior to pregnancy and want to continue or resume their medications, they should discuss treatment options with their sleep provider or neurologist regarding the risks during lactation versus the benefit of improved sleep and quality of life. Since RLS is associated with a higher incidence of depression at baseline, monitor for postpartum depression and psychosocial support or pharmacological treatment should be considered.

Infant health outcomes: There is limited data on the outcome of infants of mothers who were medically treated for RLS. For infants of mothers who were taking clonazepam or opioids long term, providers should observe for neonatal abstinence syndrome. Many agents for RLS are small molecules and transfer into breast milk with potential exposure to the nursing infant. Dopamine agonists inhibit prolactin and may decrease breast milk production, particularly if used early in the postpartum period. Once the medication is discontinued, prolactin will rebound and can re-establish lactation. Gabapentin has measurable levels in breast milk, but the infant typically has efficient renal excretion to eliminate the drug rapidly. Clonazepam has a long half-life and can infant cause sedation, particularly when used in combination with other CNS depressants. An expert consensus guideline indicates that low-dose clonazepam may be an acceptable choice for RLS during breastfeeding, though infants should be monitored for sedation, development and weight gain.

Collaborating with sleep professionals may facilitate recognizing and treating peripartum RLS can improve quality of life for women who suffer from these uncomfortable symptoms and monitoring their progress postpartum (also see Box 23.2).

INSOMNIA

Definition: Insomnia is a common sleep disorder characterized by difficulty initiating and maintaining sleep and waking up earlier than desired that results in daytime consequences.[2] Women report insomnia more frequently than men. There may be a hormonal basis because symptoms exacerbate during menstrual cycle, menopause, and pregnancy. The physical and physiological changes during pregnancy further disrupt sleep. Insomnia can occur concurrently with depression, anxiety, and other medical conditions that should be addressed simultaneously and that can be further exacerbated by poor sleep.

Improved sleep hygiene and cognitive behavioral therapy have demonstrated durability of treatment effect over medications. Hypnotics can be used for short term insomnia or if behavioral management has not been helpful. Hypnotics are sedatives which help initiate and maintain sleep by working on the gamma-aminobutyric acid (GABA) receptor. Typical agents used include benzodiazepines, hypnotic benzodiazepine receptor agonists; zolpidem, zaleplon, and eszoplicone (z-drugs). Alternatively, sedative antidepressants have been used for the co-management of depression. Over the counter antihistamines are easily accessible and have low concerns of tolerance. There are limited data about the effects of any of these medications on pregnancy, risk of malformations, impact on delivery and postpartum effects.[26] There is even less data on the recently released sleep aids such as ramelteon or suvorexant.

Issues related to pregnancy: Sleep disruption increases over the course of the pregnancy for a variety of reasons, peaking in the third trimester.[27] As estrogen and progesterone levels rise over the course of pregnancy, they bind to steroid binding proteins, which compete and increase the free cortisol levels causing decreased arousal thresholds. Near-term increased oxytocin secretion further promotes wakefulness.

For a woman who has long-standing insomnia, thorough evaluation of sleep habits can provide insight into reasons for sleep disturbance. Avoidance of certain substances and behaviors can improve sleep quality. Active cognitive behavioral therapy with a sleep mental health provider has been shown enduring benefit. Identifying and addressing comorbid disorders such as anxiety and depression are improve quality of life. None of the medications used to treat insomnia have been tested in the pregnant population. There are concerns that they may have negative consequences to both the developing fetus and the mother. Based on the National Health Insurance Database in Taiwan, 2497 women taking zolpidem had infants that were small for gestational age, preterm births, and may have had more cesarean sections compared to 12,485 women who did not use this medication.[28] Similar results in a retrospective review of 390 women who had prescriptions for hypnotics in the Swedish Medical Birth Registry found low birth weight infants that were more likely to be preterm.[29] There have not been any systematic studies of the use of benzodiazepines in the setting of insomnia.

BOX 23.2
CARE MAP FOR PREGNANCY IN THE WOMEN
WITH RESTLESS LEGS SYNDROME

BEFORE PREGNANCY/PRE-PREGNANCY/NON-PREGNANT
Review essential diagnostic criteria (see Chapter 19)
Avoid exacerbating factors
  Prolonged immobility
  Caffeine
  Tobacco
  Alcohol
Avoid certain medications
  Serotonergic antidepressants
  Sedating antihistamines
  Dopaminergic antagonists (antiemetics, antipsychotics)
Consider discontinuing or using lowest effective medication and dose

DURING PREGNANCY
Avoid exacerbating factors (see above)
Non-pharmacological options
  Moderate exercise
  Massage/pneumatic compression
  Near-infrared spectroscopy
Check hemoglobin, serum ferritin level, iron, TIBC, and % saturation
  If less than 30 mg/L → IV iron
  If less than 75 mg/L → 65 mg elemental iron once or twice a day
  If greater than 75 mg/L consider alternative therapies
Check folate and if low consider folate supplementation
Pharmacological options reserved for refractory RLS
  Carbidopa/levodopa 25/100–50/200 mg in the evening
  Clonazepam 0.25–1 mg in the evening
  Low dose oxycodone (after first trimester)

DELIVERY
Anesthesia consultation
Pain management

POSTPARTUM
Review iron status
Lactation consult—avoid dopaminergic agonists
Reassess medications within a month
Monitor for postpartum depression
Schedule neurology follow-up

Management during delivery: Women with untreated insomnia are less able to tolerate pain and have higher rates of emergent cesarean sections.

Maternal outcomes: Due to high concurrence of insomnia and depression, women with insomnia should be screened carefully for postpartum depression.

Infant health outcomes: Hypnotic medications cross the placenta and can accumulate in the fetus, but they have low rates of teratogenic effects based on registry data. None of the children of women taking zolpidem in the Taiwanese database had major congenital malformations.[28] Concerns have been raised specifically about alprazolam due to its ability to cross the placenta and teratogenic properties.[26] With prolonged exposure to benzodiazepines, an infant should be evaluated for neonatal withdrawal syndrome. There are no data on postnatal neurobehavioral effects of benzodiazepines or any other hypnotic. With some of the long-term or later use of antidepressant medications, during pregnancy for depression, there may be increased rates of major congenital malformations.[30] Specific reports suggest that providers watch for Selective Serotonin Reuptake Inhibitor (SSRI) neonatal behavioral syndrome that is characterized by respiratory, motor, central nervous system and gastrointestinal symptoms.[26] The use of antihistamines during pregnancy has not been rigorously studied.

For breastfeeding mothers, attention must be paid to sleep safety and monitoring the infant for possible sedation from any medications the mother may take. Zolpidem and zaleplon have low levels in breast milk and short half lives and are unlikely to affect the breastfeeding infant, though there is less evidence for eszoplicone. SSRIs are commonly used in breastfeeding, with a preference for sertraline and paroxetine. For benzodiazepines, a choice with low levels in breast milk and a short half life, such as lorazepam, is preferred for breastfeeding mothers.

Insomnia impacts quality of life and can change physiology especially during pregnancy, but the use of medications have been understudied and have potential consequences to pregnancy and fetal development (also see Box 23.3).

NARCOLEPSY

Definition: Narcolepsy is a disorder of central hypersomnia characterized by excessive daytime sleepiness and dysregulation of rapid eye movement (REM) sleep. The hallmark of narcolepsy, cataplexy is a sudden loss of muscle tone with retained consciousness typically triggered by strong positive emotions (laughter). The weakness can present as subtly as brief head drops, jaw sagging, or dysarthria. Additional clinical features include sleep paralysis, persistent atonia during the sleep-wake transition; hypnagogic hallucinations, dreamlike visual and/or auditory experiences in the wake to sleep transition; and sleep-onset REM periods (SOREMP). Narcolepsy affects 0.02% to 0.18% of the United States and western European populations between 15 and 40 years that overlaps child bearing age.[2]

An autoimmune mechanism of narcolepsy has been postulated as causing a deficiency of hypothalamic hypocretin-1 (orexin) neurons, which regulates sleep and appetite. The diagnosis is based on the clinical history; polysomnogram (PSG) followed by multiple sleep latency test (MSLT), and low hypocretin-1(orexin) levels for type-1 narcolepsy. The presence of HLA DQB1*0602 suggests but does not confirm the diagnosis. Narcolepsy can occur concurrently with obstructive sleep apnea, PLMS, and REM behavior disorders.[2]

Treatment for this Condition

Treatment strategies manage the symptoms of narcolepsy and are divided into behavioral techniques, wake-promoting medications, and anticataplectic medications. People with narcolepsy feel better when they have short scheduled naps. When they need to be awake for prolonged periods of time amphetamines, methylphenidate, modafinil, and armodafinil can been used. Minimizing the events of cataplexy can be achieved with antidepressants and sodium oxybate. The anticholinergic properties of antidepressants may modify motor pathways, but other medications without this mechanism have been effective also.

Issues related to pregnancy: There are no evidence based data or guidelines on the management of women with narcolepsy during pregnancy. The recommendations are based on a retrospective survey of women with narcolepsy,[31] a survey of providers caring for women with narcolepsy who became pregnant,[32] case reports and expert opinions.[33] Women taking hormonal contraception should know that as an enzyme inducer of the cytochrome P450 system modafinil may lower levels of ethinyl estradiol resulting in an increased risk of pregnancy.[34] Based on patient experience and provider survey, withdrawal of medications prior to pregnancy was recommended. The majority of the medications only have animal data to suggest harm to the fetus, but there are no controlled data in humans. Europe has organized pregnancy registries to collect these data, and the company for Nuvigil and Provigil has

---

BOX 23.3
CARE MAP FOR PREGNANCY IN THE WOMEN WITH INSOMNIA

BEFORE PREGNANCY/PRE-PREGNANCY/NON-PREGNANT

Review basic sleep hygiene
- Develop a bedtime routine.
- Maintain a regular sleep schedule.
- Avoid naps if possible.
- Establish a quiet, comfortable bedroom.
- Do not remain awake for more than 15–20 minutes.
- Do not watch TV or read in bed.
- Drink caffeinated drinks with caution.
- Avoid substances that interfere with sleep. (alcohol, smoking, etc.)
- Exercise regularly.
- If you watch the clock at night, hide it.

Consider referral to Behavioral Sleep Medicine for cognitive behavioral therapy (CBT)
Review medications use for insomnia
   Discuss potential teratogenic effects and impact on pregnancy and delivery

DURING PREGNANCY

Weight monitoring
Re-enforce sleep hygiene and CBT techniques

DELIVERY

Anesthesia consultation
Pain management

POSTPARTUM

Plan for social support to care for infant
Contraception counseling
Lactation consult
Schedule behavioral sleep medicine follow-up
Medication adjustments
Monitor for postpartum depression

---

established their own pregnancy registry.[35] Women should be advised to taper medications because abrupt withdrawal of anticataplectic medications can result in "status cataplecticus" with prolonged or repeated loss of tone.[36]

Despite the presumed autoimmune etiology, it is not clear that pregnancy exacerbates or improves the course of narcolepsy as it may in other autoimmune disorders. Based on survey data, it was noted that women with narcolepsy and cataplexy were more likely to have a higher body mass index (BMI) prior to pregnancy, have a higher rate of weight gain during the pregnancy, and impaired glucose metabolism and anemia compared to women who did not have cataplexy or the general population. Theoretically, this observation could be related to hypocretin (orexin) deficiency, which also regulates appetite. If the symptoms became intolerable, some women with narcolepsy continue on medications through their pregnancy or restart medications later in the pregnancy.

Management during delivery: The patient survey suggested that overall there were higher

---

BOX 23.4
CARE MAP FOR PREGNANCY IN THE WOMEN WITH NARCOLEPSY

BEFORE PREGNANCY/PRE-PREGNANCY/NON-PREGNANT

Contraceptive counseling

  Modafinil induction of cytochrome P450 can decrease effectiveness of hormonal
    contraception

Genetic counseling (consider HLA DQB1*0602 or orexin levels)

Behavioral treatment plan with scheduled naps

  May need to restrict driving, if falling sleep behind the wheel.

Medications adjustment, consolidation and review

  Abrupt withdrawal may precipitate increased sleepiness and cataplexy

If elevated body mass index (BMI), may consider dietary consultation

DURING PREGNANCY

Vital signs

  Height

  Weight

  Body mass index (BMI)

  Blood pressure

Modification of behavioral plan

Adjust medications for severe symptoms

Monitor for worsening of symptoms: excessive sleepiness and cataplexy

Lactation consultation, if on medications

DELIVERY

Anesthesia consultation

Prepare for cesarean section if cataplexy becomes severe

POSTPARTUM

Plan for social support to care for infant

Contraception counseling

Lactation consult

Schedule sleep medicine follow-up

Medication adjustments

Monitor for postpartum depression

---

rates of cesarean sections in women with narcolepsy and cataplexy.[31] The literature only describes 2 cases of women who had status catapleticus during delivery who were not able to progress through a normal vaginal delivery and where the decision was made to proceed to cesarean section.[36] Despite this information, the risk of cataplexy interfering with a normal vaginal delivery appears to be low.

Maternal outcomes: For women who continue the use of sodium oxybate there is a concern for potential interactions with anesthetic agents that put the woman at increased risk of apnea or sedation.

Infant health outcomes: Based on retrospective survey data, the majority of infants born to women with narcolepsy did well, but the data were subject to recall bias.[32] Recommendations for breast feeding were also conservative because of the lack of data. There have been reports of mothers with narcolepsy successfully breastfeeding while taking sodium oxybate. It is recommended that the mother abstain from breastfeeding for 4-6 hours after doses, and pumping to maintain supply or substitute a feeding may be necessary. Both the American Academy of Pediatrics and American College of Obstetrics and Gynecology do not recommend breastfeeding concurrently with the use of amphetamines as they would not recommend it for any drug of potential abuse. Animal data for modafinil suggest that levels are higher in milk than plasma but long-term effect of exposure is not known and there is no data in humans. The use of antidepressants for the treatment of narcolepsy during pregnancy also lacks data. Antidepressants have been shown to increase risk of major congenital malformations in pregnant women with depression. Although data suggests that the use of SSRI and SNRI during lactation and breastfeeding can be safe in the short term, the possible long term side consequences are not known. If needed, preferred SSRIs for breastfeeding include sertraline and paroxetine.

Narcolepsy is a condition that affects women of childbearing age. They should be counseled on family planning and that some of their medications may make their contraceptives less effective, choices regarding behavioral versus medical management during pregnancy and infant feeding and care (also see Box 23.4).

CONCLUSION

Pregnant women have disruption in their sleep as their body and physiology change, but they are also at risk for sleep disorders and should be screened for common sleep disorders. Women with prior sleep disorders should discuss management strategies with both their obstetrician and sleep provider. Collaborating with sleep professionals can improve the quality of life for the pregnant woman and potentially improve maternal and fetal outcomes.

REFERENCES

1. https://sleepfoundation.org/sites/default/files/Summary_Of_Findings%20-%20FINAL.pdf. Accessed February 14, 2017
2. American Academy of Sleep Medicine. International classification of sleep disorders. 3rd ed. Darien, IL: American Academy of Sleep Medicine; 2014.
3. Young T, Palta M, Dempsey J, Peppard PE, Nieto FJ, Hla KM. Burden of sleep apnea: Rationale, design, and major findings of the Wisconsin Sleep Cohort Study. WMJ: Official Publication of the State Medical Society of Wisconsin. 2009; 108(5): 246–249.
4. Shahar E, Whitney CW, Redline S, et al. Sleep-disordered breathing and cardiovascular disease: Cross-sectional results of the Sleep Heart Health Study. Am J Respir Crit Care Med. 2001; 163(1): 19–25.
5. O'Brien LM, Bullough AS, Chames MC, et al. Hypertension, snoring, and obstructive sleep apnoea during pregnancy: A cohort study. BJOG. 2014; 121(13): 1685–1693.
6. Bourjeily G, Fung JY, Sharkey KM, et al. Airflow limitations in pregnant women suspected of sleep-disordered breathing. Sleep Med. 2014; 15(5): 550–555.
7. Pien GW, Pack AI, Jackson N, Maislin G, Macones GA, Schwab RJ. Risk factors for sleep-disordered breathing in pregnancy. Thorax. 2014; 69(4): 371–377.
8. Facco FL, Parker CB, Reddy UM, et al. Association between sleep-disordered breathing and hypertensive disorders of pregnancy and gestational diabetes mellitus. Obstet Gynecol. 2017; 129(1): 31–41.
9. Rice JR, Larrabure-Torrealva GT, Luque Fernandez MA, et al. High risk for obstructive sleep apnea and other sleep disorders among overweight and obese pregnant women. BMC Pregnancy Childbirth. 2015; 15: 198.
10. Tantrakul V, Sirijanchune P, Panburana P, et al. Screening of obstructive sleep apnea during pregnancy: Differences in predictive values of questionnaires across trimesters. J Clin Sleep Med. 2015; 11(2): 157–163.
11. Tantrakul V, Numthavaj P, Guilleminault C, McEvoy M, Panburana P, Khaing W, Attia J, Thakkinstian A. Performance of screening questionnaires for obstructive sleep apnea during pregnancy: A systematic review and meta-analysis. Sleep Med Rev. 2017; 36: 96–106.
12. Antony KM, Agrawal A, Arndt ME, et al. Obstructive sleep apnea in pregnancy: Reliability of prevalence and prediction estimates. J Perinatol. 2014; 34(8): 587–593.
13. O'Brien LM, Bullough AS, Shelgikar AV, Chames MC, Armitage R, Chervin RD. Validation of Watch-PAT-200 against polysomnography during pregnancy. J Clin Sleep Med. 2012; 8(3): 287–294.
14. Sharkey KM, Waters K, Millman RP, Moore R, Martin SM, Bourjeily G. Validation of the Apnea Risk Evaluation System (ARES) device against laboratory polysomnography in pregnant women at risk for obstructive sleep apnea syndrome. J Clin Sleep Med. 2014; 10(5): 497–502.
15. Abdullah HR, Nagappa M, Siddiqui N, Chung F. Diagnosis and treatment of obstructive sleep apnea during pregnancy. Curr Opin Anaesthesiol. 2016; 29(3): 317–324.

16. Louis J, Auckley D, Miladinovic B, et al. Perinatal outcomes associated with obstructive sleep apnea in obese pregnant women. *Obstet Gynecol.* 2012; 120(5): 1085–1092.

17. Chen YH, Kang JH, Lin CC, Wang IT, Keller JJ, Lin HC. Obstructive sleep apnea and the risk of adverse pregnancy outcomes. *Am J Obstet Gynecol.* 2012; 206(2): 136.e1–5.

18. Fung AM, Wilson DL, Barnes M, Walker SP. Obstructive sleep apnea and pregnancy: The effect on perinatal outcomes. *J Perinatol.* 2012; 32(6): 399–406.

19. Allen RP, Picchietti DL, Garcia-Borreguero D, et al. International Restless Legs Syndrome Study Group. Restless legs syndrome/Willis-Ekbom disease diagnostic criteria: Updated International Restless Legs Syndrome Study Group (IRLSSG) consensus criteria—history, rationale, description, and significance. *Sleep Med.* 2014; 15(8): 860–873.

20. Winkelman JW, Armstrong MJ, Allen RP, et al. Practice guideline summary: Treatment of restless legs syndrome in adults: Report of the Guideline Development, Dissemination, and Implementation Subcommittee of the American Academy of Neurology. *Neurology.* 2016; 87(24): 2585–2593.

21. Srivanitchapoom P, Pandey S, Hallett M. Restless legs syndrome and pregnancy: A review. *Parkinsonism Relat Disord.* 2014; 20(7): 716–722.

22. Grover A, Clark-Bilodeau C, D'Ambrosio CM. Restless leg syndrome in pregnancy. *Obstet Med.* 2015; 8(3): 121–125.

23. Picchietti DL, Hensley JG, Bainbridge JL, et al. Consensus clinical practice guidelines for the diagnosis and treatment of restless legs syndrome/Willis-Ekbom disease during pregnancy and lactation. *Sleep Med Rev.* 2015; 22: 64–77.

24. Dostal M, Weber-Schoendorfer C, Sobesky J, Schaefer C. Pregnancy outcome following use of levodopa, pramipexole, ropinirole, and rotigotine for restless legs syndrome during pregnancy: A case series. *Eur J Neurol.* September 2013; 20(9): 1241–1246. doi: 10.1111/ene.12001.

25. http://www.aedpregnancyregistry.org/wp-content/uploads/2016-newsletter-Winter-2016.pdf. Accessed February 24, 2017.

26. Okun ML, Ebert R, Saini B. A review of sleep-promoting medications used in pregnancy. *Am J Obstet Gynecol.* 2015; 212(4): 428–441.

27. Reichner CA. Insomnia and sleep deficiency in pregnancy. *Obstet Med.* 2015; 8(4): 168–171.

28. Wang LH, Lin HC, Lin CC, Chen YH, Lin HC. Increased risk of adverse pregnancy outcomes in women receiving zolpidem during pregnancy. *Clin Pharmacol Ther.* 2010; 88(3): 369–374.

29. Wikner BN, Stiller CO, Bergman U, Asker C, Källén B. Use of benzodiazepines and benzodiazepine receptor agonists during pregnancy: Neonatal outcome and congenital malformations. *Pharmacoepidemiol Drug Saf.* 2007; 16(11): 1203–1210.

30. Bérard A, Iessa N, Chaabane S, Muanda FT, Boukhris T, Zhao JP. The risk of major cardiac malformations associated with paroxetine use during the first trimester of pregnancy: A systematic review and meta-analysis. *Br J Clin Pharmacol.* 2016; 81(4): 589–604.

31. Maurovich-Horvat E, Tormášiová M, Slonková J, et al. Assessment of pregnancy outcomes in Czech and Slovak women with narcolepsy. *Med Sci Monit.* 2010; 16(12): SR35–40.

32. Thorpy M, Zhao CG, Dauvilliers Y. Management of narcolepsy during pregnancy. *Sleep Med.* 2013; 14(4): 367–376.

33. Hoque R, Chesson AL Jr. Conception, pregnancy, delivery, and breastfeeding in a narcoleptic patient with cataplexy. *J Clin Sleep Med.* 2008; 4(6): 601–603.

34. Hoover-Stevens S, Kovacevic-Ristanovic R. Management of narcolepsy in pregnancy. *Clin Neuropharmacol.* 2000; 23(4): 175–181.

35. https://clinicaltrials.gov/ct2/show/NCT01792583. Accessed February 14, 2017.

36. Ping LS, Yat FS, Kwok WY. Status cataplecticus leading to the obstetric complication of prolonged labor. *J Clin Sleep Med.* 2007; 3(1): 56–57.

SECTION 4

Neuromuscular, Spinal Cord, and Metabolic Disorders

24

Neuromuscular Diseases

Myasthenia Gravis, Spinal Muscular Atrophy, Nondystrophic Myotonias, and Muscular Dystrophies

JOHANNA HAMEL AND EMMA CIAFALONI

ABSTRACT

Myasthenia gravis is an acquired autoimmune disorder characterized by weakness of skeletal muscle, which often affects women in the childbearing age. A number of questions arise when a woman with myasthenia gravis plans to become pregnant or presents with pregnancy, as myasthenia can affect the pregnancy, delivery and the fetus. In addition, the pregnancy can affect the course of myasthenia and worsening of the disease during pregnancy may require treatment modifications. Therefore supportive counseling, ideally preceding conception, is indicated, focusing on issues of fertility, treatment optimization and drug safety, risks of worsening of symptoms during pregnancy and delivery. Counseling on possible effects on the infant should be discussed, as such as neonatal myasthenia gravis, a treatable and transient disease. Patients with myasthenia gravis may require more intensive monitoring and care, and should be supported by a multidisciplinary team involving the obstetrician, anesthesiologist, and neurologist.

PREGNANCY IN MYASTHENIA GRAVIS

Brief Overview

Myasthenia gravis (MG) is an acquired autoimmune disorder characterized by weakness of skeletal muscle due to antibodies against the nicotinic acetylcholine receptor (AchR Ab) or other postsynaptic antigens (muscle specific tyrosine kinase [MuSK-Ab]). The weakness can involve ocular (diplopia and ptosis), bulbar (speech and swallowing) and proximal muscles of the shoulder and hip girdle. Symptoms fluctuate and the weakness is fatigable, typically worse at the end of the day or with exercise. The diagnosis is confirmed by positive antibody detection in the patient's blood sample. In seronegative patients electrodiagnostic testing (repetitive nerve stimulation test or single-fiber electromyography) confirms dysfunction of the neuromuscular junction. Treatment includes choline esterase inhibitors (pyridostigmine), which can be sufficient as symptomatic monotherapy for mild cases of generalized MG or MG involving the ocular muscles only. However, many patients with generalized MG require treatment with immunosuppressive agents (corticosteroids, azathioprine, mycophenolate mofetil, and others). Thymectomy has been shown to improve clinical outcomes and reduce use of immunosuppressive agents and is recommended for patients under the age of 65.[1] Symptoms of MG can be exacerbated by infections, medications, anesthesia, pregnancy, and postpartum. An exacerbation with weakness severe enough to necessitate intubation is considered a myasthenic crisis, which can be life threatening. The disease is more common in women than men and can occur at any age. Female incidence peaks in the third decade, affecting women in their childbearing age. When counseling and caring for the patient prior, during and after a pregnancy, knowledge of the effects of pregnancy on myasthenia gravis and vice versa, the risks of the fetus and drug safety is key. Most recommendations are based on retrospective analysis, observational or animal studies and prospective studies are rare. Safety data of medications used in MG is sparse, but information can be extracted from experience in other more common autoimmune conditions or organ transplant recipients. This article addresses questions that will occur when counseling and treating a woman with MG in the childbearing age.

Fertility

MG itself does not affect fertility. However treatment with immunosuppressive therapy can affect fertility. Most recommendations are based on retrospective analysis, observational or animal studies. Methotrexate and mycophenolate mofetil (MMF) do not seem to have repercussions on female fertility, but both drugs are contraindicated when a pregnancy is desired. MMF should be discontinued 6 weeks prior to conception.[2] Methotrexate should be discontinued 3 months prior to conception. Azathioprine and corticosteroids do not seem to have a detrimental effect on fertility.[3]

Pregnancy Planning and Counseling

Patients with MG can have a normal pregnancy and delivery.[4] However, pregnancy presents a commitment not only to physical requirements but may include the need for treatment modifications and closer monitoring through an interdisciplinary team of obstetricians, neurologists and neonatologists. Parenthood may add additional challenges for patients with MG. Therefore, counseling about pregnancy should begin early and be offered during routine clinic visits. Family planning should be part of the discussion when choosing an immunosuppressive therapy. Optimization of myasthenic status prior to conception is the goal, to minimize the need for immunosuppressive therapy. If thymectomy is indicated, this should be planned prior to the pregnancy to achieve optimal control of the disease.[5] Thymectomy was also shown to be associated with a lower likelihood of neonatal myasthenia in the infant,[4,6] but did not show an influence on other pregnancy outcome measures (such as severity of symptoms, use of medication and complications with delivery).[6]

Pregnancy

Influence of the pregnancy on MG

Pregnancy does not worsen the long-term outcome of MG.[7] The course of the disease during a pregnancy is variable and unpredictable, independent of severity of symptoms prior to conception and can change in subsequent pregnancies.[7] Approximately one-third of women experience an exacerbation of symptoms, mostly in the first trimester or postpartum.[7,8] Improvement in symptoms or even complete remission can be seen in the second or third trimester, thought to be related to the physiologic immunosuppression induced by high level of AFP that occurs during those phases of gestation.[4,9,10] Frequent emesis may interfere with absorption of oral medications.

The growing fetus may restrict the diaphragm and compromise respiratory function.[8] Myasthenia gravis can exacerbate with infections and with medications, such as certain antibiotics (eg, fluoroquinolones). Infections should be treated promptly and the patient counseled on medications that should be avoided as possible.

MG as a new diagnosis during pregnancy

The onset of MG can be triggered during pregnancy or postpartum. In one study 12% of mothers with MG developed their first symptoms or were diagnosed during their first pregnancy.[6] In a cross-sectional case controlled study from Norway, pregnancy preceded the onset of MG in 15%. The postpartum period, specifically the first 3 months after birth of the first child, was associated with a significant increase in risk for the onset of clinical symptoms of MG (relative risk 5.5)[11] and some present with myasthenic crisis.[12] The underlying mechanisms remain uncertain, fluctuations in estrogen levels or drop of alpha feto protein levels have been suggested.

During pregnancy, the diagnostic workup for suspected MG includes AChR- antibody testing. If negative, anti-muscle specific kinase (Musk) should be measured, which are positive in 38 to 50% of patients with generalized MG with negative AChR-antibodies, predominantly in females. Positive antibodies in a patient with clinically suspected MG are diagnostic. If a patient is antibody negative, electrophysiologic testing with repetitive nerve stimulation or single-fiber EMG can confirm dysfunction of the neuromuscular junction and are safely performed during pregnancy. Chest imaging to look for thymoma can be postponed until after the delivery, as thymectomy has no role during pregnancy, due to the delayed effect a benefit would unlikely occur during pregnancy.[13]

Influence of MG on the pregnancy and the fetus

The rate of spontaneous abortion is not increased in MG.[6] A study examining adverse pregnancy outcomes in 163 women with MG in Taiwan found no statistically significant difference between woman with and without MG with regards to the risk of preterm or low birth weight and births of infants small for gestational age.[14]

Treatment of MG and drug safety during pregnancy

For women who have not achieved or sustained remission, controlling symptoms and avoiding exacerbations, complications, and myasthenic crisis depends on appropriate medical therapy—with the goal of a successful and uncomplicated pregnancy. Therefore, the individualized treatment plan depends on the patient's severity and distribution of muscle weakness. Muscle weakness, involving bulbar and respiratory muscles, generally requires more aggressive treatment given the potential to be life threatening to the mother and fetus. A number of medications can be safely continued during pregnancy and patient's require reassurance and counseling on drug safety, as well as counseling on potential risk of exacerbation by discontinuing therapy. The risk of triggering a MG exacerbation by discontinuing or reducing a medication needs to be outweighed against the possible risk to the fetus. Symptomatic treatment with oral *pyridostigmine* with doses less than 600 mg/day is safe for the fetus. IV choline esterase inhibitors may produce uterine contractions and should not be used during pregnancy.[13] For mild cases, symptomatic treatment with choline esterase inhibitors may be sufficient, but the majority of patients with generalized myasthenia not in remission require immunosuppressive therapy. *Corticosteroids* (prednisone) is the treatment of choice during pregnancy. Prednisone presents little if any teratogenic risk to the fetus and only a slight increased risk of cleft palate when used in the first trimester.[9] Premature rupture of the membranes and gestational diabetes may be associated with higher doses of corticosteroids.[2] Other immunosuppressive therapies should not be initiated as a new medication during pregnancy, due to the long latency of effect. Azathioprine and cyclosporine are considered relatively safe in pregnancy. While *azathioprine* has been shown to be teratogenic in animals, no increased risk of congenital malformations has been demonstrated in humans at therapeutic dosages.[2,15] One potential explanation has been that, while azathioprine crosses the placenta, the fetus may lack the enzyme to convert azathioprine to the active 6-marcaptopurine.[2] However, fetal immunosuppression and pancytopenia, intrauterine growth restriction, and preterm delivery have been associated with azathioprine use.[2] *Cyclosporine* has not demonstrated teratogenicity, but intrauterine growth restriction may be seen. Medications that should not be used in pregnancy include *mycophenolate mofetil* (MMF) and *methotrexate*: MMF has been associated with an increased risk of miscarriage and increased number of malformations (microtia, orofacial cleft). Methotrexate has been shown to be teratogenic and associated with an increased rate of miscarriages.[2,15] There is limited data on the safe use of Rituximab in pregnancy and this medication should be replaced by alternate therapy prior to conception.[15] Immunoglobulines (IVIG) and plasmapheresis can be used to control symptoms of MG that do not respond to corticosteroids or pyridostigmine, and to manage myasthenic crisis in pregnancy. The safety of IVIG in pregnancy has not been investigated in MG but has been well documented in other disorders including neurological autoimmune conditions such as multiple sclerosis.[16] Side effects such as hyperviscosity and volume overload may be more important in pregnancy. Theoretically, plasmapheresis may induce premature delivery because of large hormonal shifts (Box 24.1).[7]

Treatment of MG and drug safety during lactation

Breastfeeding is encouraged for at least the first 6 months of an infant's life. The role of breastfeeding and its effect on MG has not been studied, although there is no evidence of a harmful effect. On the contrary, in a retrospective case controlled study examining new onset MG during pregnancy and postpartum, prolonged breastfeeding seemed to postpone the onset of new clinical symptoms of MG.[11] While it is generally recommended to avoid medications while breastfeeding, this is not an option for active MG, specifically within the vulnerable time of puerperium which is associated with an increased risk of exacerbations. Exposure to corticosteroids during breastfeeding has not been associated with negative side effects in the newborn.[17] Azathioprine exposure during breastfeeding did not reveal adverse effects on exposed children, similar to cyclosporine.[17] Data on breastfeeding safety while taking Mycophenolate mofetil are scarce. Overall, woman taking cyclosporine or azathioprine should not be discouraged from breastfeeding but should avoid breastfeeding close to peak serum concentration (ie, aim to breastfeed approximately 4 hours after the last dose).[2] If the infant is exhibiting effects of the medication, drug levels can be obtained for monitoring of exposure. Limited data exists for safety of Rituximab and breastfeeding, however, due to the large molecular weight and low oral bioavailability, it is unlikely to pass into breastmilk in sufficient quantities to affect infants. Given the lack of evidence, neonates and preterm infants should be closely monitored if their mother requires Rituximab (Table 24.1).

BOX 24.1
CARE MAP FOR PREGNANCY IN THE PATIENT WITH MG

Care Principles
- Family planning should be addressed in each patient of childbearing age and therapy modification considered prior to planning a pregnancy
- Treatment goal is minimal disease activity in the mother and minimal risk for harm to the fetus
- Risk of drug exposure for the fetus needs to be weighed against the risk of untreated maternal disease resulting in exacerbation or crisis
- Treatment decisions should be shared among neurologist, obstetrician and patient

Before pregnancy/pre-pregnancy/non-pregnant

Review of prior pregnancy complications:
- Transient muscle weakness during pregnancy, ocular or bulbar symptoms
- If history of arthrogryposis, counsel about increased risk of recurrence
- Educate about signs and symptoms of Transient Neonatal muscle weakness, difficulty feeding, hypotonia

Confirmation of neurological diagnosis:
- Positive antibody testing (AchR Ab, anti-Musk), positive electrodiagnostic testing
- Counseling on the diagnosis (medications to avoid, symptoms of crisis, triggers of exacerbation)

Assessment of myasthenic status:
- Symptoms and severity (ocular, bulbar, breathing, proximal muscle weakness)
- Evaluate fixed vital capacity (FVC) sitting and supine
- Review of current medications
- Contraceptive counseling

Optimize treatment:
- Thymectomy if not contraindicated while not pregnant
- Medication adjustment (Table 24.1) based on teratogenicity risk

During pregnancy

Clinical monitoring of the mother:
- Worsening of symptoms mostly within the first trimester
- Medication adjustment (Table 24.1)
- Monitoring and prompt treatment of infections
- Early anesthesia consult (epidural anesthesia preferred)
- No indication for C-section unless for obstetric reasons

Clinical monitoring of the fetus:
- Serial ultrasounds to monitor fetal movements/early contractures/polyhydramnios

Delivery

Multidisciplinary care
- Plan delivery with neurology, obstetrics, anesthesia, intensive care and neonatology
- Multidisciplinary discussion about delivery route and location
- C-section for standard obstetric indications only
- Convert oral pyridostigmine to parenteral equivalent if needed
- Assessment of myasthenic status, FVC monitoring
- Anesthesia consult: epidural anesthesia preferred over general anesthesia

Postpartum

Monitor newborn 12–72 hours for evidence of NMG symptoms in the baby
- Monitor for weakness, hypotonia, difficulty feeding, ptosis, respiratory distress
Maternal counseling
- Educate about possible worsening of symptoms postpartum
- Counseling on drug safety while breast-feeding (Table 24.1)

TABLE 24.1 COMMONLY USED MEDICATIONS AND THEIR SAFETY
IN PREGNANCY & LACTATION

Intervention	Pre-conception	Pregnancy	FDA*	Lactation
Safe Treatment				
Pyridostigmine	No limitations	<600 mg/day **Treatment of choice**	B/C	Larger doses can cause GI symptoms in the fetus
Corticosteroids	No limitations	**Treatment of choice** if immunosuppressive therapy is required	C	No limitations
IVIG	No limitations	**Treatment of choice** for exacerbation or myasthenic crisis	C	No limitations
Plasma exchange	No limitations	Consider, monitor fluid shifts	C	No limitations
Treatment Considered for Continuation				
Azathioprine	Contraception recommended	Continuation of therapy can be considered	D	Considered acceptable by most experts
Cyclosporine	Contraception recommended	Continuation of therapy can be considered	C	Can be considered
Unsafe During Pregnancy				
Mycophenolate mofetil	Contraception recommended until 6 weeks after discontinuation	Discontinuation recommended	D	Not recommended due to lack of information
Methotrexate	Strict contraception recommended until 3 months after discontinuation	Contraindicated	X	Contraindicated
Unknown Safety				
Rituximab	Not recommended due to lack of information	Not recommended due to lack of information	C	Not recommended due to lack of information

* The letter classifications have been replaced by new guidelines by the FDA, describing individual risk profiles, but still are known to most clinical providers. *Category B*: Animal reproduction studies showed no risk to the fetus and there are no adequate studies in pregnant women, or animal reproduction studies have demonstrated a risk; however, studies in pregnant woman have not shown an increased risk. *Category C*: Animal reproduction studies have shown an adverse effect on the fetus, there are no adequate and controlled studies in humans, and the benefits from the use may be acceptable despite its potential risks. *Category D*: Evidence of human fetal risk, but the potential benefits from the use of the drug in pregnant women may be acceptable despite its potential risks. *Category X*: Studies in animals or humans have demonstrated fetal risk, and the risk of the use of the drug in a pregnant woman outweighs any possible benefit.

Delivery and Postpartum

In a retrospective cohort study MG was associated with an increased rate of complications and interventions during delivery (40 of 135 pregnancies [30%]), the most common one being protracted labor and fetal distress.[6,18] Table 24.2 depicts a summary of reported complications with all studies with retrospective design except one.[7] The mother's clinical status does not predict complications during delivery and complications can be seen even in asymptomatic patients.[19] The first part of the delivery is usually not affected as it mainly involves smooth muscle. Within the second phase fatigue can occur due to the voluntary effort of pushing, involving striated muscles. Obstetricians may then assist with forceps or vacuum extraction, which can shorten the second labor stage.[4] During labor, parenteral anticholinesterase medications may be required, as oral absorption is limited. A dose of 60 mg oral pyridostigmine is equivalent to 1.5 mg neostigmine intramuscularly or 0.5 mg neostigmine intravenously. MG is not an indication for C-section,[4] which should be reserved for severe exacerbations or obstetric indications. On the contrary, vaginal delivery is encouraged in

TABLE 24.2 COMPLICATIONS DURING DELIVERY

	Almeida 2010	Wen 2009	Hoff 2003/2007	Djelmis 2001	Batochi 1999
Cesarean	Non urgent in 8/17 (5 due to obstetric causes)	NS (44.8% but 37.4% for all births) +	*17.3% (many elective vs. 8.6%)	17% (all but one for obstetric reasons)	30%, most for obstetric reasons
Vaginal intervention (vacuum/forceps)	NA	NS	8.7%	vacuum extraction in 9%	NA
Protracted labor	NA	NS	19%	NA	NA
Preterm rupture of membranes	NA	NS	*5.5% (vs. 1.7)	NA	NA

* statistically significant when compared to reference group, NS = not significant, NA = not assessed, + = Despite these insignificant differences, it is worth noting that a relatively high Cesarean rate in the general population can mask the possibility of an even higher rate of cesarean delivery among specific risk groups, compared to unaffected women.

patients with controlled disease.[13] Emergent C-sections should be avoided if possible as it typically involves general anesthesia and patients with MG are more sensitive to anesthetic agents. Medications to avoid in labor include non-depolarizing muscle relaxants and magnesium, which may precipitate profound weakness. In patients with eclampsia, magnesium should be avoided or used with caution because of its neuromuscular blocking effects. Barbiturates or phenytoin can be considered as alternate therapies instead.[13] Epidural analgesia is the anesthetic intervention of choice in delivery in women with MG, mainly because it can prevent or reduce the administration of potentially respiratory depressant systemic analgesics, regulate breathing and reduce fatigability.[12]

Neonatal myasthenia gravis (NMG)

NMG is caused by transplacental transmission of maternal acetylcholine receptor antibodies, described in 10–20% of children born to mothers with MG,[4,6,7] although case reports have described neonatal NMG also in women with anti-Musk antibodies.[20,21] Symptoms include difficulties in feeding, swallowing, breathing, or hypotonia of the newborn. Symptoms typically occur within 12–48 hours after birth; therefore, close monitoring of newborns of mothers with myasthenia for this time is warranted.[9] The occurrence of NMG does not correlate with maternal disease severity or anti- acetylcholine receptor antibody titer.[4,7] The severity of NMG can range from mild symptoms to respiratory distress requiring ventilation. Children with suspected NMG are more likely to show distress and signs of hypoxia during delivery.[6] For mild cases, pyridostigmine can be used, for more severe cases treatment with plasmapheresis can

be considered. Symptoms usually resolve within 1 month, can occasionally persist longer up to 4 months, and are always self-limited. Even in its milder forms, this condition is likely to affect breastfeeding by limiting milk transfer; these dyads will require additional and ongoing support to maintain maternal milk supply and the nursing relationship.

Arthrogryposis

In rare instances placental transmission of antibodies against the fetal acetylcholine receptor can cause decreased fetal intrauterine movements and result in arthrogryposis multiplex congenita (AMC), which is characterized by non-progressive contractures involving more than 2 joints. With severe manifestations, this can lead to intrauterine fetal death or neonatal death.[22] The disease occurs independent of the mother's severity of symptoms or antibody status. Serial ultrasound testing should be used to monitor for early contractures and fetal movements if there is suspicion for decreased fetal movement. The risk of developing AMC is increased in subsequent pregnancies, which is important when counseling the patient when considering future pregnancies.[23]

Conclusion

Awareness of MG as a risk factor for pregnancy and delivery, which can affect the birth process and also the newborn, should not discourage patients to become pregnant but should enforce appropriate counseling, planning, and monitoring in a multidisciplinary team involving the obstetrician, pediatrician, neurologist, and breastfeeding specialist.

PREGNANCY IN SPINAL MUSCULAR ATROPHY (SMA)

Brief Overview

Spinal muscular atrophy is a hereditary disorder with degeneration of the anterior horn cells in the spinal cord and motor nuclei in the lower brainstem. The disease severity ranges from paralysis at birth resulting in premature death (type I) to mild weakness with a normal life expectancy (type IV), with an incidence estimated of 1 in 11,000 live births and a carrier frequency of 1 in 40–67.[24] SMA is an autosomal recessive disorder, which is caused by mutations in the Survival Motor Neuron 1 (SMN1) gene. Loss of SMN1 protein function is partially compensated by SMN2 protein synthesis expressed by the SMN2 gene, which is very similar to the SMN1 gene. The presence of 3 or more copies of SMN2 is associated with a milder phenotype. Depending on severity of symptoms and age of onset, patients are classified into types I-IV. SMA II (onset between 3 and 15 months of age) and SMA III (at or after one year of age) and SMA IV even later in life. This article focuses on patients with SMA II-IV, in whom pregnancies have been described as patients with SMA I are usually too severely affected. Patients with SMA have various degrees of progressive symmetric proximal and distal muscle weakness, joint contractures, scoliosis, tongue weakness with fasciculations and reduced or absent reflexes. Weakness of the bulbar muscles can result in dysarthria and dysphagia. Progressive restrictive respiratory insufficiency results in difficulty controlling secretions and respiratory failure. There is typically no cardiac involvement. The diagnosis is confirmed by molecular genetic testing. Treatment is supportive, including (non-invasive) ventilation and cough assist devices. Since December 2016, the first disease modifying therapy has been approved by the FDA for pediatric and adult patients with SMA: Nusinersen is an antisense oligonucleotide that is administered intrathecally and targets the SMN2 gene, increasing the expression of the SMN protein with the goal to achieve a milder phenotype.[24]

Fertility

There is no known decreased fertility in women with SMA.[25]

Pregnancy Planning and Counseling

Patients with SMA should be referred for genetic counseling prior to becoming pregnant. As an autosomal recessive disorder, the risk of having a child with the disease for a woman with SMA equals roughly the carrier frequency in the population. One option for patients is to genetically screen their unaffected partner prior to conception. If the partner is a carrier, preimplantation genetic diagnosis (PGD) remains an option.[26] If the patient is already pregnant, prenatal genetic testing can be offered with amniocentesis or chorionic villus sampling (CVS).

While historically patients with SMA were counseled not to have children, recent advances in supportive care, increased life expectancy and the most recent approval of disease modifying therapy, in addition to reports of successful pregnancies in the literature, have and will further change this notion. That being said, pregnancy and parenthood present physical challenges for women with SMA that need to be understood and addressed by the patient and care providers. Available data in the literature on pregnancy in SMA patients is mostly based on retrospective analysis and case reports or series, which have shown an increased risk during pregnancy and delivery. A reporting bias with the tendency to report complicated deliveries is more likely. The risk profile depends on the patient's severity of muscle weakness, the degree of respiratory insufficiency, and the presence and degree of scoliosis and limb contractures. The goal is to establish care early on with a multidisciplinary team, which should include a neurologist, obstetrician, anesthesiologist, respiratory therapist, and pulmonologist. In a recent study, most mothers with SMA (91%) had a positive experience and chose to have more than one child, including those who experienced increased weakness during their pregnancy (Box 24.2).[25]

Pregnancy
Influence of the Pregnancy on the Course of Disease of SMA

A retrospective study of pregnancy in 25 patients with SMA was published by Awater et al and a more recent study by Elsheikh et al reported 35 pregnancies in 19 women: in each study, 4 patients had SMA type II, 20 and 14 had SMA type III and one woman in each study was affected by SMA type IV.[25,27] Thirteen of the women in these two studies were unable to walk and wheelchair-bound when becoming pregnant. Persistent worsening of symptoms, which were not further specified during or after the pregnancy, was experienced by 31% of patients in Awater et al, while Elsheikh et al reported 14 women (74%, 3 type 2; 11 type 3) with increased weakness or increased difficulty walking with persistence of weakness

BOX 24.2
CARE MAP FOR PREGNANCY IN THE PATIENT WITH SPINAL MUSCULAR ATROPHY (SMA)

Care Principles
- Family planning should be addressed in each patient of childbearing age
- The individual risk can be estimated by assessing severity of disease including muscle weakness, limb contractures, respiratory function, and scoliosis
- Care should be established and delivered by a multidisciplinary team involving neurologist, obstetrician, pulmonologist, respiratory therapist, and anesthesiologist

Before pregnancy/pre-pregnancy/non-pregnant

Review of prior pregnancy complications:
- Premature labor, non-vertex position, mode of delivery, respiratory function, thrombosis
- Education about signs and symptoms of worsening of symptoms, respiratory decompensation, CO_2 retention

Confirmation of neurological diagnosis and counseling:
- Molecular genetic testing
- Counseling on the diagnosis
- Genetic counseling with consideration of testing the partner, preimplantation genetic diagnosis or prenatal genetic testing

Assessment of neurological status:
- Symptoms and severity (bulbar and muscle weakness, breathing, scoliosis, limb contractures)
- Evaluate FVC sitting and supine
- Review of current medications which may affect respiratory function
- Consider imaging of the spine to assess anatomy for regional anesthesia
- Contraceptive counseling

During pregnancy

Clinical monitoring of the mother:
- Serial FVCs, if needed consider more invasive testing to assess CO_2 retention and hypoxia
- Worsening of weakness
- Early anesthesia consult
- Assessing need for elective C-section as a multidisciplinary decision depending on anticipated prematurity, kyphoscoliosis, fetal pulmonary maturity, anticipated cephalopelvic disproportion, and respiratory function

Clinical monitoring of the fetus:
- Assess fetal pulmonary maturity

Delivery

Multidisciplinary care
- Plan delivery with neurology, pulmonology, obstetrics, anesthesia, intensive care and neonatology
- Multidisciplinary discussion about delivery route and location
- Low threshold for C-section as a multidisciplinary decision
- FVC monitoring
- Anesthesia consult: regional anesthesia preferred over general anesthesia, but orthopedic barriers need consideration
- Increased risk of thromboembolism given immobility

Postpartum

Maternal counseling
- Educate about possible worsening of weakness postpartum
- Ensure ability to care for the child or provide additional services/support as needed

indefinitely after delivery in 6 women (42%).[25] In normal pregnancies, total lung capacity is preserved with a small reduction in residual volume. The major change in normal lung volumes is the reduction in functional residual capacity due to a reduction in chest wall compliance, starting in the early second trimester and worsening as the pregnancy progresses.[28] In Awater et al, pulmonary function was not systematically assessed, but 3 patients had restrictive lung disease during pregnancy, with reduced vital capacity (VC) values ranging from 19% to 67% and forced expiratory volume in 1 second (FEV1) values ranging from 18% to 57%.[27] Successful pregnancies have been described in case reports in patients with reduced FVCs to about 50% or below of predicted values, which remained stable throughout pregnancies.[28,29] There is no data to guide frequency of outpatient respiratory monitoring, which should be planned based on individual pulmonary function. One case report describes 2 successful pregnancies in a woman with SMA II with severe kyphoscoliosis and respiratory insufficiency (VC of 0.34 L [11% of predicted value requiring nocturnal nasal assist-control volume ventilation and cough assist device]). The patient was monitored with VC and peak cough flow rates every second week from week 10 to 22, then weekly from week 22 to 26 and respiratory function remained stable.[28] Other means of monitoring can include blood draws or if needed arterial blood gases to look for CO_2 retention. Primary treatment for hypoventilation in SMA is mechanical (preferably non-invasive) ventilation. Supplemental oxygen alone (without mechanical ventilation) when prescribed for desaturation due to alveolar hypoventilation can lead to reduced ventilatory drive, CO_2 retention, and respiratory failure and therefore should be avoided, if not in combination with non-invasive mechanical ventilation.[28] Increased back and abdominal pain as a complication during

pregnancy has been reported, which was felt to be due to the gravid uterus.[30]

Influence of SMA on the pregnancy and the fetus

Pregnant patients with SMA are at high risk for preterm delivery.[25,27,31] In the study by Awater et al, 10 of 25 patients gave birth before the 37th gestational week with a mean duration of gestational weeks resulting in live births of 36.1, with 2 late miscarriages with a slightly lower number reported by Elsheikh et al. (Table 24.3). Several case reports describe preterm births although many of them were planned electively when balancing risks related to anticipated premature delivery, maternal respiratory status, and fetal respiratory prematurity.[28,32] One patient with SMA type II with severe respiratory insufficiency (VC 19%, FEV1 17%) had a rapid deterioration after 20 gestational weeks and developed hypercapnia at 25 weeks. She was intubated but delivered a stillborn baby a week later. Apart from this patient, none of the other 24 women reported by Awater required mechanical ventilation during pregnancy.[27] The reason for premature births is unknown, although contractures, scoliosis, and respiratory insufficiency may play a role. In non-ambulatory patients, there is a theoretical increased risk of thromboembolism, although this has not been studied and while some case reports describe use of antithrombotic prophylaxis, there is no available data to generate general recommendations.[30]

Delivery and Postpartum

During delivery, women with SMA are at risk for respiratory complications, airway difficulties, and concerns related to the presence of scoliosis and lower limb and hip contractures. As mentioned previously, premature delivery presents the greatest risk. C-sections are increased in frequency in women with SMA (Table 24.3),[27,25] but successful vaginal deliveries

TABLE 24.3 COMPLICATIONS DURING PREGNANCY IN PATIENTS WITH SMA

	Miscarriage	Hypertension	Polyhydramnios	Preterm Delivery	C-Section	Instrumental Delivery	Non-vertex Presentation
Awater 2012[27]	16.3% (0.827)	6.1% (1)	3.0% (0.48)	**29.4% (<0.001)**	**42.4% (<0.001)**	**18.2% (0.029)**	18.8% (0.18)
Elsheikh 2017[25]	2.8%	2.8% (0.99)	NA	**20% (0.04)**	**34.3% (0.01)**	11% (0.31)	NA

Statistically significant values in bold. Values provided in percent, p-values in (). NA = not applicable (data not provided).

in less affected patients have been reported.[31] Eight out of 10 SMA patients who gave birth before the 37th gestational week delivered via C-section.[27] Four out of 6 women with severe scoliosis had a C-section under general anesthesia. The mode of delivery should be determined in a multidisciplinary team review of the anticipated prematurity, degree of kyphoscoliosis, anticipated cephalopelvic disproportion, and severity of respiratory dysfunction, with the goal to avoid emergency deliveries. There is no literature on breastfeeding with SMA. Given the predominantly muscular involvement, it is conceivable that the afferent spinal stimulation to the hypothalamic-pituitary axis would be functional, allowing for milk production. A mother with SMA is likely to require assistance with holding and latching the infant, and a lactation consultant should be involved early.

Anesthesia

For women who are severely affected by SMA, have spinal column deformities, and require cesarean delivery, anesthesia options can be challenging. The goals for anesthetic management include satisfactory anesthesia during surgery and postoperatively with minimal compromise of respiratory function. Regional anesthesia is preferred over general anesthesia, but epidural blockade can be difficult in patients with severe spine deformities or surgically corrected scoliosis. Several case reports describe successful use of spinal anesthesia for preterm cesarean deliveries with minimal respiratory compromise using continuous positive airway pressure. However, in some cases, this requires imaging of the spinal anatomy prior to delivery.[32] Delayed recovery from epidural anesthesia has been described in one patient.[25] Recovery after general anesthesia of a SMA patient may be delayed because of restrictive lung disease from spinal scoliosis and respiratory muscle weakness.

Conclusion

The literature on pregnancies in patients with SMA is limited and based on retrospective analysis and case reports. Management during pregnancy and delivery in patients with SMA depends on the severity of disease. Respiratory insufficiency and scoliosis represent major challenges. Prematurity is an important issue. In most women with advanced and generalized muscle atrophy, respiratory failure, and scoliosis, an elective C-section is the delivery mode of choice. Neonatal versus maternal mortality and morbidity have to be balanced when making a multidisciplinary decision regarding the optimum plan for delivery. Despite the fact that the lower limit of vital capacity (VC) in pregnancy is ill-defined, there are situations where the risk of a pregnancy with reduced lung function is considered too high, specifically when the need of invasive ventilation is anticipated.[27]

In conclusion, the management of pregnant women with SMA should include care in a multidisciplinary team with careful assessment and monitoring of pulmonary function and early assessment of the best mode of delivery and anesthesia.

PREGNANCY IN NONDYSTROPHIC MYOTONIA

Brief Overview

The nondystrophic myotonias (NDM) are rare ion channel disorders (1 in 100,000) of the skeletal muscle manifesting with muscle stiffness. Clinical severity of these disorders can range from life-threatening symptoms in a neonate with laryngeal spasms to mild late-onset symptoms in adulthood. Myotonia congenita is caused by mutations in the skeletal muscle chloride channel gene (CLCN-1) with autosomal dominant (Thomsen myotonia congenita) or recessive (Becker myotonia congenita) inheritance. Paramyotonia congenita and the sodium channel myotonias are allelic, autosomal dominant disorders caused by mutations in the skeletal muscle sodium channel gene (SCN4A). In myotonia congenita muscle stiffness is most pronounced during rapid voluntary movements following a period of rest but improves with repeated activity—the so-called "warm-up" phenomenon. In paramyotonia congenita muscle stiffness and weakness is exacerbated by cold temperature and exercise. The other sodium channel myotonias are characterized by the absence of episodic weakness but may have cold sensitivity.[33] The diagnosis is made by genetic and/or electrodiagnostic testing. The best data on treatment of myotonia is available for Mexiletine, which has been shown to effectively reduce muscle stiffness in a randomized, double-blind, placebo-controlled study.[34] Available literature on pregnancy in patients with NDM is sparse and limited to case reports and retrospective studies.

Fertility

Information is limited to one retrospective study based on patient questionnaires, which reported infertility in seven subjects (28%), which is above the US national average of 12.1%.[35]

Pregnancy Planning and Counseling

Patients should receive genetic counseling prior to becoming pregnant, which will vary depending on the underlying mutation and pattern of inheritance. Confirming the diagnosis with genetic testing is desired, but the diagnosis can be made on clinical and electrodiagnostic grounds when a pathogenic mutation cannot be identified. Patients should be counseled that often symptoms can worsen during pregnancy with resolution following delivery in most patients.[35–38] The need and safety of continued medical therapy should be reviewed prior to becoming pregnant. Myotonia can cause life-threatening laryngospasm and facial muscle stiffness in newborns affected by the disease. Therefore delivery should be planned in a multidisciplinary team with neonatal intensive care available as needed. Overall, pregnancy outcomes in NDM are favorable. In a retrospective study 87% women agreed that they supported the decision to become pregnant again (Box 24.3).[35]

Pregnancy
Influence of the Pregnancy on the Course of Disease of NDM

Case reports[36–38] and a retrospective study based on patient questionnaires[35] showed that symptoms worsened in the majority of pregnancies (76%) of patients with all types of nondystrophic myotonia and included muscle pain, worsening weakness, stiffness/spasms, and worsening fatigue. Worsening symptoms usually resolved after the pregnancy fully in 66% and partially in 32% of patients, in the majority

---

BOX 24.3
CARE MAP FOR PREGNANCY IN THE PATIENT WITH NONDYSTROPHIC MYOTONIA (NDM)

BEFORE PREGNANCY/PRE-PREGNANCY/NON-PREGNANT

Review of prior pregnancy complications:
- Worsening of myotonia or weakness, mode of delivery
- Educate about signs and symptoms of worsening of symptoms

Confirmation of neurological diagnosis and counseling:
- Molecular genetic testing
- Counseling on the diagnosis
- Genetic counseling

Assessment of neurological status:
- Symptoms and severity (myotonia, weakness, triggers)
- Review of current medications and pregnancy safety
- Contraceptive counseling

DURING PREGNANCY

Clinical monitoring of the mother:
- Worsening of weakness
- Early anesthesia consult

DELIVERY

Multidisciplinary care
- Plan delivery mode and location with neurology, obstetrics, anesthesia, and neonatology
- Anesthesia consult: avoid triggers for myotonia

POSTPARTUM

Maternal counseling
- Monitor fetus for distress and symptoms suggestive of NDM

within the first month (61%) and in most within the first 3 months (76%). Postpartum improvement is also described in case series.[36] Some patients developed their first symptoms during pregnancy.[37]

Influence of NDM on the pregnancy and the fetus

In a cross-sectional mail-out questionnaire study involving 25 women with 63 pregnancies and 53 live births, rates of preterm delivery, low birth weight, miscarriages, C-sections or instrumental assisted vaginal deliveries were not statistically different in patients with NDM compared to the national population.[35] Treatment of myotonia with mexiletine should be discussed prior to the pregnancy. No controlled data is available for mexiletine on human pregnancy (category C) but mexiletine should be considered for patients in whom myotonia is severe enough to pose a risk to mother or the fetus and especially in the second and third trimester.

Delivery and Postpartum

There was a statistically significant increased incidence of fetal distress in patients with NDM. One third of babies had difficulties after birth, most of them likely related to a diagnosis of NDM (21% of children), including difficulty feeding, spasms of face and throat, and clubfoot. Therefore the newborn requires monitoring for these symptoms and potentially treatment with mexiletine if needed. Postpartum depression was reported in 12 patients (24%), which is higher than the prevalence in the normal population (13%). A theoretical concern includes triggering of myotonia in the mother due to labor or impaired positioning during delivery due to muscle stiffness.[39] NDM is not an indication for C-section, which should be reserved for obstetric indications only. There is no literature on breastfeeding with NDM. All mother's with neuromuscular disorders are likely to require assistance with holding and latching the infant, and a lactation consultant should be involved early.

Anesthesia

There are no anesthesia guidelines, but avoiding cold temperatures, depolarizing muscle relaxants, and painful injections is recommended due to the risk of triggering myotonia.[39,40] Successful C-sections with spinal anesthesia have been reported.[40] For treatment of severe myotonia intrapartum, mexiletine should be considered.

Conclusion

Pregnancy and delivery in patients with NDM generally have a favorable outcome. The majority of patients experience worsening of symptoms during pregnancy. Intrapartum triggers that can worsen myotonia should be avoided. Postpartum monitoring of the newborn for symptoms of NDM (respiratory distress, bulbar symptoms) is recommended.

PREGNANCY IN MUSCULAR DYSTROPHIES

Brief Overview

The muscular dystrophies are an inherited group of progressive muscle disorders resulting from defects in genes required for normal muscle function. Myotonic dystrophy type 1 (DM1) and 2 (DM2) are the most common muscular dystrophies in adults with autosomal dominant inheritance caused by a tri- (DM1) and tetranucelotide (DM2) repeat expansion. As multisystemic diseases they can present with early cataracts, cardiac conduction, and endocrinologic abnormalities, cognitive deficits, and gastrointestinal involvement. Facioscapulohumeral muscular dystrophy (FSHD) is the second most common muscular dystrophy in adults, usually with an autosomal dominant inheritance; FSHD is characterized in most cases by slowly progressive muscle weakness involving the facial, scapular, upper arm, lower leg, and hip girdle muscles that can be asymmetric. Congenital myopathies (CM) are a genetically and clinically heterogeneous group of inherited muscle disorders with infantile or childhood onset of muscle weakness and hypotonia, with a static or slowly progressive course. The limb-girdle muscular dystrophies (LGMD) are a heterogenous group of genetic disorders with either autosomal dominant or recessive inheritance typically resulting in weakness of shoulder and hip girdle muscles. For most of these conditions, no disease modifying treatments are available yet and management consists primarily of supportive care. Information on pregnancy and delivery in women with these disorders is limited and restricted to retrospective studies relying on questionnaires, case reports, and series.

Fertility

Female fertility in myotonic dystrophy remains controversial. Studies with small numbers of patients, mixed methods, and patient preselection may account for some of the differences.[41]

A case-controlled study found no relationship between female fertility and the disease.[42] In a retrospective study based on patient questionnaires, 19.7% of patients with DM1 and 12.7% of patients with DM2 utilized in-vitro fertilization to become pregnant.[43] No impaired gonadal function was seen in a large cohort of women undergoing in vitro fertilization (IVF) and preimplantation genetic diagnosis (PGD).[44] Other reports showed that women with myotonic dystrophy had less responsiveness to controlled ovarian stimulation compared to controls.[45] Another study evaluating patients undergoing IV and PGD found reduced ovarian reserve, lower ovarian response to stimulation, lower clinical pregnancy, and live birth rates in women with DM1 compared to disease controls.[41] In other muscular dystrophies fertility has not been systematically studied.

Pregnancy Planning and Counseling

Genetic counseling should be offered to patients when planning a family. Counseling varies depending on genetic status and type of inheritance. For autosomal recessive disorders screening of the partner is a consideration. For most autosomal dominant inherited diseases, the 50% risk of transmitting the disorder can be nearly eliminated by a combination of IVF with intracytoplasmic sperm injection (ICSI) and PGD. A referral to a specialized center should be offered if desired by the patient. Women with myotonic dystrophy type 1 are at risk to have a child with congenital myotonic dystrophy (CDM), which is a more severe form of DM with neonatal onset. Symptoms may present late in pregnancy with reduced fetal movement and polyhydramnios. Children with CDM usually have trinucleotide (CTG) repeats with > 1,000 repeats. The repeat number of the mother is not definitively predictive of the risk to have a child with CDM, as massive intergenerational expansion can occur in asymptomatic women with only few repeats (eg, 70–90). This explains why in more than one-third of cases of DM1, the diagnosis of the mother is made after an affected child is born.[46,47]

General counseling on pregnancy depends on the manifestation and severity of the disease. Parenthood presents an additional activity of daily living that the patient may need to accomplish independently or with additional support. Care during pregnancy needs to be established in a multidisciplinary team with intensified monitoring.

In a retrospective study on women with FSHD, 90% reported that they would choose pregnancy again.[48] This is concordant with an earlier study in which all 11 patients with FSHD in retrospect supported their decision to have children.[49] Of 7 patients with CM, one advised against pregnancy, one suggested limiting the number of children and the remaining mothers supported their decision retrospectively. Of 9 patients with LGMD, most patients had a positive attitude towards their decision to become a parent (Box 24.4).[49]

Pregnancy

Influence of the Pregnancy on the Course of Disease

Worsening of symptoms during pregnancy is common in women with muscular dystrophy and can be transient (DM2) or persist after delivery (LGMD, FSHD). Most of the available data is limited due to being based on questionnaires (Table 24.4). Of 22 patients with LGMD in a retrospective study, 54% reported persistent worsening of symptoms during or after the pregnancy. Three pregnancies (8.8%) were terminated, as patients were unable to cope with increasing weakness and expected demands as a parent. Persistent worsening was also reported by patients with CM (16% of a total of 11 patients).[27] One case report describes progressive cardiac dysfunction in Bethlem myopathy, which is an unusual manifestation requiring elective C-section.[50] One-eighths of patients with FSHD reported worsening of symptoms (total n = 13). In a larger retrospective questionnaire based study of 38 women with FSHD with 105 gestations, an even larger number of women reported persistent worsening of weakness during pregnancy (24%). Most common symptoms were generalized weakness, frequent falling, difficulty carrying the infant due to shoulder weakness and increased pain.[48] The ability to walk was maintained by all women (DM, FSHD, CM, and LGMD) who were ambulatory prior to their pregnancy.[27] One case report describes transient worsening with temporary use of a wheelchair in a patient with Bethlem myopathy, with return to her pre-pregnancy functional state following delivery.[51]

Temporary or persistent worsening of the disease was not reported in patients with DM1 in the retrospective study by Awater et al, but case reports and a retrospective study describe higher prevalence and impact of symptoms after compared to prior to pregnancy, including mobility and activity limitations, pain, emotional issues, and myotonia.[27,43,52] Of 42 patients with

BOX 24.4
CARE MAP FOR PREGNANCY IN THE PATIENT WITH MUSCULAR DYSTROPHY

Care Principles
- Family planning should be addressed in each patient of childbearing age
- Genetic counseling prior to conception
- Counseling on IVF and PGD if desired
- Individual risk assessment considering severity of weakness and multi-systemic involvement

Before pregnancy/pre-pregnancy/non-pregnant

Review of prior pregnancy complications:
- Preterm labor, prematurity, polyhydramnios
- Anesthesia complications
- Worsening of symptoms

Confirmation of neurological diagnosis and counseling:
- Preferably confirmation with DNA testing
- Counseling on the diagnosis (genetic counseling, prognosis)
- Counseling on options of IVF and PGD

Assessment of disease severity:
- Symptoms and severity (bulbar, breathing, contractures, myotonia, muscle weakness)
- Multi-systemic involvement (cardiac, endocrine, gastrointestinal)
- Evaluate FVC sitting and supine and Cough Peak Flow
- Review of current medications
- Contraceptive counseling

Optimize treatment:
- Physical and occupational therapy, appropriate use of assistive devices
- Social work: assess need for additional support required to care for the child

During pregnancy

Clinical monitoring of the mother:
- Monitor for worsening of symptoms
- Monitoring and prompt treatment of infections (UTIs, respiratory)
- Early anesthesia consult (local anesthesia preferred)
- C-section for obstetrical indications

Clinical monitoring of the fetus:
- Serial ultrasounds to monitor fetal movements/early contractures/polyhydramnios
- DM1: monitor for polyhydramnios to assess for affected fetus (CDM)

Delivery

Multidisciplinary care
- Plan delivery with neurology, obstetrics, anesthesia, intensive care and neonatology
- Multidisciplinary discussion about delivery route and location
- C-section for standard obstetric indications
- FVC and cardiac monitoring
- Anesthesia consult: local anesthesia preferred over general anesthesia

Postpartum

- Monitor for weakness, hypotonia, difficulty feeding, respiratory distress in the infant
Maternal counseling
- Assess need for additional help/support to care for the child, PT, OT, Lactation consult

TABLE 24.4 COMPLICATIONS DURING PREGNANCY AND DELIVERY

	Onset or Worsening of Symptoms	Miscarriage	Hypertension/ Preeclampsia	Poly-hydramnios	Placenta Previa	UTI	Preterm Delivery	C-Section	Instrumental Delivery	Non-vertex Presentation
DM1										
[27]	NA	15.3% (0.87)	7.8% (0.8)	**17.2% (<0.001)**	**10.8% (<0.001)**	**9.4% (0.017)**	**30.7% (<0.001)**	**36.7% (<0.001)**	**15.0% (0.037)**	**34.6% (<0.001)**
[43]	yes	32.1%	7.8%	23.85%	NA	3.15%	31%++	NA	NA	NA
DM2										
[27]	21%	16.2% (0.769)	5.1% (0.512)	-	2.5% (0.065)	**7.6% (0.042)**	12.6% (0.073)	13.9% (0.749)	8.9% (0.497)	12.1% (0.533)
[43]	yes	37.1%	13.6%	-	NA	-	13.6%++	NA	NA	NA
FSHD										
[27]	13%	10.3% (0.606)	-	-	-	3.8% (0.554)	3.8% (1)	7.7% (0.411)	15.4% (0.11)	-
[48]	24%	16.2% (0.87)	3.4% *(0.51)	4.6% (0.08)	NA	3.4% (0.11)+	12.8% (0.16)	**23.8% (0.01)**	**19% (0.0002)**)**	-
CM[27,50,51]	16%, &	5% (0.34)	5.4% (1)	-	-	-	10.5% (0.639)	26.3% (0.215)	10.5% (0.639)	-
LGMD[27]	54%	5.9% (0.214)	6.9% (1)	-	-	-	3.4% (0.716)	31% (0.113)	17.2% (0.054)	**26.7% (0.04)**
Reference population[27]	NA	15%	7%	1.9%	0.4%	3%	7%	25%	7%	12.8% pre term, 4% term

Statistically significant values in bold. - = negative/not present. NA= not applicable/reported. *= preeclampsia, += confirmed infections, **= forceps only, &= case reports. ++= preterm labor.

DM2, 21% of patients experienced their first symptom (weakness, myalgia or myotonia) during pregnancy, with improvement after delivery but with worsening symptoms in subsequent pregnancies,[53] which has also been described in a case series.[54] Another study describes increased prevalence of activity limitations and increased impact of mobility and activity limitations, fatigue, communication difficulties, and sleep impairment after comparison with pre-pregnancy.[43]

The need and extent of clinical monitoring during pregnancy depends on the severity of the underlying muscular dystrophy and presence of multisystemic features. Patients with myotonic dystrophy can have respiratory insufficiency, sleep apnea, excessive daytime sleepiness, delayed gastric emptying, obstructive sleep apnea, diabetes mellitus, all of which can exacerbate during pregnancy due to physiological changes related to the growing fetus and may require additional medical attention. As a complicating factor, women with DM1 with cognitive deficits may not volunteer changes in their health and symptoms. Women with muscular dystrophies affecting respiratory muscles should be asked for symptoms such as daytime sleepiness and morning headaches, and pulmonary function testing should be carried out supine and sitting to monitor for changes in diaphragmatic function. If the muscular dystrophy affects the heart, questions and examination should be tailored to monitor for heart failure and cardiac arrhythmias. Patients with DM should be monitored for gestational diabetes.

Influence of MD on the pregnancy and the fetus

Table 24.4 depicts available data on complications during pregnancy and delivery comparing FSHD, DM1, DM2, LGMD, and CM. Obstetric complications have been described in DM1 and may suggest involvement of the smooth muscle and genitourinary tract: placenta previa was significantly more frequent in DM1 (10.8%). An increased risk of ectopic pregnancy has been described in DM1 (4%)[46] and urinary tract infections are more common in both DM1 and DM2.[27] Pulmonary function was not systematically assessed,[27] but respiratory insufficiency has been reported in a single patient postpartum with DM1.[46] Premature labor prior to the 36th week of gestation was significantly increased in both DM1 and DM2 (DM1 36.9%, DM2 17.7%), but preterm deliveries were more frequently seen only in DM1

(Table 24.4). Polyhydramnios was seen only in patients with DM1 and exclusively when the fetus is affected with CDM (17%, typically detected in seventh month). In DM2, late miscarriages (16–26th week of gestation) were seen in patients who had experienced first onset or worsening of symptoms during pregnancy. In this subgroup of patients preterm labor and prematurity were also more likely (50 and 27% respectively). Abnormalities of labor and the frequency of operative deliveries in DM2 were within the normal range. There is no congenital form of DM2, and neonatal outcomes were normal without increased mortality or incidence of polyhydramnios.[53] In patients with FSHD, there was no increased risk of prematurity, but low birth weight rate was increased.[48] For CM, the risk of pregnancy and delivery complications is not significantly greater compared to reference data. However, effects may be missed due to the heterogenousity of the group and small number of patients. Neonatal outcomes in women with DM1 are generally favorable, with exception of the babies born with CDM, which is mostly responsible for an increased perinatal loss rate of 15%.[46] Other muscular dystrophies have not been associated with increased fetal risks.

Delivery and Postpartum

Table 24.4 summarizes the complications seen in women with muscular dystrophy during delivery. Women with DM1 are at higher risk for prolonged labor affecting all stages of delivery, which might be related to uterine dysfunction affecting smooth muscle but also maternal skeletal muscle weakness affecting pushing in the later stages. Intervention is also more commonly needed in women with fetuses with CDM. As a consequence, women with DM1 are more likely to deliver with C-section[27] or have instrumentally assisted vaginal deliveries.

In LGMD, 26.7% of babies presented with a breech position at term, which is higher than the normal population (4%).[27] The risk of operative vaginal delivery (cesarean delivery and forceps deliveries) is significantly higher in women with FSHD.[48] This effect was not seen in a study with smaller sample size.[27] In FSHD, a higher incidence of low birth weight was noted (<2500 g).[48] A case of Bethlem myopathy, a form of congenital myopathy, required assistance with vacuum extraction resulting in a successful delivery.[51] The limitation of questionnaires is illustrated by the study of Ciafaloni et al on women with FSHD: While fetal distress and frequent infections were reported, review of the medical records did not provide confirmation.[48] Recently more information has become available of patients with DM1 undergoing ICSI and IVF: A large cohort of 31 women with DM1 delivered healthy children without reported complications with even successful delivery of twin pregnancies in 19.2%.[44] However, this data provides limited use as patients undergoing this procedure present a preselected cohort (eg, patients with overt uterine abnormalities are excluded). There is no literature on breastfeeding with muscular dystrophies. All mothers with neuromuscular disorders are likely to require assistance with holding and latching the infant, and a lactation consultant should be involved early.

Treatment and anesthesia

There is currently no disease modifying treatment available for patients with muscular dystrophies. Mexiletine is used for symptomatic treatment of myotonia. No controlled data is available for mexiletine on human pregnancy (category C). Severe myotonia has only been described in one pregnant woman[52] who was treated with acetaminophen for pain. Mexiletine should be considered for patients in whom myotonia is severe enough to pose a risk to mother or the fetus.

Anesthesia considerations depend on the underlying muscular dystrophy, involvement of respiratory and cardiac function, bulbar muscles (risk of aspiration), bony deformities, contractures, and risk for malignant hyperthermia. Local or regional anesthesia is generally preferred over general anesthesia. There is no risk for malignant hyperthermia in DM or FSHD, but in some CM such as central core disease or in disease caused by mutations of the ryanodine receptor there is. Patients with muscular dystrophies may be more sensitive to anesthetic drugs and have more difficulty with extubation, specifically with use of hypnotics and opioids. Muscle relaxants and succinylcholine should be avoided.[55]

Conclusion

Pregnancy and delivery risks differ between the different muscular dystrophies and clinical monitoring should be guided by the pattern and degree of muscle weakness and the degree of respiratory and cardiac involvement. Worsening of symptoms during pregnancy is seen in most muscular dystrophies. Women with DM1 experience the most complications, although primarily when the fetus is affected with CDM. Women with FSHD and DM2 have a relatively benign course

with good outcomes. Small number of patients and heterogenousity of diseases of patients with LGMD and CM make a generalized assessment of pregnancy and delivery risk challenging.

REFERENCES

1. Wolfe GI, Kaminski HJ, Sonnett JR, Aban IB, Kuo HC, Cutter GR. Randomized trial of thymectomy in myasthenia gravis. *J Thorac Dis.* 2016; 8(12): E1782–E1783.
2. Durst JK, Rampersad RM. Pregnancy in women with solid-organ transplants: A review. *Obstet Gynecol Surv.* 2015; 70(6): 408–418.
3. Leroy C, Rigot JM, Leroy M, et al. Immunosuppressive drugs and fertility. *Orphanet J Rare Dis.* 2015; 10:136.
4. Djelmis J, Sostarko M, Mayer D, Ivanisevic M. Myasthenia gravis in pregnancy: report on 69 cases. *Eur J Obstet Gynecol Reprod Biol.* 2002; 104(1): 21–25.
5. Norwood F, Dhanjal M, Hill M, et al. Myasthenia in pregnancy: Best practice guidelines from a U.K. multispecialty working group. *J Neurol Neurosurg Psychiatry.* 2014; 85(5): 538–543.
6. Hoff JM, Daltveit AK, Gilhus NE. Myasthenia gravis in pregnancy and birth: identifying risk factors, optimising care. *Eur J Neurol.* 2007; 14(1): 38–43.
7. Batocchi AP, Majolini L, Evoli A, Lino MM, Minisci C, Tonali P. Course and treatment of myasthenia gravis during pregnancy. *Neurology.* 1999; 52(3): 447–452.
8. Ciafaloni E, Massey JM. The management of myasthenia gravis in pregnancy. *Semin Neurol.* 2004; 24(1): 95–100.
9. Ciafaloni E, Massey JM. Myasthenia gravis and pregnancy. *Neurol Clin.* 2004; 22(4): 771–782.
10. Ferrero S, Pretta S, Nicoletti A, Petrera P, Ragni N. Myasthenia gravis: management issues during pregnancy. *Eur J Obstet Gynecol Reprod Biol.* 2005; 121(2): 129–138.
11. Boldingh MI, Maniaol AH, Brunborg C, Weedon-Fekjaer H, Verschuuren JJ, Tallaksen CM. Increased risk for clinical onset of myasthenia gravis during the postpartum period. *Neurology.* 2016; 87(20): 2139–2145.
12. Almeida C, Coutinho E, Moreira D, Santos E, Aguiar J. Myasthenia gravis and pregnancy: Anaesthetic management—a series of cases. *Eur J Anaesthesiol.* 2010; 27(11): 985–990.
13. Sanders DB, Wolfe GI, Benatar M, et al. International consensus guidance for management of myasthenia gravis: Executive summary. *Neurology.* 2016; 87(4): 419–425.
14. Wen JC, Liu TC, Chen YH, Chen SF, Lin HC, Tsai WC. No increased risk of adverse pregnancy

outcomes for women with myasthenia gravis: a nationwide population-based study. *Eur J Neurol.* 2009; 16(8): 889–894.

15. The EULAR points to consider for use of antirheumatic drugs before pregnancy, and during pregnancy and lactation. *Annals of the Rheumatic Diseases.* 2016; 75(5): 795–810.

16. Feasby T, Banwell B, Benstead T, et al. Guidelines on the use of intravenous immune globulin for neurologic conditions. *Transfus Med Rev.* 2007; 21(2 Suppl 1): S57–107.

17. Constantinescu S, Pai A, Coscia LA, Davison JM, Moritz MJ, Armenti VT. Breastfeeding after transplantation. *Best Pract Res Clin Obstet Gynaecol.* 2014; 28(8): 1163–1173.

18. Hoff JM, Daltveit AK, Gilhus NE. Myasthenia gravis: Consequences for pregnancy, delivery, and the newborn. *Neurology.* 2003; 61(10): 1362–1366.

19. Hoff JM, Daltveit AK, Gilhus NE. Asymptomatic myasthenia gravis influences pregnancy and birth. *Eur J Neurol.* 2004; 11(8): 559–562.

20. Behin A, Mayer M, Kassis-Makhoul B, et al. Severe neonatal myasthenia due to maternal anti-MuSK antibodies. *Neuromuscul Disord.* 2008; 18(6): 443–446.

21. Niks EH, Verrips A, Semmekrot BA, et al. A transient neonatal myasthenic syndrome with anti-musk antibodies. *Neurology.* 2008; 70(14): 1215–1216.

22. Vincent A, Newland C, Brueton L, et al. Arthrogryposis multiplex congenita with maternal autoantibodies specific for a fetal antigen. *Lancet.* 1995; 346(8966): 24–25.

23. Midelfart Hoff J, Midelfart A. Maternal myasthenia gravis: A cause for arthrogryposis multiplex congenita. *J Child Orthop.* 2015; 9(6): 433–435.

24. Farrar MA, Park SB, Vucic S, et al. Emerging therapies and challenges in Spinal Muscular Atrophy. *Ann Neurol.* 2017; 81(3): 355–368.

25. Elsheikh BH, Zhang X, Swoboda KJ, et al. Pregnancy and delivery in women with spinal muscular atrophy. *Int J Neurosci.* 2017; 127(11): 953–957.

26. Tur-Kaspa I, Jeelani R, Doraiswamy PM. Preimplantation genetic diagnosis for inherited neurological disorders. *Nat Rev Neurol.* 2014; 10(7): 417–424.

27. Awater C, Zerres K, Rudnik-Schoneborn S. Pregnancy course and outcome in women with hereditary neuromuscular disorders: Comparison of obstetric risks in 178 patients. *Eur J Obstet Gynecol Reprod Biol.* 2012; 162(2): 153–159.

28. Flunt D, Andreadis N, Menadue C, Welsh AW. Clinical commentary: Obstetric and respiratory management of pregnancy with severe spinal muscular atrophy. *Obstet Gynecol Int.* 2009; 2009: 942301.

29. Yim R, Kirschner K, Murphy E, Parson J, Winslow C. Successful pregnancy in a patient with spinal muscular atrophy and severe kyphoscoliosis. *Am J Phys Med Rehabil.* 2003; 82(3): 222–225.

30. Howarth L, Glanville T. Management of a pregnancy complicated by type III spinal muscular atrophy. *BMJ Case Rep.* 2011; *BMJ Case Reports* 2011; doi:10.1136/bcr.10.2010.34022011.

31. Argov Z, de Visser M. What we do not know about pregnancy in hereditary neuromuscular disorders. *Neuromuscul Disord.* 2009; 19(10): 675–679.

32. Maruotti GM, Anfora R, Scanni E, et al. Anesthetic management of a parturient with spinal muscular atrophy type II. *J Clin Anesth.* 2012; 24(7): 573–577.

33. Matthews E, Fialho D, Tan SV, et al. The nondystrophic myotonias: Molecular pathogenesis, diagnosis and treatment. *Brain.* 2010; 133(Pt. 1): 9–22.

34. Statland JM, Bundy BN, Wang Y, et al. Mexiletine for symptoms and signs of myotonia in nondystrophic myotonia: A randomized controlled trial. *JAMA.* 2012; 308(13): 1357–1365.

35. Snyder Y, Donlin-Smith C, Snyder E, Pressman E, Ciafaloni E. The course and outcome of pregnancy in women with nondystrophic myotonias. *Muscle Nerve.* 2015; 52(6): 1013–1015.

36. Rudnik-Schoneborn S, Witsch-Baumgartner M, Zerres K. Influences of pregnancy on different genetic subtypes of non-dystrophic myotonia and periodic paralysis. *Gynecol Obstet Invest.* 2016; 81(5): 472–476.

37. Lacomis D, Gonzales JT, Giuliani MJ. Fluctuating clinical myotonia and weakness from Thomsen's disease occurring only during pregnancies. *Clin Neurol Neurosurg.* 1999; 101(2): 133–136.

38. Gorthi S, Radbourne S, Drury N, Rajagopalan C. Management of pregnancy with Thomsen's disease. *Eur J Obstet Gynecol Reprod Biol.* 2013; 170(1): 293–294.

39. Basu A, Nishanth P, Ifaturoti O. Pregnancy in women with myotonia congenita. *Int J Gynaecol Obstet.* 2009; 106(1): 62–63.

40. Farrow C, Carling A. Successful spinal blockade in a parturient with myotonia congenita. *Int J Obstet Anesth.* 2007; 16(1): 89–90.

41. Srebnik N, Margalioth EJ, Rabinowitz R, et al. Ovarian reserve and PGD treatment outcome in women with myotonic dystrophy. *Reprod Biomed Online.* 2014; 29(1): 94–101.

42. Dao TN, Mathieu J, Bouchard JP, De Braekeleer M. Fertility in myotonic dystrophy in Saguenay-Lac-St-Jean: a historical perspective. *Clin Genet.* 1992; 42(5): 234–239.

43. Johnson NE, Hung M, Nasser E, et al. The impact of pregnancy on myotonic dystrophy: A registry-based study. *J Neuromuscul Dis.* 2015; 2(4): 447–452.
44. Verpoest W, De Rademaeker M, Sermon K, et al. Real and expected delivery rates of patients with myotonic dystrophy undergoing intracytoplasmic sperm injection and preimplantation genetic diagnosis. *Hum Reprod.* 2008; 23(7): 1654–1660.
45. Feyereisen E, Amar A, Kerbrat V, et al. Myotonic dystrophy: Does it affect ovarian follicular status and responsiveness to controlled ovarian stimulation? *Hum Reprod.* 2006; 21(1): 175–182.
46. Rudnik-Schoneborn S, Zerres K. Outcome in pregnancies complicated by myotonic dystrophy: A study of 31 patients and review of the literature. *Eur J Obstet Gynecol Reprod Biol.* 2004; 114(1): 44–53.
47. Thornton CA. Myotonic dystrophy. *Neurol Clin.* 2014; 32(3): 705–719, viii.
48. Ciafaloni E, Pressman EK, Loi AM, et al. Pregnancy and birth outcomes in women with facioscapulohumeral muscular dystrophy. *Neurology.* 2006; 67(10): 1887–1889.
49. Rudnik-Schoneborn S, Glauner B, Rohrig D, Zerres K. Obstetric aspects in women with facioscapulohumeral muscular dystrophy, limb-girdle muscular dystrophy, and congenital myopathies. *Arch Neurol.* 1997; 54(7): 888–894.
50. Flock A, Kornblum C, Hammerstingl C, Claeys KG, Gembruch U, Merz WM. Progressive cardiac dysfunction in Bethlem myopathy during pregnancy. *Obstet Gynecol.* 2014; 123(2 Pt. 2 Suppl 2): 436–438.
51. Nunes C, Barros J, Centeno M, Pinto L, Graca LM. Bethlem myopathy: Pregnancy and delivery. *Arch Gynecol Obstet.* 2014; 289(1): 219–220.
52. Benito-Leon J, Aguilar-Galan EV. Recurrent myotonic crisis in a pregnant woman with myotonic dystrophy. *Eur J Obstet Gynecol Reprod Biol.* 2001; 95(2): 181.
53. Rudnik-Schoneborn S, Schneider-Gold C, Raabe U, Kress W, Zerres K, Schoser BG. Outcome and effect of pregnancy in myotonic dystrophy type 2. *Neurology.* 2006; 66(4): 579–580.
54. Newman B, Meola G, O'Donovan DG, Schapira AH, Kingston H. Proximal myotonic myopathy (PROMM) presenting as myotonia during pregnancy. *Neuromuscul Disord.* 1999; 9(3): 144–149.
55. Veyckemans F, Scholtes JL. Myotonic dystrophies type 1 and 2: Anesthetic care. *Paediatr Anaesth.* 2013; 23(9): 794–803.

25

Charcot-Marie-Tooth Disease and Pregnancy

PETER D. CREIGH AND DAVID N. HERRMANN

Hereditary neuropathies (HN) represent the most common hereditary neuromuscular conditions worldwide.[1,2] The most common HN are the Charcot-Marie-Tooth neuropathies (CMT), a large group of genetically distinct syndromes with peripheral neuropathy as the primary feature. CMT disease affects men and women from infancy to adulthood and, while it can lead to significant functional disability, it is not generally associated with a shortened life expectancy or infertility.[1,3,4] As such, women of childbearing age with CMT and their health care providers are often faced with questions about the risks of pregnancy on the underlying disease course and the risks of CMT on pregnancy.[4]

OVERVIEW OF CHARCOT-MARIE-TOOTH DISEASE

The population prevalence of CMT is estimated at 1 in 2500, the majority of which have an autosomal dominant inheritance pattern, although X-linked and autosomal recessive patterns also exist.[2,5-7] Traditionally, CMT has been divided into clinical groups based on electrophysiologic findings (demyelinating vs. axonal neuropathy) and inheritance patterns (AD, AR, or X-linked). CMT type 1 has an autosomal dominant demyelinating pattern, CMT type 2 has an autosomal dominate axonal pattern, CMT type 4 has an autosomal recessive inheritance, and CMT-X is X-linked (Table 25.1).[8,9] Within each of these groups, there are further subgroups based on phenotypical distinctions and specific genetic mutations (ie, CMT 1A, CMT 1B, etc.). Mutations in one of four genes (PMP22 (CMT Type 1A), GJIB1 (CMT Type 1X), MFN2 (CMT Type 2A), or MPZ (CMT Type 1B) account for the majority of CMT cases.[8-10] However, to date pathologic mutations in over 80 genes have been identified and the distinctions between the traditional subtypes are becoming more complex.[7,11]

Most patients with CMT become symptomatic between ages 5–25 and develop slowly progressive distal muscle weakness, atrophy, and sensory loss, reduced deep tendon reflexes, and foot deformities (pes cavus or planus).[9] However, some patients may develop significant disability in early childhood and in others, symptoms may not develop until adulthood. Affected children are noted to be slow runners and have difficulty with activities requiring balance. Ankle-foot orthoses are often required by the third decade due to foot drop. Hand function, such as using buttons and zippers, turning keys or typing on a keyboard, becomes affected later in the course of the disease, although to a lesser extent than the feet. Fewer than 5% of patients become wheelchair dependent and there is generally no change in lifespan in most forms of CMT.

Hereditary neuropathy with liability to pressures palsies (HNPP), due to a deletion within the PMP22 gene in approximately 90% of cases, is an autosomal dominant neuropathy that is allelic with the most common subtype of CMT, CMT1A. HNPP is characterized by recurrent focal neuropathies at common sites of nerve compression or entrapment (Table 25.1). Median neuropathies at the wrist (ie, carpal tunnel syndrome) are the most common, although peroneal, ulnar, brachial plexus and radial neuropathies can also frequently develop.[12,13] Symptoms are generally first noticed in the second decade. Patients also often develop a mild distal sensorimotor polyneuropathy and rarely cranial neuropathies.

The exact pathomechanisms of the various types of CMT are still uncertain. Not surprisingly, demyelinating forms of CMT are associated with mutations in genes involved in myelin structure or regulation and axonal forms with mutations in proteins involved in axonal structure and function.[11] However, the exact mechanisms by which these mutations cause CMT are still not well understood. Interestingly, there is evidence in animal models of CMT 1A that administration of exogenous progesterone result in a more

TABLE 25.1 COMMON CHARCOT-MARIE-TOOTH CLASSIFICATIONS

Common Types	Proportion of All CMT	Inheritance	Associated Genes	Clinical Features	NCS Findings
CMT 1A	50%	AD	PMP22 (duplication)	Typical CMT phenotype: distal weakness, atrophy, and sensory loss with foot deformities	Demyelinating (upper limb CV < 38 m/s)
CMT 1B	5–10%	AD	MPZ[x]	Typical CMT phenotype. Ambulation may be delayed	Demyelinating
CMT 2A	10%	AD	MFN2	Usually a childhood onset severe neuropathy with frequent loss of ambulation	Axonal (CV >38 m/s)
CMT 4[*]	<1%	AR	Multiple genetic subtypes	CMT phenotype may vary depending on the genetic subtype	Demyelinating or axonal
CMT 1X	10–15%	XLD	GJ1B	Usually a typical CMT phenotype: males more severely affected than women	Demyelinating (males) or axonal (females)
HNPP	5–10%	AD	PMP22 (del)	Susceptibility to focal compression neuropathies	Prolonged distal latencies and focal conduction blocks

Abbreviations: AD = autosomal dominant, AR = autosomal recessive, CV = conduction velocity, del = deletion, CMT = Charcot-Marie-Tooth, GJB1 = Gap junction beta-1 protein, HNPP = hereditary neuropathy with liability to pressure palsies, MFN2 = Mitofusin-2, MPZ = Myelin protein zero, NCS = nerve conduction studies, PMP22 = Peripheral myelin protein 22, XLD = X-linked dominant
[*] Incidence of recessive forms of CMT are greater in populations with high rates of consanguinity; [x]Selected MPZ mutations may also present with a later onset CMT2 axonal phenotype

severe neuropathy, which has prompted research into the role of progesterone receptor antagonists as a potential therapeutic intervention.[14] However, endogenous progesterone levels do not appear to influence disease severity or progression.[15]

OVERVIEW OF ROUTINE CLINICAL CARE FOR PATIENTS WITH CMT

To date, there are no effective or FDA approved pharmacologic treatments aimed at disease modification for any form of CMT. As such, the primary focus of clinical care is on symptomatic treatment, maintaining functionality, and limiting secondary injury.[1] When available, care is best managed through a multidisciplinary approach involving neurologists, physical and occupational therapists, orthotists, and orthopedic surgeons.

Frequent interventions consist of proper foot stabilization and positioning with custom insoles, ankle support with ankle-foot orthoses, and walking assistive devices. Routine physical therapy for strengthening and balance training and occupational therapy to provide tools and strategies to cope with activities of daily living are crucial. Modifications to the home and work environment are often also needed in advanced stages of the disease. Neuropathic and mechanical pain as well as muscle cramps are occasionally an issue.[16–18] Symptomatic pharmacotherapy, consisting of agents approved for the management of neuropathic and musculoskeletal pain in other disorders (eg, diabetic neuropathy), may be trialed off label in the absence of controlled trials in CMT. Additionally, appropriate foot and ankle support may provide some pain relief. Occasionally, surgical interventions to correct foot deformities or modify tendons can improve pain and functionality.

Routine screening for and management of neuropathy risk factors such as diabetes mellitus, vitamin B12 deficiency, and thyroid disease are especially important in patients with CMT. In addition, medication known to induce neuropathies should be avoided whenever possible including but not limited to certain chemotherapy agents (vincristine, cisplatin, oxaliplatin, bortezomib, thalidomide, eribulin mesylate, and paclitaxel), antibiotics (metronidazole and nitrofurantoin), antiretroviral drugs (didanosine, stavudine and zalcitabine), gold salts, leflunomide, amiodarone, colchicine, dapsone, and disulfiram.

PRE-PREGNANCY PLANNING AND COUNSELING IN PATIENTS WITH CMT

Most women with CMT who choose to become pregnant will have an uncomplicated pregnancy and deliver a healthy infant.[3,19,20] However, having CMT does increase the risk of delivery-related complications and exacerbation of neurologic symptoms during pregnancy.[3,19,20] Therefore, understanding the risks and planning appropriately are crucial to all women with CMT considering pregnancy. Rudnik-Schoneborn et al surveyed 17 women with CMT who had previously been pregnant and found that 65% of them would support the decision to have children, while the remaining 35% of women advised against having children due to inability to cope with weakness and the increased responsibilities of caring for a family.[20] Additionally, all women recommended seeking medical advice and assistance in care for the family prior to pursuing pregnancy.

Optimization of Care

Women with CMT who are interested in becoming pregnant should establish care with an obstetrician and a neurologist. The diagnosis of CMT should be confirmed through family history, neurologic examination, and nerve conduction studies. Multidisciplinary neurologic care aimed at optimizing functionality and limiting injury should be initiated as previously discussed with an emphasis on ways to cope with the physical challenges specific to pregnancy and caring for a child. Respiratory function is occasionally affected in patients with CMT and should be assessed through a clinical history and examination.

There are currently no disease modifying medications for CMT. However, patients will occasionally be taking neuropathic pain medications such as tricyclic antidepressants, duloxetine, gabapentin or pregabalin, which will need to be discussed and optimized to decrease risk of fetal exposures prior to pregnancy and postpartum for lactation.

Genetic Counseling

Genetic counseling should be offered to all patients with CMT and should consist of discussions about genetic testing to make a specific subtype diagnosis and the associated implications. Identification of the causative genetic mutation provides more accurate information about inheritance risk. Additionally, when a pathologic mutation is known in either an affected woman or male partner, prenatal diagnosis becomes a possibility.[21–23] However, chorionic villous sampling comes with its own set of risks and the option to terminate an affected fetus is difficult to cope with for parents-to-be.[24] Alternatively, pre-implantation genetic diagnosis (PGD) performed on embryos obtained through in-vitro fertilization enables couples the possibility of selecting an unaffected embryo for transfer and limits the need for termination of pregnancy.[25] However, PGD can be costly and does not entirely eliminate the risk of an affected fetus or ensure a successful pregnancy.[26] Ultimately, the decision to pursue genetic testing should always rest with the patient.

PREGNANCY IN PATIENTS WITH CMT

CMT's Influence on Pregnancy

Charcot-Marie-Tooth does not appear to affect a woman's ability to carry a pregnancy. Retrospective review of 171 pregnancies in 82 women with CMT conducted by two different groups did not reveal an increased risk of miscarriage or preterm labor compared to the general population.[3,19,20] This was true even for women who were symptomatic from CMT prior to their pregnancies. Additionally, women with CMT do not appear to be at increased risk for obstetric complications during pregnancy such as preeclampsia, hypertension, polyhydramnios, urinary tract infections, premature rupture, or placenta previa.[3,19,20]

Pregnancy's Influence on CMT

Women with CMT may be at increased risk for exacerbation of neurologic symptoms during pregnancy.[20] However, the data on this matter are limited, conflicting, and inconclusive. Either way, there does not appear to be a residual effect on overall CMT disease progression or severity.[15]

There are case reports in the literature of patients with CMT experiencing exacerbation of motor and sensory symptoms during pregnancy, which in some cases resulted in loss of ambulation and respiratory insufficiency, with eventual return to previous functional state within 3 months of delivery.[27–30] In one of these reports, a sural nerve biopsy was performed and revealed endoneurial edema.[28] The authors hypothesized that the exacerbation seen during pregnancy may be due to increased venous pooling secondary to CMT associated autonomic nervous system dysfunction leading to endoneurial edema. However, the generalizability of these single case reports is limited.

Rudnik-Schoneborn et al found in a retrospective review of 45 pregnancies in 21 women with CMT that 50% of the women with subjective CMT symptom onset prior to the age of 21 reported an exacerbation of neurologic symptoms during pregnancy (8 out of 16).[20] Symptoms primarily consisted of increased weakness in the legs. Of the women who reported an exacerbation, 35% returned to baseline within 3 months after delivery, while 65% reported persistent progression. None of the five women who first developed CMT symptoms in adulthood (>20 years of age) reported an exacerbation. Awater et el also found in a retrospective review of 63 pregnancies in 33 women with CMT that deterioration was reported in 32% of pregnancies and felt to be persistent in 68% of those.[3] Unfortunately, definitive conclusions from these studies cannot be made given the retrospective nature and susceptibly to biases.

On the contrary, Swan et al conducted a retrospective cohort study exploring the role of endogenous progesterone on CMT 1A and found that pregnancy does not alter the clinical phenotype.[15] Specifically, a validated CMT clinical severity measure (CMTNS) including signs, symptoms, and nerve conductions measurements was administered to 44 women with CMT 1A who had previously been pregnant, 15 women with CMT1A who had never been pregnant, and 47 men with CMT1A. When controlled for age, there were no differences between any of the groups. Of the women who had previously been pregnant, 52% indicated a worsening of symptoms during pregnancy. The exacerbation was felt to be temporary in 56% women, while the remainder reported permanent change. However, there were no differences in the CMTNS between any of the groups of women, suggesting that pregnancy does not have a permanent contribution to the severity of neuropathy in women with CMT 1A.

Taken together, women with CMT may have up to a 50% chance of symptom exacerbation during pregnancy. However, at least in CMT 1A, these changes will not be permanent or affect overall disease progression or severity.

Clinical Care Recommendations During Pregnancy

Pregnant women with CMT should have routine pregnancy screening and monitoring through their obstetrician. In addition, they should have detailed strength and sensory exams at their routine obstetrical visits and periodically by their neurologist to assess for neurologic progression or new functional limitations that need to be addressed. Continued consultations with physical and occupation therapists should be encouraged to address ongoing needs and anticipate future functional limitations. An anesthesia consultation and delivery plan should be initiated early with a strong recommendation for a hospital based delivery, given the slight increased risk for delivery complications.[3,19]

DELIVERY IN PATIENTS WITH CMT

Risk of an Operative Delivery

There appears to be an increased risk for operative deliveries in women with CMT.[3,19] Specifically, Hoff et al found a significantly increased operative delivery rate at 29.6% (32 of 108 births) compared to 15.3% in a match reference group. This difference was driven by an increased rate of forceps use, which was 9.3% among CMT patients compared to 2.7% in the reference group. There also appeared to be a trend towards an increased number of emergent C-sections among women with CMT (12.9% vs. 7%), although this did not reach statistical significance. There was no different in the rate of elective C-sections or vacuum deliveries. Awater et al did not find a significant difference in the operative delivery rates among women with CMT compared to the general population in their review of 63 pregnancies. The different findings between these two studies may be explained, in part, by a difference in CMT disease severity among the study populations and suggest that operative delivery risk is greatest in women manifesting symptoms of CMT earlier in life. The Norwegian study conducted by Hoff et al assessed patients who had a CMT diagnosis prior to at least one of their pregnancies, while Awater et al also included patients diagnosed with CMT later in life following their last pregnancy and therefore may have included women with a milder disease course.

Risk of Other Obstetrical Complications at Time of Delivery

Overall the rates of obstetrical complications are relatively low among women with CMT with a combined complication rate (premature rupture of amniotic membranes, functional disorder of birth, injuries in the birth canal, bleeding postpartum of

>500 mL, obstruction of birth process, presentation anomalies, and complications regarding the umbilical cord) that does not differ from the general population (42.6% in the CMT cohort vs. 36.3% in a reference group).[19] However, when considering specific complications, Hoff et al found an increased risk for fetal presentation anomalies (9.3% vs. 4.5%) and postpartum bleeding (12% versus 5.8%) among Norwegian women with CMT.[19] Among the presentations anomalies, 40% where breach and 60% where abnormal cephalic. Among women with postpartum bleeding, 15% had undergone a C-section, 30% had uterine dysfunction, 15% had retained placental fragments, and 40% did not have a clear cause identified. The authors hypothesize that the increased bleeding risk may be due to increased uterine atony secondary to abnormal uterine adrenergic innervation related to the underlying hereditary neuropathy. Despite the increased presentation anomaly and postpartum bleeding rates, there was not an increased rate of perinatal mortality.[3,19,20]

Among the many types of hereditary neuropathy, HNPP is uniquely associated with an increased risk of focal compression neuropathies. Thus, pregnant women with HNPP are at an increased risk for peripheral nerve injuries during delivery. Nerve injuries in these patients are sometimes difficult to avoid, such as compression injury to the lumbosacral plexus by the intrauterine fetus or a lumbar sensory nerve root injury following spinal anesthesia.[31,32] At other times, however, neurologic deficits develop following potentially avoidable nerve injuries such as a peroneal nerve injury at the fibular neck in the setting of insufficient leg padding while in stirrups or femoral neuropathies in the setting of excessive hip flexion while in the lithotomy position.

Risk of Fetal Complications
Despite the slight increased risk for obstetrical complications, infants born to women with CMT do not appear to have an increased risk of health complications.[3,19,20] Specifically, these infants are not at an increased risk for abnormal birth measurements, perinatal cardiac or respiratory complications, perinatal mortality, birth defects, abnormal Apgar scores, or changes in general health status.

The inheritance pattern of CMT varies based on the specific subtype and therefore the risk of transmission to the infant is variable. Nevertheless, the majority of individuals with early onset forms of CMT do not manifest significant symptoms or disabilities in infancy.[9] As such, infants of women with CMT are not likely to be at an increased risk for early health complications attributable to the risk of inheriting CMT.

Clinical Care Recommendations During Delivery
Pregnant women with CMT should be encouraged to have their delivery in a hospital setting given the slight increased risks for abnormal fetal presentation, an operative delivery, and postpartum bleeding. Otherwise, they should be provided with routine delivery care. There are rare case reports of scheduled cesarean sections being performed due to intolerable progression of neurologic symptoms with resulting neurologic improvement.[27–30] However, in general, C-sections should not be routinely performed purely on the basis of the underlying CMT diagnosis. Special care should be taken in patients with HNPP during delivery to limit the risk of compression neuropathies through appropriate padding and conscientious limb positioning Box 25.1.

Anesthesia Considerations
Regional anesthesia (epidural or spinal) is recommended over general anesthesia when possible and the use of succinylcholine is discouraged on a theoretical basis.[33] However, there are many case reports documenting routine regional and general anesthesia and postoperative pain management in patients with CMT without complications.[27,29,30,34–37] Additionally, Antognini et al conducted a retrospective review of 161 surgical procedures in 86 patients with CMT and did not find an increased risk of anesthesia related complications despite 90% of the patients receiving succinylcholine and/or a potent inhalation anesthetic.[38]

POSTPARTUM PERIOD IN PATIENTS WITH CMT
The postpartum period should consist of routine neonatal and maternal care. Standard postoperative pain medications including opioids and NSAIDS are safe. Women who experience an exacerbation of neurologic symptoms during pregnancy, will generally return to their previous neurologic baseline within 3 months of delivery.[3,20] Furthermore, pregnancy does not appear to affect the overall disease progression or severity in the majority of women with CMT and routine neurologic care can be continued with a focus on addressing the challenges associated with raising

BOX 25.1
CARE MAP FOR PREGNANCY IN THE PATIENT WITH CHARCOT-MARIE-TOOTH NEUROPATHIES

1. Before Pregnancy

Confirmation of CMT diagnosis
- Based on neurologic exam, nerve conduction studies, and family history

Establish multidisciplinary care and optimize clinical management
- Establish care with an obstetrician and a neurologist
- Neurologic evaluation of weakness, balance, ambulation, and overall functionality
- Physical therapy and orthotics consultations for optimization of foot and ankle support, assistive walking devices, and strength and balance training
- Occupational therapy to provide tools and strategies to cope with activities of daily living and the challenges of pregnancy and caring for an infant
- Respiratory assessment: symptoms and signs (FVC as needed)
- Review of current medications

Genetic counseling
- Consideration of genetic testing to assist with family planning
- Prenatal and pre-implantation genetic diagnosis counseling

2. During Pregnancy

Clinical monitoring of mother
- Routine pregnancy screening and monitoring
- Detailed strength and sensory exams at routine visits: patients at increased risk for transient worsening of symptoms during pregnancy
- Continued PT and OT evaluation to monitor for functional changes and provide adaptive interventions as needed
- Early anesthesia consultation and delivery plan

Clinical monitoring of fetus
- Routine screening and monitoring: no significant increased risk to the fetus

3. Delivery

Multidisciplinary approach
- Obstetrics, anesthesia, pediatrics, neurology
- Hospital based delivery given slight increased risk for operative delivery, abnormal fetal presentation, and postpartum bleeding
- C-section for standard obstetrical indications and in the setting of intolerable progression of neurologic disease

Anesthesia and other considerations
- Regional anesthesia (epidural or spinal) preferred, but general anesthesia appears generally safe and appropriate when indicated
- Limit risk of focal compression neuropathies in patients with HNPP through appropriate limb padding and conscientious limb positioning

4. Postpartum

Pain Management
- Routine post-operative NSAID and narcotic use is safe

Maternal monitoring
- Routine obstetrical follow up
- Neurologic follow up and evaluation within three months of delivery

a child.[15] Weakness may make breastfeeding difficult. If a mother wishes to breastfeed, help with positioning, holding, or pumping may be needed depending on degree or weakness Box 28.1.

REFERENCES

1. Saporta MA. Charcot-Marie-Tooth disease and other inherited neuropathies. *Continuum (Minneapolis, Minn)*. 2014; 20(5 Peripheral Nervous System Disorders): 1208–1225.
2. Dyck PJ, Oviatt KF, Lambert EH. Intensive evaluation of referred unclassified neuropathies yields improved diagnosis. *Annals of Neurology*. 1981; 10(3): 222–226.
3. Awater C, Zerres K, Rudnik-Schoneborn S. Pregnancy course and outcome in women with hereditary neuromuscular disorders: Comparison of obstetric risks in 178 patients. *Eur J Obstet Gynecol Reprod Biol*. 2012; 162(2): 153–159.
4. Argov Z, de Visser M. What we do not know about pregnancy in hereditary neuromuscular disorders. *Neuromuscul Disord*. 2009; 19(10): 675–679.
5. Skre H. Genetic and clinical aspects of Charcot-Marie-Tooth's disease. *Clin Genet*. 1974; 6(2): 98–118.
6. Braathen GJ. Genetic epidemiology of Charcot-Marie-Tooth disease. *Acta Neurol Scand Suppl*. 2012(193): iv–22.
7. Timmerman V, Strickland AV, Zuchner S. Genetics of Charcot-Marie-Tooth (CMT) Disease within the Frame of the Human Genome Project Success. *Genes*. 2014; 5(1): 13–32.
8. England JD, Gronseth GS, Franklin G, et al. Practice parameter, evaluation of distal symmetric polyneuropathy: Role of autonomic testing, nerve biopsy, and skin biopsy (an evidence-based review). Report of the American Academy of Neurology, American Association of Neuromuscular and Electrodiagnostic Medicine, and American Academy of Physical Medicine and Rehabilitation. *Neurology*. 2009; 72(2): 177–184.
9. Saporta AS, Sottile SL, Miller LJ, Feely SM, Siskind CE, Shy ME. Charcot-Marie-Tooth disease subtypes and genetic testing strategies. *Annals of Neurology*. 2011; 69(1): 22–33.
10. Murphy SM, Laura M, Fawcett K, et al. Charcot-Marie-Tooth disease: Frequency of genetic subtypes and guidelines for genetic testing. *J Neurol Neurosurg Psychiatry*. 2012; 83(7): 706–710.
11. Gutmann L, Shy M. Update on Charcot-Marie-Tooth disease. *Current Opinion in Neurology*. 2015; 28(5): 462–467.
12. Mouton P, Tardieu S, Gouider R, et al. Spectrum of clinical and electrophysiologic features in HNPP patients with the 17p11.2 deletion. *Neurology*. 1999; 52(7): 1440–1446.
13. Potulska-Chromik A, Sinkiewicz-Darol E, Ryniewicz B, et al. Clinical, electrophysiological, and molecular findings in early onset hereditary neuropathy with liability to pressure palsy. *Muscle & Nerve*. 2014; 50(6): 914–918.
14. Sereda MW, Meyer zu Horste G, Suter U, Uzma N, Nave KA. Therapeutic administration of progesterone antagonist in a model of Charcot-Marie-Tooth disease (CMT-1A). *Nat Med*. 2003; 9(12): 1533–1537.
15. Swan ER, Fuerst DR, Shy ME. Women and men are equally disabled by Charcot-Marie-Tooth disease type 1A. *Neurology*. 2007; 68(11): 873.
16. Johnson NE, Sowden J, Dilek N, et al. Prospective study of muscle cramps in Charcot-Marie-tooth disease. *Muscle & Nerve*. 2015; 51(4): 485–488.
17. Li J. Inherited neuropathies. *Seminars in Neurology*. 2012; 32(3): 204–214.
18. Carter GT, Jensen MP, Galer BS, et al. Neuropathic pain in Charcot-Marie-Tooth disease. *Archives of Physical Medicine and Rehabilitation*. 1998; 79(12): 1560–1564.
19. Hoff JM, Gilhus NE, Daltveit AK. Pregnancies and deliveries in patients with Charcot-Marie-Tooth disease. *Neurology*. 2005; 64(3): 459–462.
20. Rudnik-Schoneborn S, Rohrig D, Nicholson G, Zerres K. Pregnancy and delivery in Charcot-Marie-Tooth disease type 1. *Neurology*. 1993; 43(10): 2011–2016.
21. Navon R, Timmerman V, Lofgren A, et al. Prenatal diagnosis of Charcot-Marie-Tooth disease type 1A (CMT1A) using molecular genetic techniques. *Prenat Diagn*. 1995; 15(7): 633–640.
22. Bernard R, Labelle V, Negre P, et al. Prenatal detection of a 17p11.2 duplication resulting from a rare recombination event and novel PCR-based strategy for molecular identification of Charcot-Marie-Tooth disease type 1A. *Eur J Hum Genet*. 2000; 8(3): 229–235.
23. Dello Russo C, Padula F, Di Giacomo G, et al. A new approach for Next Generation Sequencing in prenatal diagnosis applied to a case of Charcot-Marie-Tooth syndrome. *Prenat Diagn*. 2015; 35(10): 1018–1021.
24. Bernard R, Boyer A, Negre P, et al. Prenatal detection of the 17p11.2 duplication in Charcot-Marie-Tooth disease type 1A: necessity of a multidisciplinary approach for heterogeneous disorders. *Eur J Hum Genet*. 2002; 10(5): 297–302.
25. De Vos A, Sermon K, Van de Velde H, et al. Pregnancy after preimplantation genetic diagnosis for Charcot-Marie-Tooth disease type 1A. *Mol Hum Reprod*. 1998; 4(10): 978–984.
26. Gui B, Yang P, Yao Z, et al. A new Next-Generation Sequencing-based assay for concurrent

preimplantation genetic diagnosis of Charcot-Marie-Tooth disease Type 1A and aneuploidy screening. *Journal of Genetics and Genomics = Yi chuan xue bao.* 2016; 43(3): 155–159.

27. Brian JE, Jr., Boyles GD, Quirk JG, Jr., Clark RB. Anesthetic management for cesarean section of a patient with Charcot-Marie-Tooth disease. *Anesthesiology.* 1987; 66(3): 410–412.

28. Pollock M, Nukada H, Kritchevsky M. Exacerbation of Charcot-Marie-tooth disease in pregnancy. *Neurology.* 1982; 32(11): 1311–1314.

29. Reah G, Lyons GR, Wilson RC. Anaesthesia for caesarean section in a patient with Charcot-Marie-Tooth disease. *Anaesthesia.* 1998; 53(6): 586–588.

30. Greenwood JJ, Scott WE. Charcot-Marie-Tooth disease: Peripartum management of two contrasting clinical cases. *Int J Obstet Anesth.* 2007; 16(2): 149–154.

31. Chilvers RJ, Salman MM. Hereditary neuropathy with a liability to pressure palsies presenting as a case of sensory neuropathy following spinal anaesthesia for caesarean delivery. *Int J Obstet Anesth.* 2011; 20(1): 95–96.

32. Peters G, Hinds NP. Inherited neuropathy can cause postpartum foot drop. *Anesth Analg.* 2005; 100(2): 547–548.

33. Errando C, Pasha T, D P. Anaesthesia recommendations for patients suffering from Charcot-Marie-Tooth disease. *Orphan Anesthesia;* http://www.orphananesthesia.eu.

34. Scull T, Weeks S. Epidural analgesia for labour in a patient with Charcot-Marie-Tooth disease. *Can J Anaesth.* 1996; 43(11): 1150–1152.

35. Schmitt HJ, Muenster T, Schmidt J. Central neural blockade in Charcot-Marie-Tooth disease. *Can J Anaesth.* 2004; 51(10): 1049–1050.

36. Kapur S, Kumar S, Eagland K. Anesthetic management of a parturient with neurofibromatosis 1 and Charcot-Marie-Tooth disease. *J Clin Anesth.* 2007; 19(5): 405–406.

37. Brock M, Guinn C, Jones M. Anesthetic management of an obstetric patient with Charcot-Marie-Tooth disease: A case study. *AANA J.* 2009; 77(5): 335–337.

38. Antognini JF. Anaesthesia for Charcot-Marie-Tooth disease: A review of 86 cases. *Can J Anaesth.* 1992; 39(4): 398–400.

Guillain-Barré Syndrome and Chronic Inflammatory Demyelinating Polyradiculoneuropathy in Pregnancy

PARIWAT THAISETTHAWATKUL AND ERIC LOGIGIAN

ABSTRACT

Guillain-Barré syndrome (GBS) and chronic inflammatory demyelinating polyradiculoneuropathy (CIDP) are both immune-mediated diseases of the peripheral nervous system that typically present with symmetric, progressive muscle weakness, areflexia, and sensory symptoms or signs. GBS evolves rapidly with a nadir at 2–4 weeks usually with an antecedent viral illness, while CIDP progresses more slowly over months to years. GBS is sometimes complicated by life-threatening respiratory failure or dysautonomia. Onset of GBS and relapse of CIDP can occur during pregnancy or postpartum. But with appropriate supportive care and immunotherapy, maternal and fetal outcome in both conditions is typically excellent. The exception is fetal outcome in GBS triggered by maternal CMV or Zika infection transmitted to the fetus. Full-term vaginal delivery and regional anesthesia are preferred in maternal GBS and CIDP, but if C-section and general anesthesia are indicated, non-depolarizing agents such as succinylcholine should be avoided.

GUILLAIN-BARRÉ SYNDROME

Guillain-Barré syndrome (GBS) is an acute inflammatory polyneuropathy resulting in progressive, symmetric, typically ascending muscle weakness, hypo- or -areflexia, prominent sensory symptoms including pain but relatively mild sensory loss, variable autonomic, respiratory or cranial nerve dysfunction, and albuminocytologic dissociation (increased protein and normal cell count) in cerebrospinal fluid.[1–3] The evolving neurologic deficits reach a nadir over about 2–4 weeks, and are followed by a plateau and recovery phase.[1–3] In a prospective study of 100 GBS patients, limb weakness was present in all patients (mostly proximal weakness in 49%), followed by areflexia (83%), loss of vibration sense

at the toes (59%), facial weakness (53%), loss of joint position sense at the toes (52%), respiratory compromise requiring ventilation in 33%, and weakness of extraocular muscles (13%).[4] GBS variants with different clinical phenotypes have also been described with a similar time course and with albuminocytologic dissociation in CSF. These GBS variants include the Miller-Fisher syndrome (ophthalmoplegia, ataxia, areflexia),[5] and several forms of the disease with segmental weakness patterns: pharyngeal-cervical-brachial and paraparetic variants, severe ptosis without ophthalmoplegia,[6] ophthalmoplegic, and lower cranial nerve variants.[7]

Antecedent immunologic "triggers" in the weeks prior to onset of GBS occur in the majority of patients: respiratory tract infection (38%), gastrointestinal infection (17%), immunizations and surgery.[8] In those with preceding infections, causative serological evidence was present in about 31% including *Campylobacter jejuni* (14%), cytomegalovirus (11%), mycoplasma (1%), Epstein Barr virus (1–2%), and parvovirus B 19 (1%).[8] More recently, antecedent Zika virus infection has been implicated in GBS. In a recent outbreak in French Polynesia, 98% of GBS patients (42 cases in 7 months) were found to have elevated anti- Zika IgM or IgG antibody titers.[9]

While GBS is a clinical diagnosis, spinal fluid and electrophysiologic testing (nerve conduction studies and needle electromyography) are helpful for diagnostic confirmation. Elevated cerebrospinal fluid (CSF) protein is seen in 67–100% of patients.[1] CSF protein is often normal within the first week after onset of symptoms, but by the second or the third week is typically elevated.[1] CSF protein can be as high as 1000 mg/dL and may remain elevated for as long as 2 months before declining.[1] The majority of GBS patients have a normal cell count, but a CSF pleocytosis (5–50 cells/mm^3) occurs in a minority of patients

(14–24%), and when present may be a clue to an alternate trigger for the illness (eg, HIV, Lyme disease, sarcoidosis).[1,3] On nerve conduction studies, most European and North American GBS patients have demyelinative features on motor nerve conduction studies, particularly when tested by the second week of the illness, including conduction block, dispersion, or significant slowing of conduction that evolves over time,[10–16] hence the term acute inflammatory demyelinating polyneuropathy (AIDP). By contrast, in Asian and Central or South American GBS, nerve conduction studies often disclose predominantly motor axon loss physiology without apparent demyelination, illnesses referred to as acute motor axonal neuropathy (AMAN) or acute motor and sensory axonal neuropathy (AMSAN). Conduction block and axon loss in motor nerves are the physiological mechanisms of neurogenic muscle weakness in GBS,[17] and severe axon loss as indicated by marked reduction in distal motor response amplitudes is a prognostic factor for poor functional recovery.[18]

The differential diagnosis of GBS includes other diseases that cause rapidly progressive paralysis, such as CNS disorders (transverse myelitis, basilar artery occlusion, poliomyelitis, West Nile virus, carcinomatous meningitis), neuromuscular junction disorders (myasthenia gravis, botulism, Lambert Eaton myasthenic syndrome), other acute neuropathies (porphyria, nutritional deficiency, critical illness, arsenic poisoning, vasculitis), diseases of muscle (periodic paralysis, poly- or dermato-myositis), and rarer conditions (tick paralysis, neurotoxic fish poisoning).[3] Clinical and laboratory evaluation including spinal fluid analysis, electrodiagnostic testing and neuroimaging studies help differentiate GBS from these other disorders.

The pathogenesis of GBS is immune-mediated attack of the myelin sheath (in AIDP) or of axolemmal gangliosides at the Node of Ranvier (in AMAN).[19] The role of autoimmunity and inflammation in AIDP is supported by two large pathologic studies.[20,21] One study showed edema in the nerve roots early in the course of illness followed by swelling and irregularity of myelin sheaths and disintegration of myelin associated with macrophages and lymphocytes.[20] The other study showed peri-venular mononuclear inflammatory infiltrates seen mainly in proximal nerve segments, and associated with myelin destruction.[21] On the other hand, the axonal forms of GBS, such as AMAN,[22,23] have predominantly axonal degeneration with minimal lymphocytic infiltration[22] and have severely reduced motor response amplitudes on nerve conduction studies.[24] They are often associated with a preceding *Campylobacter jejuni* gastrointestinal infection and, in AMAN, with formation of antibodies against *C. jejuni* ganglioside-like epitopes that appear to cross react with peripheral nerve axolemmal gangliosides (anti GM-1 and anti GD-1A).[25,26] The immune-pathogenesis of AIDP is less well understood as the target antigens on the myelin or Schwann cells are not well defined.[27] Experimental allergic neuritis (EAN), a laboratory model of GBS, is associated with perivascular lymphocytic infiltrates, demyelination and axonal degeneration, and albuminocytologic dissociation[28] (similar to AIDP), and can be passively transferred to naïve animals by injecting them with lymphocytes.[29]

Optimal management of GBS requires timely immunotherapy and comprehensive supportive care. It is important to admit and observe GBS patients to monitor disease progression, particularly for respiratory failure and dysautonomia, with transfer to an intensive care unit (ICU) if necessary. Respiratory status should be monitored at least every 3 hours.[27] The Erasmus GBS respiratory insufficiency score (EGRIS) calculated from the summation of scores from days between the onset of weakness and hospital admission, presence or absence of facial or bulbar weakness and Medical Research Council sum score at admission has been proposed to predict the need for intubation and mechanical ventilation for an accuracy of up to 90%.[30] This score can also be used to determine the need for ICU admission or transfer. The other important issues are cardiac rhythm and blood pressure monitoring, management of bowel and bladder dysfunction, prophylaxis for venous thrombosis, prevention (eg, decubitus) and treatment of infection (eg, pneumonia), pain management, rehabilitation and psycho-social support.

With regard to disease-modifying immunotherapy, in 6 randomized controlled clinical trials comparing plasma exchange (PE) versus supportive care, and in 3 trials comparing intravenous immunoglobulin (IVIg) with PE, both PE and IVIg were found to shorten recovery in patients with GBS.[31] For example, in two of the largest initial PE trials in GBS patients with moderate to severe disease (eg, walking with aid or worse),[32,33] PE significantly decreased the number of patients who needed mechanical ventilation[33] and shortened the time to onset of motor recovery,[33] to improve one grade on the Hughes scale,[32] the time on ventilator,[32] or to begin weaning,[33] and the time to walk assisted[33] or unassisted.[32,33] PE can be accomplished by exchanging 2 plasma volumes on each of 5 sessions performed on alternate days, or 200–250 cc of plasma/kg over 7–14 days.[32,33] In mild GBS cases, 2 PE sessions is effective and in severe GBS cases, 4 PE sessions were not more effective than 6.[34] The beneficial effects of PE are maximal when begun in the first 1–2 weeks after symptoms onset[32,33] but have been documented even at one-year follow-up.[35] Complications related to PE include reactions to the replacement fluid (eg, fever, chills, rash; less with diluted albumin than with fresh frozen plasma), hemodynamic changes (bradycardia, hypotension) and catheter-related complications (venous thrombosis, hematoma, pneumothorax, septicemia).[32] Subsequently, IVIg 0.4 gm/kg/day X 5 days was shown to be as effective in GBS as PE.[36] Short-term use of IVIg in GBS is typically well tolerated but rarely may cause mild decline or increase in blood pressure; mild fever and dyspnea were also observed.[36] Other side effects of IVIg include skin rash, nausea, vomiting, aseptic meningitis, myalgia, renal failure, and venous or arterial thrombosis.[10] Patients with IgA deficiency can develop anaphylaxis when receiving IVIg and checking IgA levels in GBS patients before IVIg infusion is preferred, although is not always practical.[10] Combined treatment of IVIg and PE does not give a better result than IVIg or PE alone and is not recommended.[37] Intravenous methylprednisolone does not have benefit in GBS either alone[38] or in combination with IVIg[39] and is therefore not recommended. Prognosis of GBS is variable. Even though improvement after progression of symptoms is almost invariable, mortality is still 2–10%, 20% of patients are unable to walk at 6 months and many experience long term fatigue and pain.[40]

GBS in pregnancy has similar clinical manifestations as in the general population.[41] The incidence of GBS in pregnancy is unknown but is estimated to be similar to the incidence of GBS in general population (0.75–2 per 100,000 per year) with an increased risk in the first 30 days postpartum.[42] During pregnancy, most cases occur in either the second (47%) or the third (40%) trimester.[43] Diagnosis may be delayed as initial GBS complaints such as weakness or numbness can be misinterpreted as non-specific, commonly encountered symptoms in pregnancy.[43] In contrast to GBS in the general population where *Campylobacter jejuni* is the most common preceding infectious organism identified, GBS in pregnancy is more often related to preceding cytomegalovirus (CMV) infection.[43] It is therefore important to identify the causative organism in pregnancy-related GBS as CMV can affect the mother, cause placentitis, as well as congenital infection causing fetal death.[44] The diagnosis of CMV in the mother requires the presence of anti-CMV-specific IgM and IgG antibodies or positive PCR for CMV in maternal blood.[44] Recently the mosquito-borne Zika virus was reported as a causative agent for GBS during pregnancy and microcephaly in the newborn.[45,46] Therefore, if Zika virus is suspected, antibody or PCR testing for this organism should be considered as well as performance of fetal ultrasound. Miller Fisher syndrome, a more benign GBS variant, has also been reported during pregnancy associated with elevated anti GQ 1B antibody.[47]

Management of GBS is similar in pregnant and non-pregnant patients.[48] Hospitalization is strongly advised to monitor for and treat complications, the most worrisome being respiratory or airway compromise, cardiac rhythm disturbances, and hyper- or hypotension. Given the high risk of hypoxemia to the fetus and mother, timely elective intubation is paramount if required,[49] particularly around labor and delivery when respiratory demands are greater. As both pregnancy and GBS can predispose to venous thromboembolism, prophylactic anticoagulation is recommended.[43] Management of neuropathic pain in GBS during pregnancy requires the use of acetaminophen, and if necessary, opioid medications as anti-epileptic, non-steroidal anti-inflammatory or anti-depressant neuropathic pain medications are contraindicated,[43,48] recognizing that ileus or bladder distension from GBS-associated dysautonomia may be exacerbated by narcotics.

With regard to immunotherapy, both IVIg and plasma exchange have been used safely in pregnancy and lactation for GBS (and other conditions),[43,48] and should be strongly considered in AIDP, AMAN, or AMSAN patients who are, or who appear to be progressing, to the point of significant disability (eg, walking with aid or worse: bedbound, ventilated). After informed consent, treatment should be started as soon as possible. The dose of IVIg and number of plasma exchanges for GBS in pregnancy are similar to GBS in non-pregnant patients. Because IVIg is less likely to affect the patient's hemodynamics, IVIg is considered preferable during pregnancy.[43,48] But both IVIg and plasma exchange for GBS in pregnancy are associated with good maternal and fetal outcome.[50–52]

Pregnancy does not affect the course or severity of intra-partum GBS[49] while the risk of GBS does increase in the postpartum period. Termination of the pregnancy does not hasten the recovery of GBS and is not recommended.[43] Conversely, GBS does not generally affect the outcome of pregnancy either,[49] but the immunologic trigger for GBS may (eg, CMV or Zika infection). Otherwise, newborn survival in maternal GBS is excellent, 96% in one report.[43] Fetal movement is generally unaffected even in the presence of marked maternal muscle weakness, and therefore the risk of neonatal hypotonia, respiratory failure, or arthrogryposis is minimal. Only one case of neonatal GBS born from a mother with GBS in the third trimester has been reported.[53] In that case, serum from both the mother and the infant was shown to have blocking antibodies against the neuromuscular junction suggesting that there could have been transplacental transfer of antibody from the mother to the infant.[54]

GBS in pregnancy does not mandate caesarean section,[43,48] as uterine contraction is intact, even in a case of complete tetraplegia.[53] Vaginal delivery is encouraged, but vacuum or forceps assisted delivery may be required, as weakness of abdominal muscles, if present, may impair the mother's ability to push. In a severe case of GBS in the third trimester, premature labor was reported.[49]

With regard to anesthetic management of delivery in pregnant patients with GBS, one report raised concerns that spinal anesthesia can cause worsening, or a relapse, of GBS in the postpartum period.[56] However, this observation has not been confirmed,[43,57] and may be explained in part by the expected increased incidence of GBS in the postpartum period.[42] Overall, the benefit of regional anesthesia probably outweighs the risk,[43] but it is important to record a patient's neurological examination before and after the procedure.[43] Finally, if general anesthesia is employed for cesarean section, succinylcholine should be avoided as it has been reported to cause cardiac arrest due to hyperkalemia.[55] Postpartum, weakness may make breastfeeding difficult. If a mother wishes to breastfeed, help with positioning, holding, or pumping may be needed depending on degree or weakness/paralysis remaining. If the antecedent infection is known and not cleared (ie, still acute), transmission through the breast milk may need to be addressed (also see Box 26.1).

CHRONIC INFLAMMATORY DEMYELINATING POLYRADICULO-NEUROPATHY

Chronic inflammatory demyelinating polyradiculoneuropathy (CIDP) is a subacute or chronic inflammatory neuropathy characterized by progressive, stepwise, or relapsing weakness and sensory symptoms for at least 8 weeks' duration,[10] typically with demyelinating physiology on electrodiagnostic tests, elevated CSF protein with normal cell count and good response to treatment with immunotherapy.[58,59]

The core clinical features of CIDP have been described in detail in 3 major clinical studies.[59,60,61] Muscle weakness is the main symptom (78–94%), followed by paresthesia (64–79%) with neuropathic pain being less common (20–35%).[59,60,61] Muscle weakness may be predominantly proximal, suggestive of root involvement or distal suggestive of peripheral nerve involvement.[59] Approximately 10% are pure motor without a sensory deficit.[60] The weakness is usually symmetrical. Cranial neuropathies such as unilateral or bilateral facial weakness, extraocular muscle weakness (mostly third or sixth cranial nerve), bulbar weakness with difficulty swallowing, hearing loss, and difficulty chewing have also been described.[59,60] In contrast to GBS, life-threatening respiratory failure and dysautonomia are rare in CIDP. Both monophasic and slowly chronic progressive or remitting-relapsing course can be seen in CIDP.[60,61] All age groups are affected, ranging from 2 to 92 years of age.[61] The prevalence of CIDP has been estimated to be between 1.24[62] to 1.9[63] per 100,000 population with male predominance.[63] About 32% of CIDP have a history of preceding infection within 6 weeks before the symptom onset, most commonly upper respiratory tract infection.[61] In addition to the typical, idiopathic, symmetric, generalized, motor > sensory form, several other CIDP variants have been described including: (1) an asymmetric, focal or multifocal motor and sensory form; (2) a predominantly distal symmetric motor and sensory ataxic variant; (3) a pure sensory ataxic variant; (4) a generalized, symmetric pure motor form; (5) multi-focal motor neuropathy; and (6) CIDP associated with systemic disease including HIV, Lymphoma, MGUS, POEMS syndrome, Sjogren's, or Lupus.[64]

CIDP is a clinical diagnosis with confirmatory lab testing, the most important being the presence of demyelinative findings on motor nerve conduction studies.[65] There have been 16

BOX 26.1
CARE MAP FOR GBS IN PREGNANCY

CARE PRINCIPLES

- Comprehensive supportive care and timely immunotherapy
- Treatment decisions made by patient with neurologist, obstetrician and anesthetist
- No requirement to deliver early or choose C-section over vaginal delivery

BEFORE PREGNANCY/PRE-PREGNANCY/NON-PREGNANT
Principles of diagnosis and medical therapy same as during pregnancy

DURING PREGNANCY
Confirmation of diagnosis:

- Neurologic consultation
- Testing: EMG/NC, CSF exam if required
- Consider testing for CMV, Zika and fetal US in appropriate clinical setting
- Counseling

Supportive management:

- Admission to hospital; consider transfer to ICU for careful monitoring
- Serial monitoring of VS, FVC, O2 saturation, swallowing, cough, progression of weakness
- Elective intubation if necessary
- Prophylaxis for DVT, neuropathic pain control, antibiotics for infection, psychosocial support

Disease modifying therapy:

- IVIg, or Plasma Exchange (see text)

Delivery

- Multidisciplinary discussion about delivery route and location
- C-section for standard obstetric indications only
- Anesthesia consult: epidural anesthesia preferred over general anesthesia
- If general anesthesia required: avoid depolarizing agents such as succinylcholine

POSTPARTUM
Counseling:

- Risk of GBS higher in Postpartum than Intrapartum period
Principles of diagnosis and medical therapy same as during pregnancy

---

proposed electrophysiologic criteria to differentiate demyelinative from axonal neuropathies; all utilize prolongation in distal motor or F wave latency, slow conduction velocity, the presence of conduction block or dispersion, or a combination of these features.[65,66] Albuminocytologic dissociation on CSF analysis is another important diagnostic test, and is present in about 90–100% of CIDP patients.[59,60,61] CSF analysis also helps exclude other CIDP mimics such as sarcoidosis, Lyme radiculoneuropathy, carcinomatous meningitis that typically have a CSF pleocytosis. A sensory nerve biopsy can be useful diagnostically particularly with atypical clinical presentations, or with negative or indeterminate nerve conduction and CSF results.[67] Typical nerve biopsy findings in CIDP include perivascular mononuclear cell infiltrates in the epineurium or the endoneurium,

BOX 26.2
CARE MAP FOR CIDP IN PREGNANCY

CARE PRINCIPLES

- Treatment goal is minimal maternal disease activity and minimal risk to the fetus
- Treatment decisions made by patient with neurologist, obstetrician, and anesthetist
- No requirement to deliver early or choose cesarean over vaginal delivery

BEFORE PREGNANCY/PRE-PREGNANCY/NON-PREGNANT
Prior pregnancies:

- Review prior CIDP exacerbations

Assessment of current clinical status:

- Document neurologic deficits, functional disability

Confirmation of clinical diagnosis:

- Electrodiagnostic testing, CSF evaluation

Counseling:
- Review of immunosuppressive medications and potential adverse effects on germ cells and fetus
- Avoidance of higher risk immunosuppressive medications if contemplating pregnancy
- Discuss contraception if on higher risk immunosuppressive meds

Optimize treatment (see text):

- Medical therapy (IVIg, or corticosteroid preferred over plasma exchange)

DURING PREGNANCY
Clinical monitoring of the mother:

- Observe for relapse of symptoms, most common in third trimester and postpartum
- Medication adjustment with relapse (corticosteroids, IVIg preferred over plasma exchange)

Clinical monitoring of the fetus:

- CIDP poses no significant risk to fetus in absence of maternal hypotension, infection, high risk immunosuppressive agents

DELIVERY
Multidisciplinary care

- Plan delivery with neurology, obstetrics, anesthesia
- No indication for C-section unless for obstetric reasons
- Anesthesia consult: local anesthesia preferred over general
- If general anesthesia required, avoid non-depolarizing agents (succinylcholine), dose reduction for non-depolarizing agents

POSTPARTUM
Maternal counseling:

- Educate about possible exacerbation
- Principles of diagnosis and management (see text for non-pregnant patients)

edema in the endoneurium or between the endo- and –peri-neurium, onion bulb formation, and demyelinative abnormalities in the teased fiber preparation.[59]

Immunotherapy is the mainstay of therapy for CIDP.[68] Corticosteroids,[69] plasma exchange,[70,71] and intravenous immunoglobulin[72–75] are all effective and have been shown in prospective controlled clinical trials to improve motor disability, functional capacity, and the disease course over time. Pulse, rather than daily, or alternate day, prednisone (eg, high-dose monthly oral dexamethasone[76] or, high-dose weekly intravenous methylprednisolone[77]) has also been found to be effective in CIDP, the advantage being fewer side effects (weight gain, Cushingoid features, hypothalamic pituitary suppression). Comparing treatment with corticosteroids versus IVIg, oral prednisolone and IVIg were found to be no different in efficacy,[78] while pulse intravenous methylprednisolone was more often discontinued due to treatment failure than was IVIg.[79] Plasma exchange and IVIg were equally effective,[80] but there have been no studies comparing corticosteroids with plasma exchange.[68] Finally, other immunotherapies such as azathioprine, mycophenolate, cyclosporine, methotrexate, cyclophosphamide, rituximab, Interferon alpha or beta have been shown in open observational studies to be of possible benefit in CIDP[81] and are sometimes used in conjunction with, or after failure of, the 3 therapies of proven efficacy.

CIDP has a similar clinical presentation in pregnant and non-pregnant patients except that there appear to be more relapses in the former, particularly in the third trimester and in the 3-month postpartum period.[82] This is different from GBS in which pregnancy does not affect the course of intrapartum GBS. While pregnancy can affect the course of CIDP, CIDP does not typically adversely affect the course or the outcome of pregnancy and there is no increased risk of spontaneous fetal loss, or premature labor.[49]

Treatment of CIDP during pregnancy with the immunotherapies of proven efficacy is not substantially different from that of CIDP in the general population.[49] IVIg, plasma exchange and corticosteroids can all be used safely during pregnancy,[83] and should be strongly considered in pregnant CIDP patients who are functionally impaired with respect to ADLs including the workplace, walking, etc. Corticosteroids are class B drugs and are considered safe during pregnancy while use of other immunosuppressive therapies with unproven benefit are either contraindicated (eg, methotrexate class X; azathioprine, mycophenolate, and cyclophosphamide: class D) or best avoided if possible (eg, rituximab, cyclosporine, interferons: class C).[84] Since plasma exchange can be problematic with respect to IV access, and risk of hypotension, the authors prefer the use of IVIg or corticosteroids for immunomodulatory treatment of pregnant patients with CIDP. The choice between the two depends on several factors such as success of prior treatments or potential side effects, risk of weight gain, or diabetes support use of IVIg, while the presence of or high risk for thromboembolism support use of corticosteroid.

The recommendation for anesthetic management during delivery in CIDP is based on case reports given the rarity of the condition. Regional anesthesia such as spinal block or epidural anesthesia has been shown to be safe in CIDP patients during delivery.[85,86,87] and has been recommended as a procedure of choice.[85] General anesthesia, if needed, should be undertaken with caution. Depolarizing muscle relaxants such as succinylcholine have been reported to cause fatal hyperkalemia in GBS[55] and should be avoided.[88] Non-depolarizing muscle relaxants such as vecuronium were reported to have a prolonged effect in a CIDP patient undergoing gastrectomy[88] suggesting that dose reduction is required. Finally, due to unpredictability of changes in neurological condition in CIDP, a pre-anesthetic and post-anesthetic neurologic evaluation is recommended (also see Box 26.2).[85]

REFERENCES

1. Ropper AH, Wijdicks EF, Traux BT. Guillain-Barre syndrome. Philadelphia: FA Davis Company; 1991.
2. Hahn AF. Guillain-Barré syndrome. *Lancet*. 1998; 352: 635–641.
3. Ropper AH. The Guillain-Barré syndrome. *N Engl J Med*. 1992; 326: 1130–1136.
4. Winer JB, Hughes RA, Osmond C. A prospective study of acute idiopathic neuropathy. I. Clinical features and their prognostic value. *J Neurol Neurosurg Psychiatry*. 1988; 51: 605–612.
5. Fisher M. An unusual variant of acute idiopathic polyneuritis (syndrome of ophthalmoplegia, ataxia and areflexia). *N Engl J Med*. 1956; 255: 57–65.
6. Ropper AH. Unusual clinical variants and signs in Guillain-Barré syndrome. *Arch Neurol*. 1986; 43: 1150–1152.
7. Ter Bruggen JP, van der Meché FG, de Jager AE, Polman CH. Ophthalmoplegic and lower cranial nerve variants merge into each other and into

classical Guillain-Barré syndrome. *Muscle Nerve.* 1998; 21: 239–242.

8. Winer JB, Hughes RA, Anderson MJ, Jones DM, Kangro H, Watkins RP. A prospective study of acute idiopathic neuropathy. II. Antecedent events. *J Neurol Neurosurg Psychiatry.* 1988; 51: 613–618.

9. Cao-Lormeau VM, Blake A, Mons S, Lastère S, Roche C, Vanhomwegen J, et al. Guillain-Barré Syndrome outbreak associated with Zika virus infection in French Polynesia: A case-control study. *Lancet.* 2016; 387: 1531–1539.

10. Barohn RJ, Saperstein DS. Guillain-Barré syndrome and chronic inflammatory demyelinating polyneuropathy. *Semin Neurol.* 1998; 18: 49–61.

11. Albers JW, Kelly JJ Jr. Acquired inflammatory demyelinating polyneuropathies: clinical and electrodiagnostic features. *Muscle Nerve.* 1989; 12: 435–451.

12. Cleland JC, Malik K, Thaisetthawatkul P, Herrmann DN, Logigian EL. Acute inflammatory demyelinating polyneuropathy: Contribution of a dispersed distal compound muscle action potential to electrodiagnosis. *Muscle Nerve.* 2006; 33: 771–777.

13. Al-Shekhlee A, Hachwi RN, Preston DC, Katirji B. New criteria for early electrodiagnosis of acute inflammatory demyelinating polyneuropathy. *Muscle Nerve.* 2005; 32: 66–72.

14. Gordon PH, Wilbourn AJ. Early electrodiagnostic findings in Guillain-Barré syndrome. *Arch Neurol.* 2001; 58: 913–917.

15. Brown WF, Snow R. Patterns and severity of conduction abnormalities in Guillain-Barré syndrome. *J Neurol Neurosurg Psychiatry.* 1991; 54: 768–774.

16. Miller RG, Peterson C, Rosenberg NL. Electrophysiologic evidence of severe distal nerve segment pathology in the Guillain-Barré syndrome. *Muscle Nerve.* 1987; 10: 524–529.

17. Brown WF, Feasby TE. Conduction block and denervation in Guillain-Barré polyneuropathy. *Brain.* 1984; 107: 219–239.

18. Miller RG, Peterson GW, Daube JR, Albers JW. Prognostic value of electrodiagnosis in Guillain-Barré syndrome. *Muscle Nerve.* 1988; 11: 769–774.

19. Esposito S, Longo MR. Guillain-Barré syndrome. *Autoimmun Rev.* 2017; 16: 96–101.

20. Haymaker WE, Kernohan JW. The Landry-Guillain-Barré syndrome: A clinicopathologic report of 50 fatal cases and a critique of the literature. *Medicine* (Baltimore). 1949; 28: 59–141.

21. Asbury AK, Arnason BG, Adams RD. The inflammatory lesion in idiopathic polyneuritis. Its role in pathogenesis. *Medicine* (Baltimore). 1969; 48: 173–215.

22. Griffin JW, Li CY, Ho TW, Xue P, Macko C, Gao CY, et al. Guillain-Barré syndrome in northern China.

The spectrum of neuropathological changes in clinically defined cases. *Brain.* 1995; 118: 577–595.

23. Nachamkin I, Arzarte Barbosa P, Ung H, Lobato C, Gonzalez Rivera A, Rodriguez P, et al. Patterns of Guillain-Barre syndrome in children: Results from a Mexican population. *Neurology.* 2007; 69: 1665–1671.

24. McKhann GM, Cornblath DR, Griffin JW, Ho TW, Li CY, Jiang Z, et al. Acute motor axonal neuropathy: A frequent cause of acute flaccid paralysis in China. *Ann Neurol.* 1993; 33: 333–342.

25. Yuki N, Ho TW, Tagawa Y, Koga M, Li CY, Hirata K, et al. Autoantibodies to GM1b and GalNAc-GD1a: relationship to Campylobacter jejuni infection and acute motor axonal neuropathy in China. *J Neurol Sci.* 1999; 164: 134–138.

26. Sheikh KA, Ho TW, Nachamkin I, Li CY, Cornblath DR, Asbury AK, et al. Molecular mimicry in Guillain-Barré syndrome. *Ann N Y Acad Sci.* 1998; 845: 307–321.

27. Willison HJ, Jacobs BC, van Doorn PA. Guillain-Barré syndrome. *Lancet.* 2016; 388: 717–727.

28. Waksman BH, Adams RD. Allergic neuritis: an experimental disease of rabbits induced by the injection of peripheral nervous tissue and adjuvants. *J Exp Med.* 1955; 102: 213–236.

29. Astrom KE, Waksman BH. The passive transfer of experimental allergic encephalomyelitis and neuritis with living lymphoid cells. *J Pathol Bacteriol.* 1962; 83: 89–106.

30. Walgaard C, Lingsma HF, Ruts L, Drenthen J, van Koningsveld R, Garssen MJ, et al. Prediction of respiratory insufficiency in Guillain-Barré syndrome. *Ann Neurol.* 2010; 67: 781–787.

31. Hughes RA, Wijdicks EF, Barohn R, Benson E, Cornblath DR, Hahn AF, et al. Practice parameter: immunotherapy for Guillain-Barré syndrome: report of the Quality Standards Subcommittee of the American Academy of Neurology. *Neurology.* 2003; 61: 736–740.

32. The Guillain-Barré syndrome Study Group. Plasmapheresis and acute Guillain-Barré syndrome. *Neurology.* 1985; 35: 1096–1104.

33. French Cooperative Group on Plasma Exchange in Guillain-Barré Syndrome. Efficiency of plasma exchange in Guillain-Barré syndrome: Role of replacement fluids. *Ann Neurol.* 1987; 22: 753–761.

34. The French Cooperative Group on Plasma Exchange in Guillain-Barré Syndrome. Appropriate number of plasma exchanges in Guillain-Barré syndrome. *Ann Neurol.* 1997; 41: 298–306.

35. French Cooperative Group on Plasma Exchange in Guillain-Barré Syndrome. Plasma exchange in

Guillain-Barré syndrome: One-year follow-up. *Ann Neurol.* 1992; 32: 94–97.

36. van der Meché FG, Schmitz PI. A randomized trial comparing intravenous immune globulin and plasma exchange in Guillain-Barré syndrome. Dutch Guillain-Barré Study Group. *N Engl J Med.* 1992; 326: 1123–1129.

37. Plasma Exchange/Sandoglobulin Guillain-Barré Syndrome Trial Group. Randomised trial of plasma exchange, intravenous immunoglobulin, and combined treatments in Guillain-Barré syndrome. *Lancet.* 1997; 349: 225–230.

38. Guillain-Barré Syndrome Steroid Trial Group. Double-blind trial of intravenous methylprednisolone in Guillain-Barré syndrome. *Lancet.* 1993; 341: 586–590.

39. van Koningsveld R, Schmitz PI, Meché FG, Visser LH, Meulstee J, van Doorn PA et al. Effect of methylprednisolone when added to standard treatment with intravenous immunoglobulin for Guillain-Barré syndrome: Randomised trial. *Lancet.* 2004; 363: 192–196.

40. Verboon C, van Doorn PA, Jacobs BC. Treatment dilemmas in Guillain-Barré syndrome. *J Neurol Neurosurg Psychiatry.*2017; 88: 346–352.

41. Massey EW, Guidon AC. Peripheral neuropathies in pregnancy. *Continuum (Minneap Minn).* 2014; 20: 100–114.

42. Cheng Q, Jiang GX, Fredrikson S, Link H, de Pedro-Cuesta J. Increased incidence of Guillain-Barré syndrome postpartum. *Epidemiology.* 1998; 9: 601–604.

43. Chan LY, Tsui MH, Leung TN. Guillain-Barré syndrome in pregnancy. *Acta Obstet Gynecol Scand.* 2004; 83: 319–325.

44. Lupo J, Germi R, Jean D, Baccard-Longère M, Casez O, Besson G. Guillain-Barré syndrome and cytomegalovirus infection during pregnancy. *J Clin Virol.* 2016; 79: 74–76.

45. Krauer F, Riesen M, Reveiz L, Oladapo OT, Martínez-Vega R, Porgo TV, et al. Zika virus infection as a cause of congenital brain abnormalities and Guillain-Barré syndrome: Systematic review. *PLoS Med.* 2017; 14: e1002203. doi: 10.1371/journal.pmed.1002203. eCollection 2017.

46. Lozier M, Adams L, Febo MF, Torres-Aponte J, Bello-Pagan M, Ryff KR, et al. Incidence of Zika virus disease by age and sex—Puerto Rico, November 1, 2015-October 20, 2016. *MMWR Morb Mortal Wkly Rep.* 2016; 65: 1219–1223.

47. Ono M, Sato H, Shirahashi M, Tomioka N, Maeda J, Watanabe K, et al. Clinical features of Miller-Fisher syndrome in pregnancy. *Case Rep Obstet Gynecol.* 2015; 2015: 840680. doi: 10.1155/2015/840680.

48. Pacheco LD1, Saad AF, Hankins GD, Chiosi G, Saade G. Guillain-Barré Syndrome in pregnancy. *Obstet Gynecol.* 2016; 128: 1105–1110.

49. Parry GJ, Heiman-Patterson TD. Pregnancy and autoimmune neuromuscular disease. *Semin Neurol.* 1988; 8: 197–204.

50. Yamada H, Noro N, Kato EH, Ebina Y, Cho K, Fujimoto S. Massive intravenous immunoglobulin treatment in pregnancy complicated by Guillain-Barré Syndrome. *Eur J Obstet Gynecol Reprod Biol.* 2001; 97: 101–104.

51. Matsuzawa Y, Sakakibara R, Shoda T, Kishi M, Ogawa E. Good maternal and fetal outcomes of predominantly sensory Guillain-Barré syndrome in pregnancy after intravenous immunoglobulin. *Neurol Sci.* 2010; 31: 201–203.

52. Kuller JA, Katz VL, McCoy MC, Hansen WF. Pregnancy complicated by Guillain-Barré syndrome. *South Med J.* 1995; 88: 987–989.

53. Luijckx GJ, Vles J, de Baets M, Buchwald B, Troost J. Guillain-Barré syndrome in mother and newborn child. *Lancet.* 1997; 349: 27.

54. Buchwald B, de Baets M, Luijckx GJ, Toyka KV. Neonatal Guillain-Barré syndrome: Blocking antibodies transmitted from mother to child. *Neurology.* 1999; 53: 1246–1253.

55. Feldman JM. Cardiac arrest after succinylcholine administration in a pregnant patient recovered from Guillain-Barré syndrome. *Anesthesiology.* 1990; 72: 942–944.

56. Steiner I, Argov Z, Cahan C, Abramsky O. Guillain-Barré syndrome after epidural anesthesia: Direct nerve root damage may trigger disease. *Neurology.* 1985; 35: 1473–1475.

57. Kocabas S, Karaman S, Firat V, Bademkiran F. Anesthetic management of Guillain-Barré syndrome in pregnancy. *J Clin Anesth.* 2007; 19: 299–302.

58. Austin JH. Recurrent polyneuropathies and their corticosteroid treatment; with five-year observations of a placebo-controlled case treated with corticotrophin, cortisone, and prednisone. *Brain.* 1958; 81: 157–192.

59. Dyck PJ, Lais AC, Ohta M, Bastron JA, Okazaki H, Groover RV. Chronic inflammatory polyradiculoneuropathy. *Mayo Clin Proc.* 1975; 50: 621–637.

60. Bouchard C1, Lacroix C, Planté V, Adams D, Chedru F, Guglielmi JM, et al. Clinicopathologic findings and prognosis of chronic inflammatory demyelinating polyneuropathy. *Neurology.* 1999; 52: 498–503.

61. McCombe PA, Pollard JD, McLeod JG. Chronic inflammatory demyelinating polyradiculoneuropathy: A clinical and electrophysiological study of 92 cases. *Brain.* 1987; 110: 1617–1630.

62. Lunn MP, Manji H, Choudhary PP, Hughes RA, Thomas PK. Chronic inflammatory demyelinating polyradiculoneuropathy: A prevalence study in south east England. *J Neurol Neurosurg Psychiatry*. 1999; 66: 677–680.

63. McLeod JG, Pollard JD, Macaskill P, Mohamed A, Spring P, Khurana V. Prevalence of chronic inflammatory demyelinating polyneuropathy in New South Wales, Australia. *Ann Neurol*. 1999; 46: 910–913.

64. Saperstein DS, Katz JS, Amato AA, Barohn RJ. Clinical spectrum of chronic acquired demyelinating polyneuropathies. *Muscle Nerve*. 2001; 24: 311–324.

65. Bromberg MB. Review of the evolution of electrodiagnostic criteria for chronic inflammatory demyelinating polyradiculoneuropathy. *Muscle Nerve*. 2011; 43: 780–794.

66. Bromberg MB. Comparison of electrodiagnostic criteria for primary demyelination in chronic polyneuropathy. *Muscle Nerve*. 1991; 14: 968–976.

67. Vallat JM, Tabaraud F, Magy L, Torny F, Bernet-Bernady P, Macian F, et al. Diagnostic value of nerve biopsy for atypical chronic inflammatory demyelinating polyneuropathy: Evaluation of eight cases. *Muscle Nerve*. 2003; 27: 478–485.

68. Oaklander AL, Lunn MP, Hughes RA, van Schaik IN, Frost C, Chalk CH. Treatments for chronic inflammatory demyelinating polyradiculoneuropathy (CIDP): An overview of systematic reviews. *Cochrane Database Syst Rev*. January 13, 2017; 1: CD010369. doi: 10.1002/14651858.CD010369.pub2.

69. Dyck PJ, O'Brien PC, Oviatt KF, Dinapoli RP, Daube JR, Bartleson JD, et al. Prednisone improves chronic inflammatory demyelinating polyradiculoneuropathy more than no treatment. *Ann Neurol*. 1982; 11: 136–141.

70. Dyck PJ, Daube J, O'Brien P, Pineda A, Low PA, Windebank AJ, et al. Plasma exchange in chronic inflammatory demyelinating polyradiculoneuropathy. *N Engl J Med*. 1986; 314: 461–465.

71. Hahn AF, Bolton CF, Pillay N, Chalk C, Benstead T, Bril V, et al. Plasma-exchange therapy in chronic inflammatory demyelinating polyneuropathy. A double-blind, sham-controlled, cross-over study. *Brain*. 1996; 119: 1055–1066.

72. Vermeulen M, van Doorn PA, Brand A, Strengers PF, Jennekens FG, Busch HF. Intravenous immunoglobulin treatment in patients with chronic inflammatory demyelinating polyneuropathy: a double blind, placebo controlled study. *J Neurol Neurosurg Psychiatry*. 1993; 56: 36–39.

73. Hahn AF, Bolton CF, Zochodne D, Feasby TE. Intravenous immunoglobulin treatment in chronic inflammatory demyelinating polyneuropathy. A double-blind, placebo-controlled, crossover study. *Brain*. 1996; 119: 1067–1077.

74. Mendell JR1, Barohn RJ, Freimer ML, Kissel JT, King W, Nagaraja HN, et al. Randomized controlled trial of IVIg in untreated chronic inflammatory demyelinating polyradiculoneuropathy. *Neurology*. 2001; 56: 445–449.

75. Hughes RA, Donofrio P, Bril V, Dalakas MC, Deng C, Hanna K, et al. Intravenous immune globulin (10% caprylate-chromatography purified) for the treatment of chronic inflammatory demyelinating polyradiculoneuropathy (ICE study): A randomised placebo-controlled trial. *Lancet Neurol*. 2008; 7: 136–144.

76. van Schaik IN, Eftimov F, van Doorn PA, Brusse E, van den Berg LH, van der Pol WL, et al. Pulsed high-dose dexamethasone versus standard prednisolone treatment for chronic inflammatory demyelinating polyradiculoneuropathy (PREDICT study): a double-blind, randomised, controlled trial. *Lancet Neurol*. 2010; 9: 245–253.

77. Lopate G1, Pestronk A, Al-Lozi M. Treatment of chronic inflammatory demyelinating polyneuropathy with high-dose intermittent intravenous methylprednisolone. *Arch Neurol*. 2005; 62: 249–254.

78. Hughes R, Bensa S, Willison H, Van den Bergh P, Comi G, Illa I, et al. Randomized controlled trial of intravenous immunoglobulin versus oral prednisolone in chronic inflammatory demyelinating polyneuropathy. *Ann Neurol*. 2001; 50: 195–201.

79. Nobile-Orazio E, Cocito D, Jann S, Uncini A, Beghi E, Messina P, et al. Intravenous immunoglobulin versus intravenous methylprednisolone for chronic inflammatory demyelinating polyradiculoneuropathy: A randomized controlled trial. *Lancet Neurol*. 2012; 11: 493–502.

80. Dyck PJ, Litchy WJ, Kratz KM, Suarez GA, Low PA, Pineda AA, et al. A plasma exchange versus immune globulin infusion trial in chronic inflammatory demyelinating polyradiculoneuropathy. *Ann Neurol*. 1994; 36: 838–345.

81. Mahdi-Rogers M, van Doorn PA, Hughes RA. Immunomodulatory treatment other than corticosteroids, immunoglobulin and plasma exchange for chronic inflammatory demyelinating polyradiculoneuropathy. *Cochrane Database Syst Rev*. June 14, 2013; (6): CD003280. doi: 10.1002/14651858.CD003280.pub4.

82. McCombe PA, McManis PG, Frith JA, Pollard JD, McLeod JG. Chronic inflammatory demyelinating polyradiculoneuropathy associated with pregnancy. *Ann Neurol*. 1987; 21: 102–104.

83. Sax TW, Rosenbaum RB. Neuromuscular disorders in pregnancy. *Muscle Nerve*. 2006; 34:559–571.

84. Danesi R, Del Tacca M. Teratogenesis and immunosuppressive treatment. *Transplant Proc*. 2004; 36: 705–707.

85. Richter T1, Langer KA, Koch T. Spinal anesthesia for cesarean section in a patient with chronic inflammatory demyelinating polyradiculoneuropathy. *J Anesth*. 2012; 26: 280–282.

86. Schabel JE. Subarachnoid block for a patient with progressive chronic inflammatory demyelinating polyneuropathy. *Anesth Analg*. 2001; 93: 1304–1306.

87. Velickovic IA, Leicht CH. Patient-controlled epidural analgesia for labor and delivery in a parturient with chronic inflammatory demyelinating polyneuropathy. *Reg Anesth Pain Med*. 2002; 27: 217–219.

88. Hara K, Minami K, Takamoto K, Shiraishi M, Sata T. The prolonged effect of a muscle relaxant in a patient with chronic inflammatory demyelinating polyradiculoneuropathy. *Anesth Analg*. 2000; 90: 224–226.

27

Entrapment Neuropathy and Pregnancy

PARIWAT THAISETTHAWATKUL AND ERIC LOGIGIAN

ABSTRACT

Entrapment neuropathy is a focal mononeuropathy caused by compression, angulation, distortion or stretch of a peripheral nerve as it passes through a fibrous or fibro-osseous canal, or less commonly by other structures. In addition to true entrapment neuropathies, individual nerves can be injured at vulnerable anatomical locations. Pregnancy causes a wide variety of physiological changes related to reproductive hormone secretion that can affect peripheral nerve including weight gain, salt and water retention, edema and hyperglycemia. Two entrapment neuropathies that occur commonly in pregnancy are carpal tunnel syndrome and meralgia paresthetica. In addition to these true entrapment neuropathies, this chapter will address other common focal mononeuropathies: femoral, obturator and fibular neuropathies that may occur as a consequence of obstetrical procedures or of fetal or maternal positioning during delivery or in the postpartum period. Most entrapment neuropathies occurring during pregnancy or postpartum period have good prognosis with recovery or functional improvement after delivery. Rarely does a surgical intervention is required to treat entrapment neuropathy during pregnancy and therefore conservative management approaches are preferred during pregnancy.

INTRODUCTION

Entrapment neuropathy is caused by compression, angulation, or stretch of a peripheral nerve as it passes through a fibro-osseous canal such as the carpal or the cubital tunnel (in the case of the median or the ulnar nerves). In addition to true entrapment neuropathies, individual nerves can be injured at vulnerable anatomical locations such as the fibular head (in case of the fibular nerve). Pregnancy causes a wide variety of physiological changes related to reproductive hormone secretion that can affect peripheral nerve. These include weight gain, salt and water retention, edema and hyperglycemia[1]. Two entrapment neuropathies that occur commonly in pregnancy are carpal tunnel syndrome and meralgia paresthetica[2]. Most entrapment neuropathies occurring during pregnancy or postpartum period have good prognosis with recovery or functional improvement after delivery requiring conservative approach for management (please also see Box 27.1).

CARPAL TUNNEL SYNDROME (CTS)

CTS results from entrapment of the median nerve as it passes through the carpal tunnel in the wrist. The pathology of idiopathic CTS is considered to be tenosynovitis of the carpal ligament but in fact inflammation is rarely present[3]. It is the most common entrapment neuropathy and is most frequently primary or idiopathic[4]. Secondary CTS may occur as a result of focal structural changes that reduce the space within the carpal tunnel (eg, ganglion cysts)[4]. In addition, pregnancy and various systemic medical conditions[5] such as diabetes mellitus, hypothyroidism, acromegaly, amyloidosis, gout, rheumatoid arthritis are risk factors for CTS.

Typical symptoms are numbness, tingling, or pain in the hand, particularly in the palmar surface of the index, middle and the radial aspect of ring finger. Symptoms are often bilateral, but the dominant hand is usually affected initially. Frequently, a patient reports paresthesia of the whole hand or shooting pain from the wrist up to the elbow. The symptoms most often come on at night or upon waking in the morning prompting the patient to shake the hand to ease the symptoms (flick sign)[4]. As the condition advances, neurologic deficits

---

BOX 27.1
CARE MAP FOR ENTRAPMENT NEUROPATHY IN PREGNANCY

CARE PRINCIPLES

- Treatment goal is conservative treatment with surgery as a last resort
- Preventive during parturition to avoid injury of lower extremity nerves

BEFORE PREGNANCY/PRE-PREGNANCY/NON-PREGNANT

- Review prior symptoms related to entrapment neuropathy

DURING PREGNANCY
Assessment of clinical status:

- Document neurologic deficits, functional disability
- Review risk factors: weight gain, occupation

Confirmation of clinical diagnosis (if required):

- Neurologic consultation
- Electrodiagnostic or ultrasound testing

Clinical monitoring of the mother:

- Monitor weight gain, fluid retention, physical activities, pain level

Optimize treatment (see text):

- Emphasize conservative over surgical treatment
- Modification of risk factors
- Avoid higher risk pain medications

DELIVERY

- Best practices (see text) to minimize potential for lower extremity nerve injury

POSTPARTUM

- Symptoms typically improve after delivery
- Conservative management (bracing, physical therapy, pain management) usually suffices
- If pain medications are required consider fetal transfer of medications if breastfeeding

---

develop with persistent sensory loss in the lateral 4 fingers and weakness and atrophy of the thenar muscles.

The diagnosis is usually straightforward. Occasionally, patients with C6 or C7 cervical radiculopathy can present with lateral hand numbness but typically also have radicular neck pain, weakness of biceps, triceps, or wrist flexion or pronation, or a reduced biceps or triceps reflex. Similarly, patients with a lower cervical radiculopathy or lower trunk brachial plexopathy (eg, neurogenic thoracic outlet syndrome) may have thenar muscle weakness but typically have sensory loss in in the medial hand or forearm. Proximal median neuropathies are rare and can be distinguished by the presence of weakness in median-innervated forearm muscles. Finally, painful musculoskeletal conditions can be distinguished by the absence of neurologic signs or symptoms and the presence of focal tenderness over the respective tendon or joint. Electrodiagnostic testing[6] and ultrasonography[7] can confirm the diagnosis, exclude competing diagnoses, and quantitate the degree of median motor and sensory axon loss.[6,8]

Treatment of CTS depends on the severity of symptoms, signs, functional disability, and of median nerve injury on electrodiagnostic testing. In mild cases, a conservative approach using a neutral-position wrist splint is recommended.[9] The splint can be worn mainly at night for a minimum of 6 weeks as improvement in symptoms may take several weeks. Nonsteroidal anti-inflammatory medications are often recommended to relieve pain. Diuretics may be considered when there is significant wrist or finger swelling. This conservative approach is effective in about 90% of mild cases.[10] If the symptoms continue despite a conservative approach for 3–6 months, injection with corticosteroid into the carpal tunnel may be considered but the procedure may need repetition in some cases.[9] If bothersome symptoms persist despite conservative methods, or if electrodiagnostic studies reveal significant median motor or sensory axonal loss, open or endoscopic decompressive surgery may be indicated.[9]

CTS is the most common entrapment neuropathy during pregnancy[11] with an incidence that ranges widely from 0.34%[12] to 62%[13,14] depending on study methodology. In women with clinically diagnosed CTS, electrophysiologic confirmation of the diagnosis also varies widely from 7% to 43%.[15] Edema, fluid retention, excessive maternal weight (pre-pregnancy body mass index $\geq$ 30 kg/m²), excessive gestational weight gain, smoking, and alcohol use are the major risk factors for CTS in pregnancy.[13,16,17] The major cause of CTS in pregnancy is likely related to edema within the carpal tunnel given that the major risk factor is fluid retention[11] and weight gain.

Symptoms of CTS in pregnancy and in the general population are similar except that swelling of wrist, hand, or fingers or peripheral edema is more often present in the pregnant patient. Paresthesia and pain in the hands are common, particularly at night. Symptoms are more often bilateral but when unilateral, left and right hand involvement is comparable.[12,14,16] Symptoms most often begin in the third trimester[14,16,18], but if they begin earlier,[12] symptoms escalate by the third trimester.[16]

Spontaneous improvement in symptoms can be expected in most pregnant CTS patients based on data from two long-term follow-up studies.[14,19] However, if required, decompressive surgery for severe cases of CTS can be performed without complications during pregnancy.[20] Because many (if not most) patients with CTS during pregnancy have spontaneous remission of symptoms after delivery, a conservative approach to treatment is advised. Our recommendation is that all pregnant women who experience typical symptoms of carpal tunnel syndrome be treated presumptively with nocturnal neutral-position wrist splints. If symptoms are severe, atypical, are accompanied by a neurologic deficit, or do not improve within 2–3 weeks of splinting, then evaluation by a neurologist should be considered to confirm the diagnosis and stage the severity. In the evaluation process, nerve conduction studies (or ultrasonography if available) are recommended with needle EMG testing as needed to exclude alternative diagnoses (eg, cervical radiculopathy) and quantitate median motor and sensory axon loss. Thiazide diuretics are a treatment option, particularly if there is prominent swelling and weight gain, although concerns for fetal oligohydramnios exist. Nonsteroidal anti-inflammatory agents should not be used for pain control after the first trimester. If symptoms do not abate with splinting, local injection with corticosteroid into the carpal tunnel can be considered. If injection does not relieve the symptoms or the patient develops median distribution weakness or persistent sensory disturbance with electrophysiologic evidence of significant median axon loss, decompressive surgery may be required. Postpartum, help will be needed with positioning and feeding of the baby, for the breastfeeding mother with hand weakness and pain (see also Section 5, Chapter 35).

LATERAL FEMORAL CUTANEOUS SENSORY MONONEUROPATHY (MERALGIA PARESTHETICA)

Meralgia paresthetica is caused by mononeuropathy of the lateral femoral cutaneous nerve and is the most common sensory mononeuropathy in the lower extremity.[21] The lateral femoral cutaneous nerve is a pure sensory nerve formed by the ventral rami of the L2 and L3 roots. It sub-serves cutaneous sensation over the lateral thigh. It emerges into the upper thigh underneath the inguinal ligament medial to the anterior superior iliac spine.[22]

The lateral femoral cutaneous nerve has a sharp bend at the apex of which is the inguinal ligament, predisposing the nerve to compression or traction.[23]

The incidence has been estimated to be 4.3 per 10,000 persons annually.[24] The symptoms consist of unpleasant numbness and pain usually located at the lateral thigh, not going below the knee and usually not crossing the anterior or posterior midline of the thigh.[21] Symptoms are usually unilateral but can be bilateral, are typically worse with standing or walking, and are relieved by sitting.[4] There is no motor weakness. Most cases are idiopathic, but the neuropathy is often associated with diabetes mellitus, pregnancy, obesity, and advancing age.[21] Other risk factors include external compression (eg, wearing tight trousers or belts),[4] or prolonged lithotomy (flexed hips) position.[21] The diagnosis is usually straightforward with sensory loss over the lateral thigh, normal strength of hip and knee musculature, and normal knee reflexes. Electrodiagnostic testing may help in clarifying the diagnosis,[25] mainly by excluding conditions that can cause similar symptoms such as upper lumbar radiculopathy or plexopathy.[21]

Treatment is usually conservative with symptom resolution once precipitating factors are addressed.[21] Pain and numbness typically subside with weight loss, control of diabetes mellitus, or after delivery in a case with pregnancy. In non-pregnant patients with intolerable pain, antidepressants (such as tricyclic antidepressants), or anticonvulsants (such as gabapentin or pregabalin) can be used.[21] Local injection with corticosteroid or anesthetic agents can be helpful in patients that do not respond to oral pain medications. Finally, surgical treatment for pain such as neurectomy or neurolysis is effective in up to 95% of cases.[4,21]

In the Rotterdam study, the risk factor with the highest odds ratio (12.0) for meralgia paresthetica was pregnancy.[24] Meralgia paresthetica occurs quite commonly during pregnancy[26] although the incidence is unknown. Most cases occur in the third trimester[27] when the tension on the abdominal muscles and fascia is greatest. Fluid retention and laxity of the inguinal ligament may also play a role.[26] The symptoms of meralgia paresthetica during pregnancy are similar to cases without pregnancy, being aggravated by standing and walking.[23] The course based on case report data appears to be benign.[23,26,27] Most patients have spontaneous remission of pain symptoms after delivery even though some sensory loss over the thigh

may persist.[23,26,27] Most cases require only reassurance and, if needed, mild analgesics.[27] Only rarely are the symptoms severe enough to warrant nerve decompression surgery.[23,28] In pregnant patients in whom pain becomes bothersome (eg, interferes with sleep), our recommendation is escalating treatment first with acetaminophen, then local application of a lidocaine patch, and finally local injection with corticosteroid or an anesthetic agent at the inguinal ligament if pain is otherwise uncontrolled. Heat and ice applications are safe in pregnancy as well. Anti-epileptic agents for neuropathic pain are contraindicated during pregnancy,[28] and we prefer to avoid even low dose amitriptyline, as it is a Class C drug, but it may be preferable over prolonged narcotic use. Postpartum, the safety of medications in lactation should also be considered (see Section 5, Chapter 35) for a list of commonly used medications and lactation safety.

Meralgia paresthetica can also occur postpartum[29–32] in the setting of prolonged second stage of labor (especially with extreme hip flexion),[30] injury from local injection of anesthetic agents,[29] and traction of the nerve during cesarean section.[31] In all cases, however, spontaneous recovery was observed within 4 weeks after delivery.

FEMORAL MONONEUROPATHY

The femoral nerve originates from the posterior divisions of the ventral rami of the L2-4 spinal nerves. It innervates the iliopsoas, pectineus, sartorius, and quadriceps muscles[24] and provides cutaneous sensation over the medial calf (saphenous nerve) and anterior medial thigh (anterior cutaneous nerve of the thigh).[24] The proximal segment of the femoral nerve traverses the retroperitoneal pelvic space within the iliacus compartment and the distal segment passes below the inguinal ligament.[21] In the retroperitoneal space, the femoral nerve can be injured by traction or pressure from retractor blades used in pelvic surgeries (ie, abdominal hysterectomy), from retroperitoneal hematoma or ruptured aortic aneurysm.[21] At the inguinal ligament, the nerve is vulnerable to angulation/stretch during a prolonged procedure in the lithotomy position, or from compression by an inguinal hematoma or other mass.[21] Clinical features depend on the site of the lesion. A proximal lesion in the pelvis causes weakness in hip flexion, in addition to knee extension and lateral thigh rotation, sensory loss along the anteromedial thigh and the medial lower leg whereas a lesion distal to the inguinal ligament causes similar symptoms but spares hip flexion.[22] In either case, patients typically report knee weakness or buckling resulting in falls, difficulty ascending and descending stairs, numbness over the anterior thigh and the medial calf,[4] and on examination have an unevocable knee reflex in addition to the sensory and motor findings above. The diagnosis, severity, and prognosis of femoral neuropathy can be confirmed by electrodiagnostic testing,[33] which is also helpful in excluding lumbar radiculopathy or plexopathy that can cause similar symptoms. The key clinical point in differentiating femoral neuropathy from lumbar radiculopathy or plexopathy is that hip adduction is spared in femoral neuropathy and typically affected in lumbar radiculopathy or plexopathy.

Femoral mononeuropathy is seen in the immediate postpartum period in pregnancy, and has an incidence of 2.8 in 100,000.[32] While virtually all reported cases of femoral mononeuropathy occur in the postpartum period,[34–39] bilateral femoral neuropathy in the third trimester has been reported, which progressed after caesarean section but completely recovered at 3 months.[40] Femoral mononeuropathy can be unilateral[35,37,38] or bilateral,[34,36,39] can follow vaginal delivery[35–38] or cesarean section,[34,39] typically with spinal or epidural anesthesia.[34,35,37,38,39] The causes remain speculative but are thought to be due to difficult labor with prolonged lithotomy position,[35,36,37,39] use of retractors during cesarean section,[34] compression of the fetal head,[28] or rarely from retroperitoneal hematoma during cesarean section.[39] All patients should be treated conservatively with a knee splint if necessary, muscle strengthening exercises, passive range-of-motion exercises, and pain control. The prognosis of postpartum femoral mononeuropathy is good with functional recovery of muscle strength in virtually all cases.[34–39]

OBTURATOR MONONEUROPATHY

The obturator nerve originates from the anterior divisions of the ventral rami of L2-4 spinal nerves. It descends along the edge of psoas muscle and traverses the obturator foramen to supply thigh adductors and provides sensory supply to the skin of the medial thigh. Injury to the obturator nerve is rare due to its protected location in the pelvis and the medial thigh[41] but can occur as a complication of hip or pelvic surgery, femoral artery procedures, or from pelvic trauma.[41] Most surgery-related cases have acute onset and a good prognosis. Other cases associated with systemic disorders such as diabetes mellitus, or metastasis to the pelvis[41] have a chronic course and a poorer prognosis. Most cases of obturator neuropathy present with pain or paresthesia, and less frequently sensory loss over the medial thigh. Weakness of hip adductors may not be apparent,[41] or be incomplete as the adductor magnus receives a dual supply from both the obturator and sciatic nerves. The diagnosis can be confirmed by denervation of thigh adductors on electromyography, sparing iliopsoas, and quadriceps muscles. Treatment depends on the cause.[21] In most cases, conservative management with pain control is sufficient. In more chronic, intractable cases, laparoscopic neurolysis[4], or obturator nerve block[21] may be considered.

Obturator mononeuropathy associated with pregnancy typically comes to light in the postpartum period, with onset from one day to 8 weeks after delivery,[42–45] and can be unilateral or bilateral. Most cases occur in the setting of a difficult and prolonged labor after caesarean section[43–45] or rarely after vaginal delivery with forceps extraction.[42] The proposed mechanisms of postpartum obturator neuropathy include compression by the fetal head against the pelvic brim, injury from forceps, and a prolonged lithotomy position.[28] The few reported cases have significant weakness in the medial thigh and difficulty walking.[43,44,45] One patient developed a snapping hip (audible snapping sound during flexion and extension of the hip while walking).[45] Treatment recommendations include physical therapy,[44] pain control including obturator nerve block for severe pain,[42] and corticosteroid local injection to the iliotibial band for snapping hip.[45] As in most patients with acute obturator neuropathies,[41] the prognosis for full functional recovery appears to be excellent.

FIBULAR MONONEUROPATHY

The fibular nerve branches from the sciatic nerve slightly above the popliteal fossa. It gives off a motor branch to supply the short head of biceps muscle in the posterior thigh and the lateral cutaneous nerve of the knee at the level of the popliteal fossa.[46] It then winds around the fibular head and divides into the superficial and deep fibular nerves. The deep fibular nerve innervates ankle and toe extensors and subserves cutaneous sensory perception in the web space between the first and the second toes.[46] The superficial fibular nerve innervates ankle everters and subserves cutaneous sensation over the mid and lower lateral calf and dorsum of the foot.[46] Injury or compression of the fibular nerve occurs most commonly at the fibular head,[47] where the fibers destined for the deep fibular nerve are located medially adjacent to the fibular bone and those for the superficial fibular nerve more laterally.[46] The deep fibular nerve is thereby more prone to compression than the superficial fibular nerve.[47] Compressive fibular neuropathy occurs most commonly as a peri-operative complication (improper positioning of the legs, inadequate knee padding), from prolonged squatting (crop harvesting, prolonged Yoga session, childbirth) or intrapartum (excessive force applied to the knees to keep the knees and hips flexed during labor or "pushing palsy").[21] Equally frequent is fibular nerve compression at the fibular head from habitual leg crossing, or from hard mattresses in thin, bedridden patients. Less common causes include direct penetrating trauma, anterior compartment syndrome, fibular tunnel entrapment, or mass lesions (eg, Baker's cyst).[21] The core clinical symptoms are foot drop (resulting in a steppage gait) and numbness over the calf, foot or first webspace. The muscles supplied by the deep fibular nerve (foot and toe dorsi-flexors) are typically more affected than those supplied by the superficial fibular nerve (ankle everters).[47] The diagnosis can be confirmed by electrodiagnostic testing, which can also exclude competing causes of foot drop (ALS, L5 radiculopathy, lumbar plexopathy, sciatic mononeuropathy, or distal myopathy). Neuroimaging may identify structural causes of fibular mononeuropathy (eg, intra-neural ganglia) or confirm other competing diagnoses (L5 root compression).

Management depends on the severity, likely cause, and physiological type of the lesion. For example, in a neurapraxic or demyelinating lesion in the setting of external compression of the nerve at the fibular head (eg, cross-leg palsy), the prognosis is good, can be treated conservatively with ankle-foot orthosis to stabilize the ankle and prevent falls, and recovery can be expected within 3 months.[47] If it does not improve, imaging should be performed to exclude a mass lesion. By contrast, in a penetrating injury (eg, laceration) with significant axon loss, the recovery of foot drop is slow and often incomplete. In the case of marked fibular motor axon loss without clinical improvement, surgical exploration and repair of the fibular nerve is recommended.[21,47]

Fibular mononeuropathy in pregnancy occurs during childbirth[48-52] following vaginal deliveries with forceful hand pressure over the lateral part of the knees to draw the knees and the hips into a flexed position,[50,52] or following deliveries in a prolonged squatting position[48,51] during which the common fibular nerve is compressed between the biceps femoris tendon and the lateral head of the gastrocnemius muscle.[51] The neuropathy may be unilateral[48,49,52] or bilateral,[50,51] is noted immediately or within 2 days of delivery, and with symptoms and signs similar to fibular mononeuropathy in general. It is important to establish that there are no neurologic deficits in the gluteal, sciatic and tibial nerve distributions since a number of patients with peri-partum foot drop may actually have a lumbosacral plexus lesion[53,54] (likely due to compression of the lumbosacral trunk by the fetal head) or rarely a partial sciatic neuropathy[55,56] (in the setting of C-section with prolonged lateral tilt positioning and pressure over the ipsilateral buttock). Overall, the prognosis is good with spontaneous recovery in 2–4 months after delivery.[49-52] Similarly, foot drop from plexus[53,54] and sciatic[55,56] neuropathies is also good with recovery noted over the same time frame.

Many if not most cases can be prevented (see Box 27.1). During vaginal delivery, the hands should be placed behind the posterior thighs, not over the lateral part of the knees, and use of leg holders should be avoided.[49] Prolonged squatting should be minimized,[48] and the patient should squat only during contraction and sit or stand in between.[57] Should a fibular neuropathy develop, an ankle foot or foot-up orthosis can be used until foot drop recovers. In patients undergoing cesarean section under spinal anesthesia, risk of compressive sciatic neuropathy can be minimized by shortening the time in the lateral tilt position intra-operatively and postpartum.

REFERENCES

1. Gordon MC. Maternal physiology. In: Gabbe SG, Nirbyl JR, Simpson JL, et al, eds. *Obstetrics: Normal and Problem Pregnancies*. Philadelphia: Elsevier Saunders; 2012: 42–65.

2. Aminoff MJ. Pregnancy and disorders of the nervous system. In Aminoff MJ, ed. *Neurology and General Medicine*. 4th ed. Philadelphia: Churchill-Livingstone Elsevier; 2008: 673–693.

3. Preston D. Compressive and entrapment neuropathies of the upper extremities. In: Katirji B, Kaminski HJ, Ruff RL, eds. *Neuromuscular Disorders in Clinical Practice*. 2nd ed. New York. Springer; 2014: 871–902.

4. Bouche P. Compression and entrapment neuropathies. *Handb Clin Neurol*. 2013; 115: 311–366.

5. Smith G. Median mononeuropathies. In Bromberg MB, Smith AG, eds. *Handbook of Peripheral*

Neuropathy. Boca Raton, FL: Taylor & Francis; 2005: 467–480.

6. Herrmann DH, Logigian EL. Electrodiagnostic approach to the patient with suspected mononeuropathy of the upper extremity. *Neurol Clin N Am.* 2002; 20: 451–478.

7. Chen YT, Williams L, Zak MJ, Fredericson M. Review of ultrasonography in the diagnosis of carpal tunnel syndrome and a proposed scanning protocol. *J Ultrasound Med.* 2016; 35: 2311–2324.

8. Goldberg G, Zeckser JM, Mummaneni R, Tucker JD. Electrosonodiagnosis in carpal tunnel syndrome: A proposed diagnostic algorithm based on an analytic literature review. *PMR.* 2016; 8: 463–474.

9. Freimer M, Brushart TM, Cornblath DR, Kissel JT. Entrapment neuropathies. In: Mendell JR, Kissel JT, Cornblath DR, eds. *Diagnosis and Management of Peripheral Nerve Disorders.* New York. Oxford University Press; 2001: 592–632.

10. The Quality Standards Subcommittee for the American Academy of Neurology. Practice parameters for carpal tunnel syndrome: Summary statement. *Neurology.* 1993; 43: 2406–2409.

11. Massey EW, Guidon AC. Peripheral neuropathies in pregnancy. *Continuum (Minneap Minn).* 2014; 20: 100–114.

12. Stolp-Smith KA, Pascoe MK, Ogburn PL, Jr. Carpal tunnel syndrome in pregnancy: Frequency, severity, and prognosis. *Arch Phys Med Rehabil.* 1998; 79: 1285–1287.

13. Padua L, Aprile I, Caliandro P, et al. Symptoms and neurophysiological picture of carpal tunnel syndrome in pregnancy. *Clin Neurophysiol.* 2001; 112: 1946–1951.

14. Mondelli M, Rossi S, Monti E, et al. Long term follow-up of carpal tunnel syndrome during pregnancy: A cohort study and review of the literature. *Electromyogr Clin Neurophysiol.* 2007; 47: 259–271.

15. Padua L, Di Pasquale A, Pazzaglia C, Liotta GA, Librante A, Mondelli M. Systematic review of pregnancy-related carpal tunnel syndrome. *Muscle Nerve.* 2010; 42: 697–702.

16. Meems M, Truijens S, Spek V, Visser LH, Pop VJ. Prevalence, course and determinants of carpal tunnel syndrome symptoms during pregnancy: A prospective study. *BJOG.* 2015; 122: 1112–1118.

17. Wright C, Smith B, Wright S, Weiner M, Wright K, Rubin D. Who develops carpal tunnel syndrome during pregnancy: An analysis of obesity, gestational weight gain, and parity. *Obstet Med.* 2014; 7: 90–94.

18. Mondelli M, Rossi S, Monti E, Aprile I, Caliandro P, Pazzaglia C, et al. Prospective study of positive factors for improvement of carpal tunnel

syndrome in pregnant women. *Muscle Nerve.* 2007; 36: 778–783.

19. Padua L, Aprile I, Caliandro P, et al. Carpal tunnel syndrome in pregnancy: Multiperspective follow-up of untreated cases. *Neurology.* 2002; 59: 1643–1646.

20. Stahl S, Blumenfeld Z, Yarnitsky D. Carpal tunnel syndrome in pregnancy: Indications for early surgery. *J Neurol Sci.* 1996; 136: 182–184.

21. Katirji B. Compressive and entrapment neuropathies of the lower extremity. In: Katirji B, Kaminski Hj, Ruff RL, eds. *Neuromuscular Disorders in Clinical Practice.* 2nd ed. New York. Springer; 2014: 903–952.

22. Felice KJ. Focal neuropathies of the femoral, obturator, lateral femoral cutaneous nerve and other nerves in the thigh and pelvis. In: Bromberg MB, Smith AG, eds. *Handbook of Peripheral Neuropathy.* Boca Raton, FL: Taylor & Francis; 2005: 541–557.

23. Pearson MG. Meralgia paraesthetica, with reference to its occurrence in pregnancy. *J Obstet Gynaecol Br Emp.* 1957; 64: 427–430.

24. van Slobbe AM, Bohnen AM, Bernsen RM, Koes BW, Bierma-Zeinstra SM. Incidence rates and determinants in meralgia paresthetica in general practice. *J Neurol.* 2004; 251: 294–297.

25. Preston D, Shapiro BE. Lumbosacral plexopathy. In: *Electromyography and Neuromuscular Disorders: Clinical-Electrophysiologic Correlations.* 3rd ed. Philadelphia. Elsevier Saunders; 2013: 501–517.

26. Petersen PH. Meralgia paresthetica related to pregnancy. *Am J Obstet Gynecol.* 1952; 64: 690–691.

27. Rhodes P. Meralgia paraesthetica in pregnancy. *Lancet.* 1957; 273: 831.

28. Sax TW1, Rosenbaum RB. Neuromuscular disorders in pregnancy. *Muscle Nerve.* 2006; 34: 559–571.

29. Schnatz P, Wax JR, Steinfeld JD, Ingardia CJ. Meralgia paresthetica: An unusual complication of post-cesarean analgesia. *J Clin Anesth.* 1999; 11: 416–418.

30. Van Diver T, Camann W. Meralgia paresthetica in the parturient. *Int J Obstet Anesth.* 1995; 4: 109–112.

31. Paul F, Zipp F. Bilateral meralgia paresthetica after cesarian section with epidural analgesia. *J Peripher Nerv Syst.* 2006; 11: 98–99.

32. Vargo MM, Robinson LR, Nicholas JJ, Rulin MC. Postpartum femoral neuropathy: Relic of an earlier era? *Arch Phys Med Rehabil.* 1990; 71: 591–596.

33. Preston D, Shapiro B. Routine lower extremity nerve conduction techniques. In: *Electromyography and Neuromuscular Disorders: Clinical-Electrophysiologic Correlations,*

3rd ed. Philadelphia. Elsevier Saunders; 2013: 115–124.

34. Adelman JU, Goldberg GS, Puckett JD. Postpartum bilateral femoral neuropathy. *Obstet Gynecol.* 1973; 42: 845–850.

35. Montag TW, Mead PB. Postpartum femoral neuropathy. *J Reprod Med.* 1981; 26: 563–566.

36. Donaldson JO, Wirz D, Mashman J. Bilateral postpartum femoral neuropathy. *Conn Med.* 1985; 49: 496–498.

37. Cohen S, Zada Y. Postpartum femoral neuropathy. *Anaesthesia.* 2001; 56: 500–501.

38. Peirce C, O'Brien C, O'Herlihy C. Postpartum femoral neuropathy following spontaneous vaginal delivery. *J Obstet Gynaecol.* 2010; 30: 203–204.

39. Chao A, Chao A, Wang CJ, Chao AS. Femoral neuropathy: A rare complication of retroperitoneal hematoma caused by cesarean section. *Arch Gynecol Obstet.* 2013; 287: 609–611.

40. Kofler M, Kronenberg MF. Bilateral femoral neuropathy during pregnancy. *Muscle Nerve.* 1998; 21: 1106.

41. Sorenson EJ, Chen JJ, Daube JR. Obturator neuropathy: Causes and outcome. *Muscle Nerve.* 2002; 25: 605–607.

42. Warfield CA. Obturator neuropathy after forceps delivery. *Obstet Gynecol.* 1984; 64(3 Suppl): 47S–48S.

43. Nogajski JH, Shnier RC, Zagami AS. Postpartum obturator neuropathy. *Neurology.* 2004; 63: 2450–2451.

44. Hong BY, Ko YJ, Kim HW, Lim SH, Cho YR, Lee JI. Intrapartum obturator neuropathy diagnosed after cesarean delivery. *Arch Gynecol Obstet.* 2010; 282: 349–350.

45. Oh J, Kang M, Park J, Lee JI. A possible cause of snapping hip: Intrapartum obturator neuropathy. *Am J Phys Med Rehabil.* 2014; 93: 551.

46. Preston D, Shapiro B. Peroneal neuropathy. In: *Electromyography and Neuromuscular Disorders: Clinical-Electrophysiologic Correlations.* 3rd ed. Philadelphia. Elsevier Saunders; 2013: 346–356.

47. Sbei AM. Sciatic neuropathy. In: Bromberg MB, Smith AG, eds. *Handbook of Peripheral Neuropathy.* Boca Raton, FL: Taylor & Francis; 2005: 527–539.

48. Babayev M, Bodack MP, Creatura C. Common peroneal neuropathy secondary to squatting during childbirth. *Obstet Gynecol.* 1998; 91: 830–832.

49. Qublan HS, al-Sayegh H. Intrapartum common peroneal nerve compression resulted in foot drop: A case report. *J Obstet Gynaecol Res.* 2000; 26: 13–15.

50. Sahai-Srivastava S, Amezcua L. Compressive neuropathies complicating normal childbirth: Case report and literature review. *Birth.* 2007; 34: 173–175.

51. Hashim SS, Adekanmi O. Bilateral foot drop following a normal vaginal delivery in a birthing pool. *J Obstet Gynaecol.* 2007; 27: 623–624.

52. Radawski MM, Strakowski JA, Johnson EW. Acute common peroneal neuropathy due to hand positioning in normal labor and delivery. *Obstet Gynecol.* 2011; 118: 421–423.

53. Katirji B, Wilbourn AJ, Scarberry SL, Preston DC. Intrapartum maternal lumbosacral plexopathy. *Muscle Nerve.* 2002; 26: 340–347.

54. Brusse E, Visser LH. Footdrop during pregnancy or labor due to obstetric lumbosacral plexopathy. *Ned Tijdschr Geneeskd.* 2002; 146: 31–34.

55. Roy S, Levine AB, Herbison GJ, Jacobs SR. Intraoperative positioning during cesarean as a cause of sciatic neuropathy. *Obstet Gynecol.* 2002; 99: 652–653.

56. Postaci A, Karabeyoglu I, Erdogan G, Turan O, Dikmen B. A case of sciatic neuropathy after caesarean section under spinal anaethesia. *Int J Obstet Anesth.* 2006; 15: 317–319.

57. Reif ME. Bilateral common peroneal nerve palsy secondary to prolonged squatting in natural childbirth. *Birth.* 1988; 15: 100–102.

28

Neurocutaneous Disorders in Pregnancy

ASHA N. TALATI AND DAVID N. HACKNEY

INTRODUCTION

Neurocutaneous disorders, or *phakomatoses*, are hereditary and sporadic conditions that feature lesions of the skin, nervous system, and often the internal viscera. This chapter provides an overview of such conditions and their management in the setting of pregnancy, with focuses on preconception counseling and antepartum care, as well as specific considerations for anesthesia, delivery, and postpartum care. Care plans for each condition are featured at the end of each section summarizing current recommendations for best practice.

NEUROFIBROMATOSIS TYPE 1

Neurofibromatosis type 1 (NF1), also called *von Recklinghausen disease*, is an autosomal dominant condition characterized by café au lait spots and tumors of the peripheral nerves called neurofibromas. Central neurologic findings are limited but include iris hamartomas known as Lisch nodules that are pathognomonic of NF1. This condition occurs in approximately 1 in 3,000 people.[1]

Prior to conception, women with NF1 should be offered consultation with maternal fetal medicine, genetics, neurology, and anesthesiology to discuss maternal and fetal issues associated with pregnancy (Table 28.1). Similarly, men considering biologic fatherhood should meet with a genetic counselor to discuss the transmission risks.

Genetic counseling may include NF1 specific molecular genetic testing for the parents as well as the possibility of preimplantation genetic diagnosis (PGD) if the couple does not desire offspring affected by NF1. Successful live births have been reported amongst couples that have undergone PGD in which one partner has NF1.[2]

Specific maternal risks include an increased incidence of hypertensive disease, cardiovascular events, preterm labor, and cesarean delivery. Fetal considerations include an increased risk of preterm birth and intrauterine growth restriction.

It has been demonstrated that maternal and fetal outcomes worsen among with women with large numbers of peripheral lesions, with worst reported outcomes occurring among women with greater than 200 peripheral lesions.[3–5] There are currently no recommendations for timing or mode of delivery and no evidence that suggests improved outcomes with cesarean section over vaginal birth. Careful review of maternal and fetal factors as well as coordination by multidisciplinary team should assist in determination of delivery timing and means.

Retrospective evidence of patients followed with NF1 through pregnancy suggests pregnancy stimulates growth of peripheral neurofibromas, likely secondary to increased vascularity and hormonal changes. Thus, preconception and antepartum CNS imaging may be required to screen for existing CNS lesions or new growths and determine whether a patient is a candidate for neuraxial anesthesia. If general anesthesia is required, patients should be evaluated for neurofibroma formation surrounding oral structures of the airway or chest wall deformities.[6–8]

NEUROFIBROMATOSIS TYPE 2

Neurofibromatosis type 2 (NF2) is an autosomal dominant condition that typically presents with central neurologic tumors in the second decade of life, most characteristically bilateral vestibular schwannomas. Other tumors that may occur include ependymomas, meningiomas, and astrocytomas. Overall, the condition is rare, occurring in approximately 1 in 35,000–1 in 50,000 people. Cutaneous manifestations that are common in type 1 are rarely present with type 2.[1] NF1 has been associated with vascular lesions, hypertension and in some reports, pheochromocytoma.[3]

Like NF1, women with NF2 should be offered multispecialty preconception counseling including

TABLE 28.1 DIAGNOSTIC CRITERIA FOR NEUROFIBROMATOSIS TYPE 1

Any two or more:
- Six or more café-au-lait lesions more than 5 mm in diameter before puberty and more than 15 mm in diameter afterward
- Freckling in the axillary or inguinal areas
- Optic glioma
- Two or more neurofibromas or one plexiform neurofibroma
- A first degree relative with neurofibromatosis type 1
- Two or more Lisch nodules
- A characteristic bony lesion (sphenoid dysplasia, thinning of the cortex of long bones, with or without pseudoarthrosis)

From: Neurofibromatosis. Conference statement, 1988 National Institutes of Health Consensus Development Conference (1)

maternal fetal medicine, neurology, anesthesia, and both men and women with NF1 offered genetic counseling (Table 28.2). Genetic counseling including molecular genetic testing for parents and, if desired, PGD can be offered (6). However, given rarity of NF2, there are no current reports of live births after PGD among couples with this condition.

Women with NF2 are at increased risk of hypertensive disease of pregnancy, need for general anesthesia, and cesarean delivery.[4] The greatest morbidity stems from the presence of central nervous system lesions and the possibility of continued growth during pregnancy—affecting approximately 10% of women with NF2. Coordinated care between obstetrics and neurology should be undertaken to determine need for repeat imaging throughout pregnancy and close screening for symptoms of increased intracranial pressure. There is no evidence to support improved outcomes with a particular mode of delivery, (ie, vaginal birth or cesarean delivery) in the presence of NF2.[9] However, the presence of neuraxial lesions or increased intracranial pressure may increase the risk of hemorrhage or herniation with spinal anesthesia (see also Chapters 32 and 33). In this setting, general endotracheal anesthesia may be required. Valsalva and prolonged second stage may also increase maternal morbidity requiring assisted second stage.[6-8] Delivery method and timing should be determined through multispecialty recommendations based on location and size of lesions and risks associated with each mode of delivery (see also Chapter 31). NF1 and 2 patients have no contraindications to breastfeeding and are likely to be successful.

EHLERS DANLOS SYNDROME
Ehlers Danlos syndrome is a set of connective tissue disorders leading to fragile or hyperelastic skin, hyperextensible joints, vascular lesions, easy bruising, poor wound healing, and excess scarring. It is inherited in autosomal dominant fashion, however about 50% of mutations are de-novo. It can also be associated with neurodegenerative features including peripheral neuropathy due to

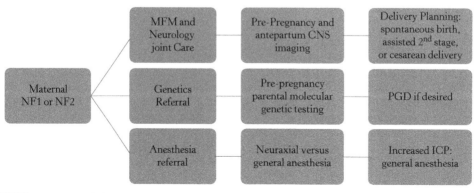

FIGURE 28.1 Care path for management of NF1 or NF2

TABLE 28.2 DIAGNOSTIC CRITERIA FOR NEUROFIBROMATOSIS TYPE 2

Any of the below criteria:
- Bilateral eight nerve tumor (shown by magnetic resonance imaging, computed tomography, or histological confirmation)
- A first-degree relative with neurofibromatosis type 2 and a unilateral eighth nerve tumor
- A first-degree relative with neurofibromatosis type 2 and any two of the following lesions: neurofibroma, meningioma, schwannoma, glioma, or juvenile posterior subcapsular lenticular opacity

---

From: Neurofibromatosis. Conference statement, 1988 National Institutes of Health Consensus Development Conference (1)

---

ligamentous laxity. Early severe disease may present with neonatal hypotonia or weakness. Severe vascular complications may also occur with Ehlers Danlos type IV including arterial aneurysm or arterial dissection. The most common site of aneurysm formation is the internal carotid artery just beyond the cavernous sinus. Severe morbidity may occur in the setting of spontaneous rupture.[1]

Pregnancy with hypermobility type EDS is relatively benign with little added risk in pregnancy. The primary adverse pregnancy outcomes is an increased risk of preterm birth with incidence ranging from 13–21%, based on retrospective single-institution studies.[10] Management of pregnancy and labor may require further care if peripheral neuropathy and weakness are present, however for the vast majority of patients, traditional prenatal care and labor management can be followed.[10] In the setting of severe peripheral weakness or neuropathy, neurological follow up is important to monitor for worsening neurologic symptoms. Assisted second stage may also be required; however, this should be determined on a case-by-case basis. Patients with hypermobility type EDS also have an increased incidence of dural ectasia and scoliosis; as such, anesthesia consultation and spine imaging may be beneficial prior to delivery to determine optimal mode of anesthesia administration.[11]

By contrast, maternal risks associated with EDS types IV (vascular EDS) are far greater, including uterine rupture, extensive perineal trauma, severe bleeding, and aortic dissection. Fetal complications can include miscarriage, fetal demise, and prematurity. Morbidity is highest when these events occur during labor at term. Given significant risk of mortality, pregnancy is not recommended in the setting of vascular EDS.[11-12] However, if pregnancy is pursued, coordinated care between maternal fetal medicine and cardiology should be established. Maternal cardiac evaluation may include echo every 4-12 weeks during pregnancy with continuation 6 months postpartum. Beta-blockers

may also be recommended to prevent progression of aortic root dilation if present. Delivery timing to precede labor may be considered if there is confirmed vascular EDS with history of arterial tears or bleeding, however there is no consensus on optimal timing of delivery.[13,14] Mode of delivery is dependent on the presence of aortopathy. In the setting of aortic root dilation greater than 45 mm, general anesthesia with cesarean delivery is often performed. However, consideration for labor and assisted second stage can be made in the setting of aortic root dilation less than 45 mm and good cardiac status. Unfortunately, perineal trauma can be common with instrumental delivery. Epidural anesthesia can be offered to patients with vascular EDS; however, such patients are at increased risk of epidural hematoma and should be carefully counseled.[11] Anesthesia consultation is necessary prior to any delivery (also see Fig. 28.2).

TUBEROUS SCLEROSIS

Tuberous sclerosis (TS) is an autosomal dominant condition with variable penetrance and is the second most common neurocutaneous condition. However, up to 50–80% of childhood cases are due to sporadic mutations. TS affects approximately 1/6000–1/9000 individuals, caused by mutation of the hamartin (TSC1) or tuberin (TSE) tumor suppressor genes on chromosomes 9 and 16, respectively. Classic cutaneous manifestations of TS include hypomelanotic macules called ashleaf spots, shagreen patches, ungula fibromas, and facial angiofibromas. Systemic hamartomas (tubers) begin developing between 14–16 weeks gestation and can affect the brain parenchyma, eyes, cardiac structure, kidneys, and lungs. Malignant transformation may also occur including subependymal giant cell astrocytomas, cardiac rhabdomyomas, and renal angiomyolipomas.[1]

Women with TS pursuing pregnancy should be offered preconception counseling with maternal fetal medicine, genetics, anesthesiology, and neurology (Table 28.3). Both men

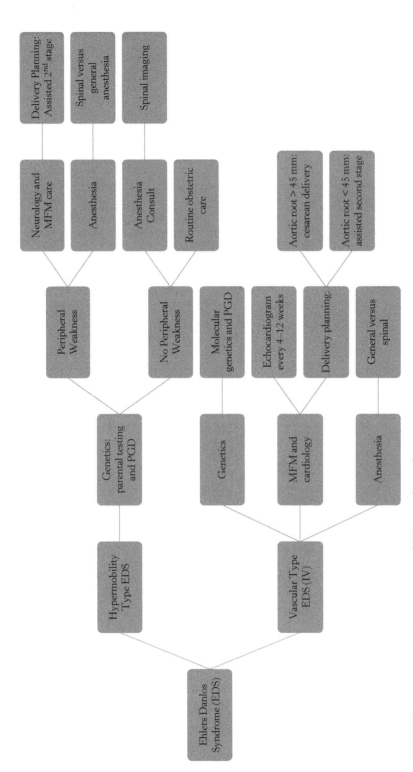

FIGURE 28.2 Care path for management of Ehlers Danlos syndrome

TABLE 28.3 DIAGNOSTIC CRITERIA FOR TUBEROUS SCLEROSIS

Genetic Diagnostic Criteria
- Mutation in TSC1 or TSC2

Clinical Diagnostic Criteria: Major Features
- Hypomelanotic macules (≥3, at least 5 mm diameter)
- Angiofibromas (≥3) or fibrous cephalic plaque
- Ungual fibromas (≥2)
- Shagreen patch
- Multiple renal hamartomas
- Cortical dysplasia
- Subependymal nodules
- Supependymal giant-cell astrocytoma
- Cardiac rhabdomyoma
- Lymphangioleiomyomatosis (LAM)
- Antiomyolipomas (≥2)

Clinical Diagnostic Criteria: Minor Features
- "Confetti" skin lesions
- Dental enamel pits (≥3)
- Intraoral fibromas (≥2)
- Retinal achromic patch
- Multiple renal cysts
- Nonrenal hamartomas

Definite Diagnosis
- Two major features or one major features with ≥2 minor features
- Possible diagnosis: either one major feature or ≥2 minor features

From: Northrup, H., Kruger, D.A., 2013. Tuberous sclerosis complex diagnostic criteria update: recommendations from the 2012 international tuberous sclerosis complex consensus conference: *Pediatric Neurology.* 49: 243–254 (1).

and women with TS should be offered genetic counseling and discussion of transmission risk. They should also consider care and delivery at a tertiary care center given risks associated with pregnancy. Molecular genetic testing and PGD are available for patients with established or suspected disease, or significant family history.[16]

Maternal risk of pregnancy is primarily dependent on location and size of hamartomas; larger lesions may have vascular involvement and increase maternal risk of bleeding. Highest risk lesions include astrocytoma, cardiac rhabdomyoma, and renal angiomyolipoma; however, all large visceral lesions incur some risk of internal hemorrhage.[15] Women with presence of astrocytoma will require close monitoring for symptoms of elevated intracranial pressure and CNS imaging to determine safety of neuraxial anesthesia. Similarly, women with presence

of cardiac rhabdomyoma may require cardiac function monitoring throughout pregnancy. Renal angiomyolipomas pose the greatest risk during pregnancy; however, they are a rare manifestation of TS. In the presence of this lesion, women should be aware of high risk of retroperitoneal hemorrhage, likelihood of continued growth of the mass, and the recommendation for scheduled cesarean delivery with simultaneous mass resection. Given risk of rupture and hemorrhage, labor and vaginal birth are contraindicated in this scenario.[15,16] There is no evidence for optimal timing and mode of delivery among women with tuberous sclerosis; delivery planning should occur in coordination with multispecialty team and depend on the patient's specific disease manifestations. TS patients have no contraindications to breastfeeding and are likely to be successful (see Figure 28.3).

Fetal TS is often caused by a sporadic mutation and can be diagnosed prenatally using ultrasound—and in some cases, MRI. Initial finding may be a cardiac rhabdomyoma, seen in approximately 1 in 10,000 pregnancies. This finding often prompts further workup including fetal echo to demonstrate location of other tubers, with some providers using MRI also.[15] Cardiac rhabdomyoma significantly increases fetal risk of arrhythmia, heart failure, and hydrops fetalis.[15,16] The presence of cardiac, central nervous, or renal tubers significantly increase the risk of perinatal morbidity and mortality. Affected infants demonstrate a high risk of miscarriage and intrauterine fetal demise. Based on case reports, neonatal survival is estimated to be 21% with high lifetime likelihood of seizure disorder, developmental delay, and residual cardiac disease.[17]

VON HIPPEL LINDAU

Von Hippel Lindau (VHL) is an autosomal dominant condition with variable expression. It causes a mutation of a tumor suppressor gene on chromosome locus 3p25–26, allowing for hemangioblastoma formation throughout the central nervous system and peripheral viscera. Common locations of lesions include the cerebellum, spine, medulla, retina, kidneys, adrenals, and pancreas. Morbidity stems from mass effect or rupture. CNS tumors may results in headache, ataxia, and progressive nystagmus depending on location of lesions. Ocular lesions may cause retinal injury, glaucoma, and macular edema. Renal cell carcinoma occurs in 70% of patients with renal tumors and is the leading cause of death among patients with VHL. An estimated 7 to 19% of patients may also have pheochromocytoma.[1]

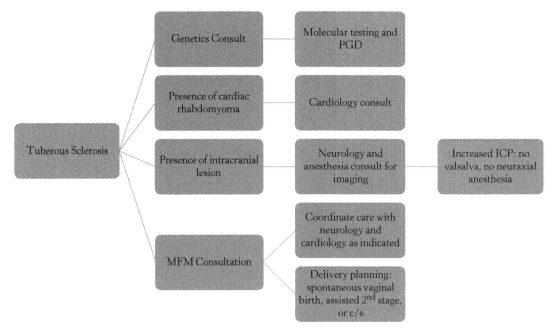

FIGURE 28.3 Care path for management of tuberous sclerosis complex

Women with VHL pursuing pregnancy or presenting with new diagnosis of pregnancy should receive multispecialty care and consider delivery at a tertiary care center. Prior to pregnancy, genetic counseling for both men and women affected by VHL including molecular diagnostic testing of parents and, if desired, PGD, should be offered. Although rare, there are case reports of successful live birth after use of PGD among women with VHL.[18]

Pregnancy has been demonstrated to stimulate growth in size and number of tumors, likely due to circulatory changes and hormonal milieu. Further, edema surrounding intracranial tumors can increase, resulting in increased risk of elevated intracranial pressure throughout pregnancy.[19–21] Given this, it is recommended that women with VHL receive pre-pregnancy imaging with MRI to assess location and size of CNS lesions and surveillance throughout pregnancy at 16 and 28 weeks, and prior to delivery.[19] Women with VHL may also have an increased incidence of hypertensive disease in pregnancy; however, this may also be related to pheochromocytoma.[20] We recommend baseline assessment of proteinuria, blood pressure, and preeclampsia labs at the start of pregnancy to help differentiate between adrenal tumor development and preeclampsia later on.

Delivery timing and method are usually related to presence and extent of maternal disease. Primary fetal risk is preterm birth, usually secondary to early delivery from a maternal indication.[19] In the presence of extensive neural tumors, anesthesiology consultation is required to determine safest route of pain control. Several case reports suggest an increased risk of herniation and hemorrhage with placement of neuraxial anesthetic in the presence of CNS lesions; however, it is not strictly contraindicated.[19] There are also case reports of successful vaginal births and epidural anesthesia.[19] In the setting of small CNS lesions and no symptoms of increased intracranial pressure, current recommendations include spinal anesthesia placement and assisted second stage.[19] Timing of delivery primarily depends on maternal condition, although one retrospective study suggested 32 weeks to prevent worsening neurologic status with advancing pregnancy (also see Fig. 28.4).[20–22]

HEREDITARY HEMORRHAGIC TELANGIECTASIA (OSLER WEBER RENDU)

Hereditary hemorrhagic telangiectasia (HHT), or *Osler Weber Rendu* syndrome, is an autosomal dominant condition with high penetrance. It presents with cutaneous telangiectasia of the face, lips, and hands typically first occurring in the teenage years. Morbidity typically occurs from vascular dysplasia of the lungs, gastrointestinal, and genitourinary tract. Arteriovenous malformations (AVM) may also occur, most commonly in the

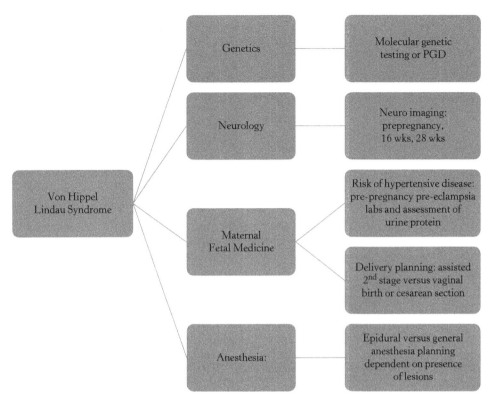

FIGURE 28.4 Care path for management of Von Hippel Lindau syndrome

liver. Diagnosis is made through clinical features such as recurrent epistaxis, cutaneous features, visceral vascular malformation, and affected first-degree family members with at least 3 of the 4 criteria present.[1]

Women with HHT and pregnancy should be offered multidisciplinary care at a tertiary care center given high risk of maternal morbidity (Figure 28.5). Prior to pregnancy, genetic testing and counseling can be offered to parents with suspected or confirmed clinical diagnosis. Once molecular abnormality is known, PGD can be utilized.[23] Counseling on specific risks of pregnancy associated with disease manifestations should be offered. Overall, highest risk of maternal morbidity due to hemorrhage stems from lung and liver vascular lesions. However, the majority of pregnancies amongst women with HHT progress normally.[24–27] Retrospective reviews demonstrate bleeding complications occurred in approximately 13% of women with HHT, exclusively amongst women who did not receive antepartum screening and management of vascular lesions.[26–28] Rates of adverse maternal/fetal outcomes overall such as prematurity, cesarean birth, low birth weight, miscarriage, and fetal demise, are similar to the general population.[29]

Amongst women with high-risk lung, liver, and cerebral AVMs, screening prior to and surveillance during pregnancy greatly assist in prevention of shunting and bleeding. Women with such lesions should be referred to appropriate vascular specialist for possible embolic therapy prior to pursuing pregnancy or during early pregnancy as risk of inappropriate shunting and rupture increase due to hemodynamic changes of pregnancy.[25] The presence of spinal and cerebral lesions is rare, occurring among 0–0.6% of patients with HHT. Given the low incidence, pre-pregnancy imaging for spinal lesions is not uniformly recommended; however, lack of imaging should not contraindicate placement of spinal anesthesia if indicated.[26] Optimal timing of delivery has not been reported and should be determined on a case-by-case basis from maternal and fetal status. There is no maternal or fetal benefit to delivery via cesarean delivery.[29] Among women with pulmonary or hepatic disease, delivery method should be determined after consultation with maternal fetal medicine, vascular, and anesthetic team. Often, valsalva during maternal expulsive efforts may be contraindicated, requiring use of an assisted second stage (also see Fig. 28.5).[26]

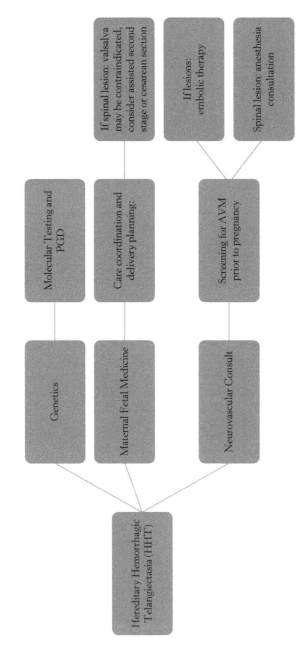

FIGURE 28.5 Care path for management of hereditary hemorrhagic telangiectasia

CONCLUSIONS

Neurocutaneous disorders have a variety of multi-organ system manifestations, most notably skin, neurologic system, and at times, internal visceral structures. In the setting of pregnancy, such disorders can lead to increased maternal and fetal risk requiring a coordinated care plan between neurology, high-risk obstetrics, anesthesiology, and other sub-specialists. Pre-conception and genetic counseling are often offered in the setting of such conditions in order to discuss pregnancy considerations and fetal impact, respectively. Establishing and coordinating care at a tertiary care center early in pregnancy can assist in creation of a maternal-fetal care plan and providing best outcomes for mother and child.

REFERENCES

1. Islam MP, Roach ES. Volume 132: Neurocutaneous syndromes. In: Aminoff MJ, Francois, B, Swaab DF, eds. *Handbook of Clinical Neurology*. 1st ed. Elsevier, 2015.
2. Merker V., Murphy T., Hughes J., Muzikansky A., Hughes, M., Souter I., Plotkin S. Outcomes of pre-implantation genetic diagnosis in neurofibromatosis type 1. *Fertility and Sterility*, 2015; 103: 761–768.
3. Sharma J., Gulati N., Malik, S. Maternal and perinatal complications in 4. Neurofibromatosis during pregnancy. *Int. J Gynecol.Obstet*. 1991; 34: 221–227.
4. Terry A., Merker V., Barker, F., Leffert L., Souter I., Plotkin S. Pregnancy complications in women with rare tumor suppressor syndromes affecting central and peripheral nervous system. *American Journal of Obstetrics and Gynecology*, 2015; 213: 108–109.
5. Terry A., Merker V., Barker, F., Leffert L., Souter I., Plotkin S. Neurofibromatosis type 1 and pregnancy complications: Population-based study. *American Journal of Obstetrics and Gynecology*, 2013; 209: 46–48.
6. Sakai T., Vallejo M., Shannon K. A parturient with neurofibromatosis type 2: anesthesia and obstetric considerations for delivery. *International Journal of Obstetric Anesthesia*, 2005; 14: 332–335.
7. Kapur S., Kumar S., Eagland K. Anesthetic management of parturient with Neurofibromatosis I and Charcot-Marie-Tooth disease. *Journal of Clinical Anesthesia*, 2007; 19: 405–407.
8. Spiegel J., Hapgood A., Hess P. Epidural anesthesia in a parturient with neurofibromatosis type 2 undergoing cesarean section. *International Journal of Obstetric Anesthesia*, 2005; 14: 336–339.
9. Segal, D. Holcberg G., Sapir O, Sheiner E., Mazor M., Katz M. Neurofibromatosis in pregnancy maternal and perinatal outcome. *European Journal of Obstetrics and Gynecology*, 1999; 84: 59–61.
10. Sundelin H., Stephansson, O., Johansson, K., Ludvigsson, J. Pregnancy outcome in joint hypermobility syndrome and Ehlers-Danlos syndrome. *Acta Obstetrica et. Gynecologica Scandinavica*, 2017; 96: 114–119.
11. Wanga S., Silverside C., Dore A., de Waard V., Mulder B. Pregnancy and Thoracic Aortic Disease: Managing the Risks. *Canadian Journal of Cardiology*, 2016; 32: 78–85.
12. Fedoruk, K., Chong K., Sermer M., Carvalho J. Anesthetic management of a parturient with hypermobility phenotype but possible vascular genotype Ehlers-Danlos syndrome. *Canadian Journal of Anesthesia*, 2015; 62: 1308–1312.
13. Murray, M.; Pepin M., Peterson, S. Byers P. Pregnancy related deaths and complications in women with vascular Ehlers-Danlos syndrome. *Genetics in Medicine*, 2014; 16: 874–880.
14. Pepin M., Schwarze U., Superti-Furga, A., Byers P. Clinical and genetic features of Ehlers-Danlos syndrome type IV, the vascular type. *New England Journal of Medicine*, 2000; 342: 673–680.
15. Gabor, M., Ferianec, V, Meciarova I., Papcun P., Holoman K. Tuberous sclerosis and pregnancy. *Ceska Gynekologie*, 2014; 79: 186–189.
16. Chao, AS., Chao A., Wang TH, Chang YC, Chang YL, Hsieh CC, Lien R, Su WJ. Outcome of antenatally diagnosed cardiac rhabdomyoma: case series and meta analysis. *Ultrasound Obstet Gynecol*, 2008; 31: 289–295.
17. Isaacs, H. Perinatal (fetal and neonatal) tuberous sclerosis: A review. *American Journal of Perinatology*, 2009; 26: 755–760.
18. Frantzen, C., Klasson, T, Links, T., Giles, R. Von Hippel-Lindau syndrome. In: Pagon RA, Adam MP, Ardinger HH et al., eds. *Gene Reviews*. 1st ed. Seattle: University of Washington; 2017.
19. Hallsworth, D., Thompson, J., Wilkinson, D., Kerr RSC., Russell R. Intracranial pressure monitoring and cesarean section in a patient with von Hippel-Lindau disease and symptomatic cerebellar hemangioblastoma. *International Journal of Obstetrics and Gynecology*, 2015; 9: 73–76.
20. Hayden, M., Gephart, R., Kalanithi, P., Chou, D. Von Hippel-Lindau disease in pregnancy: A brief review. *Journal of Clinical Neuroscience*, 2009; 16: 611–613.
21. Shaw, A., Chiocca, A., Editorial: Von Hippel-Lindau disease and pregnancy. *Journal of Neurosurgery*. 2012; 117: 815–817.
22. Kolomeyevskaya, N. Van den Veyver, I., Aagaard-Tillery, K. Pheochromocytoma and von Hippel-Lindau in Pregnancy. *American Journal of Perinatology*. 2010; 27: 257–263.
23. McDonald, J. Pyeritz, RE. Hereditary Hemorrhaic Telangiectasia. In: Pagon RA, Adam MP, Ardinger HH et al, eds. *Gene Reviews*. 1st ed. Seattle: University of Washington; 2017.

24. Goussous, T., Haynes, A., Najarian, K., Daccarett, M., David, S. Hereditary hemorrhagic telangiectasia presenting as high output cardiac failure during pregnancy. *Cardiology Research and Practice*, 2009; Article ID 437237, 3 pages, 2009. doi:10.4061/2009/437237.

25. El Shobary, H., Schricker, T., Kaufman, I. Anesthetic management of parturients with hereditary hemorrhagic telangiectasia for cesarean section. *International Journal of Obstetric Anesthesia*, 2009; 18: 176–181.

26. De Gussem, E., Lausman, A, Beder, A., et al. Outcomes of pregnancy in women with hereditary hemorrhagic telangiectasia. *Obstetrics and Gynecology*, 2014; 123: 514–520.

27. Shovlin, C., Sodhi, V., McCarthy, A., Lasjaunias, P., Jackson, JE, Sheppard, MN. Estimates of maternal risks of pregnancy from women with hereditary hemorrhagic elangiectasia (Osler-Weber-Rendu syndrome): Suggested approach for obstetric services. *British Journal of Obstetrics and Gynecology*, 2008; 1108–1115.

28. Lomax, S., Edgcombe, H. Anesthetic implications for the parturient with hereditary hemorrhagic telangiectasia. *Canadian Journal of Anesthesia*, 2009; 56: 374–384.

29. Wain K, Swanson K, Watson W, Jeavons E, Weaver A, Lindor N. 2012. Hereditary hemorrhagic telangiectasia and risks for adverse pregnancy outcomes. *Am J Med Genet Part A* 158A: 2009–2014.

29

Spinal Cord Injury in Pregnancy

KATHRYN J. DRENNAN AND MARIA VANUSHKINA

INTRODUCTION

In the United States, there are ~20,000 women living with spinal cord injury (SCI).[1] Despite the initial period of amenorrhea, SCI does not appear to impair long-term fertility in women.[2,3] In the United States, only 8 to 14% of women with SCI undertake pregnancy[1,4,5] despite the fact that most women with new SCIs are generally young,[4] with upwards of 44% of women surveyed endorsing a desire for motherhood.[6] Women with higher-level injuries, older age at time of injury and higher parity at the time of injury are less likely to become pregnant.[6,7] In contrast, married women or those with a live-in significant other, patients with sports-related SCI, greater amount of time (15+ years) since injury, as well as higher functional and emotional well-being on standardized assessment scales are more likely to become pregnant.[6,7]

Obstetric management of women with SCI is determined by the level and completeness of their injury[8,9] and requires management of associated psychosocial and physical complications and barriers. Potential non-obstetric complications of the underling injury are numerous and can become exacerbated during pregnancy, but childbearing is possible and does not carry an unacceptable risk to mother or infant.[9,10] Lower and upper urinary tract infections, autonomic dysreflexia, bowel, bladder, and/or respiratory dysfunction, worsening spasticity, impaired skin integrity and subsequent breakdown, unattended birth, and low birth weight have been repeatedly identified by several small case series as the most prevalent maternal and fetal complications, respectively.[4,7-9,11-13] The goal of this chapter is to provide an evidence-based review of the management of spinal cord injuries in women throughout the pregnancy and delivery, highlighting special considerations and precautions in this unique population. A care map specific to this patient population can be seen in Box 29.1.

BRIEF OVERVIEW OF SPINAL CORD INJURIES

The spinal cord is the major conduit through which all communications between the central nervous system and the three subdivisions of the peripheral nervous system (somatic, autonomic, and enteric) are relayed. Injuries and disorders affecting the spinal cord can be acute or chronic, congenital (eg, spina bifida) or acquired (trauma or medical illness) but will present with varying degree of multisystem impairment. The terms tetraplegia and paraplegia, which are directly related to the neurologic level of injury (NLI), are frequently encountered. Tetraplegic patients have partial or complete loss of motor and/or sensory function in the cervical segments of the spinal cord due to damage of the neural elements within the spinal canal itself. This injury pattern results in functional impairments in all four extremities and often affects chest and pelvic organs potentially leading to respiratory failure, arrhythmias, autonomic instability, and bowel and bladder complications.[14] Paraplegic patients have partial or complete loss of motor and/or sensory function in the thoracic, lumbar, or sacral but not cervical segments of the spinal cord. Upper extremity function is typically spared with pelvic organs and lower extremity involvement determined by the injury level. The underlying etiology of a chronic SCI should not be dismissed during an assessment as many diagnoses or their treatments carry specific risks and precautions that may impact maternal or fetal health. However, for most SCI patients, functional prognosis and medical complications are determined by the location and severity of the lesion.

An internationally standardized assessment exists for most patients with acquired SCIs that

BOX 29.1
CARE MAP FOR PREGNANCY IN WOMEN WITH SPINAL CORD INJURY

Pre-Conception	Pregnancy	Labor and Delivery

Creation of multidisciplinary care team
  Clearly identify team member roles
  Establish reliable communication
  Integrate patient and family in care
	Review normal physiologic changes associated with pregnancy
	  Overlaps in symptoms between normal and abnormal conditions
		Careful planning and selection of optimal location for L&D
		  Address issues with accessibility
		  Chose location with SCI specialists
		  Tour hospital early, talk to staff

Social and physical barriers to accessibility of medical facilities
  Musculoskeletal limitations to care
  Transportation issues
  Wheelchair accessible rooms
  In-office Hoyer availability
  Special table/stirrups for pelvic exam
	Obstetric management
	  Frequent monitoring especially in 3rd trimester
	  Impact of unrecognized labor
	  Potential for premature delivery
	  Impact of scoliosis, kyphosis and other orthopaedic conditions on uterine growth
	  Discuss potential for early hospitalization
		Recognition of Labor
		  Monitor for labor starting at 28 weeks
		  Frequent OB appointments
		  In-home contraction monitor
		  Teach paraplegics to feel uterus to assess for labor
		  Patients with injuries about T10 may not feel labor
		  Uterine contractions may be felt if below T10

Sexual and reproductive health education
  Contraception
  Sexual function and adaptation post injury
  Maternal and fetal outcomes
  Screen for domestic abuse
	Early Anesthesia Evaluation
	  Goal to minimize risk of AD and pain
	  Discuss role of spinal/epidural anesthesia
	  Note presence of spinal hardware/devices
	  Scar tissue in epidural space may impact dosing
		Anesthesia
		  Continuous epidural anesthesia x 48–72 hrs
		  Consider peripheral nerve blocks in all patients
		  Assistance with pain management

Medication safety assessment
  Botox
  Antispasmodics
  Cannabinoids
  Anticoagulants
  Non-steroidal anti-inflammatories
  Narcotics
  Neuromodulators/Neuroleptics
  Anti-depressants
  Anxiolytics
  Antihypertensives
  Antibiotics
  Antifungals
  Anti-emetics
  Meclazine
  Bowel program (castor oil)
  Disease modifying agents for MS, RA
	Secondary medical condition prevention, monitoring and treatment
	  Autonomic Dysreflexia
	  Bladder incontinence
	  Bladder spasms
	  Increased spasticity
	  Compromised skin integrity
	  Pressure ulcer formation
	  Bowel management
	  Respiratory function (injuries about T4 may need ventilator assessment/support)
	  Autonomic instability
	  Orthostasis
	  Weight management
	  Increased fall risk
	  VTE prophylaxis
	  Anemia
		Delivery and Monitoring
		  Risk of malpresentation at term above T12
		  Most women deliver vaginally
		  Increased risk of compilations post episiotomy
		  Increased risk of forceps/vacuum use
		  Note location of abdominal implantable devices in the event of elective or emergent c-section
		  Monitor for neurologic decompensation
		  Potential for intracerebral hemorrhage due to poorly controlled AD, image if neuro changes
		  Potential increased risk of LE fractures due to osteoporosis, may present as increased spasticity, should have low threshold for imaging

Pre-Conception	Pregnancy	Labor and Delivery
		Effects of anesthesia on bowel and bladder PM&R consultation during hospitalization for positioning, spasticity, bowel, bladder, and AD management
Safety assessment of implantable device use Intrathecal baclofen pumps Spinal cord stimulators	Early lactation consultation and education Encouraged to breastfeeding but warn of difficulty with milk production especially if above T10	**Postpartum**
PM&R evaluation Osteoporosis assessment (DXA q2yrs) Hydronephrosis assessment (US q1yr) Confirm NLI and AIS grade Syringomyelia screen (consider MRI) Bowel and bladder management plan Spasticity management plan Positioning/offloading instructions Caregiver training and education Review of community resources Facilitation of peer counselors Home set up modification Car/transportation modifications Review of durable medical equipment Splinting/orthotics/prosthetics Review of autonomic dysreflexia Written AD handout for providers PT/OT referral Respiratory function optimization	Mitigation and compensation for increasing mobility/functional limitations Home exercise program Assessment of transfers Assessment of current wheelchair Adjustments to wheelchair propulsion Monitoring for shoulder complications Caregiver training on PROM exercise On-going physical therapy On-going occupational therapy Trial of adaptive aides (eg: reachers) Positioning modifications Increased reliance on caregiver Prevention of caregiver burnout Maternity and paternity leave timing Social work assistance with costs of new DME, etc Referral to visiting nurse services/home aides Avoid bedrest whenever possible and safe	Psychosocial and Parental Support High anxiety and fear about parenting is common Baseline increased levels of stress and depression Child and family development outcomes are not impacted by SCI or physical disability Despite stressors, motherhood in SCI is associated with overall improvement in QOL Careful monitoring for postpartum depression Acknowledge and address concerns regarding impact of physical limitations on parenting Creative multidisciplinary problem solving to promote independent parenting through use of adaptive equipment and strategies On-going PT/OT support to expedite recovery and mitigate deconditioning from decreased mobility Re-initiation of contraceptive use Guidance on further family planning if interested Encourage networking to share knowledge Connect patients with local and online resources

Pre-Conception	Pregnancy	Labor and Delivery

Dietician consult
  Calcium, vitamin D
    supplementation
  Iron supplementation
  Medication-related
    deficiencies
  Weight management
		Perineal care
		  Frequent monitoring of skin and
		    incision/repair
		  Avoid heat or ice use for post epi-
		    siotomy care on insensate skin
		    to prevent thermal damage
		  Resume home bowel and bladder
		    program as soon as possible
		    post-delivery
		  Avoid digital stimulation for
		    bowel program in event of
		    third or fourth degree lacera-
		    tion repair to promote healing

Pre-conception Urologic
  evaluation
  Facilitate sexuality
    preconception
  Urodynamic studies
  Medication optimization
  UTI prophylaxis (WOCA)
		Lactation
		  Increased extremity and bladder
		    spasticity common
		  Need for adaptive equipment for
		    positioning
		  Review safety of medications be-
		    fore restarting use

provides prognostic information on injury severity and expected functional recovery. This standardized assessment was developed over many years as a collaborative project between American Spinal Injury Association (ASIA) and the International Spinal Cord Society (ISCoS).[14] The standardized physical exam can be seen in Figure 29.1. ASIA Impairment Scale (AIS) is illustrated in Table 29.1, and the step by step approach in assigning the neurologic level of injury (NLI) and an AIS grade are reviewed in Figure 29.2. Patients with high NLI and injury severity (eg, a patient classified as C5 AIS A versus a patient classified as T12 AIS D) are more severely impaired, have higher rates of morbidity and mortality, and worse prognosis for functional recovery.[14]

PRE-CONCEPTION COUNSELING

Care for women with pregnancy complicated by SCI requires co-management with providers with expertise in maternal-fetal medicine and rehabilitation.[4,12,15] Special consideration should be given to collaboration, integration of care, care coordination, and proper communication to avoid confusion, misinformation, and unintentional harm.[4,5] Both specialties face challenges with providing counseling and care for this population: there are no high-quality, prospective, well-powered studies relevant to pregnant women with SCI to date[4,10,16]; and recommendations based on clinical trials do not exist. Creating a multidisciplinary consensus of best practices for this population and engaging all groups is a potential solution for this problem. Further consideration should be given to women who do not live near large medical centers with experienced specialists. In these cases, concurrent management by a local obstetrician may be appropriate.[17]

Women with SCI benefit from close follow up and care coordination.[9,13] Unfortunately, women with SCI appear to be significantly impacted by barriers to perinatal health services, emphasizing the need for expanded availability of providers with knowledge of pregnancy and SCI related issues.[12] Only 20% of women reported receiving information regarding pregnancy during their inpatient rehabilitation following acute SCI, and only 9% of those receiving information found it adequate.[12,18]

Psychosocial Support

Future parents should be provided with a list of global and local resources, including SCI forums and relevant websites, to help with planning, expectations, and practical adjustment to parenthood as a disabled individual. An abridged list of SCI specific resources can be seen in Table 29.2.

TABLE 29.1 ASIA IMPAIRMENT SCALE

AIS	Clinical Description
A	*Complete.* No sensory or motor function is preserved in the sacral segments S4-S5.
B	*Sensory Incomplete.* Sensory but not motor function is preserved below the neurological level and includes the sacral segments S4-S5, AND no motor function
C	*Motor Incomplete.* Motor function is preserved below the neurological level**, and more than half of key muscle functions below the single neurological level of injury have a muscle grade less than 3 (Grades 0–2).
D	*Motor Incomplete.* Motor function is preserved below the neurological level**, and at least half(half or more) of key muscle functions below the NLI have a muscle grade >3.
E	*Normal.* If sensation and motor function as tested with the ISNCSCI are graded as normal in all segments, and the patient had prior deficits, then the AIS grade is E. Someone without a SCI does not receive an AIS grade.

**For an individual to receive a grade of C or D (ie, motor incomplete status) they must have either voluntary anal sphincter contraction or sacral sensory sparing (at S4/5 or deep anal pressure) with sparing of motor function more than three levels below the motor level for that side of the body. The Standards allow even non-key muscle function more than 3 levels below the motor level to be used in determining motor incomplete status (AIS B versus C).
Table adapted from: Kirshblum SC, Burns SP, Biering-Sorensen F, Donovan W, Graves DE, Jha A, et al. International standards for neurological classification of spinal cord injury (revised 2011). *J Spinal Cord Med.* 2011; 34(6): 535–546.

Patients should be made aware that increased assistance from caregivers and/or home services is often required. An experienced social worker can provide assistance for financial costs associated with pregnancy and new equipment.

Maternal and Fetal Outcomes

Providers should reinforce the fact that SCI does not reduce long-term fertility in women and that both intentional and unintentional pregnancies occur.[10] With careful management, pregnancy does not carry unacceptable medical risks to the mother or the fetus.[8] Patients should be informed that in addition to the standard physiologic changes and complications associated with all stages of pregnancy for all women, they are be at increased risk of secondary complications related to their SCI. These women will require more intensive and frequent medical follow-up, adjustments to many aspects of their daily routines and to their home setup and durable medical equipment, as well as temporary discontinuation of certain medications and treatment options. In addition, many women require hospitalization during pregnancy as a direct result of medical complications.[13] Complications are commonly seen in women with SCI. Urinary tract complaints are by far the most common with UTIs experienced by 45–100%[13] as well as recurrent UTIs (up to 75%),[13,19,20] pyelonephritis (23–31%),[13,19,20] urosepsis (1%),[21] and an increase in frequency of intermittent catheterization program.[13,19,22] Up to 60% of women

with injuries above T6 will experience autonomic dysreflexia.[13,23,24] Additionally, new pressure ulcers are seen in 6–15%,[13,19,23–25] increased spasticity in 12%,[17,19] constipation,[3,13,19,24] and thromboembolic events.[13,26]

Prospective parents should be reassured that there does not appear to be an increased risk of fetal malformations, miscarriage, stillbirth, or mortality in to children born to women with SCI.[27,28] There is a trend toward an increased risk for prematurity[3,13,19,23,25] but not consistently reproduced.[17,29] This discrepancy may be due to improved surveillance and improved management of secondary compilations in mothers over time.[17]

Accessibility Issues

Patients with SCI face physical barriers to routine obstetric care, such as pelvic exams and obstetric ultrasound, due to underlying musculoskeletal deformities or secondary conditions such as spasticity and autonomic dysreflexia (AD). Providers should be mindful of these issues and make efforts to accommodate the patient's physical limitations. Ensuring availability of trained staff and appropriate equipment to facilitate transfers is crucial. Women should be encouraged to tour clinics and hospital units as well as meet with staff to ensure their needs can be met.

Medical and Functional Optimization

In addition to standard obstetric care, multiple expert consultations are often needed prior to

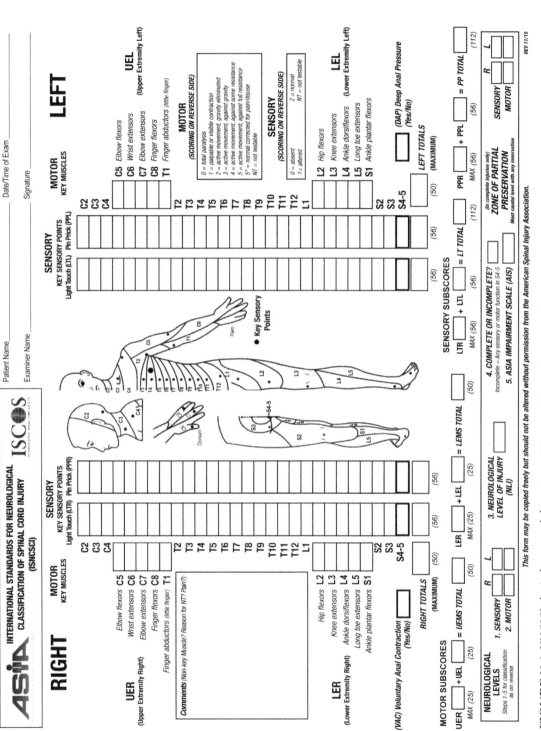

FIGURE 29.1 ISNCSCI physical exam worksheet. This worksheet is used during the recommended international standards physical examination for spinal cord–injured patients. This examination is consistently performed and interpreted by providers trained in its proper administration, such as spine surgeons and physiatrists. It can be used in an acute critical-care setting, outpatient follow-up of chronic injuries and at times points in between as a means to monitor injury recovery or complications (such as syrinx formation). Worksheet accessible online at: http://asia-spinalinjury.org/wp-content/uploads/2016/02/International_Stds_Diagram_Worksheet.pdf

Muscle Function Grading

0 = total paralysis

1 = palpable or visible contraction

2 = active movement, full range of motion (ROM) with gravity eliminated

3 = active movement, full ROM against gravity

4 = active movement, full ROM against gravity and moderate resistance in a muscle specific position

5 = (normal) active movement, full ROM against gravity and full resistance in a functional muscle position expected from an otherwise unimpaired person

5* = (normal) active movement, full ROM against gravity and sufficient resistance to be considered normal if identified inhibiting factors (i.e. pain, disuse) were not present

NT = not testable (i.e. due to immobilization, severe pain such that the patient cannot be graded, amputation of limb, or contracture of > 50% of the normal ROM)

Sensory Grading

0 = Absent

1 = Altered, either decreased/impaired sensation or hypersensitivity

2 = Normal

NT = Not testable

When to Test Non-Key Muscles:

In a patient with an apparent AIS B classification, non-key muscle functions more than 3 levels below the motor level on each side should be tested to most accurately classify the injury (differentiate between AIS B and C).

Movement	Root level
Shoulder: Flexion, extension, abduction, adduction, internal and external rotation	**C5**
Elbow: Supination	
Elbow: Pronation	**C6**
Wrist: Flexion	
Finger: Flexion at proximal joint, extension.	**C7**
Thumb: Flexion, extension and abduction in plane of thumb	
Finger: Flexion at MCP joint	**C8**
Thumb: Opposition, adduction and abduction perpendicular to palm	
Finger: Abduction of the index finger	**T1**
Hip: Adduction	**L2**
Hip: External rotation	**L3**
Hip: Extension, abduction, internal rotation	**L4**
Knee: Flexion	
Ankle: Inversion and eversion	
Toe: MP and IP extension	
Hallux and Toe: DIP and PIP flexion and abduction	**L5**
Hallux: Adduction	**S1**

ASIA Impairment Scale (AIS)

A = Complete. No sensory or motor function is preserved in the sacral segments S4-5.

B = Sensory Incomplete. Sensory but not motor function is preserved below the neurological level and includes the sacral segments S4-5 (light touch or pin prick at S4-5 or deep anal pressure) AND no motor function is preserved more than three levels below the motor level on either side of the body.

C = Motor Incomplete. Motor function is preserved at the most caudal sacral segments for voluntary anal contraction (VAC) OR the patient meets the criteria for sensory incomplete status (sensory function preserved at the most caudal sacral segments (S4-S5) by LT, PP or DAP), and has some sparing of motor function more than three levels below the ipsilateral motor level on either side of the body.

(This includes key or non-key muscle functions to determine motor incomplete status.) For AIS C – less than half of key muscle functions below the single NLI have a muscle grade ≥ 3.

D = Motor Incomplete. Motor incomplete status as defined above, with at least half (half or more) of key muscle functions below the single NLI having a muscle grade ≥ 3.

E = Normal. If sensation and motor function as tested with the ISNSCSI are graded as normal in all segments, and the patient had prior deficits, then the AIS grade is E. Someone without an initial SCI does not receive an AIS grade.

Using ND: To document the sensory, motor and NLI levels, the ASIA Impairment Scale grade, and/or the zone of partial preservation (ZPP) when they are unable to be determined based on the examination results.

Steps in Classification

The following order is recommended for determining the classification of individuals with SCI.

1. Determine sensory levels for right and left sides.
The sensory level is the most caudal, intact dermatome for both pin prick and light touch sensation.

2. Determine motor levels for right and left sides.
Defined by the lowest key muscle function that has a grade of at least 3 (on supine testing), providing the key muscle functions represented by segments above that level are judged to be intact (graded as a 5).
Note: in regions where there is no myotome to test, the motor level is presumed to be the same as the sensory level, if testable motor function above that level is also normal.

3. Determine the neurological level of injury (NLI)
This refers to the most caudal segment of the cord with intact sensation and antigravity (3 or more) muscle function strength, provided that there is normal (intact) sensory and motor function rostrally respectively.
The NLI is the most cephalad of the sensory and motor levels determined in steps 1 and 2.

4. Determine whether the injury is Complete or Incomplete.
(i.e. absence or presence of sacral sparing)
If voluntary anal contraction = **No** AND all S4-5 sensory scores = **0** AND deep anal pressure = **No**, then injury is **Complete**.
Otherwise, injury is **Incomplete.**

5. Determine ASIA Impairment Scale (AIS) Grade:

Is injury Complete? If YES, AIS=A and can record ZPP (lowest dermatome or myotome on each side with some preservation)

NO ↓

Is injury Motor Complete? If YES, AIS=B
NO ↓
(No=voluntary anal contraction OR motor function more than three levels below the motor level on a given side, if the patient has sensory incomplete classification)

Are at least half (half or more) of the key muscles below the neurological level of injury graded 3 or better?

NO ↓ AIS=C
YES ↓ AIS=D

If sensation and motor function is normal in all segments, **AIS=E**
Note: AIS E is used in follow-up testing when an individual with a documented SCI has recovered normal function. If at initial testing no deficits are found, the individual is neurologically intact; the ASIA Impairment Scale does not apply.

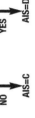

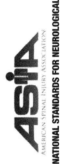

INTERNATIONAL STANDARDS FOR NEUROLOGICAL CLASSIFICATION OF SPINAL CORD INJURY

FIGURE 29.2 ISNSCI guide to injury classification based on Exam findings. This worksheet is used as a step-by-step guide to interpret the results of the international standards exam. The exam findings are used to grade the neurologic level of injury and an overall injury severity. This classification is useful for standardizing communication between providers, building databases for research purposes, and providing clinically relevant prognostic information for future functional recovery. Accessible on-line at: http://asia-spinalinjury.org/wp-content/uploads/2016/02/International_Stds_Diagram_Worksheet.pdf

TABLE 29.2 ONLINE COMMUNITIES AND RESOURCES FOR PATIENTS WITH SCI

Organization	Link	Description
United Spinal Association	www.spinalcord.org	An online resource center covering a variety of useful topics for individuals with SCI. Patients may submit questions to the staff, who will assist with resolving the situation. Includes links to additional resources.
Spinal Cord Injury BC	www.scisexualhealth.ca	Website run by a local Sexual Health Rehabilitation Service Center curated by sexual health clinicians and sexual medicine physicians with evidence based patient education regarding a variety of topics including sexuality, medical complications, partner support, and parenting. Includes topic-specific links to peer and professional run support groups, blogs, forums, books, magazines, articles, etc.
Victorian Spinal Cord Injury Program: SpinalHub	www.spinalhub.com.au	Website created as part of a multi-organizational initiative to progress works focusing on community integration post SCI. Notable components include a forum and educational resources covering a broad range of topics.

pregnancy for medical optimization in this population including but not limited to maternal-fetal medicine (MFM), urology, physical medicine and rehabilitation, anesthesiology, lactation, physical therapy, occupational therapy, nutritionist, respiratory therapy, and social work. Traditional prenatal laboratory and imaging testing should be combined with SCI specific risk factor surveillance. Current SCI health maintenance practices are detailed in Table 29.3. Given overall low rates of counseling on childbearing and planning for pregnancy, we recommend that intention for childbearing, possible planning for childbearing,

contraception, and sexual well-being be added to this schedule.

Pregnancies should be planned and indicated evaluations should be completed prior to conception. Baseline evaluation consists of renal function (including calcium, phosphorus, and creatinine), liver function, pulmonary function (including OSA screening), and urodynamic parameters. Some providers also recommend pre-conception spinal cord magnetic resonance imaging (MRI) to document the presence of a syringomyelia.[13] Thorough medication reconciliation should be performed to assess for potential teratogenic or

TABLE 29.3 HEALTH MAINTENANCE IN SPINAL CORD INJURY[30]

Assessment	Interval
Screening for Hydronephrosis	Annually for three years, then biennially
Bone density (DEXA)	Biennially
Blood pressure/postural hypotension	Yearly
Obstructive Sleep Apnea	At least yearly
Mental health assessment	Yearly
Review and counseling on physical activity and restriction	Yearly
Assessment of contraceptive plans and/or desire for childbearing	Yearly*

*: proposed
Note: A timeline for routine health assessment in spinal cord injury patients. We propose that yearly assessment for appropriate contraceptive plans and/or desire and planning for childbearing be added to the routine health maintenance of female patients with spinal cord injury.

abortifacient effects or interactions with common medications used in pregnancy. Medication risks and benefits as well as appropriate substitutions should be assessed and discussed between the obstetric team and the patient's physiatrist team. Many women benefit from a physical and occupational therapy functional assessment including review of current assistive devices and medical equipment as they will often require adjustment during pregnancy. Caregivers should be involved in this process and receive adequate support and training, as women will likely become more dependent in aspects of self-care with increasing gestational age due to limitations in mobility, especially with transfers. Secondary musculoskeletal deformities are common in SCI patients. Exam rooms need to be equipped with assistive devices to facilitate transfers, and medical staff will need to be trained on proper techniques. Providers should support and empower patients to carefully evaluate local medical facilities to ensure they are accessible and able to accommodate their needs.

MEDICAL COMPLICATIONS OF PREGNANCY IN PATIENTS WITH SCI

Urinary Tract Infections

Urinary tract infections are the most common complication in this patient population that can be reduced with proper management.[21] In a general SCI population, the risk for asymptomatic bacteriuria ranges from 75 to 100% and does not require prophylaxis as it is usually inconsequential when low-pressure storage and complete emptying are achieved.[30] Pregnancy increases the risk of urinary retention and higher intravesical pressures. Up to 40% of these women develop a UTI during pregnancy.[31] Without adequate precautions, the rate of UTIs in women with SCI during pregnancy is up to 100%.[13] The American College of Obstetricians and Gynecologists (ACOG) suggests that frequent urine cultures or antibiotic suppression are indicated because of increased risks and consequences of pyelonephritis and progression to maternal sepsis in this population requiring increased rates of hospitalization compared to the general population.[32] For the former strategy, cultures can be done monthly or per trimester, depending on the patient's prior history. Caution should be used when selecting antibiotics in women receiving oral treatment for spasticity with certain agents such as tizanidine as concurrent use of tizanidine with medications that are moderate or potent CYP1A2 inhibitors (such as cimetidine, famotidine,

verapamil, and many other medications)[33] is contraindicated.

Voiding and Renal Dysfunction

Historically, renal failure was the most common cause of death in patients with spinal cord injury.[34] Today, management of urologic dysfunction has both improved and lengthened the lives of patients with spinal cord injury.[34] The nature of voiding dysfunction will depend on the specific characteristics of the spinal cord lesion in question and can include hypotonia, detrusor overactivity, impaired bladder wall compliance, high leak point detrusor pressure and vesicoureteral reflux, as well as detrusor-sphincter dyssynergia.[34] An elevated storage pressure due to low bladder compliance or neurogenic detrusor overactivity are the major risk factors for renal deterioration.[21] Bladder management promotes social continence, low pressure storage and efficient bladder emptying; helps avoid stretch injury to the bladder from over-distention, prevents upper and lower urinary tract injury from high intravesical pressures and recurrent UTIs.[34]

In general, continence in the SCI population is maintained by a combination of pharmacological treatments to manage bladder spasms and emptying with methods such as intermittent, urethral, or suprapubic catheterization or operative interventions such as augmentation cystoplasty or continent urinary diversions using the ileocecal valve.[17,21] The risks and benefits of the available options should be addressed, including concerns about sexual function, medical complications, costs, and patient preferences. Intermittent catheterization is often recommended in women with adequate upper extremity function and dexterity, as it reduces the risk of UTIs compared to indwelling catheters. In women with tetraplegia, indwelling urethral or suprapubic catheters are used more often. MFM consultation should be initiated when deciding on initiation, continuation, or dose adjustment of pharmacologic options to reduce risk of iatrogenic complications.[13]

Changes in bladder function (including increased spasticity) changes in volume status requiring increased frequency of catheterization and leakage around indwelling catheters are common.[17,19] Limitations in mobility and increasing incontinence with advancing gestation may require use of indwelling catheters instead of intermittent catheterization protocols in one-fourth of patients.[17] For pregnant women with augmentation cystoplasty procedures, interdisciplinary cooperation between urologists and obstetricians is crucial in the event of C-sections to ensure patient safety,[13,35] although the reported complication rates are low. Improper bladder management increases the risk of AD in susceptible individuals.

Autonomic Dysreflexia (AD)

After SCI, dramatic increases in blood pressure (BP) can develop in response to sensory input entering the spinal cord below the level of the injury.[36] This hypertension, part of a condition termed AD, occurs in 50–90% of people with tetraplegia or high paraplegia over the lifetime of their injuries.[37,38] Although most susceptible individuals will experience AD soon after their injuries, there are reports of first incidence as far as 15 years post-injury.[28] These episodes are usually brief and resolve quickly with treatment, but they may last for periods ranging from day to weeks in some individuals.[11] AD occurs after injury at or above T6, because injury at these levels leaves the sympathetic control of the abdominal circulation amenable to unrestrained spinal excitatory reflexes.[9,28,36,38,39] Below the injury, sensory nerves transmit impulses that stimulate sympathetic neurons creating a large, unopposed sympathetic outflow that presents clinically with sudden elevation in BP by at least 20mmHg above baseline systolic up to as maximum of 300 mmHg systolic, piloerection, skin pallor, and severe vasoconstriction below the NLI. The inhibitory response, from cerebral vasomotor centers, causes vasodilation above the level of injury, presenting with pounding headache, flushing, blotching of skin, nasal congestion, nausea, anxiety, malaise, prickling sensation in the skull, piloerection, sweating, blushing, twitching, and increased spasticity in all limbs. Cardiac rhythm disturbances occur, including bradycardia, extra systoles, bigeminy, prolonged PR interval, and AV block. AD can result in debilitating headaches, seizures, cerebral hemorrhages, strokes, hypertensive encephalopathy, intraventricular hemorrhages, retinal hemorrhages, retinal detachment, cardiac arrest, and even death.[8,9,11,27,28] In pregnant patients experiencing AD, the fetal status should be monitored.[11]

The rate of AD in partrurients with SCI is reported as 15–85% and can occur in those with complete and incomplete injuries.[8,13,28,37] AD is a critical care emergency. Understanding the extensive list of potential triggers for AD is crucial to prevention and management. Common AD triggers include: bladder over-distension, inflammation, or infection; inflammation or distension of bowels such as seen in constipation or

diverticulitis; innocuous or noxious stimulation of the skin including tight garments and pressure sores; ingrown toenails; stimulation of visceral organs such as renal colic or biliary colic; pelvic exams or transvaginal sonography[40]; routine daily procedures such as bladder catheterization and bowel evacuation; temperature variation (including placement of feet into cold stirrups); labor, delivery, and postpartum—all three of which are particularly potent stimuli.[11,13,28,36,38] Strategies used to prevent AD in pregnancy include: early regional analgesia prior to onset of spontaneous labor[8,11,27,28]; use of local anesthetic gel for routine catheterizations[28]; limiting pelvic examination and minimizing speculum use whenever possible or the use of topical anesthetic or pudendal block for pelvic exams in severe or frequent cases.[28] Patients, their caregivers, and their multidisciplinary medical team should be provided with extensive education and reference material on AD. Patients should have a medical emergency card for AD to carry in their wallet or overnight bag.[11]

The initial management involves placing the patient in an upright position to take advantage of orthostatic reduction in BP. The next step must be to loosen any tight clothing and remove constrictive devices while also eliminating peripheral sensory triggers. It is critical that blood pressure is checked at least every 5 minutes throughout the episode of AD until the individual is stable. Providers should search for and eliminate the precipitating stimulus. In 85% of cases, AD is related either to bladder distention or bowel impaction.[11] The use of antihypertensive drugs should be considered a last resort, but may be necessary if SBP remains 150mmHg or greater following the non-pharmacologic steps described above to avoid the complications associated with uncontrolled hypertension.[11] Nifedipine, nitrates, and captopril are the most commonly used and recommended agents for the management of acute AD in the general SCI population, but captopril is contraindicated in pregnancy. Expert opinion suggests that hydralazine, labetalol sublingual nifedipine or intramuscular clonidine are safe and effective,[9] and there is some evidence magnesium sulfate may be helpful in AD.[9,37]

Venous Thromboembolism (VTE)

SCI increases the risk of deep venous thrombosis by a factor of 6.[41] While the frequency of VTE appears to be 67–100% in patients with an acute SCI, more than 80% of these events occur within the first 3 months of injury.[41] Following this, the risk is similar to that in the general population due to vessel remodeling and other physiological changes occurring below the level of SCI during the process of adaptation and recovery.[17] Low molecular weight heparin (LMWH) appears to have more efficacy with fewer bleeding episodes than heparin for this indication.[41] Insufficient data exists to comment on risk or strategies for prophylaxis in pregnant women with acute or chronic SCIs, although data suggests VTE occurs more frequently than expected in this population.[6] The greatest period of pregnancy related thromboembolic risk is the postpartum period, and thromboprophylaxis could reasonably be considered.

Impaired Skin Integrity

Decubitus ulcers are a common but often preventable complication of SCI. Factors that increase the risk of decubitus ulcers include gestational weight gain, degree of immobility, inappropriately sized medical equipment, and edema.[28] Prenatal visits should include routine skin examination for evidence of breakdown and caregivers should be encouraged to assess skin at home on a daily basis. If decubitus ulcers occur, they should be treated meticulously, including nutritional optimization and physical therapy to prevent further deterioration or additional decubiti formation.[28]

Thermoregulation

Thermoregulation is impaired in patients with SCI. The degree of thermoregulation impairment is proportional to the level of the lesion.[42] Low-level paraplegics have core temperature increases similar to those of able-bodied athletes, while those with higher lesions, particularly when exercising in warm weather are vulnerable to hyperthermia.[42] In addition, patients with SCI are vulnerable to hypothermia due to a large surface area of insensate skin and inability or diminished ability of the body to initiate heat-conserving processes such as vasoconstriction and shivering.[43] Due to increased vulnerability to both hyperthermia and hypothermia, attention should be paid to maintaining a cool but not cold temperature in the labor room and monitoring temperature with vital signs. If the temperature starts to drift to the edges of euthermic, interventions to cool or warm the patient as indicated should be undertaken.

Pulmonary Function

Respiratory complications are the leading cause of death in spinal cord injury patients.[44] Oxygen consumption increases in pregnancy by approximately 20%, and this demand is typically primarily met through an increase in minute ventilation.

Patients with injuries above T5 are at risk for varying degrees of pulmonary dysfunction, due to damage to the innervation of the diaphragm and intercostal muscles resulting in a combination of alterations in lung and chest wall compliance, decreased performance of respiratory muscles, and impaired cough. These complications act together to decrease respiratory performance and increase vulnerability to respiratory infections.[28,45] The standard of care for patients with high spinal cord lesions who are unable to adequately mobilize the diaphragm is tracheostomy and mechanical ventilation.[45,46] A variety of strategies have been developed to assist with pulmonary insufficiency due to SCI. Additionally, patients and their caregivers can be taught maneuvers to improve clearance of secretions.

Some patients with SCI may not be able to increase oxygen delivery to correspond with the increased oxygen demand of pregnancy. Supine positioning may worsen respiratory insufficiency[8,28,45] and should be avoided where possible. Additionally, respiratory status should be monitored during pregnancy and decreases in minute volume and vital capacity may help to identify patients who will need ventilatory assistance as the pregnancy continues.[8,28] Chest physiotherapy is safe to be continued through pregnancy.[45] For a SCI patient who is ventilator dependent or has significant respiratory insufficiency, these issues coupled with pregnancy depends represent a high-risk pregnancy state, with high likelihood of poor maternal/fetal outcomes. This should only be undertaken after careful consultation and discussion, and careful attention should be paid to maternal ventilation and oxygenation requirements which are altered by pregnancy.

Autonomic Instability

Injury to autonomic pathways in the spinal cord causes disruption in cardiovascular function. Orthostasis is a prominent manifestation of autonomic instability in this patient population.[8,28] Orthostatic hypotension is caused by disruptions of sympathetic outflow in areas caudal to the level injury resulting in an increase in intravascular volume and decreased systemic vascular resistance, sometimes resulting in exquisite sensitivity to afterload reducing agents.[28] Orthostasis increases fall risk in this population. Initial management includes the use of abdominal binders and compression stockings, with addition of salt tablets, increased fluid intake, and caffeine if response is inadequate. Pharmacologic treatment options may be required.

Acute Spinal Cord Injury in Pregnancy

The primary goal of acute SCI management is maternal stabilization. Fetal monitoring should be undertaken only at viable gestational ages and after emergent delivery poses an acceptable risk to the mother. Fetal monitoring should occur serially during the maternal ICU stay at a frequency determined by the severity of maternal injury/illness. The risk for fetal anomaly or loss with acute SCI in pregnancy has been estimated at 11%.[47]

Initially, care should be taken to maintain adequate uterine profusion during the initial period of spinal shock.[28] Other cardiovascular findings will depend on the level of the injury and presence and severity of other complications. For example, patients with lower spinal cord injuries will exhibit compensatory tachycardia in response to loss of sympathetic tone, and patients with higher injuries (above T1) are more likely to exhibit bradycardia because the only intact sympathetic pathway may be the vagus nerve.[28] The use of inotropic pressors to counteract neurogenic shock is not contraindicated in pregnant patients.[47] Other considerations for the care of pregnant women with critical illness and severe trauma apply, including the possibility of ARDS and need for mechanical ventilation.[47]

While a comprehensive look at the management of spinal cord injuries is outside the scope of this chapter, intact sensation for sacral pinprick (as tested between 72 hours to 1 week after injury) is an important prognostic indicator.[39] A variety of imaging studies are used to assess the spine in patients after spinal cord injury,[39] and despite the inability to shield the fetus during a CT scan of the spinal cord, the radiation exposure with CT scans and plain radiographs is significantly lower than the dose associated with fetal harm, and they should not be withheld[48] (see also Chapter 7). MRI and ultrasound are not associated with fetal risk and also should not be withheld.[48] Gadolinium contrast use has been controversial in pregnancy but has shown no fetal risk in a single prospective study,[48] and concern for fetal injury likely only exists with high and repeated doses.[48] If a venous thromboembolic event is suspected, CT pulmonary angiography is preferred imaging modality to make this diagnosis in pregnancy.[48]

Pregnancy is not a contraindication to treatment with glucocorticoids, when indicated. The only steroids known to cross the placenta are dexamethasone and betamethasone. Oral corticosteroids are generally considered acceptable for use in breastfeeding, though they may affect the milk supply. Pregnancy should not be considered a contraindication to surgical care aimed at limiting secondary injury and reducing the degree of long-term disability. Fetal monitoring during surgery could be considered if the following prerequisites are met: viable fetus, obstetric provider willing and able to intervene, the nature of the surgery would allow safe emergent delivery, the consent of her patient or her health care proxy has been obtained, and fetal monitoring is physically feasible with the operative field. Unless major hemodynamic instability is likely, fetal monitoring undertaken pre- and post-operatively is likely adequate.[49] If a prolonged surgery is necessary in the postpartum period, pumping the mother's breasts in surgery can prevent breast engorgement.

LABOR AND DELIVERY

Labor Identification

Symptoms associated with the perception of labor are dependent on the level of spinal cord injury.[17] Uterine contractions travel via Frankenhauser's plexus and into the spinal cord at T10, cervical dilatation is perceived at T11 to T12, and sensation in the perineum and vagina reach the spinal cord via lumbosacral root afferents.[17] Women with lesions caudal to T10 should have painful contractions, but perception of labor pains is impaired in higher lesions. Therefore, patients with higher SCIs are at risk for silent labor. Patients should be educated about potential concurrent symptoms of labor, such as scalp tingling, AD symptoms, an increase in the frequency of spasms, abdominal discomfort, or changes in breathing.[8,9,27,28] Women with adequate dexterity and sensation should be taught to monitor for labor using abdominal self-palpation, or caregivers can also be taught to assess the uterus for contractions.[17] To reduce the risk of unattended delivery,[28] frequent outpatient cervical examinations (if this is not an AD trigger for the patient), non-stress testing to assess contraction frequency and/or inpatient monitoring should be considered.[17] Others recommend home contraction/labor monitors with provider surveillance.[17] On admission, a urinary catheter should be placed to decrease the risk of AD and continuous fetal monitoring should be undertaken. Abnormalities in fetal monitoring may be due to AD.

Anesthesia

Women with spinal cord injury in pregnancy should have anesthesia consultation prior to delivery.[8,27,28] The concept of regional anesthesia is often anxiety provoking in this patient population as women worry about damage to their spinal cord.[17,50] No studies have specifically addressed this concern, but there has been no evidence of risk in the spinal cord injured population. Patient's anxiety should be addressed and supported, and the benefits of regional anesthesia discussed during pre-conception counseling and throughout pregnancy. For all women with SCI, including those without innervation to pertinent dermatomes, regional anesthesia has been shown to reduce episodes of AD associated with labor, delivery, and postpartum hospital stay.[9,11,13,17] Anesthesia should be initiated early, ideally as soon as labor is diagnosed or prior to induction.[17] A block height of T8–10 is adequate.[17] The effectiveness of epidural analgesia is determined by the absence of AD, as it is not possible to test the level of the block in women with a complete lesion of the spinal cord.[17] The type of regional anesthesia used varies, with literature reporting use of epidural only, spinal only, combined spinal epidural, and pudendal blocks. The optimum dosage, duration of drugs administered, and method selection are still under investigation. Case reports have suggested that spinal anesthesia may be superior to epidural anesthesia in providing hemodynamic stability against AD during deliveries via C-section.[9,17] The use of prolonged epidural anesthesia to control AD in the postpartum period for up to five days has also shown favorable results,[9] and most authors recommend use for at least 2 to 3 days postpartum due to ongoing AD triggers including fundal checks, perineal bruising/stitches, and contractions from uterine involution (commonly called afterbirth pains).[13] Epidurals may be difficult to insert in this population due to prior surgery, and scar tissue may prevent adequate spread of local anesthesia in the epidural space—continuous spinal epidurals may be helpful. It is worthwhile to note that pregnancy increases the risk of failed intubation and complications from general anesthesia, which is often compounded in patients with prior SCI of the cervical spine.[17] Further discussion of anesthesia care in neurologic disease and SCI is in Chapter 29.

Delivery Method

For women with varying degrees of SCI, the ability to push may be limited to varying degrees based on injury location. It is well documented in the literature that vaginal delivery is possible for both paraplegic and tetraplegic patients.[9,13,17] However, tetraplegic patients have increased rates of instrumented deliveries compared to paraplegic patients.[9] Regardless, a trial of labor is recommended for all SCI patients without other precautions or contraindications.[8,28] SCI specific concerns regarding vaginal delivery include presence of syringomyelia[27] and worsening urinary stress incontinence.[13] Spasms may complicate delivery and are best prevented or relieved by optimizing positioning. It is important not to force flexion during these episodes. If AD symptoms are occurring and are difficult to control, expedited delivery may be helpful to reduce triggers. Some studies report C-section rates as high as 65%, although most are elective.[13] There is no evidence that patients with preexisting syringomyelia benefit from cesarean delivery,[8,28] and no evidence that vaginal delivery results in functional deterioration.

POSTPARTUM CARE

Perineal Care

Suturing of episiotomies or lacerations must utilize standard methods of analgesia for all women with SCI, regardless of sensation in the sacral dermatomes, because pain fibers are stimulated during this procedure and can potentially lead to AD.[17] The evidence on increased risks of perineal wound breakdown above the general population is controversial,[17] but likely evaluation of perineum daily during the hospitalization and by caregivers (if the woman is unable to evaluate this herself) is good practice. Additionally, some standard practices for pain management are relatively contraindicated. Direct application of ice or heat on areas of impaired sensation confers risks of thermal damage, and patients should be advised to avoid this practice.

Lactation

Breastfeeding should be encouraged whenever feasible.[17] SCI patients frequently experience difficulties with breastfeeding due to worsening spasticity, worsening bladder spasms, AD (rarely complicates lactation), inhibition of the milk ejection reflex due to underlying neurologic lesions, and problems with infant handling[9] (see also Chapter 35). In women with complete SCI above T4, breastfeeding initiation may require visual stimulation or oxytocin nasal spray[17] because the afferent pathway of the milk ejection reflex is initiated by infant suckling and is carried from tactile receptors in the breast via the dorsal roots of T4 to T6.[17] As with many new mothers, adequate and early breastfeeding support is essential.

Adaptive Parenting

Women with SCI can parent independently with accommodations. However, they will generally require adaptation, support, rearrangement of equipment, and home modification to facilitate nursing, dressing, bathing, and handling of infants.[17] For example, special harness and straps for the wheelchair to allow easier and more secure handling of the neonate. Occupational therapy as well as trained orthoptists can assist with creative problem solving for issues as they arise. Evaluation of the home environment and assessment of options and assistance needs should be completed during the pregnancy, and postnatal follow up as the infant grows may also be needed. In addition, peer resources and equipment vendor recommendations are available through many SCI parenting websites including those in Table 29.2.

REFERENCES

1. Iezzoni LI, Yu J, Wint AJ, Smeltzer SC, Ecker JL. Prevalence of current pregnancy among US women with and without chronic physical disabilities. *Med Care.* June 2013; 51(6): 555–562.
2. Bughi S, Shaw SJ, Mahmood G, Atkins RH, Szlachcic Y. Amenorrhea, pregnancy, and pregnancy outcomes in women following spinal cord injury: A retrospective cross-sectional study. *Endocrine Practice: Official Journal of the American College of Endocrinology and the American Association of Clinical Endocrinologists.* May-June 2008; 14(4): 437–441.
3. Charlifue SW, Gerhart KA, Menter RR, Whiteneck GG, Manley MS. Sexual issues of women with spinal cord injuries. *Paraplegia.* March 1992; 30(3): 192–199.
4. Bertschy S, Pannek J, Meyer T. Delivering care under uncertainty: Swiss providers' experiences in caring for women with spinal cord injury during pregnancy and childbirth—an expert interview study. *BMC Pregnancy and Childbirth.* July 22, 2016; 16(1): 181.
5. Camune BD. Challenges in the management of the pregnant woman with spinal cord injury. *Journal of Perinatal & Neonatal Nursing.* July-September, 2013; 27(3): 225–231.
6. Ghidini A, Healey A, Andreani M, Simonson MR. Pregnancy and women with spinal cord injuries. *Acta Obstetricia et Gynecologica Scandinavica.* 2008; 87(10): 1006–1010.
7. Iezzoni LI, Chen Y, McLain AB. Current pregnancy among women with spinal cord injury: Findings from the US national spinal cord injury database. *Spinal Cord.* November 2015; 53(11): 821–826.
8. Cesario SK. Spinal cord injuries. Nurses can help affected women & their families achieve pregnancy birth. *AWHONN lifelines.* June-July 2002; 6(3): 224–232.
9. Skowronski E, Hartman K. Obstetric management following traumatic tetraplegia: Case series and literature review. *Australian & New Zealand Journal of Obstetrics & Gynaecology.* October 2008; 48(5): 485–491.
10. Bertschy S, Bostan C, Meyer T, Pannek J. Medical complications during pregnancy and childbirth in women with SCI in Switzerland. *Spinal Cord.* March 2016; 54(3): 183–187.
11. Krassioukov A, Warburton DE, Teasell R, Eng JJ. A systematic review of the management of autonomic dysreflexia after spinal cord injury. *Archives of physical medicine and rehabilitation.* Apr 2009;90(4):682–695.
12. Bertschy S, Geyh S, Pannek J, Meyer T. Perceived needs and experiences with healthcare services of women with spinal cord injury during pregnancy and childbirth—a qualitative content analysis of focus groups and individual interviews. *BMC Health Services Research.* June 16, 2015; 15: 234.
13. Le Liepvre H, Dinh A, Idiard-Chamois B, et al. Pregnancy in spinal cord-injured women, a cohort study of 37 pregnancies in 25 women. *Spinal Cord.* February 2017; 55(2): 167–171.
14. Kirshblum SC, Burns SP, Biering-Sorensen F, et al. International standards for neurological classification of spinal cord injury (revised 2011). *Journal of Spinal Cord Medicine.* November 2011; 34(6): 535–546.
15. Burns AS, Jackson AB. Gynecologic and reproductive issues in women with spinal cord injury. *Phys Med Rehabil Clin N Am.* February 2001; 12(1): 183–199.
16. Lipson JG, Rogers JG. Pregnancy, birth, and disability: Women's health care experiences. *Health Care Women Int.* January-February 2000; 21(1): 11–26.
17. Dawood R, Altanis E, Ribes Pastor MP, Ashworth F. Pregnancy and spinal cord injury. *Obstetrician & Gynecologist.* 2014; 16: 99–107.
18. Personal experiences of pregnancy and fertility in individuals with spinal cord injury. *Sex Disabil.* March 1, 2014; 32(1): 65–74.
19. Jackson AB, Wadley V. A multicenter study of women's self-reported reproductive health after spinal cord injury. *Archives of Physical Medicine and Rehabilitation.* November 1999; 80(11): 1420–1428.
20. Guerby P, Vidal F, Bayoumeu F, Parant O. Paraplegia and pregnancy. *J Gynecol Obstet Biol Reprod (Paris).* March 2016; 45(3): 270–277.
21. Pannek J, Bertschy S. Mission impossible? Urological management of patients with spinal cord injury during pregnancy: A systematic review. *Spinal Cord.* October 2011; 49(10): 1028–1032.
22. Galusca N, Charvier K, Courtois F, Rode G, Rudigoz RC, Ruffion A. Antibioprophylaxy and urological management of women with spinal

cord injury during pregnancy. *Prog Urol.* June 2015; 25(8): 489–496.

23. Cross LL, Meythaler JM, Tuel SM, Cross AL. Pregnancy, labor and delivery post spinal cord injury. *Paraplegia.* December 1992; 30(12): 890–902.

24. Baker ER, Cardenas DD, Benedetti TJ. Risks associated with pregnancy in spinal cord-injured women. *Obstetrics and Gynecology.* September 1992; 80(3 Pt. 1): 425–428.

25. Westgren N, Hultling C, Levi R, Westgren M. Pregnancy and delivery in women with a traumatic spinal cord injury in Sweden, 1980-1991. *Obstetrics and Gynecology.* June 1993; 81(6): 926–930.

26. Baker ER, Cardenas DD. Pregnancy in spinal cord injured women. *Archives of Physical Medicine and Rehabilitation.* May 1996; 77(5): 501–507.

27. Liepvre HL, Dinh A, Idiard-Chamois B, et al. Pregnancy in spinal cord-injured women, a cohort study of 37 pregnancies in 25 women. *Spinal Cord.* 2017; 55: 161–171.

28. Pereira L. Obstetric management of the patient with spinal cord injury. *Obstetrical and Gynecological Survey.* October 2003; 58(10): 678–687.

29. Hughes SJ, Short DJ, Usherwood MM, Tebbutt H. Management of the pregnant woman with spinal cord injuries. *Br J Obstet Gynaecol.* June 1991; 98(6): 513–518.

30. Reid G. Potential preventive strategies and therapies in urinary tract infection. *World J Urol.* December 1999; 17(6): 359–363.

31. Gilstrap LC, 3rd, Ramin SM. Urinary tract infections during pregnancy. *Obstet Gynecol Clin North Am.* September 2001; 28(3): 581–591.

32. ACOG Committee Opinion: Number 275, September 2002. Obstetric management of patients with spinal cord injuries. *Obstetrics and Gynecology.* September 2002; 100(3): 625–627.

33. Wagstaff AJ, Bryson HM. Tizanidine. *Drugs.* 2012; 53(3): 435–452.

34. Samson G, Cardenas DD. Neurogenic bladder in spinal cord injury. *Physical Medicine and Rehabilitation Clinics of North America.* 2007; 18: 255–274.

35. Greenwell TJ, Venn SN, Creighton S, Leaver RB, Woodhouse CR. Pregnancy after lower urinary tract reconstruction for congenital abnormalities. *BJU Int.* November 2003; 92(7): 773–777.

36. Weaver LC, Marsh DR, Gris D, Brown A, Dekaban GA. Autonomic dysreflexia after spinal cord injury: central mechanisms and strategies for prevention. *Autonomic Dysfunction After Spinal Cord Injury.* 2006; 152: 245–263.

37. Maehama T, Izena H, Kanazawa K. Management of autonomic hyperreflexia with magnesium sulfate during labor in a woman with spinal cord injury. *American Journal of Obstetrics and Gynecology.* August 2000; 183(2): 492–493.

38. Rabchevsky AG. Segmental organization of spinal reflexes mediating autonomic dysreflexia after spinal cord injury. *Prog Brain Res.* 2006; 152: 265–274.

39. McDonald JW, Sadowsky C. Spinal-cord injury. *Lancet.* February 2, 2002; 359(9304): 417–425.

40. Strine AC, Mellon MJ. Autonomic dysreflexia: Evaluation and management. *Current Bladder Dysfunction Reports.* 2013; 8(4): 319–325.

41. Ploumis BA, Ponnappan RK, Maltenfort MG, et al. Thromboprophylaxis in patients with acute spinal injuries: An evidence-based analysis. *J Bone Joint Surg Am.* 2009; 91: 2568–2576.

42. Price MJ, Campbell IG. Effects of spinal cord lesion level upon thermoregulation during exercise in the heat. *Medicine & Science in Sports & Exercise.* 2003; 35(7): 1100–1107.

43. Khan S, Plummer M, Martinez-Arizala A, Banovac K. Hypothermia in patients with chronic spinal cord injury. *Journal of Spinal Cord Medicine.* 2007; 30: 27–30.

44. Hagan EM, Lie SA, Rekand T, Gilhus NE. Mortality after traumatic spinal cord injury: 50 years of follow-up. *Journal of Neurology and Neurosurgical Psychiatry.* 2010; 81: 368–373.

45. Brown R, DiMarco AF, Hoit JD, Garshick E. Respiratory dysfunction and management in spinal cord injury. *Respiratory Care.* 2006; 51(8): 853–870.

46. Dalal K, DiMarco AF. Diaphragmatic pacing in spinal cord injury. *Physical Medicine and Rehabilitation Clinics of North America.* 2014; 25: 619–629.

47. Gilson GJ, Miller AC, Clevenger FW, Curet LB. Acute spinal cord injury and neurogenic shock in pregnancy. *Obstetrical and Gynecological Survey.* July 1995; 50(7): 556–560.

48. Copel J, El-Sayed Y, Heine P, Wharton KR. Guidelines for diagnostic imaging during pregnancy and lactation. Committee Opinion No. 656. *Obstetrics and Gynecology.* 2016; 127: e75–80.

49. Gynecology ACoOa. Non-obstetric surgery during pregnancy. Committee Opinion no. 696. *Obstetrics and Gynecology.* 2017; 129: 777–778.

50. Consortium for Spinal Cord M. Acute management of autonomic dysreflexia: individuals with spinal cord injury presenting to health-care facilities. *Journal of Spinal Cord Medicine.* Spring 2002; 25(Suppl 1): S67–88.

30

Inherited Metabolic Diseases (IMDs) and Pregnancy

AHMED I. AHMED, SARAH ALDHAHERI, AND ALLISON BANNICK

INTRODUCTION

Inherited metabolic diseases (IMDs) are rare genetic disorders; they are clinically heterogeneous and can present at any age. It affects various body organs through different mechanisms.

One mechanism of body organ damage is the result of accumulation of toxic compounds proximal to a metabolic block (eg, disorders of amino acid metabolism such as phenylketonuria (PKU), the organic acidurias such as methylmalonic acidemia (MMA), and urea cycle defects such as ornithine transcarbamylase (OTC) deficiency). Another mechanism is associated with disorders of energy metabolism resulting in energy deficiency: for example, mitochondrial respiratory chain defects, fatty acid oxidation defects, and glycogen storage disorders (GSDs).[1] Lastly, disorders of complex molecules can cause a disturbance in the synthesis or catabolism of complex molecules: for example, the lysosomal storage disorders and the peroxisomal disorders.[2] Most of these conditions are associated with neurologic implications.

With the expanded newborn screening panels, many of the IMDs have been successfully screened for since the mid-2000s in the United States.[3,4] Early diagnosis and treatment of these conditions have led to improved neurological outcomes and overall survival of these individuals, and now many of them are reaching childbearing age. Despite treatment, the potential presence of preexisting organ involvement may not only impact their fertility potential but also may impose a higher risk of adverse maternal and fetal outcomes.[5]

GENERAL PRINCIPLES

- Pregnancy leads to extra strain on maternal metabolism, this may result in the manifestation of symptoms of a previously unknown disease or a progression of a known disease.[6]
- Neurological manifestations due to adult onset IMDs during pregnancy should be considered in the differential diagnosis of acute neurological conditions in pregnancy such as mitochondrial disorders or hyperhomocystinuria in the differential of cerebrovascular stroke. Other clinical presentations of neurometabolic disorders include ataxias, movement disorders, epilepsies, encephalopathy (eg, urea cycle disorders) or peripheral neuropathy.[6]
- New onset abnormal deep tendon reflexes or dysdiadochokinesia should raise a suspicion of underlying metabolic conditions. Additionally, physicians should consider IMDs in cases of hyperemesis that are resistant to treatment or in cases of new onset hypoglycemic seizures in pregnant women.
- Once an IMD is suspected, prompt consultation with a metabolic specialist should be done followed by appropriate screening tests (in addition to routine tests, such as comprehensive metabolic panel) that include plasma amino acids, plasma acylcarnitine profile, urine organic acids, and plasma ammonia and lactate. It is important to collect samples for testing at the time of the metabolic decompensation crisis if possible, since some IMDs may have normal laboratory findings during times of wellness.
- Plan of care of an IMD during pregnancy when the woman has a molecularly confirmed metabolic diagnosis prior to pregnancy may be different than when she presents for the first time during pregnancy with a metabolic crisis.
- The physiological or pathological changes during pregnancy can easily trigger a life-threatening metabolic decompensation.

Therefore, it is crucial to take an effective interdisciplinary approach in managing metabolic decompensation during pregnancy. This should include metabolic specialist, maternal fetal specialist, metabolic dietitian, intensive care unit specialist, and neurologist. Limited information exists about reference ranges for metabolite concentrations in pregnancy.[7,8]

- Maternal metabolism changes substantially during pregnancy. Early gestation is usually characterized as an anabolic state,[7] while during the third trimester, a maternal catabolic state develops. It is prudent to consider an increased maternal caloric intake to achieve an optimal metabolic outcome particularly during the third trimester. In addition, increased protein requirements during pregnancy must also be considered.
- Most of the IMDs are autosomal recessive genetic disorders. Therefore, if the mother is affected with identified disease-causing mutations, then her partner's carrier status should be determined to establish the risk of the fetus being affected. If the fetus is affected it may cause adverse effects, ranging from structural fetal malformations of the brain to fetal cardiomyopathy, hydrops fetalis or isolated ascites, and/or fetal demise.[4,9]
- Early referral to the genetic/metabolic clinic is essential so that timely diagnosis can allow for close monitoring of potential adverse outcomes for the mother and fetus, and genetic counseling can be provided. Information regarding the expected maternal and/or fetal outcomes is critical for many patients to make their reproductive choices.
- The literature is lacking formal guidelines for managing IMDs during pregnancy (except for phenylketonuria). Data are mainly obtained from isolated case reports or small cases series.[6]

In this chapter, by sharing our experience at large tertiary metabolic and maternity centers, we will address the possible complications of some inherited disorders of metabolism that are associated with maternal neurological manifestations with emphasis on the available potential treatments.

In general, management of IMDs is challenging, especially during pregnancy. We found the following websites are helpful for both providers and patients to have access to quality care and appropriate genetics expertise, disease-specific care plans, and management protocols; www.msgrcc.org/factsheet.html and http://newenglandconsortium.org.

PRECONCEPTION COUNSELING

Screening for IMDs should begin with any prior history of modified diet or of clinical patient follow-up with other specialties such as neurology or endocrinology. In the past, treatment for IMDs may have been initiated only in early childhood years, and access to genetic or metabolic specialists may have been limited.

Women with IMD desiring pregnancy should meet with an IMD specialist to be counseled about the importance of optimizing of their metabolic control prior to conception to decrease not only the maternal risks of metabolic decompensation but also the fetal risks, including possible fetal demise. Women with an inherited disorder of amino acid or energy metabolism should continue treatment through pregnancy with strict compliance to a modified diet. While the specialized diet varies according to the specific metabolic condition, it may be low in protein, high in carbohydrate, low in fat, or high in fat.[2] Baseline evaluations through detailed clinical examination and appropriate investigations, including imaging, should be adopted to assess the appropriateness of the pregnancy timing.

There is limited knowledge in most metabolic disorders about the possibility of an IMD causing infertility. This is mostly due to the limited number of individuals with IMDs reaching reproductive age. However, with expanded newborn screening and advances in treatments for IMDs more individuals will reach reproductive age, and we may then learn more about possible infertility in IMDs. There are well-documented concerns for infertility in females with classic galactosemia, a disorder of carbohydrate metabolism. There is no known risk for infertility in males with classic galactosemia. Regardless of treatment for the IMD, females with classic galactosemia often have primary ovarian insufficiency (POI) with hypergonadotropic hypogonadism.[10] Monitoring of hormone levels (including follicle-stimulating hormone, luteinizing hormone, and estradiol) should be part of routine surveillance for females affected with classic galactosemia. Referral to reproductive endocrinology to discuss possible ethinyl estradiol replacement therapy early, and to discuss future reproductive options should occur around 10–12 years of age. Some possible reproductive options for females with classic galactosemia include embryo banking, egg banking, and ovarian tissue banking. There have been case reports of females with classic galactosemia having successful pregnancies. Infants born to those individuals seem to be asymptomatic, despite those infants at birth having elevated metabolites that are usually seen in classic galactosemia.

Contraception safety should be considered especially for hormonal contraception, which can pose an additional significant risk for the patient. For example, oral contraceptive pills should be avoided in homocystinuria due to the increased risk of blood clot and stroke. Some metabolic disorders in the infant can impact the ability and safety of the woman to breastfeed, while for others this may be possible with diet modification in the mother.

Pre-pregnancy plan of care will vary depending on the type of the IMD and should be established in conjunction with the metabolic/genetic clinic. Many general pregnancy guidelines remain important, such as initiating folic acid supplementation and lifestyle modifications (eg, smoking cessation, limiting caffeine and alcohol intake and optimizing weight, diet and general physical health).[11]

Egg or sperm donations, or adoption should be presented to all families affected by mitochondrial disease in an attempt to reduce or prevent transmission of the disease, and to facilitate the process of informed reproductive choice for the patient.[12]

PRENATAL DIAGNOSIS

Measuring Metabolites

In cases where a metabolic block occurs; either a buildup or a decrease of particular metabolites within a pathway can result. When the fetus exchanges this metabolite with the amniotic fluid, measuring that metabolite in amniotic fluid will allow the diagnosis of the metabolic defect.[1]

If risk of an IMD for the fetus is known prenatally, there are several options for prenatal diagnosis with different routes and multiple techniques of testing depending on the type of the IMD (eg, chorionic villous sampling [CVS], amniocentesis, and cordocentesis).[13] Referral to genetics for prenatal diagnosis is helpful, as they will have the best knowledge of currently available testing for a particular IMD.

ENZYMATIC ASSAY

In a small number of IMDs, such as the organic acidemias, measurement of enzyme activity may help to confirm a diagnosis. However, enzyme analysis must be determined in the index case before performing such invasive prenatal diagnostic procedures.

Analysis of some enzymes may only be available in cultured cells, where they are expressed, versus other enzymes that may not be measurable in cultured cells. In some cases the enzymatic assay can be done directly on the uncultured CVS,[14] with an obtainable result in 2 to 3 days, however this may require a relatively large tissue sample size (20–30 mg). Sometimes CVS or amniotic fluid cells may need to be cultured before enzymatic analysis, with an obtainable result in 2–4 weeks. This delay may cause a deferral in counseling the patient about the available reproductive options, including termination of pregnancy.

Interpretation of enzyme analysis results can be difficult. Care should be taken to compare the enzyme activity to the appropriate gestational age reference levels. Some patients may have only moderately low levels, which can make antenatal results difficult to interpret because of problems of distinguishing heterozygous from homozygous fetuses.

Additionally, some enzymes can also show extremely low levels (~10%) in healthy persons. This so-called pseudo deficiency state could be due to an artifact of the in vitro assay or a genuine low level. In such cases antenatal testing cannot be offered because a low result could be found in an affected fetus or a pseudo deficient but unaffected fetus. Prior to attempting to diagnose the fetus, the parents should also be tested to exclude this condition for them and to assess the presumed levels of enzyme activity in heterozygotes in that particular family. Contamination of the sample with maternal cells can also cause problems, particularly in cultured CVS cells.

MOLECULAR TESTING

Many disorders of metabolism are autosomal recessive in inheritance. Thus, there will be a higher risk of having an affected child in consanguineous families or groups with a high founder effect. Genetic counseling should be offered, and prenatal testing should be discussed as needed.

Molecular DNA testing with targeted mutation analysis is more accurate and reliable than enzymatic assay. However, DNA analysis can only be used when both disease-causing mutations have been identified in the index case, and the other parent is confirmed as a carrier of a mutation in the same gene. If a molecular fetal DNA testing is pursued; it is very important to exclude the presence of any contaminating DNA from the mother, particularly when the test result revealed heterozygous state for the maternal mutation.

Recently, preimplantation genetic diagnosis is available for a number of (usually) X-linked inherited disorders of metabolism (eg, OTC deficiency, adrenoleukodystrophy, and Fabry disease).[2]

In cases where the mitochondrial disease is inherited in an autosomal recessive manner (nuclear mitochondrial DNA), the carrier status should be confirmed in each parent with an additional evidence provided from functional studies supporting pathogenicity. When a mitochondrial DNA (mtDNA) mutation is responsible for familial heteroplasmic mtDNA mutations, the mtDNA mutation load in offspring is often variable. Thus, prenatal diagnosis (PND) is technically possible but usually not applicable because of the limitations in predicting the phenotype.[15]

A fairly new option for preventing the transmission of mtDNA diseases is preimplantation genetic diagnosis (PGD), in which embryos with a mutant load below a mutation-specific or general expression threshold of 18% can be transferred. PGD is currently the best reproductive option for familial heteroplasmic mtDNA point mutations.

Nuclear genome transfer and genome editing techniques are currently being investigated and might offer additional reproductive options for specific mtDNA disease cases.[16]

Pronuclear transfer and metaphase II spindle transfer continue to be developed but are not yet available. The present availability of PGD and the future possibility of nuclear transfer mark an exciting phase in preventing the transmission of mitochondrial disease.[12]

CARE DURING PREGNANCY, DELIVERY, AND POSTPARTUM PERIODS

In many situations, especially during early gestation, important reproductive decisions are being made by the mother (eg, termination of pregnancy). The presence of significant maternal neurocognitive deficits from long-term poorly controlled metabolic status, should be taken into high consideration regarding the mother's ability to make such important decisions.

Women with a neurocognitive impairment may need additional social and psychological support during pregnancy and after birth. These women's IMD may be difficult to manage since they are not always compliant with treatment plans, which may place them at an increased risk of acute metabolic decompensation during pregnancy, or increased risk to their health or fetal development.

During pregnancy, prolonged periods without a source of glucose (fasting state or persistent vomiting) should be discouraged and monitored for. Should a pregnant woman be on a metabolic formula that contains multivitamins; adjustment of prenatal vitamin dosing should be considered. Medications to treat IMDs should be used during pregnancy after consultation with genetic/metabolic specialist. Most medications for IMDs do not have clinical trial data on pregnant women. Direct benefit of the medication to the mother and/or fetus, along with prevention of metabolic decompensation, should outweigh the risks (known or unknown). Patients should be counseled on known or unknown risks, and be made aware of reports of medication use during pregnancy in medical literature. Providers should document counseling the patient on use of the medication during pregnancy.

Referral to other medical specialties in an interdisciplinary team approach should be adopted during pregnancy and tailored according to the type of the IMD. Antenatal monitoring such as detailed anatomy scan and fetal echocardiogram may be necessary for some IMDs especially in poor maternal adherence to the metabolic disease treatment plan. In Table 30.1, we have enlisted some of the IMDs that can cause potential maternal and/or fetal neurological complications during pregnanacy and their managments.

Pregnancy may add additional risk to any preexisting co-morbidities that are related to the primary IMD for example, cardiomyopathy in Glycogen storage disorder (GSD) type IIIa or mitochondrial disorders. Therefore, close monitoring would be appropriate to avoid maternal complications.

Acute stressful conditions such as vomiting, anorexia or acute illness (eg, acute pyelonephritis) can precipitate an acute metabolic crisis in a pregnant woman with IMD. Women with disorders of energy metabolism such as mitochondrial disorders or fatty acid oxidation defects are at risk of decompensation due to reduced calorie

TABLE 30.1 POTENTIAL MATERNAL/FETAL COMPLICATIONS AND SUGGESTED TREATMENT OF SOME IMDS ASSOCIATED WITH NEUROLOGICAL MANIFESTATIONS DURING PREGNANCY

Specific IMD	Potential Maternal Complications	Potential Fetal Complications	Treatment
Urea cycle disorders[11,28,29]	• Encephalopathy • Cerebral edema • Death		1. Protein restriction 2. Specific amino acids supplementation and a high-energy intake to suppress a tendency for catabolism 3. Nitrogen scavenger drugs 4. Serial biochemical laboratory monitoring 5. Avoid stressors 6. Emergency protocol for hyperammonemia crisis 7. Care of liver transplanted patients
Hyperhomocysteinaemia[36-38]	• Thromboembolic events (Pre—and postpartum) • Ischemic strokes • Pre-eclampsia	• Recurrent miscarriage • Placental infarction and insufficiency • Fetal demise • Placental abruption • Dysmorphic features • Congenital cardiac defects and NTD (neural tube defects)	1. Folic acid, vitamin B6, B12 2. Restriction of natural protein, if necessary
Methylmalonic acidaemia[39]	Encephalopathy due to high protein load especially after delivery due to squeeze of maternal blood from the uterus into the circulation	• Intrauterine growth restriction (IUGR) • Hypoplasia of the corpus callosum • Postnatal growth restriction • Mental retardation • Postnatal dehydration and coma	1. Special metabolic formula with restriction of isoleucine, valine, methionine, and threonine 2. Supplementation of carnitine 3. Vitamin B12 supplementation when responsive
Glycogen storage disease type I[40]	• Increasing Glucose requirement • Decreased awareness of hypoglycemia; • Hypoglycemia induced seizures • Increased risk of renal impairment due to cessation of angiotensin converting enzyme inhibitors		1. Strict control; continuous enteral nutrition 2. Avoid Angiotensin converting enzymes inhibitors in pregnancy 3. Hypoglycemia awareness
Glycogen storage disease type III[41]	• Increasing requirement of glucose; • Progressive (cardio) myopathy		1. Strict control; continuous enteral nutrition 2. Echocardiogram

TABLE 30.1 CONTINUED

Specific IMD	Potential Maternal Complications	Potential Fetal Complications	Treatment
Disorders of energy metabolism			
Mitochondrial respiratory chain defects[42–45]	• Variable course. • Asymptomatic[46] • Mitochondrial cardiomyopathy or arrhythmias • Seizures • Hypoglycemia • Gestational diabetes mellitus • Preterm contractions • Increased risk of magnesium toxicity • Exercise intolerance or muscle weakness[24,47] • Wolff–Parkinson–White syndrome,[48] persistent paresthesia[49] and focal segmental glomerulosclerosis[50] • Stroke–like episodes e.g. MELAS • Labor dystocia[51] increased caesarean section rate[48] • Uterine atony and postpartum hemorrhage	• Stillbirth • Fetal contractures • Pontocerebellar hypoplasia, • Delayed myelination, • Facial dysmorphic features	1. High dose folate if on Antiepileptic medications. 2. Supplementation of Coenzyme Q10 (ubiquinone). 3. Low dose aspirin to prevent preeclampsia 4. Serial fetal growth scan and antenatal fetal surveillance 5. Maternal echocardiogram for possible mitochondrial cardiomyopathy 6. EKG for possible cardiac arrhythmias 7. First trimester screening glucose challenge test screen 8. Close monitoring of magnesium sulfate therapy
Gaucher type I[5, 52, 53]	Thrombocytopenia, anemia, portal hypertension risk of spontaneous abortion bleeding during delivery and postpartum		Enzyme replacement treatment
Lysosomal storage disease[54]	• Gastrointestinal symptoms • Acroparesthesias • Proteinuria • Headaches • Postpartum depression	• Dysmorphic features • Hydrops fetalis and stillbirth • Hepatosplenomegaly • Placental changes: pale and bulky • Lysosomal vacuolisation	
Peroxisomal disorders[55]		• Dysmorphic features (including rhizomelic extremities) • Cardiac defects, renal cysts, defective neuronal migration, and agenesis of corpus callosum • Hepatosplenomegaly • Fetal hypokinesia • Renal hyperechogenicity • Cerebral ventricular enlargement	

intake. Women with urea cycle disorders, glycogen storage diseases, or organic acidemias can be easily decompensated due to inability to take the appropriate medications and supplementations. According to some reports, metabolic decompensation during pregnancy can be fatal to the mother and the fetus.[11,17]

It is essential to promptly and appropriately treat these maternal illnesses, with additional close monitoring of the mother and the fetus. Emergency metabolic protocols should be immediately initiated according to the type of the IMD. In our practice, all patients with IMDs are provided with multiple copies of the emergency IMD management protocol and an additional copy will be flagged in the patients' electronic medical records. The emergency protocol is a plan of care during acute conditions, which includes the delivery period. However, a separate delivery protocol may be issued by the genetic/metabolic specialist. Providers should ascertain before the delivery when the genetic/metabolic clinic needs to be notified of the delivery, which may be before, during, or after the delivery.

In certain circumstances, a fetus affected with an IMD may cause risk of harm to the mother during pregnancy. For example, the mothers of fetuses affected with Long-chain 3-hydroxyacyl-CoA dehydrogenase (LCHAD) deficiency may develop acute fatty liver of pregnancy (AFLP) or maternal HELLP syndrome (haemolysis, elevated liver enzymes, and low platelets).[18]

A protocol for testing the neonate for the IMD in the immediate neonatal period may be issued by the genetic/metabolic specialist. Depending on the state and the IMD in question, the newborn screen for the infant may be flagged to assure prompt reporting of results. If the infant is affected, breastfeeding may or may not be possible depending on the disorder and its specific manifestations. For example, the Duarte variant of galactosemia may allow partial breastfeeding even though the classic galactose-1-phosphate uridyltransferase deficiency makes breastfeeding contraindicated.

SPECIFIC DISORDERS WITH NEUROLOGICAL IMPACT ON THE MOTHER OR THE FETUS

Disorders of Energy Metabolism

Mitochondrial disorders affect tissues with the highest energy requirements. Features of these disorders can include: deafness, diabetes, proximal myopathy, external ophthalmoplegia, visual loss, gastrointestinal dysmotility, cardiomyopathy, cardiac conduction defects, epilepsy and in rarer cases encephalopathy and stroke-like episodes.[19]

Mitochondrial diseases are categorized into mitochondrial encephalomyopathy with lactic acidosis and stroke-like episodes (MELAS), myoclonic epilepsy with ragged-red fibers (MERRF), chronic progressive external ophthalmoplegia (CPEO), maternal inherited diabetes-deafness syndrome (MIDD), and others.

The course of symptoms of mitochondrial disease during pregnancy is variable among affected individuals. There are reports of complications with threatened preterm labor, fetal growth restriction, and preeclampsia.[20,21] In those who already have impaired mitochondrial function, it may be predicted that the increased respiratory and energy demand during pregnancy and particularly at the onset of labor may lead to the development of serious complications.

Mitochondrial dysfunction of the placenta may induce trophoblastic apoptosis, which may play a role in increasing the risks of fetal growth restriction and preeclampsia.[22] This requires close maternal and fetal monitoring.

Women with diabetes mellitus associated with mitochondrial disease have been reported to be at high risk for preeclampsia and threatened premature labor.[23] Myometrial contractictility secondary to disturbed energy production due to mitochondrial dysfunction might be related to uterine atony and postpartum hemorrhage in some cases.[24]

Magnesium sulfate is a widely used medication in obstetric practice. Because magnesium ions may compete with calcium ions in the mitochondria, which impairs the phosphorylation, toxic symptoms may arise from administration of magnesium sulfate. Toxicity has been reported at rate of 20% and may be encountered at therapeutic plasma levels.[25]

Those affected with MELAS syndrome in particular tend to have poor outcomes during pregnancy. There may be progressive dementia and neurological deterioration related to stroke-like episodes and recurrent seizures.

Adult-Onset Urea Cycle Disorders

Due to the rarity of these disorders, most obstetricians have little experience with the clinical management. Treatment for acute hyperammonemia should be started before the precise diagnosis is made to reduce the production of nitrogenous waste and to lower plasma ammonia levels quickly to avoid the irreversible maternal and fetal adverse effects.

Ornithine transcarbamylase (OTC) deficiency is the most common urea cycle disorder. Although OTC is an x-linked genetic disorder, it can be manifested for the first time as hyperammonemia crisis in pregnant women with elevated serum ammonia level in the setting of normal liver enzymes. Acute stressors can precipitate an acute metabolic crisis in otherwise asymptomatic pregnant women, such as infection, trauma, medications (e.g. sodium valproate), surgery, excessive protein intake, and physiological stress such as labor and delivery.[26,27] Encephalopathy, resulting in cerebral edema and consequently in death, may be the primary manifestation of the urea cycle defects such as OTC and carbamoylphosphate synthetase deficiency during or directly after pregnancy.[11,28,29]

Acute management of hyperammonemia is variable depending upon the ammonia levels and symptomatology of the patient. Management may also be different depending on whether the woman is known to have a diagnosis that causes hyperammonemia or not. General principles of management generally include: protein-free diet for 24 to 48 hours, increasing the caloric intake with high glucose infusion (addition of insulin may be necessary) and lipid administration to reverse catabolism,[30] intravenous arginine infusion, and initiation of nitrogen scavenger medications. Hemodialysis should be considered in patients with persistently high ammonia levels.[31]

In a woman with a known UCD diagnosis, nitrogen-scavenger medications should be used during pregnancy only if the potential benefit justifies the potential risk to the fetus. Use of these medications should be discussed with a metabolic specialist prior to pregnancy if possible.

Amino Acidopathies

One of the most common and well-studied IMDs is phenylketonuria (PKU). PKU is characterized by elevated phenylalanine (phe) levels due to deficiency of phenylalanine hydroxylase enzyme from genetic mutations in the phenylalanine hydroxylase gene. It has been well-documented that prolonged elevated blood phe levels causes neurological damage to those individuals affected with PKU. Elevated phe levels can also cause teratogenic effects for the fetus, often termed maternal PKU syndrome. These effects can include microcephaly, cognitive impairment (at times to the degree of mental retardation), low birth weight, congenital malformations (congenital heart defects, dysmorphology), and behavioral problems.[32] There have also been reports of elevated maternal phe levels causing spontaneous abortion. However, fetal effects can be ameliorated or decreased by the lowering and maintenance of maternal blood phe levels in the recommended goal range. This can be accomplished through a phenylalanine-restricted diet, supplementation with metabolic formula, and proper caloric intake. Information about the use of sapropterin dihydrochloride in pregnancy is limited. However, the majority of case reports cite better outcomes when use of this medication works to lower maternal blood phe levels.[33] It is imperative that consultation with a metabolic specialist and dietitian be implemented during pregnancy for a woman with PKU. Ideally, the blood phe levels should be in the recommended range prior to conception for best possible outcomes for the child. Postnatally, an echocardiogram for the neonate is recommended to assess for effects of maternal PKU syndrome.

Maple Syrup Urine Disease (MSUD) is a disorder of branched-chain amino acid metabolism. Accumulation of amino acids and subsequent ketoacids can, in combination with physiological stress, cause significant metabolic crisis that can progress to seizures and life-threatening cerebral edema. Timely and proper emergency management during times of physiologic stress is imperative to prevent lifelong complications of the disorder. Routine treatment for MSUD includes a protein-restricted diet, metabolic formula, proper caloric intake, and avoidance of physiologic stressors when possible. While MSUD is similar to PKU in some ways, there are only a few case reports at this time of pregnancies for women affected with MSUD and outcomes for their children. There are case reports of good outcomes for the mother with MSUD and her child when there is adherence to the treatment plan throughout the pregnancy, and extra precautions are initiated around the time of labor and delivery.[34] These precautions could include routine biochemistry monitoring and additional intravenous fluids and dextrose. Labor and delivery in particular should be managed in conjunction with a metabolic/genetic specialist and dietitian to prevent and treat possible complications.

Impaired Fatty Acid Oxidation

For women with hypoketotic hypoglycemia, hypotonia, unexplained cardiomyopathy, exercise or activity intolerance, or syncope episodes, a disorder

BOX 30.1
CARE MAP FOR PREGNANCY IN IMD PATIENT

PRE-PREGNANCY

- Genetic counseling: confirm the diagnosis or carrier status for the parents.
- Establish a care in metabolic/Genetic clinic.
- Review the degree of metabolic control including diet, special metabolic formula, medications, and laboratory investigations.
- Discuss the potential reproductive risk and teratogenic effects of the medications.
- Review of prior pregnancy complications, prior imaging studies, and prior labs
- Assessment of disease specific maternal risk factors:
  - Basic metabolic panel: PAA, ACP, UOA, Ammonia, and Lactate.
  - Degree of disability if any
  - Neurocognitive evaluation
  - Baseline body organ functions e.g. maternal echocardiogram
- Contraceptive counseling
- Medications adjustment, consolidation and review
- Pre-conception MFM consult

DURING PREGNANCY

- Order Metabolic labs every trimester
- Continue multidisciplinary approach
- Adjust medications, diet, and special dietary formulas
- Genetic counseling and parental diagnosis testing as indicated
- Monitor for worsening metabolic signs and symptoms
- Counsel regarding the warning signs of metabolic decompensation
- Monitor caloric requirements and avoid prolonged fasting
- Monitor for fetal structural malformations or fetal growth abnormalities
- Monitor for worsening of specific maternal risk factors
- Early anesthesia consult
- Multidisciplinary discussion to plan best delivery route and location

DELIVERY

- Alert the metabolic, MFM, and ICU teams.
- Follow the metabolic treatment plan during delivery implemented by the metabolic clinic; it varies according to the expected metabolic decompensation (eg, hyperammonemia)
- Commonly used approach: start IV Dextrose 10% with the appropriate electrolytes to prevent catabolism and decompensation
- Anesthesia consultation and pain management
- Notify the neonatologist/NICU team: if any neonatal decompensation is anticipated
- Notify pediatrician if any anticipated developmental difficulties or physical abnormalities

POSTPARTUM

- Encourage continued follow-up in the metabolic/genetic clinic
- Consider consultation with specialists as needed for comorbidities prior to discharge
- Plan for social support to care for infant and the mother (if needed)
- Lactation consult
- Medication adjustments
- Venous thromboembolism prophylaxis as indicated
- Monitor for postpartum depression
- Contraception counseling

of fatty acid oxidation should be in consideration.[35] Primary carnitine deficiency or other disorders of fatty acid oxidation, such as medium-chain acyl-CoA dehydrogenase (MCAD) deficiency, can be undiagnosed until a physiologic stressor such as pregnancy or labor and delivery causes symptoms for the woman. These symptoms include those list above but can also include sudden death. Biochemical testing can diagnose these disorders, and testing should include plasma free and total carnitine, plasma acylcarnitine profile, and urine organic acids. Supplementation with levocarnitine and intravenous dextrose, along with management of any electrolyte imbalances, can resolve most acute symptoms in these disorders. Referral to a metabolic/genetic specialist for follow-up of the new diagnosis would be needed. Infants of these women have been found to be asymptomatic from their mother's IMD. Routine newborn screening has also helped to diagnose other maternal IMDs, such as glutaric acidemia and 3-methylcrotonyl Co-A carboxylase deficiency, by detecting low carnitine levels on the infant's newborn screen (Box 30.1).

REFERENCES

1. Brassier A, Ottolenghi C, Boddaert N, et al. Prenatal symptoms and diagnosis of inherited metabolic diseases. *Archives de Pediatrie: Organe Officiel de la Societe Francaise de Pediatrie.* 2012; 19(9): 959–969.
2. Murphy E. Pregnancy in women with inherited metabolic disease. *Obstet Med.* 2015; 8(2): 61–67.
3. Lee PJ. Pregnancy issues in inherited metabolic disorders. *J Inherit Metab Dis.* 2006; 29(2–3): 311–316.
4. Walter JH. Inborn errors of metabolism and pregnancy. *J Inherit Metab Dis.* 2000; 23(3): 229–236.
5. Rosenbaum H. Management of women with Gaucher disease in the reproductive age. *Thrombosis Research.* 2015; 135(Suppl 1): S49–51.
6. Spronsen FJ, Smit GP, Erwich JJ. Inherited metabolic diseases and pregnancy. *BJOG.* 2005; 112(1): 2–11.
7. Talian GC, Komlosi K, Decsi T, Koletzko B, Melegh B. Determination of carnitine ester patterns during the second half of pregnancy, at delivery, and in neonatal cord blood by tandem mass spectrometry: Complex and dynamic involvement of carnitine in the intermediary metabolism. *Pediatr Res.* 2007; 62(1): 88–92.
8. Winter SC, Linn LS, Helton E. Plasma carnitine concentrations in pregnancy, cord blood, and neonates and children. *Clin Chim Acta.* 1995; 243(1): 87–93.
9. Paupe A, Bidat L, Sonigo P, Lenclen R, Molho M, Ville Y. Prenatal diagnosis of hypoplasia of the corpus callosum in association with non-ketotic hyperglycinemia. *Ultrasound Obstet Gynecol.* 2002; 20(6): 616–619.
10. Blau N HG, Leonard J. Physician's guide to the treatment and follow-up of metabolic diseases. In: Beat Thöny GFH, Leonard JV, Clarke JTR, eds. Springer-Verlag Berlin Heidelberg; 2006.
11. Schimanski U, Krieger D, Horn M, Stremmel W, Wermuth B, Theilmann L. A novel two-nucleotide deletion in the ornithine transcarbamylase gene causing fatal hyperammonia in early pregnancy. *Hepatology.* 1996; 24(6): 1413–1415.
12. Nesbitt V, Alston CL, Blakely EL, et al. A national perspective on prenatal testing for mitochondrial disease. *Eur J Hum Genet.* 2014; 22(11): 1255–1259.
13. Diukman R, Goldberg JD. Prenatal diagnosis of inherited metabolic diseases. *The Western Journal of Medicine.* 1993; 159(3): 374–381.
14. Verma J, Thomas DC, Sharma S, et al. Inherited metabolic disorders: prenatal diagnosis of lysosomal storage disorders. *Prenatal Diagnosis.* 2015; 35(11): 1137–1147.
15. Thorburn DR, Dahl HH. Mitochondrial disorders: Genetics, counseling, prenatal diagnosis and reproductive options. *Am J Med Genet.* 2001; 106(1): 102–114.
16. Smeets HJ, Sallevelt SC, Dreesen JC, de Die-Smulders CE, de Coo IF. Preventing the transmission of mitochondrial DNA disorders using prenatal or preimplantation genetic diagnosis. *Ann N Y Acad Sci.* 2015; 1350: 29–36.
17. Langendonk JG, Roos JC, Angus L, et al. A series of pregnancies in women with inherited metabolic disease. *J Inherit Metab Dis.* 2012; 35(3): 419–424.
18. Wilcken B, Leung KC, Hammond J, Kamath R, Leonard JV. Pregnancy and fetal long-chain 3-hydroxyacyl coenzyme A dehydrogenase deficiency. *Lancet.* 1993; 341(8842): 407–408.
19. McFarland R, Turnbull DM. Batteries not included: Diagnosis and management of mitochondrial disease. *J Intern Med.* 2009; 265(2): 210–228.
20. Mando C, De Palma C, Stampalija T, et al. Placental mitochondrial content and function in intrauterine growth restriction and preeclampsia. *Am J Physiol Endocrinol Metab.* 2014; 306(4): E404–413.
21. Group Tgd. Newcastle mitochondrial disease guidelines. 2012. http://www.newcastle-/mitochondria.com/wp-content/uploads/2012/09/Pregnancy-Guidelines.pdf
22. Li HZ, Li RY, Li M. A review of maternally inherited diabetes and deafness. *Front Biosci (Landmark Ed).* 2014; 19: 777–782.
23. Say RE, Whittaker RG, Turnbull HE, McFarland R, Taylor RW, Turnbull DM. Mitochondrial disease in pregnancy: A systematic review. *Obstet Med.* 2011; 4(3): 90–94.
24. Dessole S, Capobianco G, Ambrosini G, Battista Nardelli G. Postpartum hemorrhage and

emergency hysterectomy in a patient with mito-chondrial myopathy: A case report. *Arch Gynecol Obstet.* 2003; 267(4): 247–249.

25. Moriarty KT, McFarland R, Whittaker R, et al. Pre-eclampsia and magnesium toxicity with ther-apeutic plasma level in a woman with m.3243A>G melas mutation. *J Obstet Gynaecol.* 2008; 28(3): 349.

26. Gordon N. Ornithine transcarbamylase defi-ciency: A urea cycle defect. *Eur J Paediatr Neurol.* 2003; 7(3): 115–121.

27. Ellaway CJ, Bennetts B, Tuck RR, Wilcken B. Clumsiness, confusion, coma, and valproate. *Lancet.* 1999; 353(9162): 1408.

28. Wong LJ, Craigen WJ, O'Brien WE. Postpartum coma and death due to carbamoyl-phosphate synthetase I deficiency. *Ann Intern Med.* 1994; 120(3): 216–217.

29. Arn PH, Hauser ER, Thomas GH, Herman G, Hess D, Brusilow SW. Hyperammonemia in women with a mutation at the ornithine carbamoyltransferase locus. A cause of postpartum coma. *N Engl J Med.* 1990; 322(23): 1652–1655.

30. Singh RH. Nutritional management of patients with urea cycle disorders. *J Inherit Metab Dis.* 2007; 30(6): 880–887.

31. Enns GM, Berry SA, Berry GT, Rhead WJ, Brusilow SW, Hamosh A. Survival after treatment with phenylacetate and benzoate for urea-cycle disorders. *N Engl J Med.* 2007; 356(22): 2282–2292.

32. Waisbren SE, Hanley W, Levy HL, et al. Outcome at age 4 years in offspring of women with maternal phenylketonuria: The Maternal PKU Collaborative Study. *JAMA.* 2000; 283(6): 756–762.

33. Grange DK, Hillman RE, Burton BK, et al. Sapropterin dihydrochloride use in pregnant women with phenylketonuria: an interim report of the PKU MOMS sub-registry. *Mol Genet Metab.* 2014; 112(1): 9–16.

34. Brown J, Tchan M, Nayyar R. Maple syrup urine disease: Tailoring a plan for pregnancy. *The Journal of Maternal-fetal & Neonatal Medicine.* 2017:1–4, online published 5/2017: 1–4.

35. Schimmenti LA, Crombez EA, Schwahn BC, et al. Expanded newborn screening identifies maternal primary carnitine deficiency. *Mol Genet Metab.* 2007; 90(4): 441–445.

36. Ray JG, Laskin CA. Folic acid and homocyst(e)ine metabolic defects and the risk of placental abruption, pre-eclampsia and spontaneous preg-nancy loss: A systematic review. *Placenta.* 1999; 20(7): 519–529.

37. Wong WY, Eskes TK, Kuijpers-Jagtman AM, et al. Nonsyndromic orofacial clefts: association with maternal hyperhomocysteinemia. *Teratology.* 1999; 60(5): 253–257.

38. Rosenquist TH, Ratashak SA, Selhub J. Homocysteine induces congenital defects of the heart and neural tube: effect of folic acid. *Proc Natl Acad Sci U S A.* 1996; 93(26): 15227–15232.

39. Diss E, Iams J, Reed N, Roe DS, Roe C. Methylmalonic aciduria in pregnancy: A case report. *Am J Obstet Gynecol.* 1995; 172(3): 1057–1059.

40. Rake JP. Glycogen storage disease type I: clinical, biochemical and genetic aspects, and implications for treatment and follow-up (management of gly-cogen storage disease type I). 2003. http://www.rug.nl/research/portal/files/3014584/c6.pdf.

41. Dagli A, Sentner CP, Weinstein DA. Glycogen Storage Disease Type III. In: Pagon RA, Adam MP, Ardinger HH, et al., eds. *GeneReviews(R).* Seattle: University of Washington; 1993.

42. Lincke CR, van den Bogert C, Nijtmans LG, Wanders RJ, Tamminga P, Barth PG. Cerebellar hypoplasia in respiratory chain dysfunction. *Neuropediatrics.* 1996; 27(4): 216–218.

43. Bamforth FJ, Bamforth JS, Applegarth DA. Structural anomalies in patients with inherited metabolic diseases. *J Inherit Metab Dis.* 1994; 17(3): 330–332.

44. Samson JF, Barth PG, de Vries JI, et al. Familial mitochondrial encephalopathy with fetal ultra-sonographic ventriculomegaly and intracerebral calcifications. *Eur J Pediatr.* 1994; 153(7): 510–516.

45. Benardis PG, Ikomi AA, Bateman SG, Bowyer JJ. An inborn error of metabolism imitating hypoxic-ischaemic encephalopathy. *BJOG.* 2000; 107(7): 941–942.

46. Hosono T, Suzuki M, Chiba Y. Contraindication of magnesium sulfate in a pregnancy compli-cated with late-onset diabetes mellitus and sen-sory deafness due to mitochondrial myopathy. *Journal of Maternal-fetal Medicine.* 2001; 10(5): 355–356.

47. Berkowitz K, Monteagudo A, Marks F, Jackson U, Baxi L. Mitochondrial myopathy and pree-clampsia associated with pregnancy. *Am J Obstet Gynecol.* 1990; 162(1): 146–147.

48. Rosaeg OP, Morrison S, MacLeod JP. Anaesthetic management of labour and delivery in the par-turient with mitochondrial myopathy. *Canadian Journal of Anaesthesia.* 1996; 43(4): 403–407.

49. Yanagawa T, Sakaguchi H, Nakao T, et al. Mitochondrial myopathy, encephalopathy, lactic acidosis, and stroke-like episodes with deteriora-tion during pregnancy. *Internal medicine (Tokyo, Japan).* 1998; 37(9): 780–783.

50. Lowik MM, Hol FA, Steenbergen EJ, Wetzels JF, van den Heuvel LP. Mitochondrial tRNALeu(UUR) mu-tation in a patient with steroid-resistant nephrotic syndrome and focal segmental glomerulosclerosis.

Nephrology, Dialysis, Transplantation: Official Publication of the European Dialysis and Transplant Association—European Renal Association. 2005;20(2): 336–341.

51. Kovilam OP, Cahill W, Siddiqi TA. Pregnancy with mitochondrial encephalopathy, lactic acidosis, and strokelike episodes syndrome. *Obstetrics and Gynecology.* 1999; 93(5 Pt. 2): 853.

52. Fasouliotis SJ, Ezra Y, Schenker JG. Gaucher's disease and pregnancy. *American Journal of Perinatology.* 1998; 15(5): 311–318.

53. Torloni MR, Franco K, Sass N. Gaucher's disease with myocardial involvement in pregnancy. *Sao Paulo Medical Journal.* 2002; 120(3): 90–92.

54. Wraith JE. Lysosomal Disorders. *Seminars in Neonatology: SN.* 2002; 7(1): 75–83.

55. Nissenkorn A, Michelson M, Ben-Zeev B, Lerman-Sagie T. Inborn errors of metabolism: A cause of abnormal brain development. *Neurology.* 2001; 56(10): 1265–1272.

SECTION 5

Delivery and Postpartum

31

Approach to Delivery in the Patient with Neurologic Disease

HEATHER M. LINK AND EVA K. PRESSMAN

While management of pregnancy in patients with underlying neurologic conditions can be challenging and require a coordinated effort from multiple subspecialties, planning for and accomplishing a safe delivery of mother and infant is critical. This chapter will focus on the optimal approach to delivery planning and peripartum considerations for a variety of neurological disorders that are most likely to have an effect on mode of delivery and potentially related risk of neurologic complications. Specifically, delivery related issues in patients with intracranial masses, spinal cord injuries, central nervous system vascular abnormalities, and neuromuscular disorders will be addressed.

INTRACRANIAL MASSES

Intracranial masses include both benign and malignant conditions, and the approach to peripartum care will differ based on the diagnosis. Specifically, the risk for increased intracranial pressure and herniation, obstruction of the ventricular system, and the risk of hemorrhage will need to be considered. While many of these issues are addressed in detail in Chapter 18, this chapter will address the factors most closely related to the delivery and immediate postpartum period.

Pre-delivery Planning

Planning the delivery for a patient with an intracranial mass requires close interdisciplinary collaboration with neurosurgery, maternal fetal medicine, anesthesia, pediatrics, and oncology. Patients should be delivered at a tertiary care facility with neurosurgical services available.

For patients with malignant intracranial masses, the timing of delivery will need to be carefully balanced between the competing needs of maternal treatment and the neonatal risks of prematurity. Patient stability and progression of disease should be the key factors determining the timing of delivery. Treatment during pregnancy with neurosurgery, radiation, and chemotherapy has been successfully documented in the literature, and it is recommended that surgery and radiation be initiated in the second trimester to minimize fetal risks.[1,2] Verheecke et al. reviewed 27 cases of intracranial malignancy during pregnancy and found that among 12 women who received treatment during pregnancy, 7 delivered at or after 37 weeks; however, among the 9 women who deferred treatment until after delivery, 8 of 9 women delivered preterm.[3] For women who have been treated during pregnancy with stable disease course, or for women with less aggressive disease, it is reasonable to plan for delivery as close to 37 weeks as possible. Chemotherapy timing should allow for recovery of fetal immune system prior to delivery if possible. If treatment has been delayed until the pregnancy is delivered, or the indication for treatment develops after 32 weeks, iatrogenic preterm delivery should be considered after completion of betamethasone for fetal lung maturity.[4]

Admission Assessment

Upon presentation to labor and delivery initial assessment of maternal stability should be conducted including a full neurologic exam to establish a patient baseline. Consultant services should be notified of the patient's arrival. Care should be taken to avoid excessive hydration during labor or cesarean section due to the increased risk of cerebral edema with postpartum fluid shifts.[5]

For patients who are clinically unstable and at risk for brain herniation presenting after fetal viability, delivery by cesarean section under general anesthesia with concomitant neurosurgical decompression is recommended.[6] For patients who are clinically unstable and periviable, a multidisciplinary approach, including both NICU and neurosurgery, to discuss the risks of extreme prematurity in the setting of overall maternal prognosis is recommended to assist families with this decision-making process.

Mode of Delivery

There is no consensus in the literature regarding the preferred mode of delivery for patients in intracranial masses: each case should be assessed individually. Proponents of delivery by cesarean section advocate this approach due to concerns for possible herniation and decompensation with increased intracranial pressure associated with the second stage of labor.[7,8] Similar concerns exist regarding the use of epidural anesthesia in the event of a wet tap,[9] while others argue for epidural placement by experienced anesthesia staff and support reserving cesarean delivery only to those patients with concern for increased intracranial hypertension.[10] Owing to the rarity of brain tumors in pregnancy, information regarding delivery outcomes is limited to case series that report both delivery by scheduled cesarean section and vaginal delivery with and without the use of epidurals. Given the risk of increased intracranial pressure associated with valsalva during the second stage of labor, operative vaginal delivery may need to be considered.[8] We recommend an interdisciplinary approach to determining delivery method. In stable patients without concern for mass effect or significantly increased baseline intracranial hypertension, vaginal delivery should be considered after in-depth discussion with anesthesia regarding epidural placement or consideration of alternative pain control methods including paracervical or pudendal blocks or IV patient controlled analgesia as appropriate. If operative delivery is planned, adequate pain management should be provided.

Postpartum Considerations

Postpartum patients should be monitored for signs of volume overload and cerebral edema. Patients with highly vascular tumors such as meningiomas and acoustic neuromas are more susceptible to rapid tumor swelling from fluid shifts. Women with prolactinomas should be encouraged to breastfeed, as there is little evidence that breastfeeding increases tumor size.[11] In one observational study, 143 women with hyperprolactinemia who had cabergoline-induced pregnancy were followed for 60 months after birth. No difference in prolactin levels was observed between patients nursing for less than 2 months or more than 2–6 months. No tumor mass enlargement was seen.[12] Regardless, all patients with intracranial masses will need close follow-up in the postpartum period.[5]

SPINAL CORD INJURIES

Since general considerations regarding pregnancy and spinal cord injury are addressed elsewhere (see Section 4, Chapter 29) this chapter will focus on planning and outcome data specific to delivery and the immediate postpartum period.

Pre-delivery Planning

Planning the delivery for a patient with a spinal cord injury requires close interdisciplinary collaboration with anesthesia and obstetric providers. Patients should be delivered at a facility capable of providing 24-hour in house anesthesia coverage and preferably a tertiary care facility should the need for intensive monitoring of ICU level care become apparent.[13]

The most serious potential complication to occur during delivery among women with spinal cord injury is autonomic dysreflexia (ADR). Most commonly occurring in patients with spinal cord lesions at T6 or above, stimulus and resultant sympathetic hyperactivity occurring below the level of the lesion is uninhibited by hypothalamic feedback.[14] Symptoms of ADR include malignant hypertension, headache, diaphoresis, piloerection, nasal obstruction, loss of consciousness and arrhythmias.[15] Uterine contractions are a known stimulus for ADR making labor a particularly vulnerable time. Additional stimuli that are commonly encountered during pregnancy include bladder distention, constipation, and speculum exams.[16]

The incidence of pregnancy among women with spinal cord injuries is relatively low so information in the literature is confined to case reports and small case series. Among reports of women who experienced ADR during pregnancy, spinal cord lesions were above a T7 level, and most women had a history of ADR prior to pregnancy.[17] Additionally the presence of spinal instrumentation can make placement of regional anesthesia more difficulty. A thorough history, including available imaging, should be obtained prior to delivery and reviewed during pre-delivery planning with an experienced anesthesiologist.

Women with spinal cord injury can have difficulty identifying signs of labor, which puts them at increased risk for out of hospital birth.

Because of this, women should be counseled on how to palpate uterine contractions and recognize non-painful stimuli of labor such as increased respirations and diaphoresis. Initiating routine cervical exams after 28 weeks as a potential screening for preterm birth risk among spinal cord injury patients has been suggested.[13] Interventions such as this should be tailored to each patient's particular obstetric history and risks for preterm labor. Consideration needs to be made that vaginal exams and cervical manipulation can be potential triggers for ADR, and patients should be assessed accordingly.

Initial Assessment

Upon presentation to labor and delivery, assessment of maternal stability should be conducted. Anesthesia consultant services should be notified of patient presence and for patients with high spinal cord lesions and those considered to be at risk for ADR regional anesthesia should be initiated early. Local anesthetics are recommended, as narcotic-only neuraxial medications have not been shown to be effective in minimizing noxious stimuli from reaching the spinal cord. Episodes of ADR are accompanied by significant diaphoresis, and the traditional taping method of an epidural catheter may not be sufficient. Suturing the catheter in place to prevent inadvertent dislodgment has also been recommended.[17] The bladder should remain drained during labor to further reduce the risk of bladder distention and ADR. Invasive blood pressure monitoring with arterial lines should be considered for high-risk patients.

For patients whose ability to sweat has been disrupted by their spinal cord injury, maternal hyperthermia can result. Providers should be aware of this as maternal hyperthermia occurring during labor could be confused with chorioamnionitis, making diagnosis difficult.[13]

Mode of Delivery

The mode of delivery for patients with spinal cord injury should be based on prior obstetric history, obstetric indications for cesarean section and risk of severe ADR. The largest case series in the literature of 37 pregnancies documented a 33% vaginal delivery rate and greater than 60% rate of cesarean section in the cohort.[18] The majority of cesarean deliveries were planned, with elective and repeat listed as the most common indications. Spinal cord injury is not a contraindication to vaginal delivery, and vaginal delivery should be attempted for most patients. If a patient were to develop ADR

during labor that is not responsive to medical management with epidural or antihypertensive therapy, cesarean section may be necessary. If ADR develops during the second stage of labor the provider can consider expedited delivery with an assisted second stage.[13]

Postpartum Considerations

Patients with an uncomplicated antepartum and intrapartum course are expected to do well during delivery. Sharpe and colleagues reported on a small cohort of patients, 4 of which experienced ADR during the pregnancy, and 3 patients had symptoms postpartum. For women who experience ADR during pregnancy or intrapartum, consideration should be made to continue neuraxial analgesia for a few days postpartum to decrease the risk of ADR. Providers and patients should also be aware that lactation can also be a potential trigger for ADR in the postpartum period, and initiation of breastfeeding should be accompanied by close maternal monitoring.[17]

While immobility in pregnancy is generally considered to place patients at an increased risk for venous thromboembolism, there are not consistent recommendations in the literature regarding prophylactic use of anticoagulant medication. Use should be individualized to a patient's particular risk profile with consideration given to the general increase in thrombotic risk associated with the postpartum period.

CENTRAL NERVOUS SYSTEM VASCULAR ABNORMALITIES

Vascular abnormalities of the central nervous system include arteriovenous malformations (AVM) of the brain and spinal cord, aneurysms, cavernous malformations, venous angiomas, and telangiectasias. Autosomal dominant genetic etiologies have been described for cavernous malformations, telangiectasias, and possibly arteriovenous malformations; so family history of these disorders may prompt investigation. Most vascular abnormalities present with signs and symptoms of increased intracranial pressure or bleeding. These include headache, seizure, or stroke (see also Section 2, Chapters 12–17). For patients with these disorders delivery considerations are based on: the potential effects of increased intracranial pressure during the second stage causing bleeding from the vascular abnormality, implications of regional analgesia, or anesthesia and the potential effects of peripartum fluid shifts. While the effects of intracranial or spinal bleeding can be devastating, the risks of such an event are generally low and often essentially eliminated by treatment prior to pregnancy.

Pre-delivery Planning

Patients with known CNS vascular abnormalities should ideally plan pregnancies to optimize their outcome. With preconception consultation, patients can decide if treatment prior to pregnancy is indicated and would decrease the risks of neurologic sequellae related to hormonal effects or increases in vascular volume related to pregnancy or increases in intracranial pressure or fluid shifts inherent to delivery. In general, complete treatment of a vascular abnormality prior to pregnancy eliminates related risks and subsequent prenatal care and method of delivery should be based on the usual obstetric indications. If treatment is not possible, not recommend or not completed prior to pregnancy, several additions to pregnancy care and delivery management are recommended.

For patients with diagnoses made before pregnancy, imaging prior to pregnancy will likely have already identified the location and extent of the vascular abnormality. Some lesions are more likely to change over time or change due to the effects of increases in estrogen or progesterone during pregnancy. Though data are limited, arteriovenous malformations, aneurysms less than 5 mm, venous angiomas, and telangectasias have been shown to remain unchanged through pregnancy, and repeat imaging is not needed.[19] Larger aneuryms, especially those in high-risk locations or with blebs, do warrant imaging in late pregnancy. Similarly, cavernous malformations have been shown to increase in size during pregnancy.[20] For patients with known hereditary telangiectasia, imaging of the lungs and spine in addition to the brain is important due to the risks of telangiectasias in these area and their potential complications. If patients have not been thoroughly evaluated, additional imaging may be needed.

Outside of pregnancy, CNS vascular malformations are imaged using CT, MRI, and angiography. While it is appropriate to minimize radiation exposure particularly in the first trimester, diagnostic levels of radiation are generally safe in later pregnancy and should be utilized if they are needed to make accurate diagnoses and clinical plans. CT and angiographic contrast is considered safe in pregnancy, but gadolinium-based MRI contrast is generally avoided due to concerns for inflammatory conditions in the offspring as well as increased rates of stillbirth and neonatal deaths.[21]

Management of patients with CNS vascular abnormalities requires a team approach. Input from the neurologist or neurosurgeon (and perhaps the radiologist) on the stability of the malformation and the clinical history is needed to determine the risks of intracranial bleeding or other complications. The primary obstetrician or maternal fetal medicine specialist should assess the alterations needed during prenatal care and potential impact of labor, vaginal delivery, or cesarean delivery.

Initial Admission Assessment

Patients with known CNS vascular abnormalities should have a thorough neurologic exam on admission for delivery. Any neurologic symptoms or physical exam findings related to the vascular abnormality should be fully documented so that if symptoms or signs change over the peripartum period the extent of such changes can be determined.

Mode of Delivery

Considerations for mode of delivery in patients with intracranial vascular malformations include the potential effects of hypertension or repeated valsalva on intracranial pressure, the impact of dural puncture and CSF leakage from spinal anesthesia or complications of epidural analgesia/anesthesia, and the effects of intubation on intracranial pressure. In addition, for patients with spinal cord vascular abnormalities, the risk of epidural hematoma due to regional anesthesia/analgesia also needs to be considered.

For all conditions in which repeated valsalva or pushing may be contraindicated, the option of passive descent and assisted vaginal delivery with either forceps or vacuum should be considered. In general, this is more likely to be accomplished if epidural analgesia is used but systemic narcotics and local/pudendal anesthesia may also allow delivery in this way.

Limited data exists on the effects of mode of delivery for several CNS vascular abnormalities. There is no evidence suggesting that vaginal delivery will increase the cerebral AVM bleeding risk or that cesarean section can prevent hemorrhage from AVM.[22] Similarly, the risk of cavernous malformation hemorrhage is not significantly changed during pregnancy, delivery, or postpartum.[23] Women with hereditary hemorrhagic telangiectasia are at greater risk for pulmonary or uterine bleeding than for intracranial complications with delivery and there does not seem to be any impact from mode of delivery.[24]

Postpartum Considerations

There is limited data indicating an increased risk of hemorrhage from AVMs in the postpartum period, likely related to rapid hormonal and hemodynamic changes that occur after delivery.[25] In addition, there is the potential increased risk of postpartum hemorrhage in patients with hereditary hemorrhagic telangiectasia due to possible endomyometrial involvement. No specific postpartum risks have been identified for cavernous malformations or venous angiomas.

NEUROMUSCULAR DISORDERS

Neuromuscular disorders include a wide variety of relatively rare conditions that affect the peripheral nervous system and skeletal muscles leading to weakness or stiffness of the affected muscles. Many of these conditions are genetic, but there are also acquired disorders, often related to the immune system, such as myasthenia gravis. The impact of neuromuscular disorders on pregnancy and pregnancy on neuromuscular disorders can be found in Section 4, Chapter 24. This section will focus on the effect of these disorders on delivery and the immediate postpartum period, as well as data that can guide delivery management for optimal outcomes.

Pre-delivery Planning

Planning for delivery includes optimizing the patient's neurologic and muscular function, assessing for special needs during labor and delivery, as well as determining if additional assistance will be needed for the care of the infant both in the hospital as well as when the patient goes home. Considerations for delivery include evaluating the patient for triggers and moderators of muscle fatigue, assessing the impact of her disorder on ambulation and positioning in labor and determining the patient's ability to push and potential need for an assisted delivery.

Initial Admission Assessment

On presentation for labor and delivery, patients should be assessed for potential respiratory or airway issues, spinal deformity that may affect regional analgesia or anesthesia, and limitations of hip flexion and abduction. In addition,

certain conditions such as myasthenia gravis are exacerbated by magnesium sulfate; and for this reason, extreme caution should be used in patients with pre-eclampsia with severe features or magnesium administration for fetal neuroprotection in the setting of imminent preterm birth.

Mode of Delivery

Data for mode of delivery for many neuromuscular disorders is limited.[26] This is particularly true for the rarer inherited disorders where data comes from small retrospective studies. While some studies show increased rates of cesarean deliveries and assisted vaginal deliveries, it is not clear if this is due to actual maternal exhaustion or physician concern regarding the risks of muscle fatigue.[27,28,29] Some studies of myasthenia gravis in pregnancy suggest that assisted deliveries and cesarean sections are also more common,[30] but others have not confirmed this.[31,32] Mode of delivery does not seem to affect the incidence of myasthenic exacerbations in the postpartum period, but these patients are sensitive to nondepolarizing agents used for general anesthesia. As a result, these agents should be avoided.[30]

Postpartum Considerations

Postpartum issues include risk for thrombosis and potential issues with self-care and infant care. Similar to spinal cord injury patients, immobility is generally considered to place patients at an increased risk for venous thromboembolism; however, again, there are not consistent recommendations in the literature regarding prophylactic use of medication. Use should be individualized to a patient's particular risk profile with consideration given to the general increase in thrombotic risk associated with the postpartum period.

For neuromuscular conditions with immunologic etiologies, there is the potential for flares in the postpartum period. Guillain-Barré syndrome is reported to occur nearly 3 times more often in the period 30 days postpartum, and myasthenia gravis exacerbations can be triggered postpartum as well.[26]

REFERENCES

1. Cohen-Gadol, AA, Friedman JA, Friedman JD, Tubbs RS, Munis JR, Meyer FB. Neurosurgical management of intracranial lesions in the pregnant patient: A 36-year institutional experience and review of the literature. *Journal of Neurosurgery.* 2009; 111(6): 1150–1157.

2. Terry AR, Barker FG, Leffert L, Bateman BT, Souter I, Plotkin SR. Outcomes of hospitalization in pregnant women with CNS neoplasms: A population-based study. *Neuro-Oncology.* 2012; 14(6): 768–776.

3. Verheecke M, Halaska MJ, Lok CA, et al. Primary brain tumours, meningiomas and brain metastases in pregnancy: Report on 27 cases and review of literature. *European Journal of Cancer.* 2014; 50(8): 1462–1471.

4. Girault A, Dommergues M, Nizard J. Impact of maternal brain tumours on perinatal and maternal management and outcome: A single referral centre retrospective study. *European Journal of Obstetrics, Gynecology, and Reproductive Biology.* 2014; 183: 132–136.

5. Stevenson CB, Thompson RC. The clinical management of intracranial neoplasms in pregnancy. *Clinical Obstetrics and Gynecology.* 2005; 48(1): 24–37.

6. Jayasekera BA, Bacon AD, Whitfield PC. Management of glioblastoma multiforme in pregnancy. *Journal of Neurosurgery* 2012; 116(6): 1187–1194.

7. Johnson N, Sermer M, Lausman A, Maxwell C. Obstetric outcomes of women with intracranial neoplasms. *International Journal of Gynaecology and Obstetrics.* 2009; 105(1): 56–59.

8. Tewari KS, Cappuccini F, Asrat T, Flamm BL, Carpenter SE, Disaia PJ, Quilligan EJ. Obstetric emergencies precipitated by malignant brain tumors. *American Journal of Obstetrics and Gynecology.* 2000; 182(5): 1215–1221.

9. Ravindra VM, Braca JA, Jensen RL, Duckworth EA. Management of intracranial pathology during pregnancy: Case example and review of management strategies. *Surgical Neurology International.* 2015; 6: 43.

10. Abd-Elsayed AA, Díaz-Gómez J, Barnett GH, et al. A case series discussing the anaesthetic management of pregnant patients with brain tumours. *F1000Research.* 2013; 2: 92.

11. Maiter D. Prolactinoma and pregnancy: From the wish of conception to lactation. *Ann Endocrinol (Paris).* June 2016; 77(2): 128–134.

12. Auriemma RS, Perone Y, Di Sarno A, et al. Results of a single-center observational 10-year survey study on recurrence of hyperprolactinemia after pregnancy and lactation. *J Clin Endocrinol Metab.* January 2013; 98(1): 372–379.

13. Pereira L. Obstetric management of the patient with spinal cord injury. *Obstetrical and Gynecological Survey.* 2003; 58(10): 678–687.

14. Wanner MB, Rageth CJ, Zäch GA. Pregnancy and autonomic hyperreflexia in patients with spinal cord lesions. *Paraplegia.* 1987; 25(6): 482–490.

15. Maehama T, Izena H, Kanazawa K. Management of autonomic hyperreflexia with magnesium sulfate during labor in a woman with spinal cord injury. *American Journal of Obstetrics and Gynecology.* 2000; 183(2): 492–493.

16. Jeong S, Lee J, Do SH, Hwang JW, Ryu J. Labor analgesia and anesthetic management during emergency cesarean section of parturient with spinal cord injury (SCI). *Korean Journal of Anesthesiology.* 2013; 65: S95–96.

17. Sharpe EE, Arendt KW, Jacob AK, Pasternak JJ. Anesthetic management of parturients with pre-existing paraplegia or tetraplegia: a case series. *Int J Obstet Anesth.* 2015; 24(1): 77–84.

18. Sterling L, Keunen J, Wigdor E, Sermer M, Maxwell C. Pregnancy outcomes in women with spinal cord lesions. *Journal of Obstetrics and Gynaecology Canada.* 2013; 35(1): 39–43.

19. Tanaka H, Katsuragi S, Tanaka K, Iwanaga N, Yoshimatsu J, Takahashi JC, Ikeda T. Impact of pregnancy on the size of small cerebral aneurysm. *J Matern Fetal Neonatal Med.* 2016; 14: 1–4.

20. Pozzati E, Acciarri N, Tognetti F, Marliani F, Giangaspero F. Growth, subsequent bleeding, and de novo appearance of cerebral cavernous angiomas. *Neurosurgery.* 1996; 38(4): 662–669.

21. Ray JG, Vermeulen MJ, Bharatha A, Montanera WJ, Park AL. Association between MRI exposure during pregnancy and fetal and childhood outcomes. *JAMA.* 2016; 316(9): 952–961.

22. Lv X, Liu P, Li Y. The clinical characteristics and treatment of cerebral AVM in pregnancy. *Neuroradiol J.* 2015; 28(3):234–237.

23. Witiw CD, Abou-Hamden A, Kulkarni AV, Silvaggio JA, Schneider C, Wallace MC. Cerebral cavernous malformations and pregnancy: Hemorrhage risk and influence on obstetrical management. *Neurosurgery.* 2012; 71(3): 626–631.

24. de Gussem EM, Lausman AY, Beder AJ, et al. Outcomes of pregnancy in women with hereditary hemorrhagic Telangiectasia. *Obstet Gynecol.* 2014; 123(3): 514–520.

25. Bateman BT, Schumacher HC, Bushnell CD, et al. Intracerebral hemorrhage in pregnancy: Frequency, risk factors, and outcome. *Neurology* 2006; 67:424–429.

26. Guidon AC, Massey EW. Neuromuscular disorders in pregnancy. *Neurol Clin.* 2012; 30: 889–911.

27. Ciafaloni E, Pressman EK, Loi AM, et al. Pregnancy and birth outcomes in women with facioscapulohumeral muscular dystrophy. *Neurology.* 2006; 67(10): 1887–1889.

28. Snyder Y, Donlin-Smith C, Snyder E, Pressman E, Ciafaloni E. The course and outcome of pregnancy in women with nondystrophic myotonias. *Muscle Nerve*. 2015; 52(6): 1013–1015.

29. Rudnik-Schoneborn S, Zerres K. Outcome in pregnancies complicated by myotonic dystrophy: A study of 31 patients and review of the literature. *Eur J Obstet Gynecol Reprod Biol*. 2004; 114(1): 44–53.

30. Djelmis J, Sostarko M, Mayer D, et al. Myasthenia gravis in pregnancy: Report on 69 cases. *Eur J Obstet Gynecol Reprod Biol*. 2002; 104(1): 21–25.

31. Hoff J, Daltveit A, Gilhus N. Myasthenia gravis. *Neurology*. 2003; 61(10): 1362.

32. Wen JC, Liu TC, Chen YH, et al. No increased risk of adverse pregnancy outcomes for women with myasthenia gravis: A nationwide population-based study. *Eur J Neurol*. 2009; 16(8): 889–894.

32

Anesthetic Considerations for Neurologic Patients

MELISSA KRESO, MARJORIE GLOFF, AND RICHARD WISSLER

GENERAL APPROACH TO ANESTHESIA IN PREGNANCY COMPLICATED BY NEUROLOGIC DISEASE

Regardless of any neurologic disease or other pregnancy complications, in general, most pregnant women in the United States (60%) will choose to utilize labor and delivery analgesia.[1] Even among women who are not intending to utilize labor analgesia, the unpredictable nature of pregnancy means that many women will need analgesia for safe delivery and care of the maternal/fetal dyad. This is especially true for women with underlying medical disorders. Therefore, discussion of anesthetic options, and the review of their safety relative to a woman's preferences and concerns should be started early in the pregnancy.

Pregnant women in general can be assumed have additional anesthesia risks relative to other patient populations. They have narrower, more edematous airways, slower gastric emptying, more adipose tissue in the neck and chest: this leads to less neck extension and difficulty placing instrumentation orally and results in increased risks for failed aspiration. Additionally, pregnancy physiology results in high minute ventilation and low residual volumes, leading to intolerance of respiratory compromise and lack of respiratory reserve. Left or right uterine displacement avoids aortocaval compression.

Unless contraindicated in the pregnant population, neuraxial anesthesia is the preferred option for anesthetic delivery for both vaginal and cesarean deliveries. General anesthesia in the pregnant population carries inherent risks and many neurologic conditions have unique risks regarding administering general anesthesia. However, if spinal is contraindicated, this may also remove the option for epidural anesthesia. It is vital to understand that any epidural can become an inadvertent dural puncture with a larger gauge needle compared to a spinal anesthetic (see also Section 5, Chapter 32). Thus, in order for a patient to be a candidate for an epidural, she must be a candidate for *both* a spinal and an epidural. This importance of wording will make a difference as to whether a patient is a candidate for epidural anesthesia. If a spinal anesthetic is contraindicated, then epidural anesthesia is riskier to place.

In most neurologic conditions both neuraxial anesthesia and general anesthesia are options. In cases where there is intracranial pathology or increased intracranial pressure, care must be taken on an individualized basis to decide on optimal care with regard to delivery—including options for anesthesia techniques and for valsalva maneuvers/hemodynamic swings. Neurologic disease in pregnancy has a wide range of effect and physical manifestations. Each patient must be individually evaluated; as two patients with the same disease may have very different care plans due to variation in the expression and functional status of their disease. Early multidisciplinary care is prudent for these individuals. A risk/benefit discussion of anesthesia types is essential for each patient, and individualized care based on risk factors is important. The patient's individual neurologic manifestations, her pregnancy complications, and her planned delivery approach will help to guide the options for delivery. Often consultation from neurology, obstetrics, and anesthesia will be necessary to guide management (see Box 32.1).

SPINAL CORD INJURIES

More women are able to become pregnant after sustaining a spinal cord injury due to improvements in acute management and rehabilitation. Injuries related to the spinal cord create unique challenges for the anesthesiologist regarding labor analgesia. Spinal cord injury patients have higher incidences of hypercoagulability, decreased respiratory reserve, and sensate challenges when assessing neuraxial techniques (see also Chapter 29). Any patient

---

BOX 32.1
CARE MAP FOR ANESTHESIA CARE IN THE NEUROLOGY PATIENT

During Pregnancy

Early anesthesia consult

Optimization of disease care

Evaluation of specific neurologic manifestations:

For pulmonary disease: Pulmonary function testing each trimester

For NF1/NF2: MRI in 3rd trimester of spine

Delivery

Multidisciplinary discussion to plan best delivery route and location including discussion of anesthetic plan

Anesthesia consultation

Pain management plan, with discussion of those diseases sensitive to narcotics, or those at high risk of respiratory failure.

Planning for those at high risk prolonged anesthesia

Postpartum

Pain medication adjustments for those with respiratory manifestations

Prompt evaluation of headache, weakness, focal neurologic symptoms.

---

with a lesion above T10 is at risk for autonomic hyperrelexia (AH) (Figure 32.1).[2–4] Depending on the level of the lesion, there is a great deal of variation in the amount and quality of sensation, as well as the risk for AH. (See Table 32.1 for further details on lesion level, risk of autonomic hyperreflexia, and expected sensation during labor).[5,6]

Any patient with a lesion above T6 should be considered at high risk for AH. Physiologically, lesions below T6 typically allow enough descending inhibitory parasympathetic control to modulate the splanchnic tone and prevent the severe systemic hypertension and subsequent physiologically mediated responses (Figure 32.2). Many of the symptoms such as flushing, headaches, blurry vision, and diaphoresis are similar to pre-eclampsia presentations, which is important to rule out. Given the potential danger associated with this condition, it is important to determine which patients are at risk for AH during their prenatal care. Common obstetrical triggers are listed in Table 32.2.[4,7–10]

Patients that have not previously had AH are still at risk, although patients that have experienced previously are at higher risk for developing it in the peripartum and postpartum period.[11] All patients at risk for AH warrant close hemodynamic monitoring postpartum and possibly continuation of analgesia. AH has been reported as late as 5 days postpartum.[12]

Data on optimal care management is limited. A case series of 9 deliveries in patients with spinal cord injuries had a higher frequency of patients having AH in the first 3 days postpartum relative

Fast Facts[2]
• Seen in patients with cervical through mid-thoracic lesions

Disease Features[2]
• Extreme hypertension • Bradycardia • Headaches • Blurred vision • Flushing • Sweating • Pilomotor erection

Severity[3,4]
• Hypertensive encephalopathy • Intracranial hemorrhage • Death

FIGURE 32.1 Autonomic dysreflexia

TABLE 32.1 LEVEL SPINAL CORD LESION, RISK OF AH AND EXPECTED SENSATION DURING LABOR

Level of Spinal Cord Lesion	At Risk for AH?	Expected Sensation during Labor
Above T6	Yes, very high risk	Likely to have painless labor
Complete lesion below T6 but above T10	Yes	Will most likely detect sensation with contractions but likely to have painless labor
Incomplete lesion below T6 but above T10	Yes	More likely to have pain with labor
Below T10	No	Will most likely have pain with labor

to labor. General anesthesia, spinal anesthesia, and epidural anesthesia were all utilized in this series. Only 4 of these spinal cord injuries were above T6.[13] Another case series of 5 tetraplegic patients all with spinal cord injuries in the region of C6 were followed through 7 pregnancies. Early epidurals were utilized in all of these deliveries due to heightened awareness of AH in this population. Stimuli were promptly identified and managed including administration of sublingual nifedipine and intramuscular clonidine. Prolonged postpartum usage of epidural analgesia was not used to manage AH symptoms in this series.[14]

Clinical Implications

The risk for AH should be assessed, and if a patient is at risk, then early neuraxial analgesia with epidural, spinal, or combined spinal/epidural anesthesia should

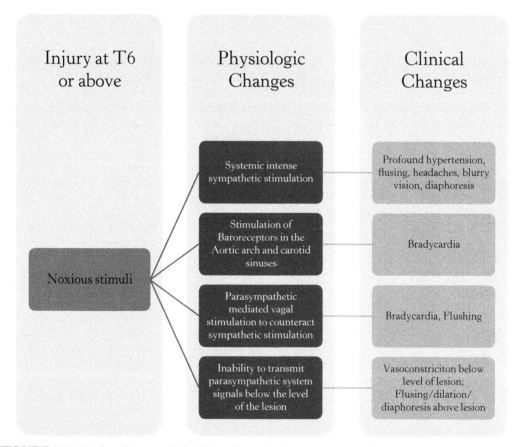

FIGURE 32.2 Spinal cord injury and physiologically mediated response to stimuli.

Adapted from Karlsoon AK, Spinal Cord. 1999. 37 (6): 383. 91 and Barard EJJ, The secularity of spinal cord injured women, physiology and pathophysiology: A review. *Paraplegia.* 1989; 27:99–112. [5–6]

TABLE 32.2 COMMON CAUSES OF AUTONOMIC HYPERREFLEXIA IN THE OBSTETRIC ENVIRONMENT[4,7-10]

Augmentation of labor with oxytocin infusions
Bladder/Bowel distension
Vaginal instrumentation, including speculum exam
Perineal distention
Amniotomy
Acute changes in blood pressure (like with contractions)
Infection

Fast Facts		
• Autoimmune		
• Women more commonly affected		
• Childbearing years		
Disease Features		
• Episodic skeletal muscle Weakness		
• Worsened with activity		
Severity[3,4]		
• Group 1 (mild) - primarily ocular symptoms		
• Group IV-V (severe) - pulmonary compromise and bulbar involvement		

FIGURE 32.3 Myasthenia gravis

be considered during labor. Local anesthetics should be utilized to block afferent noxious stimuli from reaching the spinal cord, as narcotic only neuraxial techniques are not effective in minimizing these stimuli.[15] Depending on the severity and frequency of AH symptoms in patients, invasive hemodynamic monitoring and possibly laboring in an intensive care unit may be appropriate. For most patients frequent noninvasive blood pressure monitoring is appropriate. Hemodynamics should be monitored closely while establishing the neuraxial blockade.

Determining neuraxial blockade level can be challenging if patients are insensate below their lesion. Loss of deep tendon reflexes in lower extremities and superficial reflexes of the abdominal wall can be helpful in estimating the level of the block.

If general anesthesia is needed, these patients are at additional risk. Due to the immobilization, up-regulation of acetylcholine receptors can lead to exaggerated hyperkalemic states after use of succinylcholine and therefore it should be avoided.[16] Breastfeeding is possible as soon as the patient is awake, and should not be delayed, as the cross into the colostrum and breast milk is negligible (see also Breastfeeding).

NEUROMUSCULAR JUNCTION DISORDERS

Myasthenia Gravis (MG)

Myasthenia gravis (MG) has highly variable pregnancy manifestations with one-third improving (especially in second and third trimesters), one-third worsening, and one-third unchanged.[17-18] There is a 30% risk of exacerbation postpartum, with the highest risk in the first month postpartum.[19] Symptoms occurring in one pregnancy do not predict the symptoms in another pregnancy, and the disease is highly variable and unpredictable during gestation (Figure 32.3).[20]

Clinical implications

Early antepartum consultation with anesthesiology is necessary to help assess baseline strength, respiratory, and bulbar involvement, as well as to help determine risk factors and allow for additional counseling of what to expect. Pulmonary function testing might be warranted to help with the risk assessment of peri- and postpartum respiratory compromise and failure (Table 32.3). In severe forms, especially with significant bulbar involvement, aspiration is a significant risk. General anesthesia (vs. spinal) for these patients if undergoing cesarean delivery may allow the ability to better secure the airway with an endotracheal tube.

Patients with MG are at risk for two kinds of crises: myasthenic and cholinergic. Infections and stress (both emotional and surgical) increase the risk of exacerbations. Predictors of death due to crises are old age, time to recognition, and the

TABLE 32.3 INDEPENDENT RISK FACTORS FOR REQUIRING POSTOPERATIVE VENTILATION IN THE MYASTHENIC POPULATION

Preoperative Pulmonary Function Test	Values	Percentage of Predicted
FVC (L.sec^{-1})	2.6+/− 0.8	77.8 +/-20
MEF$_{50\%}$	3.9+/−1.6	80.2+/-22
FEF$_{25-75\%}$ (L.sec^{-1})	3.3+/−1.1	85.5+/-27.2

Table adapted from Naguib et al. Multivariate determinants of the need for postoperative ventilation in myasthenia gravis. *Can J Anaesth.* 1996; 43: 1006–13.[32]

need of endotracheal intubation.[21] Labor and delivery units need to be aware of monitoring for myasthenic crises since approximately 30% of patients have exacerbations in the first month postpartum. Cholinesterase inhibitors, intravenous immunoglobulins, plasmapheresis, and possibly endotracheal intubation may be warranted.

A cholinergic crisis can occur if a patient is given too high a dose of cholinesterase inhibitors such as neostigmine (a neuromuscular-blocking reversal agent in many general endotracheal anesthetics). Excessive salivation, sweating, bradycardia, abdominal cramping, urgency of urination, muscle weakness are all symptoms. Stopping cholinesterase inhibitors, administering anticholinergics such as atropine or glycopyrrolate and possibly endotracheal intubation are all treatment options.

Regional anesthesia

Neuraxial techniques are the preferred method of anesthesia for vaginal delivery or for cesarean section if possible.[22] Spinal anesthesia, epidural anesthesia and combined spinal epidurals have all been utilized without significant harm.[23–25] Even though MG does not affect smooth muscle, it does affect striated skeletal muscle, and patients are prone to fatigue from voluntary expulsion in the second stage of labor, with a higher risk of needing assisted deliveries.[26] Lower-dose local anesthetic solutions have been recommended to facilitate maximum maternal efforts. Doses of 8mg and 10mg intrathecal bupivacaine have been quoted in the literature, which is a reduction of a fourth to a third of standard dosing.[24–25] Amide local anesthetics should be utilized since ester- based local anesthetics are metabolized through plasma cholinesterases. The cholinergic medications used to treat MG unpredictably can cause blocks to last longer. Even with cautious dosing, patients may still need ventilatory support especially if bulbar muscles are involved.

General anesthesia

General anesthesia can be utilized in patients with MG, but there are unique caveats that need to be understood. The primary concern is response to neuromuscular depolarizing (NMD) agents such as succinylcholine, which are typically utilized for general anesthesia in cesarean sections. In patients treated with cholinesterase inhibitors, plasma cholinesterase levels are limited. Since succinylcholine is metabolized by plasma cholinesterases the response to NMDs may last longer, and patients are at risk for prolonged blockades. Alternatively, if patients are

not being treated with cholinesterase inhibitors, they can have increased sensitivity and prolonged effects to non-depolarizing neuromuscular blocking agents due to lower numbers of acetylcholine receptors.[27] Therefore if these agents must be utilized, using a small amount or agents with a shorter half-life is prudent. Testing the extent of muscle relaxant is not reliably accurate due to the acetylcholine antibodies preventing full-strength contractions and therefore baseline testing prior to administration of muscle relaxants for comparison is more helpful.

Reversing neuromuscular blockade in MG patients can also be difficult since cholinesterase inhibitors are typically utilized for treatment and increase resistance to reversal agents. Sugammadex sodium is a reversal agent that selectively binds to neuromuscular blocking agents. There are case reports of 3 patients with different stages of MG undergoing surgeries showing faster reversal with sugammadex sodium after without any postoperative complications.[28–30]

Respiratory concerns

Pulmonary function testing might be warranted to help with the risk assessment of peri- and postpartum respiratory compromise and failure (Table 32.3). In patients with moderate respiratory compromise clinically, the usage of BiPAP in addition to the neuraxial blockade can improve the safety and efficacy of neuraxial anesthesia.[31] Expiratory weakness is the main determinant for postoperative ventilator support in myasthenic patients (Table 32.2).[32] In a study of surgical patients risk factors for postoperative myasthenic crisis included bulbar symptom presence, preoperative anti-acetylcholine receptor antibody serum levels higher than 100nmol/L, and/or intraoperative blood loss greater than 100 mL.[33] Given the expected blood loss associated with cesearans, MG patients requiring cesarean delivery should be considered high risk. Due to these increased risks, neuraxial techniques are the preferred method of anesthesia for these patients for both vaginal or cesarean delivery.[22] However, in patients with severe respiratory or bulbar compromise requiring cesarean delivery, securing the airway electively via general anesthesia may be more efficacious given the resultant respiratory muscle weakness from neuraxial anesthesia.

Medication concerns

When a patient has MG, care needs to be taken when providing medicines that predispose to weakness (Table 32.4).[34–35] For patients with

TABLE 32.4 MEDICATIONS
PREDISPOSING PARTURIENTS
WITH MYASTHENIA GRAVIS
TO WEAKNESS[34-35]

Magnesium
Propanolol
Aminoglycoside antibiotics (like gentamycin)
Alpha agonists (like terbutaline and ritodrine)
Quinidine
Narcotics (in those with pulmonary weakness)

Fast Facts
• Acute inflammatory demyelinating polyradiculoneuropathy
• Onset generally 1–3 weeks post acute URI or gastroenteritis
Disease Features
• Initial symptoms include distal paresthesias and followed by leg weakness
• Can impair respiration
• Can affect eye movements
• Can cause dysphagia
• Can affect autonomic function
Severity
• Treatment is generally IVIG and plasmapharesis
• Life-threatening condition
• Can cause lasting muscle weakness and difficulty with ambulation

FIGURE 32.4 Guillain-Barré syndrome

respiratory involvement there will be more susceptibility to opioid induced respiratory depression, and caution should also be utilized administering these agents for post-operative pain control. Additionally, other commonly used obstetrical medications such as gentamycin and magnesium sulfate are contraindicated in the MG patient.

CENTRAL NERVOUS SYSTEM DISORDERS

Historically regional anesthetic techniques have been avoided due to speculation that intrathecal anesthetics could exacerbate these disease processes.[36] Now, much of what we know has come from case reports or smaller studies and neuraxial anesthetic complications seem to be less common than previously thought. Epidural anesthesia has not been shown to worsen disease processes, and there is not much guidance in the literature regarding spinal anesthesia in this patient population. A retrospective study of 139 patients with preexisting CNS disorders undergoing neuraxial anesthesia were found to have no new or progressive postoperative deficits.[37] However, each disorder has specific characteristics that pose unique challenges to the anesthetic management, and all types of anesthesia have been utilized for these populations—although an individualized approach to care is important.

Guillain-Barré Syndrome

Guillain-Barré syndrome (GBS) is a life-threatening disorder with frequent deaths despite treatments with IVIG and plasmapharesis. About 10% of patient with GBS will still have severe disability despite resolution of the initial presentation (Figure 32.4).[38]

Fortunately the incidence of GBS during pregnancy is low. A review summarizing 30 case reports

of patients with GBS during pregnancy showed that 4 out of 20 had onset in the first trimester, 14 out of 30 had onset in the second trimester, and 12 out of 30 had onset in the third trimester.[39] These were similar incidences found in an earlier report from 1985.[40] However, the risk of GBS increases immediately postpartum with a rate ratio of 2.93 (9% CI 1.20–7.11) during the first 30 days after delivery.[41-42] Although the reason for this increase postpartum is unclear, many neurologic autoimmune disorders are alleviated with pregnancy and are exacerbated after delivery. During pregnancy, cytokines such as interleukin-10 are secreted that down-regulate production of other cytokines. After delivery the balance of these cytokines is shifted. This is the hypothesized cause of the increased incidence of relapses and exacerbations in the postpartum period.[43]

Clinical implications

Both regional and general anesthesia have some potential additional risk in parturients with GBS. With general anesthesia, the use of succinylcholine can lead to hyperkalemia, which can lead to cardiac arrest. This can be seen in patients even after a reported recovery of over a month.[44] Nondepolarizing muscle relaxants are a better choice but still pose risks since GBS is a demyelinating polyradiculoneuritis. Patients can also have sensitivity to nondepolarizing muscle relaxants, and lower doses may be necessary. There is also a higher need for postoperative mechanical ventilation, and the team should be aware of this possibility.

Regional anesthesia is not contraindicated in these patients. However, women may have fears of paralysis or unpleasant lumbar puncture memories, and they may benefit from early anesthetic consultation for a detailed risk discussion and options available. GBS patients are sensitive to local anesthetics and profound hypotension/bradycardia may occur and will often present more quickly.[45] As a result, these patients may require smaller doses of local anesthetics.[46–47]

Multiple Sclerosis

Multiple Sclerosis (MS) is an autoimmune demyelination disorder that tends to remit during pregnancy, especially during the third trimester; however, it is typically followed by an increased risk of flare in the first 3 months postpartum. The symptoms, severity, and progression vary widely (Figure 32.5). As these women tend to be of reproductive age, the question of regional analgesia and flare risk postpartum has been an area of considerable focus. The Pregnancy in Multiple Sclerosis (PRIMS) Study as well as others have found the risk of relapse after delivery was not affected by the use of epidural analgesia.[48–49] Further analysis showed that the only factors correlating to postpartum relapse risk were number of relapses during the pre-pregnancy year, number of relapses during pregnancy, and a higher disability burden at pregnancy onset. Cesarean delivery regardless of neuraxial technique has also been found to not increase relapse rates postpartum.[50–51] Given the risks of general anesthesia, neuraxial anesthesia is therefore the preferred method for patients with MS requiring cesarean delivery. The PRIMS data focused on epidural analgesia, whereas the most common type of anesthesia utilized for cesarean sections is spinal anesthesia. There are case reports of spinal anesthesia being utilized and given the high prevalence of MS, between 20 and 200/100,000; yet the total number of cases where a relapse has occurred appears to be low.[52–53] A survey of 592 obstetric anesthesiologists in the United Kingdom showed that spinal or combined spinal epidural is the preferred method for women diagnosed with MS, with 98.1% preferring this for elective cesarean section and 99.3% for an emergent cesarean section.[54] Regardless of the anesthesia technique chosen, it is important to monitor temperature carefully and possibly use cooling blankets or room temperature intravenous fluids if body temperature rises.[55]

NEUROECTODERMAL DISORDERS

Neurofibromatosis 1 (NF1)

Neurofibromatosis is a disease of highly variable inheritance and expressivity (Figure 32.6), but the primary risk for anesthesia considerations is related to the possible development of spinal neurofibromas leading to increased risk of hematoma formation and increased intracranial pressure. All patients with NF1 and 2 should undergo a lumbosacral non-contrast MRI with T1

Fast Facts
• Autoimmune demyelination
• Women >> Men
Disease Features
• Varied neurologic changes
• Paresthesias
• Muscle spasms
• Motor weakness
• Difficulty with balance and coordination
• Dysphagia
• Vision problems
• Pain
• Issues with Bowel, Bladder
• Impaired cognition
• Temperature Sensitivity
Severity
• Tends to remit in pregnancy
• Risk of flare in the first 3 months postpartum

FIGURE 32.5 Multiple sclerosis

Fast Facts
• Autosomal dominant inheritance
• Associated with ectodermal and mesodermal tumors
• Peripheral neurofibromas typically appear first during puberty
Disease Features
• Cafe au lait spots
• Neurofibromas express progesterone receptors which can therefore increase in size/number during pregnancy[56]
• Spinal neurofibromas can be present[56]
• Rarely, airway fibromas can occur[57]
• Can be associated with pheochromocytomas[58]
• Cutaneous and subcutaneous neurofibromas along the chest wall, kyphoscoliosis, thoracic neoplasms intersitial lung disease can occur[59]
Severity
• Dependent on number and location of neurofibromas[58]

FIGURE 32.6 Neurofibromatosis 1 (NF1)

and T2 weighted sequencing prior to regional anesthesia in late pregnancy. A MRI with contrast is optimal in viewing neurofibromas, but in pregnancy efforts are made to avoid contrast dye; and with the T1 and T2 weighted sequencing, radiologists can usually visualize the masses especially when looking for growth changes. If spinal neurofibromas exist near optimal sites for regional anesthesia, then there is a risk of puncturing the tumor and spreading tumor cells. There is also a risk of bleeding resulting in an epidural hematoma.

Embryologically, the cell types of both pheochromocytomas and neurofibromatosis have the same origin in the ectoderm of the neural crest, and these disorders can occur together. All NF1 patients should be screened for hypertension and if diagnosed, should undergo evaluation to rule out other causes such as renal artery stenosis, a catecholamine secreting nodular plexiform neurofibroma, or in about 1% of patients, a concurrent pheochromocytoma (Table 32.5).[58] Although rare, pheochromocytomas may mimic pregnancy-induced hypertension, and diagnosis assures early interventions to reduce risk of mortality and morbidity.[60]

Clinical implications

No type of anesthesia is precluded for delivery, but the decision must be made on an individual basis based on the patient's airway features, restrictive lung disease, and recent MRI imaging of the spine. Although rare, airway neurofibromas can lead to airway management difficulties and increased risk of bleeding in the airway. Only about 5% of NF1 patients have intraoral manifestations.[57] Loss of voice or dysphagia should warrant further evaluation for vocal cord involvement, which could significantly impact the pregnancy as well as anesthesia for delivery. There are case reports and association with many rare complications (Table 32.4)[61-64], as well as a

---

TABLE 32.5 COMPLICATIONS REPORTED IN PARTURIENTS WITH NEUROFIBROMATOSIS[61-64]

Renal artery rupture
Severe hypertension—Consider the following:
  Nodular plexiform neurofibroma
  Pheochromocytoma
Spontaneous hemothorax
Concomitant sarcoma
Neurofibromas of airway or spinal canal

---

case report of a previously undiagnosed NF1 parturient receiving epidural analgesia for labor pain with an inadvertent dural puncture and epidural hematoma formation.[65]

Spinal neurofibromas can also occur leading to increased risk of hematoma formation and increased intracranial pressure. Epidural and spinal anesthesia have successfully been utilized for labor in parturients with NF1 after central tumor involvement was ruled out.[66-67] All patients with NF1 and 2 should undergo a lumbosacral non-contrast MRI with T1 and T2 weighted sequencing prior to regional anesthesia in late pregnancy. A MRI with contrast is optimal in viewing neurofibromas, but in pregnancy efforts are made to avoid contrast dye. And with the T1 and T2 weighted sequencing, radiologists can usually visualize the masses, especially when looking for growth changes. If spinal neurofibromas exist near optimal sites for regional anesthesia, then there is a risk of puncturing the tumor and spreading tumor cells. There is also a risk of bleeding resulting in an epidural hematoma. However, even with MRI imaging of the spine in the third trimester to evaluate for spinal fibromas, there is some risk that tumor formation could have occurred *between the imaging and administration of neuraxial anesthesia.* Low-dose solutions with the aim to monitor for patient movement are optimal to better monitor for rapid spinal hematoma compression. General anesthesia has been used on many occasions for treatment of patients with NF1, but altered sensitivities with succinylcholine and nondepolarizing muscle relaxants has been described.[68] Neuromuscular monitoring is helpful when utilizing these agents.

Neurofibromatosis 2 (NF2)

Although NF2 is rarer than NF1, the lack of cutaneous involvement in some individuals may make it harder to identify (Figure 32.7).

Clinical implications

Spinal, epidural, and general anesthesia have all been utilized successfully.[70-72] Patchy distribution of anesthetics is more likely due to neurofibromas causing less reliable spread of local anesthesia in the epidural space. Just like NF1 patients, NF2 patients should undergo a lumbosacral non-contrast MRI with T1 and T2 weighted sequencing prior to regional anesthesia in late pregnancy to rule out spinal neurofibromas near optimal sites

Fast Facts
• Much rarer than NF1
• Primarily CNS involvement; may be devoid of cutaneous involvement
• Generally first appears in second decade of life

Disease Features
• Hearing loss is common as vestibulocochlear schwannomas are the hallmark of disease
• Given CNS involvement - spinal involvement is more likely than NF1[69]
• Rarely, airway fibromas can occur
• Spinal neurofibromas can be present
• Can be associated with pheochromocytomas

Severity
• Dependent on number and location of neurofibromas

FIGURE 32.7 Neurofibromatosis 1 (NF1)

Fast Facts
• Primary - also known as pseudotumor cerebri is idopathic
• Secondary
• From malfunctioning VP Shunt
• From space occupying lesions

Disease Features
• Dependent on disease process

FIGURE 32.8 Intracranial hypertension (ICH)

for regional anesthesia, as these can increase the risk of puncturing the tumor and spreading tumor cells and/or epidural hematoma. In order to watch for complications, use of low-dose solutions to allow monitoring of patient movement is necessary to monitor for rapid spinal/epidural hematoma compression.

Risks of general anesthesia include neurofibromas in the airway leading to airway management difficulties from compression and bleeding complications. It would be prudent to consider potential increased sensitivity to muscle relaxants in NF2 as in NF1, although data supporting this is lacking. Given the variety of risks with no guarantee that there are no neurofibromas at the time of neuraxial procedures, it is important to have a detailed risk/benefit discussion with the patient as an active participant in the decision making for analgesic management of their delivery.

INTRACRANIAL HYPERTENSION (ICH)

Primary intracranial hypertension

Idiopathic intracranial hypertension (IICH), or pseudotumor cerebri, is when increased cerebrospinal fluid pressure occurs without any intracranial pathology or secondary cause of IICH (Figure 32.8). The main symptom is headache, which is found in about 90% of cases.[73]

Clinical implications

Neuraxial anesthesia is an excellent choice for analgesia in these patients especially since CSF drainage is a treatment for IICH. Pain increases

intracranial pressure and epidural analgesia mitigates this risk:[74] however, high volumes of local anesthetic administered into the epidural space may augment the increase in intracranial pressure in patients who already have IICH.[75] It is important to note the timing of the last therapeutic lumbar puncture as recent CSF drainage can increase the risk of a high spinal blockade.[76] Despite these risks, epidural anesthesia has been used successfully in patients.[77-79]

Lumboperitoneal Shunts

Both general and neuraxial anesthesia have been utilized with success in parturients with lumboperitoneal and ventriculoperitoneal shunts, although neuraxial anesthesia is preferred.[80] There is no need for imaging studies if the selected interspace for epidural anesthesia is either above or below the prior entry scar and a midline approach is being used. Shunt catheters are placed under the skin directly lateral to the entry point. However, if there is any resistance upon removal of the catheter, imaging may be warranted due to the theoretical risk of catheter-shunt entanglement.[81]

Many shunts placed in childhood are no longer functional by the time a woman is of reproductive age. However, shunt malfunction can occur during pregnancy due to uterine enlargement or after delivery due to obstruction from blood clots, and patients could present with symptoms of ICH, which can be confused for other pregnancy complications. Prophylactic antibiotics are not necessary for uncomplicated vaginal deliveries in patients with lumboperitoneal or ventriculoperitoneal shunts based on a 16-year study of 8 patients with shunts over 25 pregnancies.[82] If administering general anesthesia, care to minimize extreme increases in intracranial pressure is important to maintain proper shunt function.

Intracranial Pathology/Secondary Intracranial Hypertension

The options for management can be quite confusing given the idiosyncrasies among different kinds of space occupying lesions. The decision tree in Figure 32.9 (adapted from Leffert et al) discusses the elements necessary to assess risks of neurologic deterioration from neuraxial anesthesia in patients with intra-cranial pathology and aid in clinical care decisions.[83] This complicated group of patients should have early multidisciplinary planning prior to delivery involving obstetrics, anesthesiology, neurology, or neurosurgery, as well as neonatal involvement to individualize management.

Intracranial Arachnoid Cysts

Arachnoid cysts are collections of CSF that develop within the arachnoid membrane. They are rare but can be found in the brain or the spine. Generally, they are asymptomatic and are generally diagnosed incidentally after a patient undergoes a CT/MRI for an unrelated reason. Occasionally patients will have signs of intracranial pressure including headaches, blurred vision, and presyncopal or syncopal episodes.[84] Complications of these cysts include expansion of focal neurological signs and acute rupture into the subarachnoid or subdural space. In these situations, surgical interventions may be necessary. Complications can occur spontaneously or secondary to trauma, infection, and sudden changes in intracranial pressure.[85]

Clinical implications

Both neuraxial and general anesthesia have been used to manage analgesia of patients with arachnoid cysts. In patients with symptoms of increased intracranial pressure, neuraxial anesthesia may be contraindicated or relatively contraindicated due to risks associated with accidental dural puncture.[86] In other patients with no modifications of the cyst and no signs of increased intracranial pressure, neuraxial anesthesia in the form of epidural anesthesia has been utilized without issues.[84-85] It is important to converse with the patient's neurologist or neurosurgeon prior to offering neuraxial anesthesia.

Space Occupying Lesions

Fortunately space occupying tumors are rare during pregnancy with an incidence of 2.6/100,000.[87] Patients with stable disease presenting early with no evidence of neurological deterioration, gestational advancement can generally be allowed to continue into the early second trimester before neurosurgery and radiotherapy are initiated. Vaginal deliveries are possible for patients whom are deemed as stable with care to minimize valsalva maneuvers.

Clinical implications

When patients are having significant symptoms, including headaches, sensitivity to light/noise, nausea/vomiting, and ataxic movements, care must be taken to avoid increases in intracranial pressure (ICP), which can further shift the brain off midline and also cause cerebellar herniation into the foramen magnum. In these patients neurosurgical decompression is needed.[88]

Care to avoid sudden changes in ICP, blood pressure, and cerebral blood flow are necessary especially during noxious stimuli such as intubation, head pinning, scalp incision, and valsalva maneuvers during labor. Opioids and infiltration of the skin with local anesthetics can help blunt these responses. The use of fluorinated gases can help reduce cerebral metabolic rates and minimally effect on ICP. High dose opioids can prevent hypertension from laryngoscopy and many anesthetic drugs act as antiepileptic medications including thiopental and propofol. Left uterine displacement should be utilized prior to delivery to avoid aortocaval compression.

Other neurosurgical and medical management of ICP in pregnancy is largely unchanged from the non-pregnant state. Mannitol is a diuretic frequently utilized in neurosurgical cases. Mannitol has been used in safely during pregnancy,[89] but animal studies have shown mannitol infusions to significantly change fetal osmolarity causing a net transfer of fluid from fetus to mother,[90] decreased fetal lung fluid production,[91] and decreasing urinary flow rate.[92] However, if necessary, can likely safely be used with monitoring of fetal amniotic fluid volumes. Hyperventilation can temporarily correct intracranial pressure swings, but this may cause a leftward shift in the maternal oxyhemoglobin dissociation curve and potentially impair fetal oxygenation. Maternal hypercarbia should be avoided. Steroids are sometimes utilized perioperatively to reduce intracranial edema. There have been some reports of low birth weight in fetuses exposed to chronic steroid usage for maternal asthma, and no studies

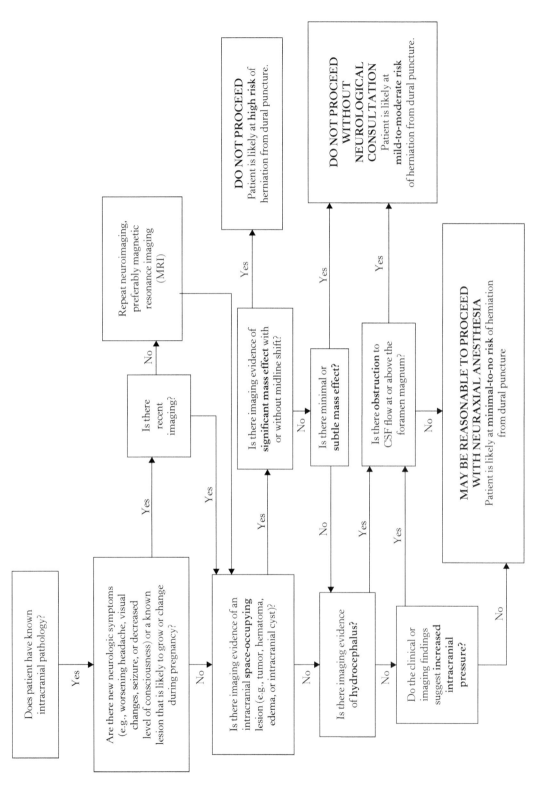

FIGURE 32.9 Decision tree summarizing the critical elements for assessing the risks of neurological deterioration from neuraxial anesthesia in patients with intracranial space-occupying lesions. CSF, cerebrospinal fluid. Leffert LR, Schwamm LH. Neuraxial Anesthesia in Parturients with Intracranial Pathology. *Anesthesiology.* 2013; 199:703–718.[83]

have evaluated it for patients with mass lesions.[93] There has been not been enough research on repeated short-term usage of steroids for reduction of peri-tumor edema; however, patients should be counseled on these risks and the proposed benefits.[94]

Arnold Chiari Malformation

Arnold Chiari Malformation (ACM) varies in symptoms and severity but is becoming increasingly diagnosed as imaging techniques improve (Figure 32.10).

Clinical implications

Neurologic consultation can be helpful in determining safety of neuraxial anesthesia. General, epidural, and spinal anesthesia were all utilized in a case series of 30 deliveries of women with Arnold Chiari without any negative long-term sequelae. One patient developed a postdural puncture headache after an intrathecal spinal catheter that resolved with an epidural blood patch.[100] In patients where general anesthesia is utilized, care must be taken to avoid hyperextension for prolonged periods due to the hypermobility of the occipitoatlantal and atlantoaxial joints that can occur with chiari malformations type I.[101]

For patients with Arnold Chiari that have undergone surgical correction, the type of anesthesia can be more complicated. Surgeries can remove the obstruction and alleviate symptoms but some associated abnormalities such as tethered spinal cord can still exist and may represent a contraindication to neuraxial anesthesia. Spinal anesthesia has been successfully utilized in parturients with surgically corrected type I Arnold Chiari malformation.[102]

There are also cases of headaches after epidural being associated with new diagnosis of Arnold Chiari. There is a case report of a patient with a failed epidural followed with repeat spinal attempts and had a persistent headache that was not responsive to an epidural blood patch. Brain magnetic resonance imaging (MRI) revealed an undiagnosed Arnold Chiari malformation.[103] Another case report of a patient with persistent headaches after dural puncture had an MRI showing cerebellar descent consistent with acquired Arnold Chiari malformation.[104]

HEREDITARY NEUROMUSCULAR DISORDERS

Spinal Muscular Atrophy (SMA)

Spinal muscular atrophy is a hereditary neurologic disease with an incidence of 1 in 10,000 and presents in one of four forms (Figure 32.11). Much of anesthesia planning has to do with how much proximal weakness and bulbar involvement is present, especially if restrictive lung disease is seen.[105] A case series found that exacerbations were noted in muscle weakness in 8 out of 12 patients during pregnancy after the second trimester.[107] This disease has an unpredictable pattern with pregnancy and has a possibility of deterioration antenataly.

Fast Facts
• 4 types -Type I-IV • Prevalence is 1:1000-1:5000; increasingly diagnosed with better imagining techniques[95–96] • Diagnosed when the cerebellar tonsils descend at least 5mm through the foramen magnum[97] • May result in disordered CSF flow that can be partial or intermittent[98]
Disease Features
• Type I -symptoms range from asymptomatic to headaches, ataxia, sensorimotor impairments, seizures[99] • Type II -diagnosed in infancy with myelomengoceles -may have associated apnea, CN abnormalities and upper extremity weakness • Type III -brainstem and cerebellum has protruded into the foramen magnum and result in severe neurologic dysfunction • Type IV-Cerebellar hypoplasia
Severity
• Dependent on type and patient

FIGURE 32.10 Arnold Chiari malformation (ACM)

Fast Facts
• SMA is inherited in a recessive pattern, and prenatal screening is available and commonly offered • Incidence: 1:10000 • 4 Types
Disease Features[105-106]
• Type 1: Bulbar muscles affected, usually prominent respiratory failure early in life • Type 2: Truncal and significant extremity weakness especially in the proximal muscles, bulbar muscles can be affected, restrictive lung disease common • Type 3: Proximal muscle weakess, eventually will become wheelchair bound • Type 4: Proximal lower extremity muscle weakness, possibly can become wheelchair bound
Severity[105-106]
• Type 1: Severe, life expectancy into toddler years • Type 2: Less severe, life expectancy into 3rd decade of life • Type 3: Milder, life expectancy into the childbearing years and beyond • Type 4: Adult onset

FIGURE 32.11 Spinal muscular atrophy (SMA)

SMA may be associated with an increased incidence of preterm labor.

Clinical implications

General anesthesia has been safely administered to patients with SMA for cesarean sections and might be the only option for patients with significant respiratory compromise, back surgeries prohibiting the use of neuraxial anesthesia, or who cannot lie flat.[108-109] Succinylcholine should be avoided due to the possibility of a hyperkalemic cardiac arrest and its use may also trigger myotonia.[110] Neuraxial anesthesia has been utilized in this patient population in the form of both spinal anesthesia and epidural anesthesia.[111-112]

Due to the increased sensitivity of opiate-related respiratory depression in this patient population, opiate usage should be minimized; however, neuraxial preservative-free morphine has not been reported to cause complications in the dose of 0.1mg intrathecally. Intravenous alfentanil while under general anesthesia and low-dose epidural solutions containing fentanyl have both been utilized for pain relief.[109,111]

Myotonic Dystrophy

Myotonic Dystrophy (MD) is a progressive myotonic disorder.[112] There are 2 types and both involve multiple systems including skeletal and smooth muscle while also affecting the cardiac, gastrointestinal, pulmonary, endocrine, and neurologic systems (Figure 32.12).

Fast Facts
• Inherited • Most common adult muscular dystrophy[113] • Two types
Disease Features[114]

• Type 1
  • More severe form
  • Can cause cardiomyopathy and pulmonary disturbances
• Type 2
  • More peripheral - affecting distal muscles first and then affecting proximal muscles much later

Severity
• Dependent on type

FIGURE 32.12 Myotonic dystrophy

Clinical implications

MD Type I patients often have narrow facies, high arched palates, and are limited in their abilities to open their mouths which can complicate airway management. The most common complications following general anesthesia are respiratory issues, including atelectasis, ventilator failure, and pneumonia.[115] Cardiac involvement is usually in the form of conduction issues or cardiomyopathies and is commonly asymptomatic. Echocardiography and arrhthymia evaluations are recommended.[116] If implantable cardiac rhythm devices are in place, these should be interrogated prior to delivery.

Both epidural and spinal anesthesia have been utilized in this population. Caution should be utilized when administering opiate medications due to increased sensitivity. Myotonia is an intrinsic process to the muscle itself and is independent of neuromuscular transmission so neuraxial blockade will not relieve symptoms.

General anesthesia should be avoided whenever possible in patients with MD. Patients with MD already have a high risk for aspiration due to delayed gastric emptying and weakness of pharyngeal muscles, which is exacerbated by the inherent aspiration risks due to the changes in pregnancy. MD Type I patients often have significant airway issues as noted above. Additionally, the temporomandibular joint has a tendency to dislocate, prompting the need for careful jaw manipulation further complicating airway management. Common general anesthesia triggers of shivering and hypothermia increase risk of myotonic dystrophic exacerbations.[114]

Retrospective studies in children and adults have both shown a higher risk of perioperative pulmonary complications including atelectasis, pneumonia, and acute ventilator failure.[115,117] It is important to assess MD patients for morbidity and mortality. A 5-point scale known as the muscular impairment rating scale (MIRS), developed by Mathieu, is helpful in determining morbidity of disease (Table 32.5).[118] Having a MIRS of 3–5 increases risk of perioperative pulmonary complications.[114,118] In the event that a MD patient receives a muscle relaxant it is imperative that a muscle relaxant reversal agent be utilized. Failure to do so has been shown to be an independent risk factor for adverse perioperative outcomes.[119] Close ventilatory monitoring in recovery is necessary, and ventilator support should be readily available.

The association of malignant hyperthermia with myotonic dystrophy has been controversial, with several case reports reporting erratic responses to succinylcholine. However in a study of 154 MD type 1 patients where volatiles were utilized there were no cases of malignant hyperthermia symptoms.[115] Another review of the literature concluded that the risk of malignant hyperthermia in the myotonic dystrophy population appears to be the same as that of the general population. Currently there are only theoretical risks of malignant hyperthermia in patients with hypokalemic periodic paralysis due to the mutational locus of both hypokalemic periodic paralysis and malignant hyperthermia both being on the same gene, although further research is needed.[120]

Epilepsy

Epilepsy is commonly encountered during pregnancy, as well as during labor and delivery, and it affects over 1 million US women of childbearing age, with only migraine, stroke, and Alzheimer's disease occurring more frequently (Figure 32.13).

Fast Facts
• Characterized by recurrent seizure activity in the absence of metabolic disorders or acute brain disease
• Seizures in pregnancy are most commonly seen in patients with pre-existing epilepsy[121]

Disease Features
• Recurrent seizures

Severity[122]
• Pregnancies and neonates of women with epilepsy are twice as likely to have adverse outcomes
• IUFD, c-section, 1 minute APGAR score <7, Low birthweight, abnormal development, perinatal death
• 4–6% risk for congenital malformations in mothers treated with antiepileptic monotherapy

FIGURE 32.13 Epilepsy

Clinical implications

Having epilepsy is not a contraindication to receiving epidural or spinal anesthesia. A retrospective review of 100 obstetric patients with epilepsy where 19 received general anesthesia, 48 received spinal anesthesia, 21 received epidural anesthesia, and 12 received a pudendal block had 5 women with postpartum seizures. Of these, 1 was in the general anesthesia group and had received enflurane, while there were 4 in the spinal anesthesia group and none in the epidural anesthesia group.[123] No abnormal clotting parameters or platelet count issue occurred preoperatively in a series of patients with epilepsy undergoing surgery.[124] Although these numbers are small, they do suggest that anesthesia itself is not a trigger for seizure in WWE.

VASCULAR DISORDERS-SUBARACHNOID HEMORRHAGE (SAH)

The diagnosis of subarachnoid hemorrhage (SAH) (Figure 32.14) may be obscured initially because symptoms such as nausea, vomiting, and headaches are common during pregnancy. The decision to treat is influenced by the site and type of lesion, clinical condition of the patient, and whether or not vasospasm is occurring (see also Chapters 15, 16).[124] Unruptured aneurysms diagnosed during pregnancy tend to be treated if they are symptomatic or enlarging.[126] Medical management of arteriovenous malformations seems to be as effective as surgical intervention during pregnancy.[127] When surgical intervention is necessary, there has been a shift to endovascular repair in recent years.[128] Cerebral angiography and/or coiling delivers a dose of 1–3 mSv to the fetus[128] which is well under the suggested maximum acceptable radiation exposure for pregnant women (10mSv) and fetuses (5mSv)[130] (see also Chapters 7, 16). If repaired, then there are no specific special anesthetic considerations for labor and delivery.

Fast Facts
• Incidence: 5.8 per 100,000 deliveries in women 15–44[125]

Disease Features
• Nausea, vomiting, headaches are key features of rupture
• Can progress to coma/death

Severity
• Dependent on location, ruptured or unruptured status, and presence of vasospasm[126]

FIGURE 32.14 Subarachnoid hemorrhage (SAH)

If unrepaired, it is prudent to avoid increases in intracranial pressure and blood pressure and excessive valsalva maneuvers should be avoided. Neuraxial analgesia and anesthesia in the form of epidural and spinal technique can provide conditions to meet these goals during vaginal delivery provided that there are no contraindications for an unintentional dural puncture. If intracranial pressure is already elevated significantly there is risk that an unintentional dural puncture can lead to herniation of the cerebellum even during neuraxial placement. Consultation with neurology or neurosurgery is often needed to obtain guidelines for whether these techniques are options for the parturient's labor and delivery.

REFERENCES

1. Osterman M, Martin J. Epidural and spinal anesthesia use during labor: 27-state reporting area, 2009. *National Vital Statistics Reports.* 2011; 59(5): 2. https://www.cdc.gov/nchs/data/nvsr/nvsr59/nvsr59_05.pdf

2. Quimby CW Jr., Williams R, Greifenstein F. Anesthetic problems of the acute quadriplegic patient. *Anesth Analg.* 1973; 52(3): 333–340

3. Abouleish E. Hypertension in a paraplegic parturient. *Anesthesiology.* 1980; 53: 348–349.

4. McGregor JA, Meeuwsen J. Autonomic hyperreflexia: a mortal danger for spinal cord-damaged women in labour. *Am J Obstet Gynecol.* 1985; 151: 330–332.

5. Berard EJJ. The sexuality of spinal cord injured women, physiology and pathophysiology: A review. *Paraplegia,* 1989; 27: 99–112.

6. Karlsoon AK. Autonomic dysreflexia. *Spinal Cord.* 1999; 37 (6): 383–391.

7. Rossier AB, Ruffieux M, Ziegler WH. Pregnancy and labour in high traumatic spinal cord lesions. *Paraplegia.* 1969; 7: 210–216.

8. Boucher M, Santerre L, Menard L, Sabbah R. Epidural and labor in paraplegics. *Can J Obstet Gynecol.* 1991; 3: 130–132.

9. Ravindran RS, Cummins DF, Smith IE. Experience with the use of nitroprusside and subsequent epidural analgesia in a pregnant quadriplegic patient. *Anesth Analg.* 1981; 60: 61–63.

10. Tabsh KMA, Brinkman DR III, Regg RA. Autonomic dysreflexia in pregnancy. *Obstet Gynecol.* 1982; 60: 119–121.

11. Crosby E, St-Jean B, Reid D, Elliott R. Obstetrical anaesthesia and analgesia in chronic spinal cord-injured women. *Can J Anaesth.* 1992; 39(5): 87–94.

12. Cross LL, Meythaler JM, Tuel SM, Cross AL. Pregnancy, labour and delivery post spinal injury. *Paraplegia.* 1992; 30: 890–902.

13. Sharpe EE, Arendt KW, Jacob AK, Pasternak JJ. Anesthetic management of parturients with pre-existing paraplegia or tetraplegia: a case series. *Int J of Obstet Anes.* 2015; 24 (1): 77–84.

14. Skowronski E, Hartman K. Obstetric management following traumatic tetraplegia: Case series and literature review. *Aust NZ J Obstet Gynaecol.* 2008; 48: 485–491.

15. Abouleish, E, Hanley E, Palmer S. Can epidural fentanyl control autonomic hyperreflexia in a quadriplegic parturient? *Anesth Analg.* 1989; 68:523–526.

16. Martyn J, Richtsfeld M. Succinylcholine-induced hyperkalemia in Acquired Pathologic States. *Anesthesiology* 2006; 104:158–169.

17. Stafford IP, Dildy GA. Myasthenia gravis and pregnancy. *Clin Obstet Gynecol.* 2005; 48: 48–56.

18. Plauche, WC. Myasthenia gravis in mothers and their newborns. *Clin Obstet Gynecol* 1991; 34: 82–99.

19. Ciafoloni E, Massey JM. The management of myasthenia gravis in pregnancy. *Semin Neurol.* 2004; 24:95–100.

20. Djelmis J, Sostarko M, Mayer D et al. Myasthenia gravis in pregnancy: report on 69 cases. *Eur J Obstet Gynecol Reprod Biol.* 2002; 104: 21–25.

21. Alshekhlee A, Milds JD, Katirji B, Preston C, Kaminski HJK. Incidence and mortality rates of myasthenia gravis and mysathenic crisis in US hospitals. *Neurology* 2009; 72: 1548–1554.

22. D'Angelo R, Gerancher JC. Combined spinal and epidural analgesia in a parturient with severe myasthenia gravis. *Reg Anesth Pain Med,* 1998; 23: 201–203.

23. Chabert L, Benhamou D. Myasthenia gravis, pregnancy and delivery: a series of ten cases. Ann Fran de Reanim. 2004; 23: 459–464.

24. Rodriguez MAP, Mencia TP, Alvarez FV, Baez YL, Perez GMS, Garcia AL. Low dose spinal anesthesia for urgent laparotomy in servere myasthenia gravis. *Saudi J Anaeth.* 2013; 7(1): 90–92.

25. Mundad S, Shah B, Atram S. Emergency cesarian section in a patient with myasthenia gravis: is nauraxial anesthesia safe? *Saudi J Anaesth.* 2012; 6(4): 430–431.

26. Midelfar J, Daltveit A, Gilhus N. Myasthenia gravis: Consequences for pregnancy, delivery, and the newborn. Neurology 2003; 61:1362–1366.

27. Blichfeldt-Lauridsen L, Hansen BD. Anesthesia and myasthenia gravis. *Aeta Anaesthesiol Scand* 2012; 56: 17–22.

28. Unterbuchner C, Fink H, Blobner M. The use of sugammadex in a patient with myasthenia gravis. *Anaesthesia* 2010; 65: 302–305.

29. De Boer HD, van Egmond J, Driessen JJ, Booij LHJD. A new approach to anesthesia management

in myasthenia gravis: reversal of neuromuscular blockade by sugammadex. *Rev Esp Anestesiol Reanim.* 2010; 57: 181–184.

30. Petrun AM, Mekis D, Kamenik M. Successful use of rocuronium and sugammadex in a patient with myasthenia. *Eur J Anaesthesiol.* 2010; 27: 917–918.

31. Warren J, Sharma S. Ventilatory support using bilevel positive airway pressure during neuraxial blockade in a patient with severe respiratory compromise. *Anesth Analg.* 2006; 102: 910–911.

32. Naguib M, el Dawlatly AA, Ashour M, Bamgboye EA. Multivariate determinants of the need for postoperative ventilation in myasthenia gravis. Can J Anaesth 1996; 43: 1006–1013.

33. Watanabe A, Watanabe T, Obama T, et al. Prognostic factors for myasthenic crisis after transsternal thymectomy in patients with myasthenia gravis. *J Thorac Cardiovasc Surg.* 2004; 127: 868–876.

34. Cohen BA, London RS, Goldstein PG. Myasthenia gravis and preeclampsia. *Obstet Gynecol.* 1976; 48: 35S.

35. Barrons RW. Drug-induced neuromuscular blockade and myasthenia gravis. *Pharmacotherapy.* 1997; 17: 1220–1232.

36. Fleiss A. Multiple sclerosis appearing after spinal anesthesia. *NY State J Med.* 1949; 49: 1076.

37. Hebl JR, Horlocker TT, Schroeder DD. Neuraxial anesthesia and analgesia in patients with preexisting central nervous system disorders. *Anesth Analg.* 2006; 103: 223–228.

38. Vassiliev D, Nystrom E, Leight C. Combined spinal and epidural anesthesia for labor and desarean delivery in a patient with Guillain Barre Syndrome. *Reg Anes Pain Med.* 2001; 26(2): 174–176.

39. Chan LY, Tsui MH, Leung TN. Guillain-Barre syndrome in pregnancy. *Acta Obstet Gunecol Scand.* 2004; 83: 319–325.

40. Nelson LH, McLean WT. Management of Landry-Guillan-Barre syndrome in pregnancy. *Obstet Gynecol.* 1985; 65: 25S-29S.

41. Jiang GX, de Pedro-Cuesta J, Strigard K. Pregnancy and Guillain-Barre syndrome: A nationwide register cohort study. *Neuroepidemiology.* 1996; 15: 192–200.

42. Cheng Q, Jiang GX, Fredrikson S. Increased incidence of Guillain-Barre syndrome postpartum. *Epidemiology.* 1998; 9: 601–604.

43. Wegmann TG, Lin H, Guilbert L, Mosmann TR. Bidirectional cytokine interactions in the maternal-fetal relationship: Is successful pregnancy a TH2 phenomenon? *Immunol Today.* 1993; 14: 353–356.

44. Feldman JM. Cardiac arrest after succinylcholine administration in a pregnant patient recovered from Guillain-Barre Syndrome. *Anesthesiology.* 1990; 72:942–944.

45. Perel A, Reches A, Davidson JT. Anaesthesia in the Guillain Barre syndrome. *Anaesthesia.* 1977; 32: 257–260.

46. McGrady EM. Management of labour and delivery in a patient with Guillain Barre Syndrome. *Anaesthesia.* 1987; 42: 899–900.

47. Willison, H, Jacobs B, van Doorn P. Guillain Barre Syndrome. *Lancet.* 2016; 388: 717–727.

48. Confavreux C, Hutchinson M, Hours M, Cortinovis-Tourniaire P, Moreau T. Rate of pregnancy-related relapse in Multiple Sclerosis. *NEJM.* 1998; 339(5): 285–291.

49. Vukusic S, Hutchinson, M Hours M, et al. Pregnancy and multiple sclerosis (the PRIMS study): Clinical predictors of post-partum relapse. *Brain.* 2004; 127(6): 1353–1360.

50. Pasto L, Portaccio E, Ghezzi A, et al. Epidural analgesia and cesarean delivery in multiple sclerosis post-partum relapses: The Italian cohort study. *BMC Neurology.* 2012; 12: 165.

51. Jalkanen A, Alanen A, Airas L, et al. Pregnancy outcome in women with multiple sclerosis: Results from a prospective nationside study in Finland. *Multiple Sclerosis,* 2010; 16(8): 950–955.

52. Bornemann-Cimenti H, Sivro N, Toft F, Halb L, Sandner-Kiesling A. Neuraxial anesthesia in patients with multiple sclerosis—a systematic review. *Rev Bras Anestesiol.* 2017 Jul—Aug; 67(4): 404–410.

53. Kingwell E, Marriott JJ, Jette N et al. Obstetrical epidural and spinal anesthesia in multiple sclerosis. *J Neurol.* 2013; 35: 109–120.

54. Drake E, Drake M, Bird J, Russell R. Obstetric regional blocks for women with multiple sclerosis: A survey of UK experience. *Int J Obstet Anesth.* 2006; 15(2): 115–123.

55. Berger J, Sheremata W. Persistent neurological deficit precipitated by hot bath test in Multiple Sclerosis. *JAMA.* 1983; 249(13): 751–1753.

56. McLaughlin M, Jacks T. Progesterone receptor expression in neurofibromas. *Cancer Research.* 2003; 63: 752–755.

57. Basen E, Pierce HE, Jackson WF. Multiple neurofibromatosis with oral lesions; review of the literature and report of a case. *Oral Surg* 1955; 8: 263–280.

58. Delgado J, Martin, M. Anaesthetic implications of von Recklinghausen's neurofibromatosis. *Paediatric Anaesthesia,* 2002; 12: 374.

59. Zamora AC, Collard HR, Wolters PJ, Webb WR, King TE. Neurofibromatosis-associated lung disease: A case series and literature review. *Eur Respir J.* 2007; 29(1): 210–214.

60. Humble RM. Phaechromocytoma, neurofibromatosis and pregnancy. *Anaesthesia.* 1967; 22: 296–303.

61. Tapp E, Hickling RS. Renal artery rupture in a pregnant woman with neurofibromatosis. *J Pathol,* 1962; 97: 398–399.

62. Edwards JNT, Fooks M, Davey DA. Neurofibromatosis and severe hypertension in pregnancy. *Br J Obstet Gynaecol.* 1983; 90: 528–531.

63. Brady DB, Bolan JC. Neurofibromatosis and spontaneous hemothorax in pregnancy: Two case reports. *Obstet Gynecol.* 1984; 63: 355–375.

64. Ginsburg DS, Hernandez E, Johnson JWC. Sarcoma complicating von Recklinghausen disease in pregnancy. *Obstet Gynecol* 1981; 58: 385–387.

65. Esler MD, Durbridge J, Kirby S. Epidural haematoma after dural puncture in a parturient with neurofibromatosis. *Br J Anaesth.* 2001; 87: 932–934.

66. Dounas M, Mercier FJ, Lhuissier C, Benhamou D. Epidural analgesia for labour in a parturient with neurofibromatosis. *Can J Anaesth.* May 1995; 42(5 Pt. 1): 420–422, 422–424.

67. Sahin A, Aypar U. Spinal anesthesia in a patient with neurofibromatosis. *Anesth Analg.* 2003; 97: 1855–1856.

68. Hirsch NP, Murphy A, Radcliffe JJ. Neurofibromatosis: Clinical presentations and anaesthetic implications. *Br J Anaesth.* 2001; 86: 555–564.

69. Mautner VF, Tatagiba M, Lindenau M, et al. Spinal tumors in patients with neurofibromatosis type 2: MR imaging study of frequency, multiplicity, and variety. *AJR Am J Roentgenol.* 1995; 165(4): 951–955.

70. Speigel JE, Hapgood A, Hess PE. Epidural anesthesia in a parturient with neurofibromatosis type 2 undergoing cesarean section. *Int J Obstet Anesth.* 2005; 14(4): 336–339.

71. Sakai T, Vallejo M, Shannon KT. A parturient with neurofibromatosis type 2: Anesthetic and obstetric considerations for delivery. *Int J Obstet Anesth.* 2005; 14(4): 332–335.

72. Blackney K, McKeen M, Lai Y. Anesthetic management of a parturient with segmental neurofibromatosis. *Journal of Anesthesiology and Clinical Science.* 2014; 3: 5. http://www.hoajonline.com/journals/pdf/2049-9752-3-5.pdf

73. Friedman DI. Pseudotumor cerebri presenting as headache. *Expert Rev Neurother.* 2008; 8: 397–407.

74. Galbert MW, Marx GF. Extradural pressures in the parturient patient. *Anestheliology.* 1974; 40: 499–502.

75. Hilt H, Gramm HJ, Link J. Changes in intracranial pressure associated with extradural anaesthesia. *Br J Anaesth.* 1986; 58: 676–680.

76. Aly EE, Lawther BK. Anaesthetic management of uncontrolled idiopathic intracranial hypertension during labour and delivery using an intrathecal catheter. *Anaesthesia.* 2007; 62: 178–181.

77. Bedson CR, Plaat F. Benign intracranial hypertension and anaesthesia for casesarean section. *Int J Obstet Anesth.* 1999; 8: 288–290.

78. Abouleish E, Ali V, Tang RA. Benign intracranial hypertension and anesthesia for cesarean section. *Anesthesiology.* 1985; 63: 705–707.

79. Kim K, Orbegozo M. Epidural anesthesia for cesarean section in a parturient with pseudotumor cerebri and lumboperitoneal shunt. *J Clin Anesth.* 2000; 12: 213–215.

80. Goulart AP, Moro ET, Rios Rde P, Pires RT. Subarachnoid blockade for cesarean section in a patient with ventriculoperitoneal shunt: case report (Portugese). *Rev Bras Anestesiol.* 2009; 59: 471–475.

81. Bedard JM, Richardson MG, Wissler RN. Epidural anesthesia in a parturient with a lumboperitoneal shunt. *Anesthesiology.* 1999; 90: 621–623.

82. Landwehr JB Jr., Isada NB, Pryde PG, Johnson MP, Evans MI, Canady AI. Maternal neurosurgical shunts and pregnancy outcome. *Obstet Gynecol.* 1994; 83: 134–137.

83. Leffert, LR Schwamm LH. Neuraxial anesthesia in parturients with intracranial pathology. *Anesthesiology.* 2013; 199:703–718.

84. Larkin C, Murphy F, Browne I. Anaesthetic management of pregnancy complicated by a symptomatic arachnoid cyst. *Int J Obstet Anesth.* 2009; 18(3): 291–292.

85. Brice A, Barnichon C, Benhamou D. Intracranial arachnoid cysts and obstetric anesthesia: Two case reports. 2010; 29: 648–650.

86. McCormick RN, Stutley JE, Green RJ. An unusual cause of postpartum collapse or a red herring? *Anaesthesia* 2003; 58(4): 398–399.

87. Bondy ML, Scheurer ME, Malmer B, Barnholtz-Sloan JS, Davis FG, Il'yasova D, et al: Brain tumor epidemiology: Consensus from the Brain Tumor Epidemiology Consortium. *Cancer.* 2008; 113(7Suppl): 1953–1968.

88. Tewari KS, Cappuccini F, Asrat T, et al: Obstetric emergencies precipitated by malignant brain tumors. *Am J Obstet Gynecol.* 2000; 182: 1215–1221.

89. Bharti N, Kashyap L, Mohan VK. Anesthetic management of a parturient with cerebellopontine-angle meningioma. *Int J Obstet Anes.* 2002; 11: 219–221.

90. Faber JJ, Green TJ. Foetal placental blood flow in the lamb. *J Physiol.* 1972; 223: 375–393.

91. Ross MG, Leake RD, Ervin MG, Fisher DA. Fetal lung fluid response to maternal hyperosmolality. *Pediatric Pulmonology.* 1986; 2(1): 40–43.

92. Lumbers ER, Stevens AD. Changes in fetal renal function in response to infusions of a hyperosmotic solution of mannitol in the ewe. *J Physiol.* 1983; 343: 429–446.

93. Schatz M, Dombroski MP, Wise R, et al. The relationship of asthma medication use to perinatal outcomes. *J Allergy Clin Immunol.* 2004; 113: 1040–1045.

94. Bodiabaduge A, Jayasekera P, Bacon A, Whitfield P. Management of glioblastoma multiforme in pregnancy. *J Neurosurg.* 2012; 116: 1187–1194.

95. Speer MC, Enterline DS, Mehltretter L, et al. Chiari type I malformation with or without syringomyelia: prevalence and genetics. *J Genet Couns.* 2003; 12: 297–311.

96. Steinbok P. Clinical features of Chiari I malformations. *Childs Nerv Syst.* 2004; 20: 329–331.

97. Penney DJ, Smallman J. Arnold Chiari malformation and pregnancy. *Int J of Obstet Anes.* 2001; 10: 139–141.

98. Oldfield E, Maraszko K, Shwker T, Patronas N. Pathophysiology of syringomyelia associated with Chiari I malformation of the cerebellar tonsils. *J Neurosurg.* 1991; 80: 3–15.

99. Iannetti P, Spalice A, De Felice Ciccoli C, et al. Seizures in paediatric Chiari type I malformation: the role of single-photon emission computed tomography. *Acta Paediatr.* 2002; 91: 313–317.

100. Chantigan R, Koehn M, Ramin K, Warner M. Chiari malformation in parturients. *J Clin Anesth.* 2002; 14: 201–205.

101. Milhorat T, Bolognese P, Nishikawa M, McDonnell N, Francomano C. Syndrome of occipitoatlantoaxial hypermobility, cranial settling, and Chiari malformation Type I in patients with hereditary disorders of connective tissue. *J Neurosurg Spine.* 2007; 7: 601–609.

102. Landau R, Giraud R, Delrue V, Kern C. Spinal anesthesia for cesarean delivery in a woman with a surgically corrected type I Arnold Chiari malformation. *Anesth Analg.* 2003; 97: 253–255.

103. Hullander RM, Bogard TD, Leivers D, Moran D, Dewan DM. Chiari I malformation presenting as recurrent spinal headache. *Anesth Analg.* 1992; 75: 1025–1026.

104. Sathi S, Stieg PE. 'Aquired' Chiari I malformation after multiple lumbar punctures: Case report. *Neurosurgery.* 1993; 32: 306–309.

105. Wessel HB. Spinal muscular atrophy. *Pediatrics.* 1989; 18: 421–427.

106. Pearn J. Classification of spinal muscular atrophies. *Lancet.* 1980; 1: 919–922.

107. Pugh CP, Healey SK, Crane JM, Young D. Successful pregnancy and spinal muscular atrphy. *Obstet Gynecol.* 2000; 95: 1034.

108. McLouglin L, Bhagvat. Anaesthesia for caesarean section in spinal muscular atrophy type III. *Int J Obstet Anes.* 2004; 13: 192–195.

109. Habib, A. Helsley S. Millar S. Devalli P, Muir H. Anesthesia for cesarean section in a patient with spinal muscular atrophy. *J Clin Anesth.* 2004; 16: 217–219.

110. Paterson IS. Generalized myotonia following suxamethonium: A case report. *Br J Anaesth.* 1962; 34: 340–342.

111. Harris SJ, Moaz K. Caesarean section conducted under subarachnoid block in two sisters with spinal muscular atrophy. *Int J Obstet Anes.* 2002; 10: 125–127.

112. Weston LA, DiFazio CA. Labor analgesia and anesthesia in a patient with spinal muscular atrophy and vocal cord paralysis. *Reg Anesth.* 1996; 21: 350–354.

113. Udd B, Karhe R. The myotonic dystrophies: Molecular, clinical, and therapeutic challenges. *Lancet Neurol.* 2012; 11(10): 891–905.

114. Rosenbaum HK, Miller JD. Malignant hyperthermia and myotonic disorders. *Anesthesiol Clin North Am.* 2002; 20(3): 623–664.

115. Mathieu J, Allard P, Potvin L, Prevost C, Begin P. A 10-year study of mortality in a cohort of patients with myotonic dystrophy. *Neurology.* 1999; 52(8): 1658–1662.

116. Petri H, Vissing J, Witting N, Bundgaard H, Kober L. Cardiac manifestations of myotonic dystrophy type 1. *Int J Cardiol.* 2012; 160(2): 82–88.

117. Sinclair JL, Reed PW. Risk factors for perioperative adverse event sin children with myotonic dystrophy. *Pediatr Anesth.* 2009; 19: 740–747.

118. Mathieu J, De Braekeleer M, Prevost C, Boily C. Myotonic dystrophy: Clinical assessment of muscular disability in an isolated population with presumed homogenous mutation. *Neurology.* 1992; 42: 203–208.

119. Veyckemans F, Scholtes JL. Myotonic Dystrophies type 1 and 2:anesthetic care. *Pediatric Anesthesia.* 20123; 23: 794–803.

120. Parness J, Bandschapp O, Girard T. The myotonias and susceptibility to malignant hyperthermia. *Anesth Analg.* 2009; 109: 1054–1064.

121. Karad DR, Guntupalli KK. Neurologic disorders in pregnancy. *Crit Care Med.* 2005; 33(S10): S362–371.

122. Borthen I, Gilhus NE. Pregnancy complications in patients with epilepsy. *Curr OPpin Obstet Gynecol.* 2012; 24: 78–83.

123. Aravapalli R, Abouleish E, Aldrete JA. Anesthesia implications in the parturient epileptic patient. *Anesth Analg.* 1998; 67: S266.

124. Manohar C, Avitsian R, Lozana S, et al. The effect of entiepileptic drugs on coagulation and bleeding in the perioperative period of epilepsy surgery: the clinical clinic experience. *J Clin Neurosci.* 2011; 18: 1180–1184.

125. Bateman BT, Olbrecht VA, Berman MF et al. Peripartum subarachnoid hemorrhage: Nationwide data and institutional experience. *Anesthesiology.* 2012; 116: 324–333.

126. Tarnaris A, Haliasos N, Watkins LD. Endovascular treatment of ruptured intracranial aneurysms during pregnancy: Is this the best way forward? Case report and review of the literature. *Clin Neurol Neurosurg.* 2012; 114: 703–706.

127. Dias MS, Sekhar LM. Intracranial hemorrhage from aneurysms and arteriovenous malformations during pregnancy and the puerperium. *Neurosurgery.* 1990; 25: 855–865.

128. Ng J, Kitchen N. Neurosurgery and pregnancy. *J Neurol Neurosurg Psychiatry.* 2008; 79: 745–752.

129. Meyers PM, Halbach VV, Malek AM, et al. Endovascular treatment of cerebral artery aneurysms during pregnancy: report of three cases. *AJNR Am J Neuroradiol.* 2000; 21: 1306–1311.

130. Shah AJ, Kilcline BA. Trauma in pregnancy. *Emerg Med Clin North Am.* 2003; 21: 615–629.

33

Neurologic Complications in Obstetric Anesthesia

MARJORIE GLOFF, MELISSA KRESO, AND RICHARD WISSLER

Obstetric anesthesiology is the practice of anesthesia that focuses on providing safe and effective anesthesia and analgesia for pregnant patients. This includes labor and vaginal or cesarean delivery, as well as related procedures such as postpartum repairs, miscarriage management, removal of retained products of conception or bilateral tubal ligation.[1] Obstetric anesthesia usually falls into two categories; neuraxial anesthesia (either spinal or epidural), or general anesthesia.

Neuraxial anesthesia is the usual option for providing anesthesia and analgesia in healthy OB patients without contraindications, since the serious risks of neuraxial anesthesia are rare, and the benefits and safety for the mother and fetus are well established.

Neuraxial anesthesia takes one of two forms-either spinal or epidural. In a spinal anesthetic, local anesthetics and adjuncts such as opioids are directly injected into the CSF within the subarachnoid space (Figure 33.1). Dense anesthesia can be obtained with small doses and small volumes of medications. It generally requires 8-fold less medication to provide the same amount of anesthesia when compared to an epidural. In an epidural anesthetic, medications are injected into the epidural space (Figure 33.1). From the epidural space the medications diffuse through the dura/arachnoid and into the CSF. Therefore, an epidural anesthetic is an "indirect" spinal anesthetic.

Relative contraindications to performing a neuraxial anesthetic are numerous but include the two basic categories- (1) abnormal hemostasis leading to an increased risk of a neuraxial hematoma, a compressive neurologic injury, and (2) systemic or local lumbar infection with an increased risk of acute meningitis or chronic epidural abscess. It is important to note that while a patient may have a relative medical/physiological contraindication to one neuraxial anesthetic technique, she may be an appropriate candidate for the other- and these concerns should be discussed with the OB anesthesiologist.

Commonly discussed risks of neuraxial anesthesia including bleeding/bruising, transient worsening of chronic back pain, infection, allergy or toxicity to medications, block failure, postdural puncture headache, hypotension and rare neurologic injury. Neurologic morbidity in obstetric anesthesia can be further classified by if these complications are systemic, central neurologic, and peripheral neurologic processes. An example of a systemic process is based on vascular uptake of local anesthesia from the epidural space. If either the epidural medication dose or the speed of vascular uptake exceeds critical values, then local anesthetic systemic toxicity (LAST) can occur with predominantly neurologic and cardiac manifestations. Central processes include postdural puncture headache, neurotoxicity from medications, physical nerve injury by block placement equipment, epidural hematoma, epidural abscess, meningitis and opioid-induced respiratory depression. Peripheral neurologic processes include peripheral nerve or plexus injuries. Each of these areas of complications (systemic, central neurologic, and peripheral neurologic) will be discussed in detail, and summarized in the care map (Box 33.1).

SYSTEMIC PROCESSES

Local anesthetic systemic toxicity (LAST) is a constellation of clinical findings that is associated with intravascular injection of local anesthetics and these symptoms can worsen with increasing doses of local anesthetic injected. Toxicity can range from symptoms of tinnitus and perioral numbness to slurred speech and altered mental status to seizures and cardiovascular collapse. Timing of onset of symptoms can be variable, and as a result, patients should be closely monitored for LAST for 30 minutes after the injection of local anesthetic finishes.[2] Mild symptoms are thought to be the result of local anesthetic passive absorption and can be seen in patients even with appropriate dosing and correctly placed local anesthesia. Severe symptoms are most commonly seen with unintentional intravascular injection.[2] In its most

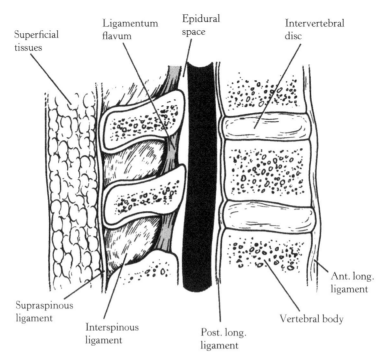

FIGURE 33.1 Spinal structures traversed for neuraxial anesthesia
Figure details the structures an epidural or spinal needle traverses to reach its destination. The epidural space is labeled. The dura and intrathecal spaces are depicted as the black-shaded structure just deep to that. Imaged used by permission of : Oxford University Press from Principles and Practice of Regional Anaesthesia 4e edited by Graeme McLeod, Colin McCartney, and Tony Wildsmith (2012): Figure 12.4 (p.116) from chapter: "Anatomy and physiology of the vertebral canal" by Ian Parkin and Alastair Chambers[10]

severe form, LAST can be fatal if not immediately treated. Treatment includes immediate ACLS and intralipid administration.

The rates of LAST are unclear, but it is rare. Fetal LAST is also possible and was implicated with fetal deaths in the 1960s and 1970s after paracervical blocks in parturients during labor.[3] In the 1970s, bupivacaine was implicated in the death of healthy patients receiving non-obstetric regional and obstetric epidural blockade.[4] As a result of these reports, bupivacaine 0.75% is now contraindicated for use in epidural anesthesia in obstetrics.[2] From more modern data, Paech et al evaluated 10,995 epidurals performed for labor and delivery in Perth, Australia, from 1989 to 1994, specifically identifying complications related to those epidurals.[5] In this cohort, LAST was seen in 1 in 3500 epidurals with all symptoms reported as mild, and none reported as severe.

CENTRAL PROCESSES

The dura mater is fused by a dense basement membrane to the underlying arachnoid membrane, forming a combined membrane structure on the deep or anterior border of the epidural space.[6] This combined membrane is referred to as the "dura." When placing a lumbar epidural block, the block needle is advanced anteriorly from the skin in the posterior lumbar midline, through the ligaments between the lumbar vertebrae and entering the epidural space just deep to the ligamentum flavum. The lumbar epidural space is approximately 6 mm in depth[7], although the actual depth encountered can be less due to the angulated shape of the lumbar epidural space both longitudinally and in cross-section.[8,9]

Therefore, even with careful block technique, the opportunity exists for an unintended puncture of the dura with the epidural block needle. The incidence of unintended dural puncture varies with different practices, but a 3% rate with labor epidural block placement is not uncommon. With a spinal anesthetic, the spinal needle traverses the epidural space, deliberately punctures the dura, and continues into the subarachnoid space. Therefore, every spinal anesthetic is associated with a deliberate dural puncture.

A postdural puncture headache (PDPH) is defined as a postural headache after instrumentation,

BOX 33.1
CARE MAP FOR NEUROLOGIC COMPLICATIONS IN OBSTETRIC ANESTHESIA

Not all central and peripheral complications are caused by neuraxial anesthesia (ie, spinals, epidurals)

SYSTEMIC
Local Anesthetic Systemic Toxicity

Subtypes:
  Mild: Perioral numbness, tingling. Occurs from absorption by nearby blood vessels
  Moderate: Slurred speech and altered mental status
  Severe: Seizures and Cardiovascular Collapse. Occurs from direction injection into vessels.
Onset: Immediately-30 minutes post-injection
Treatment: Supportive, ACLS and intralipid in severe cases
Incidence: 1/3500 reported by Paech et al and all mild[5]

CENTRAL
Post-dural puncture headache
Toxicity (also known as high spinal)

Symptoms: dyspnea and can be followed by hypoxemia, drowsiness, coma, possible death
Treatment: Supportive including ventilator, blood pressure and ACLS as indicated
Incidence: 2 in 10,000 as reported by Scott and Tunstall[19]

Central Nerve Injury

Etiology: Unknown, possibly direct trauma, ischemia, or local anesthetic toxicity
Incidence: 0–0.9 in 100,000[32]

Hematoma

Incidence: 1 in 200,000[23] to 1 in 505,000[24]
Etiology: Trauma, injury to underlying venous malformation, thrombocytopenia, medication-effect, spontaneous
Clinical Presentation: Generally within the first 48 hours, severe backache, hypoalgesia, muscle weakness and incontinence
Treatment: Emergent MRI and neurosurgical consultation, generally requires surgical decompression

Epidural Abscess

Incidence: 0.2–1 in 100,000[23,24]
Etiology: Unknown, Iatrogenic (ie, contamination of equipment or medications, nasopharyngeal droplets from placing provider), bacteremic seeding from the patient herself
Clinical Presentation: Generally delayed (>48 hours), fever, severe backache, hypoalgesia, muscle weakness and incontinence
Treatment: Emergent MRI and neurosurgical consultation, antibiotics, may require surgical decompression

Meningitis

Etiology: Septic (hematogenous spread versus contamination) and Aseptic (chemical irritation)

Clinical Presentation: fever, headache, neck pain and/or stiffness, photophobia, nausea and/or vomiting, altered mental status

Treatment: Antibiotics, supportive care

Opioid-induced Respiratory Failure

Etiology: associated with both epidural and intrathecal opioids, more commonly seen with hydrophilic compounds but can be seen with any opioid.

Clinical Presentation: Bradypnea and apnea, hypoxemia

Considerations: Close respiratory monitoring for 24 hours post neuraxial morphine; 2 hours post neuraxial fentanyl

Treatment: supportive measures, naloxone

PERIPHERAL NERVE INJURY

Incidence with neuraxial anesthesia: 0.3–7.5 in 100,000[24, 32]

Incidence of obstetric palsies: 0.2–92 in 10,000[33]

Etiologies: needle/catheter trauma to the nerve root or peripheral nerve, positioning injuries due to inability to easily reposition

Clinical presentation: parethesias pain and often associated weakness.

Treatment: Generally supportive and generally will resolve within a few weeks to months

MEDICOLEGAL CONSIDERATIONS

Individualized risk discussions should occur with the depth of risk that the patient requests explored

---

such as neuraxial block placement or attempted placement, that may have caused a hole in the dura and must occur within the first 5 days after dural puncture.[11,12] The presumed pathophysiology of PDPH is a leak of CSF through this dural hole, with immediate reabsorption by blood vessels in the epidural space. If the CSF leak and normal CSF reabsorption exceed CSF production, then there is a relative loss of CSF and a decrease in the hydraulic support of the brain and spinal cord. This concept of PDPH is consistent with clinical studies that have documented that larger block needles, in general, have higher risks of PDPH presumably due to higher rates of CSF leak. Epidural needles are larger (18 gauge) than spinal needles (25 gauge) to allow a 20-gauge epidural catheter to be threaded into the epidural space for continuing medication administration. In general, spinal anesthetics are single-dose blocks and do not require threading

an intrathecal catheter. Therefore, an inadvertent dural puncture with a standard 18-gauge epidural needle has an approximate risk of 40% for a subsequent symptomatic PDPH. In contrast, the deliberate dural puncture for spinal anesthesia with a 25-gauge spinal needle has a PDPH risk of 1–2%.

The natural history of PDPH is spontaneous resolution, as the hole in the dura heals, and the CSF leak slows and then stops. Unfortunately, it is not possible to clinically predict which patients will have rapid resolution of PDPH with time and conservative treatment and which patients will have persistent symptoms requiring an epidural blood patch. The widely accepted rate of normal CSF production in human adults is 500–600 ml/day.[13] In order to be symptomatic a PDPH patient must have a combined daily CSF loss (normal reabsorption plus the lumbar leak) greater than daily CSF production. It is useful to think of patients with iatrogenic dural punctures on a symptomatic spectrum. Patients with small CSF leaks are probably asymptomatic, and patients with large CSF leaks are likely to have longer-lasting and more intense PDPH symptoms. Symptoms of a PDPH usually are not present until 12 to 24 hours after the dural puncture. A new headache during or immediately after the placement of an epidural block is more likely related to pneumocephalus from air in the epidural placement syringe.[14] Postpartum patients with a headache that have received regional anesthesia should be evaluated by the anesthesia team for a postural headache. During this initial evaluation, the team needs to carefully exclude other serious causes of postpartum headache such as meningitis or subarachnoid hemorrhage.

The treatment of PDPH is based on the pathophysiology and natural history of the disorder.[11] Given the high probability of spontaneous resolution, most patients are treated for the first symptomatic day with rest, oral fluids, oral caffeine, and oral analgesics. While the majority (~95%) of PDPHs last for less than a week, they can negatively impact a woman's ability to perform her activities of daily living.[15] For patients with continuing symptoms on the second day, an epidural blood patch should be considered. This procedure involves a new lumbar epidural needle placement, followed by injection of 15–20 ml of sterile venous blood from the same patient. This procedure has an effectiveness of 85–90% with resolution of PDPH symptoms within 8–12 hours. The risks of an epidural blood patch include an unintended repeat dural puncture and worsening PDPH symptoms, infection, back pain and nerve damage from needle trauma. Therefore each patient should be given a clear opportunity to choose conservative therapy versus an epidural blood patch, including an individual consideration of relative risks and benefits. Despite continuing research interest in medical therapy for PDPH, there are no medical therapies to recommend for PDPH treatment at this time.

There are two areas of PDPH management that remain controversial. One is a prophylactic epidural blood patch.[16] This procedure is the same as a blood patch done for PDPH, but this preventative treatment is initiated before the patient knows if she will actually have a headache. Venous blood from the patient is injected through the epidural catheter after delivery, before the epidural catheter is removed.

The risks include back pain or infection from bacteria within the blood sample shortly after delivery. The second area of controversy is the post-delivery management of an intrathecal catheter, the term used for a catheter that electively resides in the intrathecal space after an inadvertent dural puncture. Several investigators have speculated that retention of an intrathecal catheter for a period of time may decrease the risk of a subsequent symptomatic PDPH, perhaps by accelerating the repair process in the dura at the site of injury. The existing literature is conflicting and inconclusive about the overall benefit of retaining an intrathecal catheter for 24 hours after delivery as a strategy for decreasing the risk of PDPH.[17,18] The risks of this strategy include possible infection or medication errors. Both a prophylactic epidural blood patch and the postpartum retention of an intrathecal catheter are areas of individual clinical judgment by the OB anesthesiologist for each patient.

Toxicity

Central local anesthetic toxicity can be seen with spinal and epidural anesthesia, colloquially coined "high spinals." "High spinals" can be seen with cephalad spread of local anesthetics and can occur with both types of neuraxial anesthesia. Symptoms of high spinals include dyspnea and can be followed by hypoxemia, drowsiness, coma, and if left unsupported, death. Treatment for this includes ventilatory and hemodynamic support and will resolve as the local anesthesia is metabolized. Scott and Tunstall reported an incidence of a "high spinal" to be 2/10,000 (0.02%) in their two-year prospective surveying of serious complications with neuraxial anesthesia.[19]

Central Nerve Injury

Direct central nerve injury is exceedingly rare from neuraxial anesthesia. According to the National Audit Project published by Cook et al in 2009, the risk of paraplegia and death from obstetric neuraxial anesthesia is 0–0.9/ 100,000.[22] There are, however, case reports of direct injury to the conus medullaris and spinal cord after neuraxial anesthesia. A series of case reports compiled by Reynolds suggest that direct injury can occur even after the presence of free-flowing clear CSF through the spinal needle is confirmed.[20] The hypothesized etiology of these direct injuries is from small hemorrhages or infarcts, either due to direct local anesthetic injection or trauma from the needle. In general, anesthesiologists will plan to place their neuraxial blocks below L2 as the spinal cord is thought to terminate above that level.[20] The level of puncture is determined based on anatomic landmarks and may not always be appropriately identified. However, Broadbent et al looked at MRI imaging of patients' spines after being marked by the anesthesiologist and found 13 out of 100 patients' cords ended at L2 or lower, potentially increasing the risk of cord injury.[21] This study also found that anesthesiologists with over 5 years of experience mismarked L2 too cephalad up to 70% of the time. Most often L2 was misjudged too cephalad by one vertebral level and sometimes up to four vertebral levels.[21] Despite this anatomic variability and evidence that spinals can be placed at misjudged levels, direct spinal cord injury is exceedingly rare. In fact, of the total neuraxial blocks from all obstetric comers (320,425) in the Third National Audit Project there were no reported paraplegias or deaths associated with the anesthetic technique. All paraplegias and deaths were found in patients presenting for non-obstetric perioperative care and the majority of patients were older than 50.[22]

Hematoma

Hematomas are collections of blood in and around the spinal cord, generally due to bleeding after regional anesthesia placement or after catheter removal. Although this complication is rare, the reported incidence varies between 1 in 200,000 to 1 in 505,000. Ruppen et al compiled a meta-analysis in 2006 that evaluated obstetric historical data from 1966 forward with respect to incidence of epidural hematoma, epidural infection, and nerve injury in patients with epidural anesthetics.[23] Scott and Hibbard performed a retrospective study looking at obstetric patients in the United Kingdom who received neuraxial anesthesia from 1982–1986.[24] Ruppen reported the incidence of epidural hematoma to be about 1 in 200,000 while Scott and Hibbard reported the risk to be approximately 1 in 505,000.

Risk factors for hematoma include thrombocytopenia, use of anticoagulant therapy, and bleeding disorders (both acquired and inherited) as well as traumatic neuraxial placement, spinal tumors, and spinal deformities. As co-morbidities are increasing in general, many more pregnant women require blood thinners for various underlying comorbidities. Anticoagulation does increase the

risk of hematoma formation during neuraxial anesthesia, and consultation with the anesthesiology team prior to delivery is ideal to assure appropriate anticoagulant timing for safe neuraxial placement. The American Society of Regional Anesthesia (ASRA) has defined guidelines with respect to the placement and removal of neuraxial blocks and catheters in these patients (see recommendation in Table 33.1).[25]

While not well defined in the obstetric population, thrombocytopenia is also associated with neuraxial hematomas and there are many possible etiologies for thrombocytopenia in pregnancy. The degree of thrombocytopenia at which any particular practitioner will provide a neuraxial anesthetic is a risk-benefit decision based on the clinical scenario at hand and individualized to each patient. There is no predetermined cut-off for absolute platelet count and subsequent inclusion or exclusion from neuraxial anesthesia. Importantly, the rate of platelet decline is an important factor for a safe neuraxial placement and additional studies such as thromboelastography or thromboelastometry may be utilized to help guide decision making. In general, an acceptable guideline for platelet count is 100,000 per microliter, knowing that even at this level the risk of hematoma exists. For women who acquire a bleeding disorder after epidural placement (ie, platelet counts drop after placement, disseminated intravascular coagulation [DIC], etc.), the catheter may need to remain in place even without anesthetic use or medications being given until the coagulopathy is corrected to avoid hematoma formation during removal. This, however, must be balanced against the infectious risks of long-term catheter retention with the goal of catheter removal by post-placement day 7.

Although hematoma is rare, if it occurs it can lead to permanent disabling injury if not promptly discovered and treated. The obstetric and anesthesiology teams need to be aware of the presenting symptoms including severe backache, hypoalgesia (decreased sensitivity to painful stimuli), muscle weakness, and incontinence. If these clinical symptoms are present, urgent MRI and a neurosurgical consultation are necessary as the treatment is emergent surgical decompression. If the treatment is delayed, the patient may go on to develop permanent paraplegia from compression and resultant ischemia of the cord. It is important to realize that there have been case reports of spontaneous epidural hemorrhage in parturients who have not received neuraxial anesthesia. Thus,

TABLE 33.1 TIMING OF NEURAXIAL ANESTHESIA TECHNIQUES
WITH ANTICOAGULATION

ASRA Guidelines for Anticoagulant Management in Neuraxial Blocks and Catheters

Medication	Block/Catheter Placement Considerations	Catheter Removal Considerations
Warfarin	Stop 4-5 days prior to planned procedure INR must be normalized before initiation of neuraxial block (Grade 1B)	INR <1.5 - neuraxial catheters should be removed and neuro assessment should occur for at least 24 hrs after removal (Grade 2C) INR: 1.5 - <3 - removal of indwelling catheters should be done with caution after meds reconciled for meds that influence hemostasis but not INR (eg, NSAIDs, ASA, UFH, LMWH) (Grade 2C). Neuro assessments should occur before catheter removal and continued until the INR has stabilized at the desired prophylaxis level (Grade 1C) INR: >3, dose should be held or reduced in patients with indwelling neuraxial catheters (Grade 1A). No definitive recommendation regarding the management to facilitate removal of neuraxial catheters in patients with therapeutic levels of anticoagulation during neuraxialcatheter infusion (Grade 2C)
Low Molecular Weight Heparin (LMWH) (eg, enoxaparin)	Discontinued 36 hours prior to placement and transitioned to unfractionated heparin	Low dose LMWH should start 12 hours post-delivery or 12 hours post epidural removal (whichever is later) Low dose LMWH should start 24 hours after c-section Higher dose LMWH should be restarted 24 hours after delivery or after epidural removal (whichever is later)
Fondaparinux	Avoid indwelling catheters until more clinical experience is available If single shot technique is used it should occur as a single needle pass and be atraumatic (in line with what exists in clinical trials) If not feasible, an alternate method of prophylaxis should be considered.	Avoid indwelling catheters until more clinical experience is available
Thrombin Inhibitors (ex: lepirudin, bivalirudin, argatroban)	Recommendation against neuraxial techniques (Grade 2C)	
Heparinoids (ex: danaparoid)	Not addressed in the ASRA guidelines	Not addressed in the ASRA guidelines
Aspirin	No increased risk, no specific concerns regarding timing of neuraxial block performance and last dose of aspirin	No increased risk, no specific concerns regarding timing of epidural catheter removal and last dose of aspirin

Table abstracted from Horlocker TT, Wedel DJ, Rowlingson JC, et al. Regional anesthesia in the patient receiving antithrombotic or thrombolytic therapy: American Society of Regional Anesthesia and Pain Medicine Evidence-Based Guidelines (Third Edition). *Regional Anesthesia and Pain Medicine.* January 1, 2010; 35(1): 64–101.[25]

diligence is mandatory to identify any patient whom may experience these symptoms, regardless of her exposure to neuraxial anesthesia.[26]

Infection

Epidural abscesses are infections in and around the spinal cord, generally due to infectious seeding during regional anesthesia placement. Scott and Hibbard estimate the risk of an epidural abcess to be approximately 0.2 out of 100,000.[24] Rupen estimates the risk lies closer to 1 in 110,000 and 1 in 145,000.[23]

These abscesses can compress the spinal cord much like an epidural hematoma but generally are slower to present clinically. Hematomas generally present within 0–2 days after neuraxial placement or removal of a catheter but can be delayed. It must be underscored that any symptoms concerning cord compression/compromise demand emergent imaging and neurosurgical consultation. The symptoms of back pain, hypoalgesia, and motor weakness are all similar to hematoma presentation,

but generally the onset of symptoms is three or more days after block attempt/placement. The delayed onset of symptoms and possible fever can help distinguish an abscess from a hematoma.[27] Loo et al evaluated case reports of epidural abscess in obstetric patients and found that 57% of the cases were caused by Staph aureus, but in all Staph aureus studies no identified origin of the bacteria could be found.[26] However, there are non-obstetric case reports that have found that the causative organisms can be linked to the nasopharynx of the placing provider and to contaminated multi-dose vials.[28] The American Society of Anesthesiologists has therefore assembled a practice advisory that advises aseptic techniques for the placement of neuraxial anesthesia (Figure 33.2).[29] As above, it is important to note that abscess formation can occur spontaneously and has been reported in obstetric patients who did not have any neuraxial anesthesia. Loo et al found two case reports of patients who developed epidural abscesses that were later linked to group B strep, which was thought to have

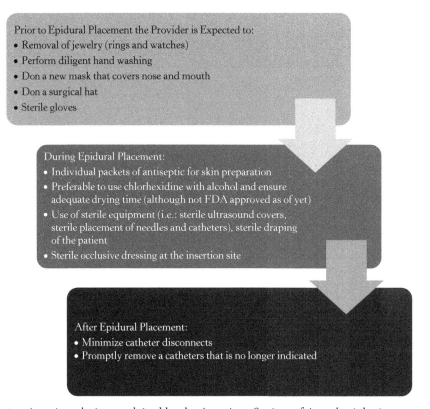

FIGURE 33.2 Aseptic techniques advised by the American Society of Anesthesiologists

Adapted from: The Practice Advisory for the Prevention, Diagnosis, and Management of Infectious Complications Associated with Neuraxial Techniques. A report by the American Society of Anesthesiologists Task Force on Infectious Complications Associated with Neuraxial Techniques. Anesthesiology 2010; 112: 000-000[29]

spread hematogenously.[26] If an epidural abscess is suspected, an urgent gadolinium-enhanced MRI and neurosurgical consultation is recommended.[26] The treatment is generally surgical decompression, antibiotics, or both.

Meningitis is another feared infectious complication, although a rare one. Presenting symptoms can include fever, headache, neck pain and/or stiffness, photophobia, nausea/vomiting, and altered mental status (see also Chapter 11). Aseptic and bacterial meningitis are more frequently seen in spinal techniques but can be seen in epidural and combined spinal-epidural techniques. Aseptic meningitis has been hypothesized to arise from chemical irritation from prepping or cleaning solutions. The presentation can be similar if not identical to bacterial meningitis; generally, patients recover quickly and have no permanent deficit.[26] Similar to epidural abscesses, cases of bacterial meningitis are broad but some have been linked to the nasopharyngeal secretions of the placing providers. In the studies that have linked cases of bacterial meningitis to nasopharyngeal secretions, the placing providers admitted to not wearing masks.[26] In each of these case reports, the patients fortunately made complete recoveries with antibiotics and supportive measures.[26] Regardless, the American Society of Anesthesiologists recommends careful aseptic techniques to avoid this complication.[29]

A relative contraindication to placing a neuraxial anesthetic is untreated or poorly controlled systemic or central nervous system infection. There is concern that by placing a foreign body into or through the epidural space then that space could become seeded by bacteria and result in an epidural abscess. One common infection seen in parturients is chorioamnionitis. Goodman et al evaluated 517 patients who had been found to have chorioamnionitis and who had received neuraxial anesthesia. Of these patients, 13 were found to be bacteremic and 4 did not receive antibiotics until after their neuraxial block was placed. None of the women in the study went on to develop epidural abscesses or bacterial meningitis.[30] Bader et al evaluated 319 patients, 3 of whom were bacteremic and received epidurals prior to any antibiotic therapy. There were again no infectious complications found in these deliveries.[31] Despite these findings, every patient deserves a thorough risk and benefit discussion when it comes to the placement of neuraxial anesthesia in the setting of infection.

Respiratory Depression

Respiratory depression can result from neuraxial opioid placement and is linked to the hydrophilic properties of the compound. In opioids that are hydrophilic (ie, morphine), the onset of respiratory depression can be delayed when compared to more lipophilic components (ie, fentanyl). The theory behind this is that hydrophilic compounds are more likely to be present in the CSF for longer periods of time and can spread rostrally. These compounds can then be absorbed by the brainstem and can cause bradypnea or apnea. Conversely, more lipophilic compounds are apt to absorb into the nervous tissue closer to the site of injection- which is generally lumbar and very distal from the respiratory centers of the brain. Certainly, systemically provided opioid analgesia in combination with neuraxial administered opioids could compound the respiratory depression risk. Although respiratory depression is a rare risk, it is a potentially catastrophic one if not immediately identified and treated. In the aforementioned study by Paech et al of 10,995 women, there were 3 cases of respiratory depression, 2 of which were linked to epidural morphine alone. The third was associated with epidural pethidine in combination with systemic methyldopa and phenytoin. All patients were treated supportively; two were provided naloxone and all recovered fully.[5] Therefore, in women receiving neuraxial morphine, close respiratory monitoring should occur for 24 hours after the last dose of morphine was received. This includes hourly respiratory rates or continuous pulse-oximetry. Also, prior to giving systemic opioids, the patient should be evaluated by the anesthesiologist and the anesthesiologist should be aware of all systemic opioids being provided to the patient for this subsequent 24 hours.

PERIPHERAL PROCESSES

Peripheral neurologic complications from neuraxial anesthesia are a concern for many patients and obstetricians and again are thankfully rare occurrences. Peripheral neurologic injury is known to be associated with both vaginal and cesarean births. There are a number of hypothesized etiologies for peripheral injuries including position of the baby or parturient during the second stage of labor, duration of the second stage of labor, parturient and infant size, use of instrumentation for delivery, and the use of neuraxial anesthesia. It is important to note that neurologic injury can therefore occur during labor and/or delivery without the use of neuraxial anesthesia and that all possible etiologies should be addressed when determining cause.

Accurate maternal morbidity data are not readily available in the United States, and thus incidence of these peripheral processes is difficult to assess.[5] There are a number of retrospective analyses published to shed light on the incidence. According to Scott and Hibbard's findings, peripheral nerve injury is the most common of the serious non-fatal complications in obstetric patients. In the 505,000 obstetric blocks they reviewed, 38 patients were found to have neuropathy involving a single spinal nerve, an incidence of 7.5 in 100,000.[24] According to the National Audit Project of the Royal College of Anaesthetists which included 320,425 obstetric patients, the risk of permanent nerve injury was 0.3–1.2 in 100,000.[32]

Hypothesized etiologies for peripheral nerve injury from neuraxial anesthesia include direct needle/catheter trauma to a single nerve root or peripheral nerve, positioning injuries due to inability to easily reposition and local anesthetic toxicity.[26] Patients usually present with lower-extremity paresthesias and may also have concomitant motor weakness. Generally, peripheral injuries are transient with the majority recovering completely but there have also been reports of permanent injuries. Scott and Tunstall looked prospectively at 122,989 neuraxial blocks placed from 1990-1991 and uncovered 128 reported complications. Of these, 46 were reported as neuropathy, which was the most common complication outside of post-dural puncture headaches. They reported that all cases resolved in 1 to 12 weeks (2 patients lost to follow-up) and no permanent disabilities were reported.[19]

As mentioned above, not all nerve injuries are related to the neuraxial anesthesia. Common obstetric palsies include femoral, obturator and common peroneal nerve injuries. Lumbosacral plexus injuries can also be seen. These injuries are much more common than neuraxial anesthesia-associated nerve injuries with a reported incidence of 0.2–92 in 10,000.[33] The causes of obstetric palsies are thought to be associated with direct pressure on the lumbosacral plexus by the fetal head, possible ischemia secondary to pressure, difficult, long and/or instrumented deliveries, legs extremely flexed during stage 2, legs positioned in stirrups for prolonged periods and are more common during vaginal births to nulliparous women.[26] These injuries also tend to recover in the majority of cases.

MEDICOLEGAL CONSIDERATIONS

The process of obtaining consent for neuraxial anesthesia or analgesia generally comes at a delicate or stressful time for the majority of parturients who desire the intervention. With the combination of stress, pain, and patient expectations, in-depth consent discussions can be difficult and given the rarity of the risks may cause more stress for the patient. However, Bethune et al found that despite the above realities, 10–14% of parturients want disclosure of even the rarest of risks associated with neuraxial anesthesia. The majority of parturients wanted to be informed if any risk of at least 1 in 10,000 patients.[34] According to Wong, the majority of the maternal closed claims in the American Society of Anesthesiologists Closed Claims Database are due to nerve injury, and payment was only made in one-third of those cases. Other claims associated with obstetric anesthesia include headache, insufficient pain management, and emotional distress.[33] As is true elsewhere in medicine, it is important to have clear communication with the patient and her health-care providers and have to adequate and patient-centered discussions of risks.

REFERENCES

1. American Society of Anesthesiologists Task Force on Obstetric Anesthesia. Practice guidelines for obstetric anesthesia: an updated report by the American Society of Anesthesiologists Task Force on Obstetric Anesthesia. *Anesthesiology.* 2007; 106: 843–863.
2. Neal JM, Bernards CM, Butterworth JF IV, et al. ASRA practice advisory on local anesthetic systemic toxicity. *Regional Anesthesia and Pain Medicine.* March 1, 2010; 35(2): 152–161.
3. Rosen MA. Paracervical block for labor analgesia: A brief historic review. *American Journal of Obstetrics and Gynecology.* May 31, 2002; 186(5):S127–130.
4. Albright GA. Cardiac arrest following regional anesthesia with etidocaine or bupivacaine. *Anesthesiology.* 1979; 51: 285–287.
5. Paech MJ, Godkin R, Webster S. Complications of obstetric epidural analgesia and anaesthesia: a prospective analysis of 10 995 cases. *International Journal of Obstetric Anesthesia.* January 1, 1998;7(1): 5–11.
6. Vandenabeele F, Creemers J, Lambrichts I. Ultrastructure of the human spinal arachnoid mater and dura mater. *J Anat.* 1996; 189: 417–430.
7. Bevacqua BK, Haas T, Brand F. A clinical measure of the posterior epidural space depth. *Reg Anesth.* 1996; 21: 456–460.
8. Hogan QH. Lumbar epidural anatomy. A new look by cryomicrotome section. *Anesthesiology.* 1991; 75: 767–775.
9. Reina MA, Lirk P, Puigdellivol-Sanches A, et al. Human lumbar ligamentum flavum anatomy for epidural anesthesia: Reviewing a 3D MR-based

interactive model and postmortem samples. *Anesth Analg.* 2016; 122: 903–907.

10. Principles and Practice of Regional Anaesthesia 4e edited by Graeme McLeod, Colin McCartney, and Tony Wildsmith (2012): Figure 12.4 (p.116) from chapter: "Anatomy and physiology of the vertebral canal" by Ian Parkin and Alastair Chambers

11. Headache Classification Committee of the International Headache Society. The international classification of headache disorders, 3rd edition, beta version. *Cephalalgia.* 2013; 33: 715–716.

12. Gaiser RR. Postdural puncture headache: an evidence-based approach. *Anesthesiology Clin.* 2017; 35: 157–167.

13. Benarroch EE. Choroid plexus-CSF system: recent developments and clinical correlations. *Neurology.* 2016; 86: 286–296.

14. Gomez-Rios MA, Fernandez-Goti MC. Pneumocephalus after inadvertent dural puncture during epidural anesthesia. *Anesthesiology.* 2013; 118: 444.

15. Chestnut DH, Wong CA, Tsen LC, Kee WD, Beilin Y, Mhyre J. Postpartum headache. In: A Macarthur,ed. Chestnut's Obstetric Anesthesia: Principles and Practice. 4th ed. Elsevier Health Sciences; 683.

16. Agerson AN, Scavone BM. Prophylactic epidural blood patch after unintentional dural puncture for the prevention of postdural puncture headache in parturients. *Anesth Analg.* 2012; 115: 133–136.

17. Russell IF. A prospective controlled study of continuous spinal analgesia versus repeat epidural analgesia after accidental dural puncture in labour. *Int J Obstet Anesth.* 2012; 21: 7–16.

18. Bolden N, Gebre E. Accidental dural puncture management: 10-year experience at an academic tertiary care center. *Reg Anesth Pain Med.* 2016; 41: 169–174.

19. Scott DB, Tunstall ME. Serious complications associated with epidural/spinal blockade in obstetrics: A two-year prospective study. *International Journal of Obstetric Anesthesia.* July 31, 1995; 4(3): 133–139.

20. Reynolds F. Damage to the conus medullaris following spinal anaesthesia. *Anaesthesia.* March 1, 2001; 56(3): 238–247.

21. Broadbent CR, Maxwell WB, Ferrie R, Wilson DJ, Gawne-Cain M, Russell R. Ability of anaesthetists to identify a marked lumbar interspace. *Anaesthesia.* November 1, 2000; 55(11): 1122–1126.

22. Cook TM, Counsell D, Wildsmith JA. Major complications of central neuraxial block: Report on the Third National Audit Project of the Royal College of Anaesthetists. British Journal of Anaesthesia. February 1, 2009; 102(2): 179–190.

23. Ruppen W, Derry S, McQuay H, Moore RA. Incidence of epidural hematoma, infection, and neurologic injury in obstetric patients with epidural analgesia/anesthesia. *Journal of the American Society of Anesthesiologists.* August 1, 2006; 105(2): 394–399.

24. Scott DB, Hibbard B. Serious non-fatal complications associated with extradural block in obstetric practice. *British Journal of Anaesthesia.* May 1, 1990; 64(5): 537–541.

25. Horlocker TT, Wedel DJ, Rowlingson JC, et al. Regional anesthesia in the patient receiving antithrombotic or thrombolytic therapy: American Society of Regional Anesthesia and Pain Medicine Evidence-Based Guidelines (Third Edition). *Regional Anesthesia and Pain Medicine.* January 1, 2010; 35(1): 64–101.

26. Loo CC, Dahlgren G, Irestedt L. Neurological complications in obstetric regional anaesthesia. *International Journal of Obstetric Anesthesia.* April 1, 2000; 9(2): 99–124.

27. Grewal S, Hocking G, Wildsmith JA. Epidural abscesses. *British Journal of Anaesthesia.* March 1, 2006; 96(3): 292–302.

28. North JB, Brophy BP. Epidural abscess: A hazard of spinal epidural anaesthesia. *ANZ Journal of Surgery.* August 1, 1979; 49(4): 484–485.

29. Horlocker TT, Birnbach DS, Connis RT, et al. Practice advisory for the prevention, diagnosis, and management of infectious complications associated with neuraxial techniques: A report by the American Society of Anesthesiologists Task Force on infectious complications associated with neuraxial techniques. *Obstetric Anesthesia Digest.* June 1, 2011; 31(2): 85.

30. Goodman EJ, DeHorta E, Taguiam JM. Safety of spinal and epidural anesthesia in parturients with chorioamnionitis. *Regional Anesthesia and Pain Medicine.* September 1, 1996; 21(5): 436–441.

31. Bader AM, Datta S, Gilbertson L, Kirz L. Regional anesthesia in women with chorioamnionitis. *Regional Anesthesia and Pain Medicine.* March 1, 1992; 17(2): 84-hyhen.

32. Cook TM, Counsell D, Wildsmith JA. Major complications of central neuraxial block: Report on the Third National Audit Project of the Royal College of Anaesthetists. *British Journal of Anaesthesia.* February 1, 2009; 102(2): 179–190.

33. Wong CA. Nerve injuries after neuraxial anaesthesia and their medicolegal implications. *Best Practice and Research Clinical Obstetrics and Gynaecology.* June 30, 2010; 24(3): 367–381.

34. Bethune L, Harper N, Lucas DN, et al. Complications of obstetric regional analgesia: How much information is enough? *International Journal of Obstetric Anesthesia.* January 31, 2004; 13(1): 30–34.

Perinatal Depression in Neurological Disease and Disability

MARTE HELENE BJØRK AND MALIN EBERHARD-GRAN

INTRODUCTION

A minor or major depressive episode that affects women during pregnancy or in the first year after delivery is often labeled perinatal depression.[1,2] Approximately 7–15% of mothers.[1,3] and 4–10% of fathers present with depressive symptoms in this period.[4] Depression is one of the most common complications of the perinatal period.[5]

When depression occurs in this period of life, it may affect the child and the family substantially.[5–9] Depressed mothers may interact with their infant differently than non-depressed women and be less sensitive to the child's needs.[9] They play less with their child face-to-face, and they often touch and talk to the child less positively than non-depressed women.[10–12] It is well documented that long-term parental depression is a risk factor for emotional and cognitive problems in children.[9,10,13–17]

The psychiatric problems that occur in the period around childbirth often relate to problems the woman had before childbirth. Individual predisposition is the main identified risk factor.[18] The principles of diagnosing depression are roughly the same as at other times in life. In the American Psychiatric Association's Diagnostic and Statistical Manual of Mental Disorders, fifth edition,[19] and the International Classification of Diseases, 10th edition[20] the criteria are similar to major depression outside of pregnancy but require an onset in the pregnancy or the puerperium (Table 34.1). The symptoms include depressed mood, diminished interest and pleasure in most activities, fatigue, feelings of guilt, psychomotor changes, and diminished ability to concentrate. Sleep problems more than what the care of the baby explain are common. Changes in appetite or body weight are part of the diagnostic criteria.[19,20] Some mothers struggle with excessive worry for the baby's health or feeding, general anxiety, or thoughts of harming themselves or the baby.

Non-pregnant patients with brain disorders have increased prevalence of depression compared to others.[21] Also during the perinatal period this group have a markedly increased risk of depression compared to other parents (Table 34.2).[22–27] In particular, women who have a history of psychiatric disease are at risk.[25,28,29] Disease-related factors that may make parenting more difficult further increase the risk for depression.[28,30]

The co-existence of perinatal depression and neurological disorders could potentially worsen the course of both diseases. Special regard is necessary when evaluating symptoms, as these may overlap between the disorders.[31,32] Anti-depressive treatment may influence neurological diseases, and medication used for neurological diseases may induce symptoms of depression.[33,34] The anti-depressant norepinephrine and dopamine blocker bupropion may, for example, have a proconvulsant effect, while the antiepileptic drugs topiramate and levetiracetam are associated with depressive symptoms.[33–35] Both neurological and psychiatric health personnel should therefore be alert to the co-existence of perinatal depression and neurological disorders, and treatment should be interdisciplinary.

EPILEPSY AND PERINATAL DEPRESSION

In women with epilepsy, the point prevalence of depression is estimated to approximately 17–19% during pregnancy[25,26] and 16–39% in the postnatal period.[22,24,25] These rates are substantially higher than the rates estimated among women without epilepsy in respective control groups (9–12%, Table 34.2).[22,25,26] The prevalence of depression is also higher in men with epilepsy than among men without epilepsy in the perinatal period (4% versus 2–3%, Table 34.2).[27]

The risk of perinatal depression in women with epilepsy is associated with high seizure activity

---

TABLE 34.1 DSM-5 AND ICD-10 DIAGNOSTIC CRITERIA FOR DEPRESSION

DSM-5[1]

Major depression

At least five symptoms present for at least 2 weeks, for most of nearly every day

A symptom must be:
- Depressed mood
- Markedly diminished interest or pleasure in all or most activities

Other symptoms:
- Substantial weight loss when not dieting or weight gain, or increase or decrease in appetite
- Insomnia or hypersomnia
- Psychomotor agitation or retardation
- Fatigue or loss of energy
- Feelings of worthlessness or excessive or inappropriate guilt
- Diminished ability to think or concentrate or indecisiveness
- Recurrent thoughts of death or suicidal ideation (with or without a specific plan)

Symptoms cause clinically significant distress or impairment in social, occupational, or other important areas of functionality

Symptoms not due to direct physiological effects of a substance or another medical condition

The occurrence of a major depressive episode is not better explained by schizoaffective disorder or other psychotic disorders and there has never been a manic or hypomanic episode

Depressive episode with insufficient symptoms*:Depressed affect and at least one other of the above symptoms associated with clinically significant distress or impairment persisting for at least 2 weeks

With peripartum onset[†]: Onset of mood symptoms happens during pregnancy or in the 4 weeks after delivery

ICD-10[2]

Severe depression

At least seven symptoms, usually present for at least 2 weeks, experienced with severe intensity for most of every day

All three key symptoms associated should be present:
- Persistent sadness or low mood
- Loss of interests or pleasure
- Fatigue or low energy

At least four associated symptoms should be present:
- Disturbed sleep
- Poor concentration or indecisiveness
- Low self-confidence
- Poor or increased appetite
- Suicidal thoughts or acts
- Agitation or slowing of movements
- Guilt or self-blame
- Individual unable to continue with social, work or domestic activities, except to a very restricted extent

Moderate depression: At least two key symptoms and three associated symptoms should be present

Minor depression: At least two key symptoms and two associated symptoms should be present, with no symptoms present to an intense degree

With peripartum onset: Disorder commencing within 6 weeks of delivery

---

ICD=international classification of diseases (published by WHO[2]). DSM=diagnostic and statistical manual of mental disorders. *Changed from minor depression in DSM-4 (2 to 4 depressive symptoms experienced for at least 2 weeks, 1 symptom should be depressed mood or loss of pleasure). † Changed from with peripartum onset in DSM-4 (onset of mood symptoms within first 4 weeks after delivery).

---

and high anti-epileptic treatment load.[24,25] Both high dosage or serum concentrations, as well as antiepileptic polytherapy, seem to be associated with depression.[24,25] Anti-epileptic drugs known to be mood stabilizing in non-pregnant populations, such as valproate and lamotrigine,[36,37] do not reduce the risk of perinatal depression when used for anti-epileptic purposes in observational

TABLE 34:2 FREQUENCY OF DEPRESSION IN EPILEPSY PATIENTS TREATED WITH ANTI-EPILEPTIC DRUGS

Author	Neurological Diagnosis	Population	Sex	Number	Diagnostic Tool	Depression Frequency	Adjusted Risk[1]
Turner et al [22]	Epilepsy	Epilepsy clinic	Female	Epilepsy: 35 Controls: 35	EDPS >9 clinical interview	*5-8 weeks postnatal* Epilepsy: 35% Controls: 11%	Not available
Turner et al [23]	Epilepsy	Epilepsy clinic	Female	Epilepsy: 35 Controls: 35	EDPS >9 clinical interview	*5-8 weeks postnatal* epilepsy: 39% Controls: 12%	Not available
Galanti et al [24]	Epilepsy	Tertiary epilepsy center	Female	Epilepsy 56	BDI ≥ 12	*Within 12 weeks postnatal* Epilepsy 25%	No controls included
Reiter et al [26]	Epilepsy	Population based cohort	Female	Epilepsy 329 Reference: 106.224	SCL-5 mean > 1.75	*Gestational week 13–17* Epilepsy 19% Reference cohort: 11%	2.0 (1.5–2.7)
Bjørk et al [25]	Epilepsy	Population based cohort	Female	Epilepsy 319 Reference: 98.282	SCL-8 mean > 1.75	*Gestational week 30* Epilepsy: 17% Reference: 9% *6 months postnatal* Epilepsy: 16% Reference: 10%	Perinatal period total 1.6 (1.2–2.2)
Reiter et al [27]	Epilepsy	Population based cohort	Male	Epilepsy 243 Reference: 75.677	SCL-8 mean > 1.75	*Gestational week 13–17* Epilepsy: 4% Reference: 3%	4.2 (0.9 – 3.3)
Razas et al [28]	Multiple sclerosis (MS)	Population registry study	Female Male	MS: Female 255, Male 105 Control: Female: 904 Male:303	Depression and/or anxiety in public health databases	*Within 4 weeks before to 12 months after delivery* MS female: 26% MS male: 26% Control female: 21% Control male: 10%	Female: 1.3 (1.0–1.7) Male: 2.7 (1.7–4.3)
Wesström et al [29]	Restless legs (RLS)	Population based cohort	Female	RLS: 134 Controls: 792	Pregnancy EDPS > 12 postnatal EDPS > 11	*Gestational week 17* RLS: 16% Controls 5% *Gestational week 32* RLS: 17% Controls 8% *6 weeks postnatal* RLS: 23% Controls 12%	*Gestational week 17* 2.9 (1.4–5.9) *Gestational week 32* 2.0 (1.1–3.8) *6 weeks postnatal* 1.9 (1.0–3.8)

1) Adjusted risk compared to non-epilepsy (95% confidence interval) if available
2) Based on hospital records from a subcohort (n=40)
EDPS: Depression diagnosed by the Edinburgh postpartum depression scale
BDI: Depression diagnosed by the Beck depression inventory
SCL-5: Hopkins symptom checklist 5 item (3 questions concerning depression, 2 concerning anxiety)
SCL-8: Hopkins symptom checklist 8 item (4 questions concerning depression)

studies.[24,25,30] Depressive symptoms in the perinatal period should therefore not be treated by adding a second anti-epileptic drug assumed to be mood stabilizing.[30] Anti-epileptic medications may also have side effects that mimic perinatal depression. Topiramate is used for generalized and focal epilepsy but can induce or worsen depressed mood, anxiety, fatigue, suicidal ideation, insomnia, weight loss, and psychomotor slowing.[33,38,39]

Compared to other women with perinatal depression, depressed women with epilepsy more often have a previous history of mood and/or anxiety disorders.[25] Pregnant women with epilepsy also more often have little contact with people other than their partners; report lower relationship satisfaction and are more likely to be single mothers than other childbearing women.[40] In addition, their pregnancies are also more frequently unintended.[40] Both during and after pregnancy, their overall quality of life is lower than for women without epilepsy.[40] Physical and sexual abuse before or during pregnancy are more common in this group than in women without epilepsy and further increase the odds of perinatal depression three to four fold.[25] Childcare is more complicated for women with epilepsy, as epileptic seizures may pose a risk to the child (eg, during bathing, changing, carrying, and breastfeeding).[41] In a single mother with low social support, these practical issues can be especially difficult.[30]

Epilepsy patients appear undertreated for depression in pregnancy. The results from a prospective cohort study show that depressed pregnant women without epilepsy are treated with antidepressive drugs more than three times as often as depressed women with epilepsy.[25] Long-term outcome from peripartum depression is less favorable for women with epilepsy who have been abused or have a pre-pregnancy history of psychiatric disease. In absence of these risk factors, their prognosis in terms of resolution of depressive symptoms after the peripartum period is similar to women without epilepsy.[25]

MULTIPLE SCLEROSIS AND PERINATAL DEPRESSION

Multiple sclerosis is common in women of childbearing age. The risk of disease onset and relapse is increased in the postnatal period.[42,43] Postnatal onset of multiple sclerosis can be intertwined with postnatal depression,[44] and the symptoms may overlapp. Fatigue, psychomotor slowing, and cognitive difficulties are symptoms of both inflammatory brain disease activity and postnatal depression. This can delay treatment for both

disorders. In a large study of parents with multiple sclerosis, 40% were registered with prior mental health morbidity compared to 22% of control parents.[45] In the perinatal period, more than a quarter were diagnosed with a mood or anxiety disorder (Table 34.2).[28] However, women were less vulnerable than men, who had a two- to three-fold increased risk compared to the population without multiple sclerosis.[28] The authours hypothesized that depression can be triggered by their new role as fathers, as physical and cognitive impairment might prevent them from actively supporting their families financially, emotionally, and in daily tasks.[28] Multiple sclerosis–related symptoms and low social support also correlate with emotional distress in mothers in the postnatal period.[46] Perinatal depression and anxiety increase the risk of psychiatric disease in children of patients with multiple sclerosis.[28] The increased risk was also present when adjusting for psychiatric disorders after the postpartum period.[28] By contrast, children of mentally stable parents with multiple sclerosis do better emotionally and developmentally than their peers of equal socioeconomic status.[45] This underlines the importance of rapidly detecting and treating emotional problems during this critical period.

HEADACHES AND PERINATAL DEPRESSION

Headaches are common among fertile women, reported in approximately 34–48% before pregnancy and 23–45% during the first year after birth.[47,48] It has been reported that women with postnatal headaches have more depressive symptoms than headache-free women.[49] The relationship between the disorders is probably bidirectional, with headaches increasing the likelihood of depression and vice versa. Both depression and headaches may prevent the mother from attending to the needs of her child.[48,50] Diagnosing and treating both disorders are of great importance and should be done in parallel.[51] Postnatal headaches can be of primary origin, the most common being tension type headaches and migraines.[48] However, the puerperium is a high-risk period for several severe disorders where headache is a prominent symptom. Cerebral venous thrombosis, pre-eclampsia, pituitary pathology, reversible cerebral vasoconstriction syndrome, and posterior reversible encephalopathy syndrome lead to headache and can cause significant maternal morbidity and mortality if left untreated.[52] Cerebrospinal fluid leakage headache after intrapartum epidural anesthesia accounts for 5% of all headache cases in the puerperium; this can be incapacitating but is easily treated.[48,51] Hence, headache co-occurring with perinatal depression should not lead to a diagnosis of tension-type headaches due to an assumption of psychological tension, without ruling out secondary causes.[51]

Psychological, physical, and sexual violence by a partner is often related to headaches in the postpartum period.[53,54] If the abused women are also depressed, the odds of having migraines increase two to three fold.[54] A headache consultation in the perinatal period should therefore always include sensitive questions concerning the psychosocial situation as well as the presence of depressive symptoms.

SLEEP, NEUROLOGICAL DISEASE, AND DEPRESSIVE SYMPTOMS

Sleep quality is of importance in pregnancy care of the neurological patient. Sleep-wakefulness disturbances occur in a wide range of disorders affecting the brain.[55] There is a strong bilateral relationship between insomnia and perinatal depressive symptoms.[56] Poor sleep quality in the perinatal period predict development of depressive symptoms as well as increased symptom severity, puerperal psychosis, and suicidal ideation.[56,57] It is possible that poor sleep represents a mediator in the development of perinatal depression in neurological disease. In a study of pregnant women with pre-gestational severe restless legs, perinatal depression was found in 16–23%, compared to 5-13% of healthy controls (Table 34.2).[29] In contrast, sleep problems caused by perinatal depression can also exacerbate neurological disorders. Sleep deprivation is a common trigger for epileptic seizures and headache attacks.[58,59] Avoiding sleep deprivation should therefore be a part of pregnancy and postnatal care in neurological patients. This includes treating neurological symptoms such as pain and spasticity that may negatively affect sleep, as well as treating comorbid sleep disorders such as insomnia. Discuss and plan strategies for ensuring sufficient sleep and rest after delivery *before* delivery. Implement these strategies at the maternity ward for these patients. After discharge from the maternity ward, the partner handling the baby at night and mobilization of psychosocial support can prevent sleep deprivation and exhaustion.

CONSEQUENCES OF PERINATAL DEPRESSION

In this period, depression may have significant ripple effects if the woman is not cared for, as it can lead to exacerbation of symptoms and prolonged depression. In the most serious cases, there may also be a risk of suicide or infanticide.[21,60,61] Death by maternal suicide occurs in 4 in 100,000 live births and is a leading cause of postnatal mortality in Western countries.[32,62] The majority of women who commit suicide in the postnatal period have a psychiatric diagnosis, usually postnatal psychosis, severe depression, bipolar disorder, and/or anxiety.[18,32,62] Postnatal psychoses are rare, occurring in about 1–2 in 1000 mothers during the first 4 weeks following delivery.[63] However, in women with pre-pregnancy bipolar disorder, schizoaffective disorder, or previous postnatal psychosis, the risk of postnatal psychosis increases dramatically.[63,64] A postnatal psychosis often develops rapidly and can be hard to recognize for non-specialized psychiatric health personnel.[32] Infanticide occurs in 2–7 out of 100,000 children in developed countries,[65] and a subset of those incidents is caused by maternal psychosis.[65] While infanticide is extremely rare in mothers with postnatal depression, these women may have frequent thoughts of harming the infant,[66] and the risk of physical child abuse is increased.[67]

The presence of depression in neurological disorders is important for several reasons. In neurological disorders, depression can exacerbate symptoms,[68] reduce treatment adherence,[69,70] diminish quality of life,[71-73] and interfere with self-management, leading to accelerated disease progression.[21,68] From the confidential inquiry into maternal deaths in the United Kingdom,[32] 18% of the deaths related to an underlying psychiatric condition in the postnatal period were due to insufficient treatment, detection, or follow-up of physical disease. These cases included inadequate treatment and follow- up of epilepsy leading to sudden unexpected death, lack of treatment for thromboembolic disorders, and misattribution of cerebral involvement of a autoimmune disorder to a functional psychiatric disorders.[32] Particular care should be taken if the only symptoms of a suggested psychiatric disorder are seemingly unexplained physical symptoms, or if the woman has no history of psychiatric illness.[32]

MANAGEMENT

Pregnancy Planning

In patients where the neurological disorder or its treatment could complicate pregnancy or be harmful to the child, it is strongly recommended that the pregnancy is planned several months ahead of conception. Evaluating the risk for

---

BOX 34.1
PREGNANCY CARE MAP[3,30,75,76]

A. Assess risk factors for pregnancy psychiatric disease during the first pregnancy-related consultation
  a. Previous severe depression/bipolar disease/psychosis
    ➤ Consult psychiatrist
    ➤ Alert patient and pregnancy caregivers[a] of risk and symptoms of postnatal psychosis
  b. Previous unipolar depressive episodes
    ➤ Alert patient (and if possible, relatives) and pregnancy caregivers[1] of risk of perinatal depression
  c. Apply sensitive questions concerning: social support, traumatic life events, psychological/physical/sexual abuse and substance abuse

B. Apply two perinatal depression screening questions at all pregnancy and postnatal visits (Figure 34.1)

C. Apply EDPS if positive answers to one or both questions in B or on suspicion of depression (Figure 34.1)

D. Patients screening positive on EDPS or clinical suspicion of depression
  a. Refer to further psychiatric evaluation
  b. Ask for thoughts of harming themselves, their infants, or anyone else. If yes → emergency referral
  c. Assess diminished ability to care for themselves, to maintain therapy of their neurological disease and ability to care for the baby. If yes → emergency referral.
  d. Measure hemoglobin and thyroid-stimulating hormone levels. Patients on antiepileptic drugs should have antiepileptic drug plasma level, folate, vitamin B12 evaluated[b]
  e. Consider relation to underlying neurological disease or medication side effects
  f. Assess need for increased social support
  g. Alert other pregnancy care givers[1]

E. Before an antidepressant drug is started:
  a. Consider interaction with the neurological disorder or treatment.
  b. If anxiety is present: choose an antidepressant with effect on anxiety.
  c. Rule out bipolar disorder

[a]Information to pregnancy care givers: Health personnel involved in pregnancy care such as the general practitioner, obstetrician, community nurse, midwife, etc. If possible, inform partner/family

[b]Anti-epileptic drug toxicity, hypothyroidism, folate- and B12 deficiency could present with depressive symptoms. Anti-epileptic drugs could interfere with B12 and folate metabolism.

EDPS: Edinburgh postpartum depression score (Figure 34.1)

---

perinatal depression should be an integral part of the neurological pregnancy care. This includes investigating all risk factors for pregnancy psychiatric disease (Box 34.1), screening for depression during consultations (see below and Figure 34.1), referring positive screens for further psychiatric evaluation and treatment, and alerting all health personnel involved in the pregnancy care of the risk of perinatal depression. In addition, consider the need for increased support after delivery at an early stage.

Diagnosis
Inadequate consultation time is a notable challenge in the provision of neurological patient care.[74] A sensible approach recommended by the United States Agency for Healthcare Research and Quality and the United Kingdom's National Institute for Health and Care Excellence (NICE), is a three-step diagnostic method.[3,75,76] This approach recommends that women should be asked, in a sensitive manner, 2 questions related to feelings of depression, hopelessness, and lack of interest or pleasure in activities (Figure 34.1).[3] Women who respond with an affirmative answer to either question should then be further screened for depression.[3,75,76] When screening for perinatal depression in general and in patient populations in particular, it is important to use diagnostic tools that exclude bodily symptoms. The Edinburgh

A : Screening questions (all women)

- During the past month, have you been bothered by feeling down, depressed or hopeless

- During the past month, have you often been bothered by little interest or pleasure in doing things?

↓ Positive answer to either question or clinical suspicion of depression

B : Edinburgh Post Partum Depression Score (EDPS)

Please check the answer that comes closest to how you have felt in the PAST 7 DAYS, not just how you feel today.

1. I have been able to laugh and see the funny side of things
   - ☐ As much as I always could
   - ☐ Not quite so much now
   - ☐ Definitely not so much now
   - ☐ Not at all

2. I have looked forward with enjoyment to things
   - ☐ As much as I ever did
   - ☐ Rather less than I used to
   - ☐ Definitely less than I used to
   - ☐ Hardly at all

*3. I have blamed myself unnecessarily when things went wrong
   - ☐ Yes, most of the time
   - ☐ Yes, some of the time
   - ☐ Not very often
   - ☐ No, never

4. I have been anxious or worried for no good reason
   - ☐ No, not at all
   - ☐ Hardly ever
   - ☐ Yes, sometimes
   - ☐ Yes, very often

*5. I have felt scared or panicky for no very good reason
   - ☐ Yes, quite a lot
   - ☐ Yes, sometimes
   - ☐ No, not much
   - ☐ No, not at all

*6. Things have been getting on top of me
   - ☐ Yes, most of the time I haven't been able to cope at all
   - ☐ Yes, sometimes I haven't been coping as well as usual
   - ☐ No, most of the time I have coped quite well
   - ☐ No, I have been coping as well as ever

*7. I have been so unhappy that I have had difficulty sleeping
   - ☐ Yes, most of the time
   - ☐ Yes, sometimes
   - ☐ Not very often
   - ☐ No, not at all

*8. I have felt sad or miserable
   - ☐ Yes, most of the time
   - ☐ Yes, quite often
   - ☐ Not very often
   - ☐ No, not at all

*9. I have been so unhappy that I have been crying
   - ☐ Yes, most of the time
   - ☐ Yes, quite often
   - ☐ Only occasionally
   - ☐ No, never

*10. The thought of harming myself has occurred to me
   - ☐ Yes, quite often
   - ☐ Sometimes
   - ☐ Hardly ever
   - ☐ Never

↓ Positive EDPS screen[1] or clinical suspicion of depression

C : Comprehensive clinical evaluation

FIGURE 34.1 Three-step algorithm for identification of parents with peripartum depression

1) Positive Edinburgh postpartum depression score (EDPS): A sum score equal to or higher than 10 points. Each item is scored 0, 1, 2 or 3 according to the severity of the response (items marked with * are scored in reverse: 3,2,1 or 0).[77]

2) All parents should be asked two questions (A) at consultations in the pregnancy or postpartum period. An affirmative response to either question should lead to the administration of the EDPS (B). Screen-positive parents should be referred for further comprehensive clinical evaluation (C).

The figure is adapted from Steward et al.[3]

Postpartum Depression Scale (EDPS) is a 10-item questionnaire developed for the pregnant and postnatal state.[77] Its efficacy in identifying women with perinatal depression has been validated,[78] and it also performs well among somatic patient populations.[79] The scale is easy to use, takes less than 5 minutes to complete, and has been translated into more than 25 languages.[18] Moreover, both the American College of Obstetricians and Gynecologists[18] and the American Academy of Pediatrics[2] recommend using the EDPS during health-care visits to detect perinatal depression cases. Women with scores above the threshold identified by the EDPS should undergo further psychiatric evaluation including a comprehensive clinical interview.[3,75,76] Neurologists should also rule out the possibility that the underlying neurological disease or its treatment cause the depressive symptoms.

Treatment

Treatment options for perinatal depression in neurological disease are derived from guidelines on perinatal depression in neurologically healthy women,[76] as well as from studies of depression in neurological disease outside pregnancy. Perinatal depression is managed with psychosocial strategies, psychotherapy (including high intensity psychological intervention with cognitive behavioral therapy [CBT]), and antidepressant medications: usually selective serotonin reuptake inhibitors (SSRI).[3,76] In most neurological patients, it is assumed that depressive symptoms respond well to treatment with SSRIs and selected serotonin-norepinephrine reuptake inhibitors (SNRIs), though few methodological adequate studies have been done.[80] However, in patients with restless legs, SSRIs can exacerbate the movement disorder. This has been reported particularly for sertraline,[81] which is often recommended for postnatal depression due to minimal transference to breast milk.[3]

The choice of drug treatment or non-pharmacological interventions depends on the severity of symptoms, potential interactions with medical treatment for the neurological disorder, potential for teratogenic effects during pregnancy,[5] breastfeeding and the patient's preference.[3,34] The use of drug therapy should be considered in women with moderate to severe symptoms, in women that presents with mild depression but has a history of severe depression, in women where psychotherapeutic therapy has been ineffective or is unavailable.[3,76] Anxiety should also be taken into account[34] as it predicts a higher risk of treatment-resistant depression, including a higher risk of suicidality.[34] In these cases, a type of SSRI or CBT effective in anxiety should be selected.[34,82]

Before beginning treatment, clinicians must rule out a bipolar disorder or a postnatal psychosis as these require different management and should be handled by psychiatrists.[3,18,34] In patients without neurological diseases, mild to moderate postnatal depression is usually managed at the primary-care level. However, as the medical and psychosocial situations of neurological patients are usually more complicated, we recommend that the patients are considered for treatment by specialists and at an earlier time. We recommend a multidisciplinary approach.

Breastfeeding is encouraged for mothers with antenatal as well as postpartum depression, and may prevent or decrease symptoms of depression in both groups. Pregnancy depression predicts shorter duration of breastfeeding.[83] Increased attention to breastfeeding goals and problems is critical. Most antidepressant medications are compatible with breastfeeding, though it is important to check each medication regimen. Combined therapies may potentiate side effects in the infant, especially in preterm infants or neonates.

Patients with Concomitant Anti-epileptic Drug Use

In patients with epilepsy, SSRIs in therapeutic doses rarely cause seizures to worsen.[34] However, this has been a concern for clomipramine, maprotiline, amoxapine, and bupropion.[34] Some anti-epileptic drugs may influence the serum concentration of anti-depressive drugs and vice versa.[37] Reduced serum levels due to interactions may cause therapy failure, while increased serum levels may increase the risk of teratogenic effects. Antiepileptic drug teratogenicity is dose dependent.[84] Serum concentration measurements of both medications are especially important when the drugs have interacting potential. Potential embryotoxic effects from polytherapy with antiepileptic and antidepressant drugs have not been investigated,[30] and caution is therefore advised. Psychotherapy is the first line treatment for mild to moderate depression in pregnant or breastfeeding women using antiepileptic drugs.

Electro Convulsive Therapy (ECT)

ECT is an effective treatment of postnatal psychosis in the general population.[63] However, in patients with epilepsy, ECT may induce status epilepticus. It should therefore not be used during pregnancy, and caution is advised in the postnatal period.[30]

SUMMARY

Both females and males with neurological disease have an increased risk of depression in the perinatal period. Perinatal depression can have severe consequences for the health and quality of life of both the patient and their family. Health personnel treating people with neurological disorders should be aware of risk factors for depression and should screen for depressive symptoms during and after pregnancy. On suspicion of depression, swift referral for diagnostic evaluation and treatment is important. Communicate clearly the risk for and symptoms of depression, consequences for child safety and need for psychosocial support to the parents and to other pregnancy caregivers. While psychotherapy is the first choice of treatment for pregnant women with low to moderate levels of depression, we recommend an SSRI if pharmacotherapy is needed. Medical personnel should be aware of interactions with other neuroactive agents, especially anti-epileptic drugs. Treat depression and neurological disease in parallel. Lastly, multidisciplinary treatment and follow up of depression during and after pregnancy in patients with brain diseases is critically important.

REFERENCES

1. Gavin NI, Gaynes BN, Lohr KN, Meltzer-Brody S, Gartlehner G, Swinson T. Perinatal depression: A systematic review of prevalence and incidence. *Obstet Gynecol.* 2005; 106(5 Pt 1): 1071–1083.

2. Earls MF. Incorporating recognition and management of perinatal and postpartum depression into pediatric practice. *Pediatrics.* 2010; 126(5): 1032–1039.

3. Stewart DE, Vigod S. Postpartum depression. *New England Journal of Medicine.* 2016; 375(22): 2177–2186.

4. Paulson JF, Bazemore SD. Prenatal and postpartum depression in fathers and its association with maternal depression: A meta-analysis. *JAMA.* 2010; 303(19): 1961–1969.

5. Howard LM, Molyneaux E, Dennis CL, Rochat T, Stein A, Milgrom J. Non-psychotic mental disorders in the perinatal period. *Lancet.* 2014; 384(9956): 1775–1788.

6. Letourneau NL, Tramonte L, Willms JD. Maternal depression, family functioning and children's longitudinal development. *Journal of Pediatric Nursing.* 2013; 28(3): 223–234.

7. Letourneau NL, Dennis CL, Benzies K, et al. Postpartum depression is a family affair: Addressing the impact on mothers, fathers, and children. *Issues in Mental Health Nursing.* 2012; 33(7): 445–457.

8. Goodman SH, Rouse MH, Connell AM, Broth MR, Hall CM, Heyward D. Maternal depression and child psychopathology: A meta-analytic review. *Clinical Child and Family Psychology Review.* 2011; 14(1): 1–27.

9. Stein A, Pearson RM, Goodman SH, et al. Effects of perinatal mental disorders on the fetus and child. *Lancet.* 2014; 384(9956): 1800–1819.

10. Dietz LJ, Jennings KD, Kelley SA, Marshal M. Maternal depression, paternal psychopathology, and toddlers' behavior problems. *Journal of Clinical Child and Adolescent Psychology.* 2009; 38(1): 48–61.

11. Field T. Postpartum depression effects on early interactions, parenting, and safety practices: A review. *Infant Behav Dev.* 2009; 33(1): 1–6.

12. O'Hara MW, McCabe JE. Postpartum depression: Current status and future directions. *Annual Review of Clinical Psychology.* 2013; 9: 379–407.

13. Avan B, Richter LM, Ramchandani PG, Norris SA, Stein A. Maternal postnatal depression and children's growth and behaviour during the early years of life: exploring the interaction between physical and mental health. *Archives of Disease in Childhood.* 2010; 95(9): 690–695.

14. Zelkowitz P, Papageorgiou A, Bardin C, Wang T. Persistent maternal anxiety affects the interaction between mothers and their very low birthweight children at 24 months. *Early Human Development.* 2009; 85(1): 51–58.

15. Skurtveit S, Selmer R, Roth C, Hernandez-Diaz S, Handal M. Prenatal exposure to antidepressants and language competence at age three: Results from a large population-based pregnancy cohort in Norway. *BJOG: An International Journal of Obstetrics and Gynaecology.* 2014; 121(13): 1621–1631.

16. Stein A, Malmberg LE, Sylva K, Barnes J, Leach P. The influence of maternal depression, caregiving, and socioeconomic status in the postnatal year on children's language development. *Child care, Health and Development.* 2008; 34(5): 603–612.

17. Rahman A, Iqbal Z, Bunn J, Lovel H, Harrington R. Impact of maternal depression on infant nutritional status and illness: a cohort study. *Archives of General Psychiatry.* 2004; 61(9): 946–952.

18. Committee on Obstetric Practice. The American College of Obstetricians and Gynecologists committee opinion no. 630: Screening for perinatal depression. *Obstet Gynecol.* 2015; 125: 1268–1271.

19. American Psychiatric Association. *Diagnostic and Statistical Manual of Mental Disorders.* 5th ed. Arlington, VA: American Psychiatric Publishing; 2013.

20. World Health Organization. *The ICD-10 classification of Mental and Behavioural Disorders: Diagnostic Criteria for Research.* Geneva: World Health Organization; 1993.

21. Bulloch AG, Fiest KM, Williams JV, et al. Depression—a common disorder across a broad spectrum of neurological conditions: A cross-sectional nationally representative survey. *General Hospital Psychiatry.* 2015; 37(6): 507–512.

22. Turner K, Piazzini A, Franza A, et al. Postpartum depression in women with epilepsy versus women without epilepsy. *Epilepsy Behav.* 2006;9(2): 293–297.

23. Turner K, Piazzini A, Franza A, Marconi AM, Canger R, Canevini MP. Epilepsy and postpartum depression. *Epilepsia.* 2009;50(Suppl 1): 24–27.

24. Galanti M, Newport DJ, Pennell PB, et al. Postpartum depression in women with epilepsy: Influence of antiepileptic drugs in a prospective study. *Epilepsy Behav.* 2009; 16(3): 426–430.

25. Bjork MH, Veiby G, Reiter SC, et al. Depression and anxiety in women with epilepsy during pregnancy and after delivery: A prospective population-based cohort study on frequency, risk factors, medication, and prognosis. *Epilepsia.* 2015; 56(1): 28–39.

26. Reiter SF, Veiby G, Daltveit AK, Engelsen BA, Gilhus NE. Psychiatric comorbidity and social aspects in pregnant women with epilepsy: The Norwegian Mother and Child Cohort Study. *Epilepsy Behav.* 2013; 29(2): 379–385.

27. Reiter SF, Veiby G, Bjork MH, Engelsen BA, Daltveit AK, Gilhus NE. Psychiatric comorbidity, social aspects and quality of life in a population-based cohort of expecting fathers with epilepsy. *PloS ONE.* 2015; 10(12): e0144159.

28. Razaz N, Tremlett H, Marrie RA, Joseph KS. Peripartum depression in parents with multiple sclerosis and psychiatric disorders in children. *Multiple Sclerosis.* 2016; 22(14): 1830–1840.

29. Wesstrom J, Skalkidou A, Manconi M, Fulda S, Sundstrom-Poromaa I. Pre-pregnancy restless legs syndrome (Willis-Ekbom Disease) is associated with perinatal depression. *Journal of Clinical Sleep Medicine.* 2014; 10(5): 527–533.

30. Bjørk MH, Veiby G, B AE, Gilhus NE. Depression and anxiety during pregnancy and the postpartum period in women with epilepsy: A review of frequency, risks and recommendations for treatment. *Seizure.* 2015; 28: 39–45.

31. Gerace C, Corsi FM, Comanducci G. Apathetic syndrome from carotid dissection: A dangerous condition. *BMJ Case Reports.* 2013; Sep 2, 2013. doi:10.1136/ bcr-2013-009686.

32. Cantwell R, Clutton-Brock T, Cooper G, et al. Saving Mothers' Lives: Reviewing maternal deaths to make motherhood safer: 2006-2008. The Eighth Report of the Confidential Enquiries into Maternal Deaths in the United Kingdom. *BJOG: An International Journal of Obstetrics and Gynaecology.* 2011; 118(Suppl 1): 1–203.

33. Mula M, Trimble MR, Lhatoo SD, Sander JW. Topiramate and psychiatric adverse events in patients with epilepsy. *Epilepsia.* 2003; 44(5): 659–663.

34. Kanner AM. The treatment of depressive disorders in epilepsy: What all neurologists should know. *Epilepsia.* 2013; 54(Suppl 1): 3–12.

35. Lafay-Chebassier C, Chavant F, Favreliere S, Pizzoglio V, Perault-Pochat MC. Drug-induced depression: A case/non case study in the French Pharmacovigilance Database. *Therapie.* 2015; 70(5): 425–432.

36. Fountoulakis KN, Grunze H, Vieta E, et al. The International College of Neuro-Psychopharmacology (CINP) treatment guidelines for Bipolar disorder in adults (CINP-BD-2017), part 3: The clinical guidelines. *The International Journal of Neuropsychopharmacology.* 2016; 20(2): 121–179.

37. Mula M, Monaco F, Trimble MR. Use of psychotropic drugs in patients with epilepsy: Interactions and seizure risk. *Expert Review of Neurotherapeutics.* 2004; 4(6): 953–964.

38. Silberstein SD. Topiramate in migraine prevention: A 2016 perspective. *Headache.* 2017; 57(1): 165–178.

39. Donegan S, Dixon P, Hemming K, Tudur-Smith C, Marson A. A systematic review of placebo-controlled trials of topiramate: How useful is a multiple-indications review for evaluating the adverse events of an antiepileptic drug? *Epilepsia.* 2015; 56(12): 1910–1920.

40. Reiter SF, Bjork MH, Daltveit AK, et al. Life satisfaction in women with epilepsy during and after pregnancy. *Epilepsy Behav.* 2016; 62: 251–257.

41. Fox C, Betts T. How much risk does a woman with active epilepsy pose to her newborn child in the puerperium? A pilot study. *Seizure.* 1999; 8(6): 367–369.

42. Coyle PK. Management of women with multiple sclerosis through pregnancy and after childbirth. *Therapeutic Advances in Neurological Disorders.* 2016; 9(3): 198–210.

43. Vukusic S, Hutchinson M, Hours M, et al. Pregnancy and multiple sclerosis (the PRIMS study): Clinical predictors of post-partum relapse. *Brain: A Journal of Neurology.* 2004; 127(Pt. 6): 1353–1360.

44. Akkaya C, Kocagoz SZ, Turan OF, Taskapilioglu O, Kirli S. Onset of multiple sclerosis following post-partum depressive and manic episodes. *Psychiatry and Clinical Neurosciences.* 2007; 61(6): 698–699.

45. Razaz N, Joseph KS, Boyce WT, et al. Children of chronically ill parents: Relationship between parental multiple sclerosis and childhood developmental health. *Multiple Sclerosis.* 2016; 22(11): 1452–1462.

46. Gulick EE, Kim S. Postpartum emotional distress in mothers with multiple sclerosis.

Journal of Obstetric, Gynecologic, and Neonatal Nursing: JOGNN. 2004; 33(6): 729–738.

47. Saurel-Cubizolles MJ, Romito P, Lelong N, Ancel PY. Women's health after childbirth: A longitudinal study in France and Italy. *BJOG: An International Journal of Obstetrics and Gynaecology.* 2000; 107(10): 1202–1209.

48. Goldszmidt E, Kern R, Chaput A, Macarthur A. The incidence and etiology of postpartum headaches: A prospective cohort study. *Canadian Journal of Anaesthesia.* 2005; 52(9): 971–977.

49. Stein G, Morton J, Marsh A, et al. Headaches after childbirth. *Acta Neurol Scand.* 1984; 69(2): 74–79.

50. Steiner TJ, Stovner LJ, Katsarava Z, et al. The impact of headache in Europe: Principal results of the Eurolight project. *Journal of Headache and Pain.* 2014; 15: 31.

51. Mezzacappa A, Isabelle N, Jean-Baptiste C, et al. Long-term Postpartum Headache: PDPH Associated with Major Depression. *Pain Physician.* 2016; 19(7): E1105–1107.

52. Lim SY, Evangelou N, Jurgens S. Postpartum headache: Diagnostic considerations. *Practical Neurology.* 2014; 14(2): 92–99.

53. Audi CA, Segall-Correa AM, Santiago SM, Perez-Escamilla R. Adverse health events associated with domestic violence during pregnancy among Brazilian women. *Midwifery.* 2012; 28(4): 356–361.

54. Cripe SM, Sanchez SE, Gelaye B, Sanchez E, Williams MA. Association between intimate partner violence, migraine and probable migraine. *Headache.* 2011; 51(2): 208–219.

55. Anderson K. Sleep disturbance and neurological disease. *Clinical Medicine (London, England).* 2011; 11(3): 271–274.

56. Okun ML. Sleep and postpartum depression. *Current Opinion in Psychiatry.* 2015; 28(6): 490–496.

57. Wolfson AR, Crowley SJ, Anwer U, Bassett JL. Changes in sleep patterns and depressive symptoms in first-time mothers: Last trimester to 1-year postpartum. *Behavioral Sleep Medicine.* 2003; 1(1): 54–67.

58. Grigg-Damberger MM, Ralls F. Sleep disorders in adults with epilepsy: Past, present, and future directions. *Current Opinion in Pulmonary Medicine.* 2014; 20(6): 542–549.

59. Rains JC, Poceta JS. Sleep-related headaches. *Neurologic Clinics.* 2012; 30(4): 1285–1298.

60. Bronnum-Hansen H, Stenager E, Nylev Stenager E, Koch-Henriksen N. Suicide among Danes with multiple sclerosis. *Journal of Neurology, Neurosurgery, and Psychiatry.* 2005; 76(10): 1457–1459.

61. Jones JE, Hermann BP, Barry JJ, Gilliam FG, Kanner AM, Meador KJ. Rates and risk factors for suicide, suicidal ideation, and suicide attempts in chronic epilepsy. *Epilepsy Behav.* 2003; 4(Suppl 3): S31–38.

62. Esscher A, Essen B, Innala E, et al. Suicides during pregnancy and 1 year postpartum in Sweden, 1980-2007. *The British Journal of Psychiatry: The Journal of Mental Science.* 2016; 208(5): 462–469.

63. Sit D, Rothschild AJ, Wisner KL. A review of postpartum psychosis. *Journal of Women's Health.* 2006; 15(4): 352–368.

64. Kendell RE, Chalmers JC, Platz C. Epidemiology of puerperal psychoses. *The British Journal of Psychiatry: The Journal of Mental Science.* 1987; 150: 662–673.

65. Porter T, Gavin H. Infanticide and neonaticide: a review of 40 years of research literature on incidence and causes. *Trauma, Violence & Abuse.* 2010; 11(3): 99–112.

66. Jennings KD, Ross S, Popper S, Elmore M. Thoughts of harming infants in depressed and nondepressed mothers. *Journal of Affective Disorders.* 1999; 54(1–2): 21–28.

67. Cadzow SP, Armstrong KL, Fraser JA. Stressed parents with infants: reassessing physical abuse risk factors. *Child Abuse & Neglect.* 1999; 23(9): 845–853.

68. Williams LS. Depression and stroke: cause or consequence? *Seminars in Neurology.* 2005; 25(4): 396–409.

69. Mohr DC, Goodkin DE, Bacchetti P, et al. Psychological stress and the subsequent appearance of new brain MRI lesions in MS. *Neurology.* 2000; 55(1): 55–61.

70. Mohr DC, Goodkin DE, Gatto N, Van der Wende J. Depression, coping and level of neurological impairment in multiple sclerosis. *Multiple Sclerosis.* 1997; 3(4): 254–258.

71. Wang JL, Reimer MA, Metz LM, Patten SB. Major depression and quality of life in individuals with multiple sclerosis. *International Journal of Psychiatry in Medicine.* 2000; 30(4): 309–317.

72. Ben-Shlomo Y, Camfield L, Warner T, Group Ec. What are the determinants of quality of life in people with cervical dystonia? *Journal of Neurology, Neurosurgery, and Psychiatry.* 2002; 72(5): 608–614.

73. Boylan LS, Flint LA, Labovitz DL, Jackson SC, Starner K, Devinsky O. Depression but not seizure frequency predicts quality of life in treatment-resistant epilepsy. *Neurology.* 2004; 62(2): 258–261.

74. Morrish P. Inadequate neurology services undermine patient care in the UK. *BMJ.* 2015; 350: h3284.

75. Myers E, Aubuchon-Endsley N, Bastian L, et al. Efficacy and safety of screening for postpartum depression.

Comparative effectiveness review 106. (Prepared by the Duke Evidence-based Practice Center under Contract No. 290-2007-10066-I.) AHRQ Publication No. 13-EHC064-EF. In: Rockville, MD: Agency for Healthcare Research and Quality; April 2013. www.effectivehealthcare.ahrq.gov/reports/final.cfm.

76. Antenatal and postnatal mental health: Clinical management and service guidance. National Institute for Health and Care Excellence (NICE) Clinical guideline [CG192] Published date: December 2014 Last updated: August 2017. https://www.nice.org.uk/guidance/cg192

77. Cox JL, Holden JM, Sagovsky R. Detection of postnatal depression. Development of the 10-item Edinburgh Postnatal Depression Scale. *British Journal of Psychiatry: The Journal of Mental Science.* 1987; 150: 782–786.

78. Owora AH, Carabin H, Reese J, Garwe T. Summary diagnostic validity of commonly used maternal major depression disorder case finding instruments in the United States: A meta-analysis. *Journal of Affective Disorders.* 2016; 205: 335–343.

79. Lloyd-Williams M, Friedman T, Rudd N. Criterion validation of the Edinburgh postnatal depression scale as a screening tool for depression in patients with advanced metastatic cancer. *J Pain Symptom Manage.* 2000; 20(4): 259–265.

80. Lin JJ, Mula M, Hermann BP. Uncovering the neurobehavioural comorbidities of epilepsy over the lifespan. *Lancet.* 2012; 380(9848): 1180–1192.

81. Hargrave R, Beckley DJ. Restless leg syndrome exacerbated by sertraline. *Psychosomatics.* 1998; 39(2): 177–178.

82. Mula M. Treatment of anxiety disorders in epilepsy: An evidence-based approach. *Epilepsia.* 2013; 54(Suppl 1): 13–18.

83. Dias CC, Figueiredo B. Breastfeeding and depression: A systematic review of the literature. *J Affect Disord.* January 15, 2015; 171: 142–154.

84. Tomson T, Battino D, Bonizzoni E, et al. Dose-dependent risk of malformations with antiepileptic drugs: An analysis of data from the EURAP epilepsy and pregnancy registry. *Lancet Neurology.* 2011; 10(7): 609–617.

35

Breastfeeding in the Context of Neurological Disorders

RUTH A. LAWRENCE AND CASEY ROSEN-CAROLE

INTRODUCTION

Lactation is the physiologic completion of the reproductive cycle. It is therefore unsurprising to note its essential impact on the optimization of maternal and infant health. Breastfeeding has been shown to have far-reaching impacts on morbidity and mortality, health-care costs, and the environment. It has been noted to decrease the risk of breast and ovarian cancers and postpartum depression in mothers, as well as risks of childhood infections, hospitalizations, sudden infant death syndrome, and childhood leukemia among other benefits[1,2] (Table 35.1). Historically, women with complex disease states or medication regimens were discouraged from breastfeeding due to concerns for the risks of worsening disease and/ or medication transfer to the infant. However, as physicians have come to understand the essential impact of breastfeeding on maternal-child health there have been more efforts to support breastfeeding for all women including those with complex disease. Research has led to advances in treatment options and improved understanding of the mechanisms of medication transfer into human milk. Together, these have led the medical community to reconsider the stance of limiting breastfeeding, and it is now possible to promote breastfeeding in women with neurological disorders while mitigating risk to themselves and their infants.

When managing pregnancy and lactation with a woman who also has a neurological disorder, it is essential to understand the disease, its impact on the mother's physiology, the progress of the pregnancy, and the development of the fetus and infant. Apart from the neurologic disease itself the possible effect of medications on lactation and the infant must be considered. Ideally medications can be chosen or altered late in pregnancy to reduce any potential negative influence on the mother and infant during lactation.

Making and Releasing Breast Milk: A Brief Review of Lactation Physiology

Understanding the impact of neurologic injury or disease on breastfeeding first requires an understanding of mammary development and the role of the nervous system on the basic mechanism of milk production and release.

Breast development occurs through puberty and then again with each pregnancy; therefore any disease process which occurs during these periods may affect milk production, especially those that are hormonal in nature. Breast architecture includes alveolar milk-producing cells, arranged into lobules and connected to a branching ductal system that ends in 4–18 ductal openings at the nipple.[3] (Figure 35.1) These are surrounded by connective and adipose tissue. Alveoli and ducts are surrounded by myoepithelial cells which are responsible for milk ejection during let-down. First colostrum is seen within acinar (secretory) cells by the third month of gestation, and by the second trimester prolactin begins to actively stimulate the secretion of colostrum.[4] After delivery with expulsion of the placenta, the rapid fall in plasma progesterone initiates lactogenesis, which is hormonally dependent during the first few days after delivery (Lactogenesis I). Ideally, the infant is put to the breast within the first hour after birth to promote the second phase of lactogenesis (Lactogenesis II), which occurs at 2 to 3 days postpartum. In this phase the maintenance of milk supply is driven by milk removal, and milk composition and volume continue to change until "mature milk" is established at approximately 10 days (Lactogenesis III, formerly called galactopoesis). A full-term healthy infant

TABLE 35.1 EXCESS HEALTH RISKS ASSOCIATED WITH
NOT BREASTFEEDING

Outcome	Excess Risk* (%)
Among full-term infants	
Acute ear infection (otitis media)[2]	100
Eczema (atopic dermatitis)[11]	47
Diarrhea and vomiting (gastrointestinal infection)[3]	178
Hospitalization for lower respiratory tract diseases in the first year[4]	257
Asthma, with family history[2]	67
Asthma, no family history[2]	35
Childhood obesity[7]	32
Type 2 diabetes mellitus[6]	64
Acute lymphocytic leukemia[2]	23
Acute myelogenous leukemia[5]	18
Sudden infant death syndrome[2]	56
Among preterm infants	
Necrotizing enterocolitis[2]	138
Among mothers	
Breast cancer[8]	4
Ovarian cancer[2]	27

Taken from: The Surgeon General's Call to Action to Support Breastfeeding. Office of the Surgeon General (US); Centers for Disease Control and Prevention (US); Office on Women's Health (US). Rockville (MD): Office of the Surgeon General (US); 2011

* The excess risk is approximated by using the odds ratios reported in the referenced studies.

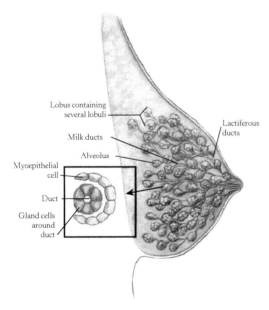

FIGURE 35.1 Female breast and ductal system with cross section of myoepitheal cells around duct opening. Myoepithelial cells contract to eject milk. Used with permission from Lawrence RA, Lawrence RM. *Breastfeeding: A Guide for the Medical Profession*, 8th ed. Figures 2–10, p. 43.

has exhibited suckling and swallowing in utero and exhibits some innate behaviors in reaching the breast of the mother and latching.[5] These normal physiologic behaviors may be interrupted by complicated deliveries, anesthetics, and separation of mothers and infants—all of which are more common in women who have medically complicated pregnancies.

The ejection reflex arc is the most important contributor to milk production and release during Lactogenesis II and III. Prolactin and oxytocin are the primary hormones released. Figure 35.2 illustrates the process of let-down through the ejection reflex arc as the primary process. When the infant suckles at the breast, mechanoreceptors in the nipple and areola are stimulated, and impulses are transmitted to the hypothalamus via somatic afferent nerves. The hypothalamus, in turn, stimulates the posterior pituitary to release oxytocin.[6] Oxytocin is carried via the bloodstream to the breast and uterus. In the breast, oxytocin stimulates myoepithelial cells to contract and eject milk from the alveolus. In women with intact chest wall sensation, this is likely to accompany a tingling, aching, or

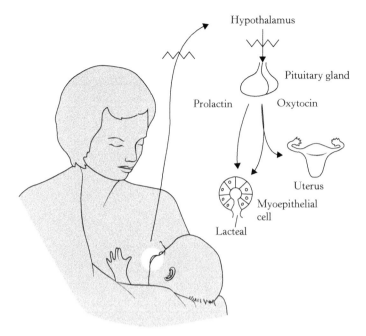

FIGURE 35.2 Milk ejection reflex: The role of the nervous system on the basic mechanism of milk production and milk release. Used with permission from Lawrence RA, Lawrence RM. *Breastfeeding: A Guide for the Medical Profession*, 8th ed., p. 261.

full sensation, which is commonly called "let-down." In the uterus, oxytocin stimulates the postpartum uterine fibers to contract, expelling the placenta (immediately after delivery) and minimizing blood loss (through the postpartum period). This signaling pathway may also be initiated by other anticipation of infant feeding, such as the infant crying or rooting. Maternal stressors such as pain and anxiety can inhibit let down.[7]

Prolactin is the initial hormone responsible for milk production in the alveolus, during pregnancy as well as later lactogenesis. Serum prolactin levels vary by individual and increase during breastfeeding or pumping episodes[8] (Figure 35.3). A rise of prolactin during nursing is indicative of optimal pituitary functioning for breastfeeding, and can be measured by pre- and post-feed prolactin levels[9] (see Table 35.2 for normal values).

Figure 35.4 shows innervation of the breast. Branches of the fourth, fifth, and sixth intercostal nerves supply the breast, whose sensory and autonomic fibers innervate the smooth muscle in the nipple and blood vessels. While the nipple-areola complex is more heavily innervated, the mammary body itself has predominantly autonomic innervation, with no parasympathetic, cholinergic, or ganglia found in mammary tissue.[10] Acinar

mammary myoepithelial cells do not appear to be innervated, suggesting that milk secretion is instead hormonally controlled after nerve stimulation of the nipple.

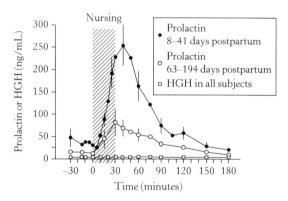

FIGURE 35.3 Plasma Prolactin and growth hormone concentrations during nursing in postpartum women. Note the rise in prolactin with nursing. This effect diminishes over time between the first 2 months of lactation and the following 3–6 months, while growth hormone levels remain stable. Used with permission from Lawrence RA, Lawrence RM. *Breastfeeding: A Guide for the Medical Profession*, 8th Figure 8–24, p. 261. Taken from: Noel GL, Suh HK, Frantz AG: Prolactin release during nursing and breast stimulation in postpartum and nonpostpartum subjects. *J Clin Endocrinol Metab.* 1974; 38: 413.

TABLE 35.2 PROLACTIN NORMAL VALUES*

	Range (ng/mL)	Average (ng/mL)
Males and prepubertal and postmenopausal females	2–8	–
Females' menstrual life	8–14	10
Term pregnancy	200–500	200
Amniotic fluid	Up to 10,000	–
Lactating women	*Response to breastfeeding*	
First 10 days	Baseline 200	Rise to 400
10-90 days	60–110	70–220
90-180 days	50	100
180 days to 1 year	30–40	45–80

Used with permission from Lawrence RA, Lawrence RM. *Breastfeeding: A Guide for the Medical Profession.* 8th ed, Table 3-2, p. 65. Prolactin Levels
* Collation of values from multiple studies and sources.

BREASTFEEDING GOALS

In general, every woman should have the opportunity and support to breastfeed. The World Health Organization (WHO), American Academy of Pediatrics (AAP), American College of Obstetrics and Gynecology (ACOG), and Academy of Family Practice (AAFP) all recommend that women breastfeed exclusively for 6 months and continue with solids added until at least 12 months and as long thereafter as the mother-baby dyad wish.[11-14]

Despite this support from all the major obstetrical and pediatric societies, the initiation and continuation of breastfeeding in the United States is nowhere near universal, though it is improving from declining rates throughout the early 20th century. The incidence of breastfeeding among new mothers was approximately 30% in the 1970s, the nadir of 60 years of decline.[15] Current breastfeeding initiation rates exceed 80% at hospital discharge, and approach Healthy People 2020 goals. This is both a result of and necessitates health-care

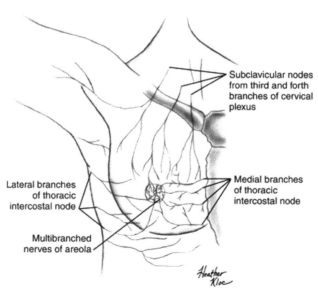

FIGURE 35.4 Innervation of mammary gland. Supraclavicular nerves and lateral and medial branches of intercostal nerves provide sensory innervation. Sympathetic and motor nerves are provided by supracervical and intercostal nerves. Used with permission from Lawrence RA, Lawrence RM. *Breastfeeding: A Guide for the Medical Profession*, 8th ed.

professionals' familiarity with breastfeeding counseling and support of the maternal-infant dyad in all clinical contexts. Breastfeeding rates are lower for women with complicated pregnancies and deliveries, who require additional support and encouragement to be successful.[16]

For women with neurologic conditions, the discussion about the pros and cons of lactation and the feasibility of lactation should occur at the onset of pregnancy, or even more ideally preconception. The physician should provide a thorough discussion of the benefits of breastfeeding for mother and infant (Table 35.1), which are extensive. Furthermore, for a mother who has struggled medically in pregnancy or childbirth, breastfeeding can provide an empowering and normalizing moment in the care of her newborn: only she can produce milk for her infant. The disadvantages of breastfeeding for the infant are minimal, with the exception of medication exposures, which may carry risks. In diseases that involve the presence of immune antibodies, there may be passage of antibodies into the breast milk, with the theoretical risk of exposure of the infant to these antibodies. However, in most cases antibodies only pass into the milk if the molecules are small tiny. No immune disease has been reported in infants exposed to these antibodies. Rather, breast milk in general appears to have a protective effect in decreasing incidence and severity of autoimmunity.[17] The disadvantages to the mother include the possible need to alter medication or treatment regimens, which may impact her symptoms or disease progression. Additionally, breastfeeding requires energy and may involve lack of sleep. In general breastfeeding mothers are found to have similar or improved sleep quality compared to bottle-feeding mothers[18,19] nevertheless, exclusively breastfed infants cannot easily be put in the care of others to be fed. For neurologic diseases that are strongly influenced by fatigue, or for mothers whose disease states involve difficulty with maintenance of an adequate weight, this may pose a risk of relapse or poor symptom control. Finally, autonomic dysreflexia has on rare reports been noted to be triggered by breastfeeding.[20] (See Chapter 29.)

General Approach to Breastfeeding

The discussion of breastfeeding for women with neurologic disease should be based on the specific neurologic disease, its impact on maternal milk production, the medications required, as well as her functional mobility and ability to put the infant to the breast. The therapeutic impact of maternal drugs, their passage into the milk and the oral absorption of the drug by the infant are additional considerations (Box 35.1). A lactation consultant or breastfeeding specialist is often helpful to the provider and patient in reviewing these considerations. Women should be encouraged to create support systems for the postpartum period and to assist with breastfeeding as well as baby care: it has been shown that women with more support are more likely to overcome challenges and meet their breastfeeding goals.[21] Women at low risk for preterm delivery and who are at a higher risk of breastfeeding problems may be encouraged to begin hand expression twice per day from 36 weeks of gestation. This practice may reduce time to lactogenesis II and makes colostrum available to the infant if supplementation is required due to mother-baby separation or low milk supply.[22]

In general, if a woman can conceive and carry a pregnancy, she should be able to lactate. Causes for failure to lactate or low milk supply in women with neurologic disorders may include direct trauma to the breasts, their innervation or blood supply (eg. with a spinal cord injury), impacts on the mammary gland or hypothalamic-pituitary hormonal axis during pubertal development or pregnancy (eg, cabergoline treatment, cranial radiation, pituitary resection, or obesity), or delivery impacts on the hypothalamic-pituitary axis (eg, severe hemorrhage or Sheehan syndrome). In addition, complicated or preterm deliveries may result in maternal-infant separation, which is a risk factor for delayed onset of breastfeeding and subsequent decreased milk supply.[23] Breast growth and development in pregnancy can serve as an indicator that the physiologic growth and development of milk ducts is occurring normally. If the breasts fail to respond to pregnancy, the prognosis of producing milk is poor. Within a few weeks of the due date, colostrum may begin to appear in small amounts when the breasts are stimulated, another indication that hormonal stimulation and growth is occurring.

After delivery if mother and infant are stable, the infant should be placed immediately skin-to-skin with the mother, and ideally the first attempt to breastfeed should occur within 1 hour. In the case of necessary separation, the mother who desires to breastfeed should be encouraged to hand express milk within 1 hour of birth, which is likely to decrease time to lactogenesis II and improves milk supply by the end of the first week.[24–26] A neurologically impaired mother may initially require

---

BOX 35.1
CARE MAP FOR BREASTFEEDING/LACTATION IN THE NEUROLOGIC DISEASE PATIENT

Before Pregnancy/Pre-pregnancy

    Review of prior pregnancies and lactation challenges

    Medication adjustment

During Pregnancy

    Assessment of adaptation of breasts for lactation—size, color, sensation

    Anatomic abnormalities—mammary hypoplasia, inverted nipples

    Review medications

    Consultant physician/lactation expert

At Delivery

    Prior to delivery:

        Multidisciplinary discussion to plan best delivery route and location

        Alert Neonatologist/NICU team; consider NICU tour for parents; Notify pediatrician if anticipated fetal involvement

        Notify pregnant woman of lactation support available

    If dyad is stable:

        Put infant to breast immediately/within one hour

        Assist mother in attaching infant

        Put infant to breast every 1–3 hours

    If dyad is not stable, or is separated:

        Assist mother in hand expression within 1 hour of delivery

        Assist mother with hand expression or breast pumping (hospital grade pump) every 4 hours

    Medication review:

        Per routine for neurologic disorder

        Temporary pain regimen

        Physician consultant is necessary

Postpartum

    Assess and assist need for physical support during breastfeeding or pumping

    Consider adjustment of medication for timing of feeding schedule

    Consult physician/lactation expert for latch

    Assess and assist fatigue

    Counsel on increased caloric intake for breastfeeding—refer as needed

---

assistance at each feeding or with hand expression, especially after the fatigue of labor. Typically, within a few weeks most infants will learn to position themselves without help, although assistance with placement, mobility, and changing positions may still be needed.

Plans for management of mother and infant after discharge should include visiting nurses, visiting lactation consultant and medical monitoring as needed, depending on the severity of the mother's neurological condition. Because of the neuroendocrine control of milk supply after lactogenesis

II, frequent milk removal is necessary to achieve and maintain a full milk supply. For this reason, replacing breastfeeding with infant formula results in decreased (and eventual loss of) milk supply. For the mother who desires to breastfeed, her goal must therefore be achieved through frequent breastfeeding or pumping. However, this practice requires time, energy, and wakefulness; thus, all mothers should be encouraged to nap during the day and seek help with other tasks in order to prevent exhaustion. If sleep problems are more severe, or neurologic symptoms worsen because of fatigue, strategies may be employed to help the mother balance breastfeeding with the goal of maintaining her energy balance. For instance, some mothers will circumvent sleep difficulties by pumping bottles for others to feed during a longer rest period at night. This is particularly helpful if medications are being used that require a longer period before nursing, such as sodium oxybate in narcolepsy management. If use of a medication is necessary for sleep, another caregiver must be available and responsible for the infant while the mother is medicated and asleep. In general, a gap between nursing episodes of more than 6 hours at night may result in return of menses, and women should be counseled to obtain appropriate birth control to prevent closely spaced pregnancy.[27] Less frequent feeding may also result in decreased milk supply.[28] Some women may choose to begin pumping early postpartum in order to store milk for sharing of feeding responsibilities. This approach is useful whenever the mother is, or may become, unavailable to feed the infant such as when the mother returns to work or has planned surgeries. It also may assist in the maintenance of a supply as it replaces a supplementary feed (of breast milk) with a pumping session (neuroendocrine signaling).

In terms of diet and nutrition, most women can self-regulate to ensure adequate intake of fluid and calories to lactate, lose intrapartum weight, and maintain their health. However, for women with neurologic disorders and wasting or poor weight gain in pregnancy, achieving the additional 500 extra calories per day may prove more of a challenge.[29] Intake less than 1,800 kcal/day is not recommended during lactation.[30] Seeing a dietician or nutritionist may be helpful.

MEDICATION SAFETY WHILE BREASTFEEDING

One of the most important topics to review in the discussion of breastfeeding in women with neurologic disease is the safety of the baby when the mother requires medication for disease control. Preconception and prenatal counseling on medication safety for lactation is essential, as the immediate postpartum period is a stressful time in which to discuss medication changes, or tell women that they may not breastfeed while taking medications essential for their health. Individual medications must be discussed on a case-by-case basis, because recommendations are dependent on the newborn's health, the possible adjustment of timing or dosages, medication alternatives, and combinations of therapies. Consultation with a breastfeeding medicine specialist or lactation pharmacist may assist in these conversations, though the mother's primary prenatal care provider and neurologist should maintain primary focus on the mother's medication list.

Most over the counter drugs for everyday complaints such as colds, headaches, and aches and pains are safe. Additionally, if the medication is one that is normally given safely to an infant, it can be assumed it is acceptable for the mother to take while breastfeeding (eg, most antibiotics, acetaminophen and ibuprofen). For other drugs, recommendations should be primarily based on whether the drug is essential or may be discontinued, whether evidence exists for the drug's safety, and the characteristics of the medication itself (Table 35.3). If evidence is lacking, medication characteristics can be used to determine risk level, such as maternal serum levels, molecular weight, protein binding, and oral bioavailability.[31] Because passage into milk is dependent on maternal serum levels, medications may be timed to avoid peak plasma times, such as dosing a medication immediately after a feed or pumping session. Drugs with a molecular weight of less than 300g/mol are more likely to pass in mother's milk, while those heavier than 600g/mol are less likely to pass. Heavyweight molecules or compounds such as insulin and heparin, as well as immunoglobulins are very large and do not pass into milk. Drugs that are highly protein bound do not typically pass into milk (eg, warfarin) and can be used with relative safety while breastfeeding. Equally important is oral bioavailability (ie, if the infant absorbs the medication in appreciable levels through the gastrointestinal tract even if milk levels are present). Many medications are poorly absorbed from the gut of the infant (eg, drugs requiring injection administration, immunoglobulins), and therefore passage through the breast milk may be of little concern. The infant should always be observed for side effects such sleepiness, irritability, poor feeding, and lack of weight gain.

TABLE 35.3 CONSIDERATIONS FOR MEDICATION USE DURING LACTATION AND SELECTED RESOURCES

Considerations	Resources
1. Most medications are safe for breastfeeding 2. If a medication is used in infants, it is generally considered safe for breastfeeding 3. Can medication be discontinued? 4. Does evidence exist for drug safety (see resources)? 5. Drugs are unlikely to reach high levels in infant serum with: 　• Low maternal serum levels 　• High molecular weight (above 600g/mol or Da) 　• Highly protein bound 　• Low lipid solubility 　• Low oral bioavailability 6. Is the mechanism of action of the medication likely to harm the infant? 7. Does the medication impact milk supply?	**Database reference:** • **LactMed**, National Library of Medicine—online. Peer reviewed and fully referenced database of drugs used during lactation. (access at: https://toxnet.nlm.nih.gov/newtoxnet/lactmed.htm) **Hotlines, Online resources and Peer-to-peer support:** • **Human Lactation Study Center**, University of Rochester, NY—telephone support for healthcare professionals. Staffed by a lactation pharmacist and breastfeeding medicine specialist. Assistance to providers attempting to assess safety and alternatives to complex medical needs during lactation (access at: 585-275-0088) • **Infant Risk Center**, Texas Tech University Health Sciences Center—telephone and online support for healthcare professionals and community. Provides information on pregnancy, breastfeeding and medications. (access at: http://www.infantrisk.com/) • **Mother to Baby**, Organization of Teratology Information Specialists—online and telephone-based resource. Provides many fact sheets for medications online (access at: https://mothertobaby.org/fact-sheets-parent/) **Textbooks:** • **Medications & Mother's Milk**, 17th Ed, 2017, T Hale and H Rowe, Springer Publishing Co, NY, NY.—referenced compendium of medication safety while breastfeeding. Originator of the categories of safety for lactation (L1-5). • **Breastfeeding, A Guide for the Medical Profession**, 8th Ed, 2016, R Lawrence and R Lawrence, Elsevier, Saunders, Mosby, Churchill.—resource on all aspects of medical management of breastfeeding.

Resources to determine safety of a medication for breastfeeding are included in Table 35.3. In general, these resources provide available maternal and infant levels of drugs, possible side effects on infants and on lactation itself, and a list of alternative drugs. Hale and Rowe in *Medications and Mother's Milk* use a classification system intended to provide clear guidance, which may be especially helpful for those who lack familiarity with weighing the risks and benefits of medications during breastfeeding. This categorization uses 5 levels of safety, L1 through L5: L1 being the safest and L5 representing medications contraindicated in breastfeeding mothers (Table 35.4). Table 35.5 has a list of commonly prescribed medications and their considerations during lactation. However, as new evidence becomes available continuously, up-to-date references should be checked each time a medication plan is created.

There are both risks and benefits to the use of herbals. In the popular literature, herbals are credited with curing a number of illnesses and are frequently used by women with low milk supply.[32] Consultation with an expert practitioner who knows both herbals and lactation is essential if mothers desire to take herbal remedies, particularly in combination with medications for neurologic conditions. Depending on their sources, may also include wide varieties in potency and contamination remains a concern.

BREASTFEEDING AND RADIOLOGIC PROCEDURES, TREATMENTS, AND SURGERIES

Women with neurologic diseases often require other diagnostic and therapeutic procedures, most of which are compatible with breastfeeding.

TABLE 35.4 LACTATION SAFETY CATEGORIES

Category	Description
L1	Safest—A large number of studies have been performed which do not demonstrate any increased risk or the possibility of neonatal harm is remote.
L2	Safer—A limited number of studies have been performed without any observed increased risk.
L3	Moderately Safe—Controlled studies have been performed and demonstrate a potential for minimal non-adverse effects.
L4	Hazardous—There is evidence of neonatal effects with breastfeeding.
L5	Contraindicated—There is significant documented harm in breastfed neonates.

Hale TW, Rowe HE. *Medications and Mother's Milk.* 17th ed. New York, NY: Springer; 2017

Breastfeeding does not need to be interrupted for imaging procedures, or most IV contrast agents (eg, Gadolinium, Iodinated X-ray Contrast Media).[33] Similarly, most anesthetic agents have low serum levels once mothers are awake and able to nurse. Therefore, prolonged pumping and discarding milk is rarely necessary. An exception to this may be if an infant is premature or less than 3 months old and the anesthetic agent used has a long half-life. In this case, pumping and storing prior to the procedure, then pumping the milk for 4 to 6 hours after the procedure may be considered. The post-procedure milk may be stored for future use, as gaseous agents are likely to diffuse out of the milk with storage and the milk may be safe for future use with an older infant. The Academy of Breastfeeding Medicine provides a protocol on the use of analgesia and anesthesia in breastfeeding mothers, which can be a useful reference for decision making.[34]

Surgery

There are several considerations for women requiring surgeries, or who may become incapacitated or require separation from their infants. For this, it is essential to understand the mother's breastfeeding goals, as they will impact the level of intervention required to assist with breastfeeding. For mothers desiring to exclusively breastfeed, encouragement and assistance should be provided to pump and store milk in preparation for a longer surgery or anticipated separation. This maintains exclusivity and will avoid exposure to cow's milk protein and any side effects in the infant at an already stressful time. An infant may also require practice with a bottle, as some exclusively breastfed babies may refuse a bottle at first. In addition, for maintenance of milk supply and avoidance of plugged ducts and mastitis, it is important for a mother who desires to breastfeed to have assistance with pumping during periods of incapacity.

This may be achieved by a nurse in the operating room pumping a mother's breasts for her, or family helping to pump a mother's breasts if she is unable to do so while awake (Guillain Barre, MS), sedated or comatose. This assistance is particularly important if a pause in breastfeeding will be longer than usual feeding spacing, such as 2 hours for the neonate, or 2-6 hours for older infants.

Lactation Recommendations for Specific Neurologic Diseases and Conditions (Alphabetically)

Depression

Depression in pregnancy and the postpartum period is common, and women with neurologic diseases may be at higher risk (see Chapter 34). [35] Postpartum depression may impact all levels of infant care and bonding, among them breastfeeding. The relationship between breastfeeding and peripartum depression is poorly understood. Depression appears to be predictive of shorter breastfeeding duration, though reviews are less clear on whether breastfeeding itself is predictive of lower rates of postpartum depression.[36] There is some evidence that negative breastfeeding experiences may increase levels of depression in the postpartum period. Therefore, an approach that encourages and supports mothers with neurologic disease to breastfeed, while providing close follow up to readily recognize and manage breastfeeding difficulties is most likely to be supportive of women's goals and minimize any negative impact. Most antidepressants are considered compatible with breastfeeding (see Table 35.5) and cessation of breastfeeding in order to treat depression is not necessary.

Headaches

Three types of headaches—common/occasional, migraine and lactational—have been associated with lactation and described in the medical

---

TABLE 35.5 COMMON MEDICATIONS UTILIZED FOR NEUROLOGIC SYMPTOMS AND THEIR SAFETY IN LACTATION

Antithrombotics

Aspirin (Salicylic Acid)	Compatible with breastfeeding at doses lower than 325mg daily. Long-term, high-dose maternal aspirin therapy was associated with infant metabolic acidosis in one case report. Theoretical risk for infant Reye syndrome with high doses and concurrent infant viral infection.
Heparin/Low Molecular weight Heparin	Compatible with breastfeeding. Large molecule, does not pass into milk
Warfarin (Coumadin)	Compatible with breastfeeding. High protein with low passage into milk. The infant should be monitored closely and given vitamin K when indicated. Possible interaction with other drugs infant may be taking.

Anti-hypertensives
General Principles: Choose preferred medications

Atenolol	Alternative agent is preferred. Excreted into the breast milk at 2–7x serum dosage. Increased risk for beta-blockade in the young infant. Infants older than 3 months of age appear to be at lower risk. Alternatives exist.
Labetolol	Compatible with breastfeeding
Nicardipine	Compatible with breastfeeding
Propanolol	Compatible with breastfeeding

Anti-Epileptics (see also Chapter 21)
General Principles: Decrease to pre-pregnancy medication dosages as soon as possible after birth. Valproate, Phenobarbital, Phenytoin and Carbamazepine may pass into milk at lower levels than others. Monitor infants for drowsiness, irritability, weight gain and development, especially when combination therapies are used.

Carbamazepine (Tegretol®)	Compatible with breastfeeding. Patients of Asian descent appear higher risk for serious dermatologic reactions due to HLAB*1502. Serum concentrations in infants are usually detectable but below therapeutic range. The medication is used in children and the American Academy of Pediatrics committee on mediations in breastfeeding lists carbamazepine as compatible with breastfeeding.
Lamotrigine (Lamictal®)	Compatible with breastfeeding but follow closely. Reports of mild thrombocytosis, withdrawal symptoms with weaning and CNS depression. Serum concentrations in nursing infants are approximately 30% of maternal serum concentrations. Neonates are at higher risk. Infants are given lamotrigine for seizures.
Levetiracetam (Keppra®)	Compatible with breastfeeding. May decrease milk supply in some women.
Oxcarbazepine (Trileptal®)	Compatible with breastfeeding.
Phenytoin (Dilantin®)	Compatible with breastfeeding. Rare idiosyncratic reactions.
Topiramate (Topamax®)	Compatible with breastfeeding.
Valproate (Depakane®)	Compatible with breastfeeding. Theoretical risk of hepatotoxicity, so monitoring for jaundice, bruising, bleeding.
Zonisamide	Alternative agent is preferred. Limited data but high levels in milk and infant serum have been seen.

Anti-Psychotics & Mood Stabilizing
General Principles: Monotherapy may be preferable. Monitor infants for drowsiness, irritability, weight gain and development, especially when combination therapies are used.

(continued)

TABLE 35.5 CONTINUED

Aripiprazole (Abilify®)	Alternative agents may be preferred. Limited data that doses up to 15mg daily produce low levels in milk. Can lower serum prolactin levels in a dose-related manner.
Lithium	Alternative agents may be preferred. Infant serum levels have ranged from 10–50% of maternal serum levels. The diminished renal clearance in neonates can elevate serum levels of lithium. Increased caution with premature infants, neonates or dehydrated infants. The American Academy of Pediatrics recommends that breast-feeding be undertaken with caution by women undergoing lithium treatment. Lithium serum concentrations, CBC, BUN/Creatinine and TSH may be monitored.
Haloperidol (Haldol®)	Likely compatible with breastfeeding. Limited data that doses up to 10mg daily produce low levels in milk and do not affect the breastfed infant. Can lower serum prolactin levels in a dose-related manner.
Olanzapine (Zyprexa®)	Compatible with breastfeeding. Maternal doses up to 20mg daily produce low levels in milk and undetectable levels in infant serum. May be a first-line agent during breastfeeding.
Quetiapine (Seroquel®)	Compatible with breastfeeding. Maternal doses up to 400mg daily produce low levels in milk. May be a first-line agent during breastfeeding.
Risperidone (Risperdal®)	Alternative agents may be preferred. Limited data that doses up to 6mg daily produce low levels in milk. Can lower serum prolactin levels in a dose-related manner.

Central Nervous System Agents
General Principles: Use after breastfeeding has been well established may lessen impact on milk production.

Bromocriptine	Alternative agents may be preferred. Potential to suppress prolactin and decrease milk production. Can cause hypertension, stroke, seizures and psychosis when used for lactation suppression.
Cabergoline	Alternative agents may be preferred. Potential to suppress prolactin and decrease milk production. Potentially is a better choice that bromocriptine. Women treated with cabergoline before pregnancy can breastfeed.
Levodopa	Compatible with breastfeeding. Potential to suppress prolactin and decrease milk production, particularly if given before breastfeeding is well established.

Headache and Pain Medications (see also antihypertensives)

Acetaminophen (Tylenol®)	Compatible with breastfeeding.
Diclofenac	Compatible with breastfeeding.
Eletriptan and Sumatriptan	Compatible with breastfeeding.
Frovatriptan	Alternative agent may be preferred. Long half-life and limited data.
Ibuprofen (Motrin®, Advil®)	Compatible with breastfeeding.
Naproxen (Aleve®)	Alternative agent may be preferred while nursing a newborn or premature infant. Long half-life and reported serious adverse reaction.

Immunomodulators and Steroids (See also Chapter 10)
General Principles: Large immunoglobulins are unlikely to pass into milk. Smaller molecules have little research.

Immunoglobulins (IVIG, Glatiramir, Interferon-B, Rituximab).	Compatible with breastfeeding. Limited data, however large molecules that have poor oral bioavailability.

TABLE 35.5 CONTINUED

Methylprednisolone	Compatible with breastfeeding. For IV administration, such as in burst treatment for Multiple Sclerosis, infants have been shown to receive a low dose. However, breastfeeding immediately preceeding an infusion and delaying next feed until 2-4h after will limit infant dose. High steroid doses may cause temporary loss of milk supply. Mother should be encouraged to prepare for pulse steroids by pumping and storing milk.
Oral agents (fingolimod, terifluonimide and di- methyl fumarate)	Alternative agent is preferred. Small molecules, likely to pass into breastmilk, little data to support safety.
Prednisone	Compatible with breastfeeding. No adverse effects have been reported. High steroid doses may cause temporary loss of milk supply. Encourage mother to prepare for pulse steroids by pumping and storing milk.

Immunosuppressants (See also Chapter 10)
General Principles: Usually large molecules and limited passage into milk. Monitor infant, may draw infant serum dose with concerns

Azathioprine	Compatible with breastfeeding. Dosages up to 200mg have found low or unmeasurable serum infant levels. Cases of mild, asymptomatic neutropenia have been reported. Consider CBC and LFT monitoring.
Cyclosporine	Likely compatible with breastfeeding. Most infants have not had detectable blood levels. No adverse events have been reported.
Mycophenolate (CellCept®)	Alternative agent is preferred. Limited data and small molecule.
Tacrolimus	Likely compatible with breastfeeding.

Muscle Relaxants
General Principles: Choose agents with a shorter half life, monitor infants for sedation. Topical and intrathecal doses are unlikely to affect infants.

Baclofen	Compatible with breastfeeding.
Tizanidine (Zanaflex®)	Alternative agent is preferred. Small molecule with a long half life, lipophilic, with CNS penetration.

Sedatives
General Principles: Choose agents with a short half life. Monitor infants for drowsiness, irritability, weight gain and development, especially when combination therapies are used.

Clonazepam (Klonopin®)	Compatible with breastfeeding at low doses for refractory restless leg syndrome. Because of longer half-life, a shorter acting drug may be preferred for other indications.
Lorazepam (Ativan®), Oxazepam	Compatible with breastfeeding. Short half life and is safely used in infants.

Misc

ACTH/Corticotropin	Compatible with breastfeeding. High molecular weight, short half life and low oral bioavailability.
Antidepressants	Most are compatible with breastfeeding. Optimal choices in- clude Sertraline (Zoloft) and Paroxetine (Paxil) due to low passage into breastmilk. Monitor infant for restlessness, crying and insomnia.
Hydroxyzine (Atarax®)	Compatible with breastfeeding. Larger or more prolonged doses may decrease milk supply or cause drowsiness in infants. Caution with neonates and preterms.
Oxybutinyn (Ditropan®)	Possibly compatible with breastfeeding. No information avail- able. Long-term use may decrease milk supply.

(continued)

TABLE 35.5 CONTINUED

Iron, Folic acid (Restless leg syndrome)	Compatible with breastfeeding.
Mannitol	Compatible with breastfeeding.
Meclizine (Meclin®)	Compatible with breastfeeding. Larger doses or prolonged use may cause sedation or decrease milk supply.

Sources
- Lactmed https://toxnet.nlm.nih.gov/newtoxnet/lactmed.htm,
- WHO http://www.who.int/maternal_child_adolescent/documents/55732/en/,
- *Breastfeeding: A Guide for the Medical Profession*, 8th ed., by Ruth A. Lawrence MD (author), Robert M. Lawrence MD (author) Figure 8–23, p 261
- Sachs HC. *Committee On Drugs of the American Academy of Pediatrics.* The Transfer of Drugs and Therapeutics Into Human Breast Milk: An Update on Selected Topics, Pediatrics, September 2013, VOLUME 132 / ISSUE 3
Harden CL, et al. Practice Parameter update: Management issues for women with epilepsy—focus on pregnancy (an evidence-based review): Vitamin K, folic acid, blood levels, and breastfeeding. Report of the Quality Standards Subcommittee and Therapeutics and Technology Assessment Subcommittee of the American Academy of Neurology and American Epilepsy Society. Apil 2009. 73(2). P142–9

literature. Considerations for headaches in the setting of lactation include ruling out other serious conditions (pre-eclampsia, sinus venous thrombosis, etc.), preventing and treating pain, and medication management to reduce the risk of impact on lactation and the infant. Each individual mother should receive counseling for headache management and should work with a lactation consultant and her providers to optimize medication choices during pregnancy and lactation.[37]

Occasional common headaches without localizing neurologic symptoms during lactation should be treated with attention to adequate hydration and prevention of fatigue. Changes in caffeine consumption in the peripartum period may put a woman at risk for headaches. In addition, the stress of managing a new baby and concomitant muscle tension of holding can result in muscular spasms of the shoulder and neck, which may result in headaches. Fatigue and postpartum depression can trigger or exacerbate headaches. If medications are needed, common over-the-counter medications such as acetaminophen and ibuprofen are well tolerated. Salicylic acid is excreted in breast milk with aspirin ingestion at doses above 325mg daily (though not at low-dose 75–325mg daily used to treat other conditions, see Table 35.5). Because of reports of metabolic acidosis, and the unknown risk of Reye syndrome, it is not recommended to use high-dose aspirin while breastfeeding.

Migraine headache is a unilateral, hormonally sensitive, episodic headache disorder that may worsen in the postpartum period. Breastfeeding may decrease the risk of recurrence of migraines after pregnancy.[38,39]

Migraine headaches differ from lactational headaches in that they were often present prior to pregnancy and have different triggers. Most migraine medications are considered compatible with breastfeeding, including electriptan and sumatriptan (see Table 35.5). Zonisamide, atenolol, and tizanidine are not appropriate. Timing of medication administration may help reduce drug transfer to infants; generally, dosing just before a nursing episode may help to avoid peak plasma times of shorter-acting agents.

Lactational headaches are headaches occurring only during suckling; they stop when the infant stops suckling and published information is limited to case reports. Additionally, one case report exists of a mother whose headache preceded latching and resolved after feeds.[40] Some authors have sought to determine a hormonal link with oxytocin or prolactin for these headaches, because of their association with breastfeeding, the finding that oxytocin levels may be high during orgasmic headaches and that prolactin levels have been found to be high during migraine headaches. Theoretically, although hyperprolactinemia does not cause headaches per se, headaches and hyperprolactinemia reflect a derangement of neurotransmitters that could result in headaches.[38,41] Only one case report measured prolactin and vasopressin during an apparent lactational headache and found little association.[42] Based on clinical experience, the headaches usually resolve about 8 to 12 weeks after delivery. Medications and therapies safe for breastfeeding should be used to alleviate pain, and any additional triggers should be avoided, such as fatigue and stress. Rarely, the mother is forced to wean if pain cannot be controlled with other therapies.

Epilepsy and anti-epileptic medications

Many medical reports have discussed the management of breastfeeding women with epilepsy—and each makes great efforts to highlight the importance of breastfeeding for maternal and infant health and infant intellectual development. Anti-epileptic drugs (AEDs) are generally considered compatible with breastfeeding, though the infant should be monitored for CNS effects (Table 35.5).[43] The American Academy of Pediatrics states that with appropriate monitoring infants can be breastfed and usually benefit by it.[44] The American Academy of Neurology and American Epilepsy Society statement indicates that small amounts of drug passes into the breastmilk for many anti-epileptics, though more studies are needed to evaluate impact on the infant.[45-48] More recently, Meador, et al followed 181 children who had been exposed to anti-epileptic drugs via breastfeeding through 6 years of life and found higher IQ and verbal abilities in breastfed children with no adverse effects.[49] However, women with epilepsy may be at risk for early breastfeeding cessation, due to seizure control or medication management issues.[50] Other management guidelines for women with mood disorders suggest the safe use of anti-epileptic agents for psychotropic needs during breastfeeding.[51] A single study suggesting a higher risk for poor neurodevelopmental outcomes with valproate, oxcarbazepine, and lamotrigine did not differentiate between exposure in utero versus breastfeeding—and therefore limits the ability to generalize this data.[52] Each mother and infant should therefore be monitored individually depending on medications, dosages, and gestational age of the infant.

Mobility limitations

Physical and mobility limitations are likely to make breastfeeding and infant care more difficult. The obstetrician, medical lactation consultant, and the physical therapy/occupational therapy teams should be involved with women with mobility limitations during the pregnancy to help them prepare for these challenges. Although breastfeeding has considerable benefit to both mother and the infant, the ability of the woman with neurologic mobility impairments to achieve this goal may be limited. Women with deceased mobility or impairment will require varying amounts of assistance depending on their degree of limitation and the gestational age of the infant. Putting a neonate to the breast requires use of one hand and arm to pick up and support the infant, while the other arm is needed to support the breast and offer it to the infant while holding or compressing the areola and nipple. Support with pillows and positioning devices can facilitate the positioning and stability of the infant. As the infant gets older, many women are able to achieve a comfortable latch with positioning devices and support of one arm.

Knowledge of the mother's neurologic limitations will determine how much assistance the mother will require to place the infant at the breast—some women will require full support from an assistant during the suckling time, burping, diapering, and settling the infant back in the crib. A neurologically impaired mother who is likely to require this level of assistance at each feeding and with child care will need to develop an appropriate care network during pregnancy. Additionally, the mother should consider having support persons from home stay with her while in the hospital so that they may learn how to best support her prior to discharge. If a mother needs help to breastfeed, she will also need help to bottle feed. Consultation with physical and occupational therapy to plan for discharge is recommended.

Multiple sclerosis

Multiple sclerosis (MS) is the most commonly recognized chronic inflammatory demyelinating disease. It is more common in women than men and typically has onset between 20 and 40 years of age. Thus, clinicians have a greater exposure to women with this disease who are pregnant and subsequently lactating than any other neurologic disease.[53] Breastfeeding may improve postpartum remission rates and symptoms, particularly if breastfeeding is exclusive in the first 6 months. (see Chapter 10 for further discussion) A mother who has MS should be encouraged to breastfeed unless there is a special contraindication such as an unusual medication being prescribed. Most medications used for MS are compatible with breastfeeding, including monoclonal antibodies, steroids, and adjunctive agents, with the exception of some oral agents (eg, fingolimod, teriflunimide, and dimethyl fumarate), which are small molecules and lack available data.

Pituitary disorders

Due to the importance of the neurogenic feedback loop, women with pituitary deficiency are at risk for lactational failure. Most syndromes involving the pituitary gland will still allow lactation if the woman is able to conceive without interventions, unless the hormonal crisis has developed during an established pregnancy. The best example of pituitary dysfunction affecting lactation is Sheehan syndrome, in which hemorrhagic collapse during delivery due to postpartum hemorrhage causes pituitary shock and thereby failure of lactation. This relationship between postpartum hemorrhage and anterior pituitary necrosis was first identified by British pathologist Harold Sheehan. Indeed, some degree of hypopituitarism has been reported in 32% of women with severe postpartum hemorrhage. The extent of damage predicts rapidity of onset as well as magnitude of the pituitary hypofunction. The gland has a large reserve so that more than 75% destruction is necessary to produce clinical symptoms.[54] Lactational failure and hyponatremia may be the first signs of this disorder and should prompt a full pituitary workup when noted in conjunction with a life-threatening hemorrhage after delivery. Women with this disorder may remain amenorrheic and require hormone replacement throughout their life. There is anecdotal evidence that a medical oxytocin trigger with oxytocin nasal spray is possible for women with deficiency due to prior pituitary infarct or washout. It is relatively well tolerated by mothers and has a low-risk profile. (Compound as 40IU synthetic oxytocin [Syntocinon] per ml. Deliver one 100μl spray 2–5 minutes before expressing milk or nursing.)[55]

Tumors or rarely vascular disorders may also affect the anterior pituitary. Most tumors are functionless but may still produce prolactin. Treatment with bromocriptine or cabergoline is typically used to shrink the tumor, and both suppress lactation. If these medications are discontinued at delivery then lactation is usually possible. If medications are necessary, cabergoline is more apt to be associated with successful lactation, particularly if started or restarted after breastfeeding is well established.

Lymphocytic adenohypophysitis (LAH) has a striking temporal association with pregnancy, often developing in the last month of pregnancy or during the first two months postpartum. Antipituitary antibodies have been demonstrated in many cases. Given advancements in obstetric care leading to fewer postpartum hemorrhages, it may represent a larger percentage of women with postpartum hypopituitarism and is seen in association with symptoms of anterior pituitary deficiencies (headache, visual changes, diabetes insipidus), hypoprolactinemia and inability to lactate.[56] Concern for this disorder should prompt a thorough evaluation which includes an MRI, as the inflammatory process may produce a mass.[57]

Cushing syndrome is caused by excess ACTH production or ACTH source such as a tumor. Cortisol secretion is controlled by the hypothalamic-pituitary axis. Pregnancy is rare due to anovulation.[58]

There is no data on breastfeeding with Cushing syndrome. Due to suppression of the hypothalamic-pituitary axis, it may potentially inhibit lactation, though galactorrhea due to hyperprolactinemia in Cushing is a well-established phenomenon as well.[59] Women and their newborns should be monitored closely for adequacy of milk supply.

Sensory loss to the chest wall/breast, spinal cord injury

Women with decreased sensation to the chest wall may lack the afferent sensation to stimulate the let-down reflexes discussed above. For this reason, neurologic disease with decreased sensation of the chest wall or breast also has the potential to lack appropriate milk production, particularly after the colostral phase. This is apparent with a spinal injury rostral to T_6, which results in partial or complete blockage of the suckling-induced afferent stimulation (Figure 35.5). In these cases, the hypothalamus is not stimulated and oxytocin is not released. If the ejection reflex does not occur, only a small amount of milk is released to the infant. Over time, feedback inhibition in the pathway leads to a reduction in milk production. In a study of women from Canada and Sweden with spinal cord injuries reported by Karolinska Institutet, 18 had injuries above T_6 and 20 below T_6.[60] Pregnancy-related problems were greater with higher lesions; however, lactation problems were similar to those of women without spinal cord injury. Women with spinal cord injury above T_6 were significantly more likely to have engorged breasts, insufficient milk production or ejection and autonomic dysreflexia, compared with those with lesions below T_6, and duration of breastfeeding was shorter.

Other stimulants of oxytocin release that have been found to cause let-down, including auditory (hearing the baby cry) or other anticipation of feeding,[7] may provide alternate pathways to achieve let-down for women with blocked afferent signaling. In these cases, mothers must be attentive to the signal and put the baby immediately to breast, as they are unlikely to have other sensations of let-down. One case series of tetraplegic women with cervical spinal cord

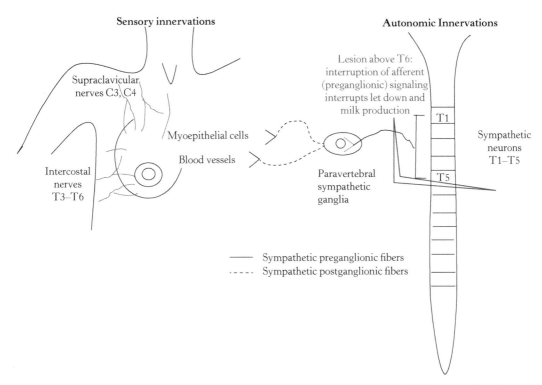

FIGURE 35.5 Sensory and autonomic breast innervations. The sensory innervations of the breast are from the C3-4 and T3-6 nerve roots, and sympathetically innervated from T1-T5. Women with spinal injury rostral to T_6 have partial or complete blockage of the suckling-induced afferent stimulation reducing hypothalamic stimulation and therefore oxytocin release and ejection reflex do not occur.

injuries reported successful breastfeeding with a combination of psychogenic stimuli and oxytocin nasal spray.[61] (Compound as 40IU synthetic oxytocin [Syntocinon] per ml. Deliver one 100μl spray 2–5 minutes before expressing milk or nursing.)[55] Using a hospital grade pump on schedule may also intensify the stimulus to the breasts and increase milk production in these difficult cases.

Viral encephalitis

Viral encephalitis can be caused by numerous different viruses including arboviruses or viruses carried by mosquitoes. The list is long: Eastern Equine, La Crosse, St. Louis, West Nile, and Western Equine—all named by geographic location. They are usually mild but can be fatal. The first report of West Nile Virus in human milk was given to the CDC in 2002,[62] in which a mother acquired the infection from a blood transfusion, and the infant remained healthy. Follow-up in the next five years by the CDC reported ten cases of maternal or infant West Nile infection while breastfeeding, though they include possible cases of vertical transmission and primary infant infection. In the 7 cases from 2002 to 2005 in which mothers were breastfeeding at the time of infection, milk samples were not consistently positive, and all but one infant remained healthy; the final infant developed only a rash. The CDC continues to seek blood and milk samples but considers that the presence of mosquito-borne viral illness does not require weaning.[63,64]

Tick-borne encephalitis is transmitted to humans by the bite of a tick or ingesting unpasteurized milk from infected goats, sheep, and cows. Disease severity increases with age, and residual symptoms and neurologic deficits vary by subtype. Association with geography, age, altitudes, climate, and ticks is well documented. Despite between 5000 and 13000 cases being reported throughout Europe and Russia, transmission human to human via milk consumption or blood transfusion has rarely been reported in encephalitis. No reference to breastfeeding is found in the published literature, and it is not considered a contraindication to breastfeeding.[65] (See Chapter 11 for further discussion of potential neurologic infections and their impact on breastfeeding.)

CONCLUSION

Breastfeeding is the natural completion of the reproductive cycle, and a dyadic process involving two patients whose health must be considered jointly. Because of this, the promotion of breastfeeding in women with neurologic disease is increasingly supported by evidence and improved understandings of the impact of maternal medications on infant health. The strong evidence of extensive benefits of breastfeeding for mothers and children is compelling, and these benefits are arguably even more important for women with neurologic disease in pregnancy. However, the impact cannot be reduced to numbers alone. Breastfeeding is a singularly empowering moment for many mothers, as it is theirs alone and assists in the secure bonding process and safe transition to motherhood that should be in every woman's reach.

REFERENCES

1. Horta BL, Victora CS: Long-term effects of breastfeeding: a systematic review. *World Health Organization*, 2013. http://apps.who.int/iris/bitstream/10665/79198/1/9789241505307_eng.pdf
2. Ip S, Chung M, Raman G, et al: Breastfeeding and maternal and infant health outcomes in developed countries. *Agency for Healthcare Research and Quality.* 2007 Apr; (153): 1–186.
3. Ramsay DT, Kent JC, Hartmann RA, Hartman PE: Anatomy of the lactating human breast redefined with ultrasound imaging. *J Anat.* 2995; 206(6): 525–534.
4. Lawrence RA, Lawrence RM: *Breastfeeding: A Guide for the Medical Profession*, 8th ed. Philadelphia: Elsevier; 2006: 60–65.
5. Righard L, Alade MO: Effect of delivery room routine on success of first breastfeed. *Birth.* 1992; 19: 185.
6. Uvnas-Moberg KU. *The Oxytocin Factor: Tapping the Hormone of Calm, Love, and Healing.* Cambridge, MA: Da Capo; 2003.
7. Lawrence RA, Lawrence RM: *Breastfeeding: A Guide for the Medical Profession.* 8th ed. Philadelphia: Elsevier; 2016: 260–264.
8. Noel GL, Suh HK, Frantz AG: Prolactin release during nursing and breast stimulation in postpartum and nonpostpartum subjects. *Journal of Clinical Endocrinology and Metabolism.* 1974; 38(3): 413–423.
9. Lawrence RA, Lawrence RM: *Breastfeeding: A Guide for the Medical Profession.* 8th ed. Philadelphia: Elsevier; 2016: 65.
10. Lawrence RA, Lawrence RM: *Breastfeeding: A Guide for the Medical Profession.* 8th ed. Philadelphia: Elsevier, 2006: 47–49.
11. World Health Organization. Infant feeding recommendation. In Global Strategy on Infant and Young Child Feeding. *Bulletin World Health Organization,* WHA55 AGG/15, paragraph 10, 2002. http://apps.who.int/gb/archive/pdf_files/WHA55/ea5515.pdf?ua=1
12. American Academy of Pediatrics. Policy statement: Breastfeeding and the use of human milk. *Pediatrics*, 2012; 129(3).
13. American Academy of Family Physicians. Position paper: Breastfeeding, family physicians supporting. *Am Fam Phys.* 2015; 91(1): 56–57.
14. American College of Obstetricians and Gynecologists. Committee opinion #658: Optimizing support for breastfeeding as part of obstetric practice. *ACOG.* 2016; 127: e86–92, 2016.
15. Hirschman C, Hendershot GE. Trends in breast feeding among American mothers. *Vital Health Stat.* 1919; 23 3: 1–39.
16. Kozhimannil KB, Jou J, Attanasio LB, et al. Medically complex pregnancies and early breastfeeding behaviors: a retrospective analysis. *PLoS One.* 2014; 9(8): e104820.
17. Lawrence RA, Lawrence RM: *Breastfeeding: A Guide for the Medical Profession.* 8th. Philadelphia: Elsevier; 2016: 217.
18. Tobback E, Behaeghel K, Hanoulle I, et al: Comparison of subjective sleep and fatigue in breast- and bottle-feeding mothers, *Midwifery.* 2017; 47: 22–27.
19. Triviño-Juárez JM, Nieto-Pereda B, Romero-Ayuso D, et al: Quality of life of mothers at the sixth week and sixth month post partum and type of infant feeding, *Midwifery.* 2016; 34: 230–238.
20. Dakhil-Jerew F, Brook S, Derry F: Autonomic dysreflexia triggered by breastfeeding in a tetraplegic mother. *J Rehabil Med.* 2008; 40(9): 780–782.
21. Rosen-Carole C, Hartman S. ABM Clinical Protocol #19: Breastfeeding promotion in the prenatal setting, academy of breastfeeding medicine, revision. *Breastfeed Med.* 2015; 10(10): 451–457.
22. Forster DA, Moorhead AM, Jacobs SE, et al: Advising women with diabetes in pregnancy to express breastmilk in late pregnancy (Diabetes and Antenatal Milk Expressing): A multicentre, unblinded, randomised controlled trial. *Lancet.* 2017; 389: 2204–2213.
23. Moore ER, Anderson GC, Bergman N, and Dowswell T: Early skin-to-skin contact for mothers and their healthy newborn infants. *Cochrane Database Syst Rev.* 2016; 16:5.
24. Parker LA, Sullivan S, Krueger C, et al. Effect of early breast milk expression on milk volume and timing of lactogenesis stage II among mothers of very low birth weight infants: A pilot study. *J Perinatol.* 2012; 32(3): 205–209.

25. Ohyama M, Watabe H, Hayasaka Y. Manual expression and electric breast pumping in the first 48 h after delivery. *Pediatr Int.* 2010; 52(1): 39–43.

26. Parker LA, Sullivan S, Krueger C, et al: Strategies to increase milk volume in mothers of VLBW infants. *MCN Am J Matern Child Nurs.* 2013; 38(6): 385–390.

27. Lawrence RA, Lawrence RM. *Breastfeeding: A Guide for the Medical Profession.* 8th ed. Philadelphia: Elsevier; 2016: 695.

28. Lawrence RA, Lawrence RM. *Breastfeeding: A Guide for the Medical Profession.* 8th ed. Philadelphia: Elsevier; 2016: 267.

29. Lawrence RA, Lawrence RM. *Breastfeeding: A Guide for the Medical Profession.* 8th ed. Philadelphia: Elsevier; 2016: 293.

30. Institute of Medicine. *Nutrition During Lactation*, Washington, DC: National Academy Press; 1991: 6, 12, 101–102.

31. Lawrence RA, Lawrence RM: *Breastfeeding: A Guide for the Medical Profession.* 8th ed. Philadelphia: Elsevier; 2016: 364–374.

32. Bazzano AN, Cenac L, Brandt AJ, et al: Maternal experiences with and sources of information on galactagogues to support lactation: A cross-sectional study, *Int J Womens Health* 2017; 9: 105–113.

33. American College of Radiology. (2017). ACR Manual on Contrast Media Version (10.3) Retrieved from https://www.acr.org/~/media/ACR/Documents/PDF/QualitySafety/Resources/Contrast-Manual/Contrast_Media.pdf/#page=106

34. Reece-Stremtan S, Campos M, & Kokajko L: ABM Clinical Protocol #15: Analgesia and anesthesia for the breastfeeding mother, revision. *Breastfeeding med.* 2017; 12(9).

35. Bulloch AG, Fiest KM, Williams JV, et al: Depression--a common disorder across a broad spectrum of neurological conditions: a cross-sectional nationally representative survey. *General Hosp Psychiatry.* 2015; 37(6): 507–512.

36. Dias CC, Figueiredo B. Breastfeeding and depression: A systematic review of the literature. *J Affect Disord.* 2015; 171: 142–154.

37. Hutchisson S, Marmura MJ, Calhoun A, et al: Use of common migraine treatments in breast-feeding women: A summary of recommendations, a review. *Headache.* 2013; 53: 614–627.

38. Hoshiyama E, Tatsumoto M, Iwanami H, et al: Postpartum migraines: A long-term prospective study. *Intern Med.* 2012; 51: 3119–3123.

39. MacGregor EA. Migraine in pregnancy and lactation: A clinical review. *J Fam Plann Reprod Health Care.* 2007; 33: 83–93.

40. Thorley V. Lactational headache: A lactation consultant's diary. *J Hum Lact.* 1997; 13(1): 51–53.

41. Sammaritana LR, Bermas BL: Rheumatoid arthritis medications and lactation. *Rheumatology.* 2014; 26: 354–360.

42. Askmark H, Lundberg PO: Lactation headache—a new form of headache? *Cephalalgia.* 1989; 9: 119.

43. Davanzo R, Bo SD, Bua N, et al: Antileptic drugs and breastfeeding. *Italien J Pediatrics.* 2013; 39: 50.

44. American Academy of Pediatrics Committee on Drugs: Transfer of drugs and other chemicals into human milk. *Pediatrics.* 2001; 108(3): 776–789.

45. Harden CL, Pennel PB, Koppel BS, et al: Practice parameter update: Management issues for women with epilepsy—focus on pregnancy (an evidence-based review): Vitamin K, folic acid, blood levels, and breastfeeding. Report of the Quality Standards Subcommittee and Therapeutics and Technology Assessment Subcommittee of the American Academy of Neurology and American Epilepsy Society. *Neurology.* 2009; 73(2): 142–149.

46. Veiby G, Engelsen BA, Gilhus NE: Early child development and exposure to antiepileptic drugs prenatally and through breastfeeding: A prospective cohort study on children of women with epilepsy. *JAMA Neurol.* 2013; 70(11): 1367–1374.

47. Veiby G, Bjørk M, Engelson BA, Gilhus NE: Epilepsy and recommendations for breastfeeding, *Seizure.* 2015; 28; 57–65.

48. Sabers A, Tomson T. Managing antiepileptic drugs during pregnancy and lactation, *Current Opinion in Neurology.* 2009; 22:157–161.

49. Meador KJ, Baker GA, Browning N, et al. Breastfeeding in children of women taking antiepileptic drugs: cognitive outcomes at age 6 years, *JAMA Pediatr.* 2014; 168(8): 729–736.

50. Hao N, Jiang H, Wu M, et al. Breastfeeding initiation, duration and exclusivity in mothers with epilepsy from South West China, *Epilepsy Res.* 2017; 135: 168–175.

51. Yonkers KA, Wisner KL, Stowe Z, et al. Management of bipolar disorder during pregnancy and the postpartum period, *Am J Psychiatry.* 2004; 161(4): 608–620.

52. Veroniki AA, Rios P, Cogo E, et al. Comparative safety of antiepileptic drugs for neurological development in children exposed during pregnancy and breast feeding: A systematic review and network meta-analysis, *BMJ Open.* 2017; 7:e017248. doi:10.1136/bmjopen–2017–017248.

53. Riley CS, Tullman MJ. Multiple sclerosis. In: Rowland LP, Pedley TA, eds. *Merritt's Neurology.* 12th ed. Philadelphia: Wolters Kluwer Lippincott Williams & Wilkins, 2010.

54. Lawrence RA, Lawrence RM: *Breastfeeding: A Guide for the Medical Profession*. Philadelphia: Elsevier; 2007: 577.

55. Lawrence RA, Lawrence RM: *Breastfeeding: A Guide for the Medical Profession*. 8th ed. Philadelphia: Elsevier; 2016: 264.

56. Patel MC, Guneratne N, Haq N, et al: Peripartum hypopituitarism and lymphocytic hypophysitis. *Q J Med*. 1995; 88: 571.

57. Ples M: Chiasmal disorders. In: *Albert & Jakobiec's Principles & Practice of Ophthalmology*. 3rd ed. Ed; Daniel AlbertJoan Miller Dimitri AzarBarbara Blodi. Elsevier; 2000: 3935–3952.

58. Lado-Abeal J, Rodriguez-Arnao J, Newell-Price JD, et al: Menstrual abnormalities in women with Cushing's disease are correlated with hypercortisolemia rather than raised circulating androgen levels. *J Clin Endocrinol Metab*. 1998; 83: 3083–3088.

59. Peña KS, Rosenfeld JA. Evaluation and treatment of galactorrhea. *Am Fam Physician*. 2001; 63(9): 1763–1771.

60. Holmgren, T. The impact of spinal cord injury on the lactation and ability to breastfeed. Karolinska Institutet. Retrieved from http://asia-mmg. societyhq.com/2016annual/guide/protected/syllabus/lectures/2016-PA-1461338977-8823.pdf. Accessed October 20, 2017

61. Cowley KC: Psychogenic and pharmacologic induction of the let-down reflex can facilitate breastfeeding by tetraplegic women: A report of 3 cases, *Arch Phys Med Rehabil*. 2005; 86(6): 1261–1264.

62. Centers for Disease Control and Prevention: Possible West Nile Virus transmission to an infant through breastfeeding, Michigan. *Morb Mortal Wkly Rep*. 2002; 51(877).

63. Centers for Disease Control and Prevention. Pregnancy & breastfeeding, In: *West Nile Virus*. Retrieved Feb 2018 from: https://www.cdc.gov/westnile/faq/pregnancy.html

64. Hinckley AF, O'Leary DR, Hayes EB: Transmission of West Nile virus through human breast milk seems to be rare. 2007; *Pediatrics*. 119(3): e666–e671.

65. Bogovic P, Franc S: Tick-borne encephalitis: A review of epidemiology, clinical characteristics, and management. *World J Clin Cases*. 2015; 3(5): 430–441.

INDEX

Note: Page numbers followed by *t* and *f* indicate tables and figures, respectively. Boxed material is indicated by *b*.

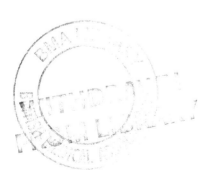